MORE PRAISE FOR *OPTIMAL WELLNESS*

"A wonderful book in every way. It is well organized and written, and immensely readable. I was especially impressed by the comprehensive discussion of topics which are relevant to anyone and everyone who wishes to enjoy good health. I highly recommend it."
> —William G. Crook, M.D.
> Author of *The Yeast Connection and the Woman*

"A valuable resource for anyone interested in maintaining good health and treating illness safely and naturally."
> —Alan R. Gaby, M.D.
> President, American Holistic Medical Association
> Author of *Preventing and Reversing Osteoporosis*

"For almost twenty years, patients in Seattle have greatly benefited from Dr. Golan's skillful blending of conventional and alternative medicine. His special insights have helped many to dramatically improve their health, especially those for whom the conventional approaches proved inadequate. This unique handbook makes available to everyone the opportunity to experience for themselves optimal wellness."
> —Joseph E. Pizzorno, Jr., N.D., President
> Bastyr University
> Coauthor of *Encyclopedia of Natural Medicine*

"An ideal book to have in the home library as well as for the physician who is interested in alternative medicine. The book has obviously taken a tremendous effort and reflects the unique and careful observations and treatment that take place in an intelligent and innovative physician's practice."
> —David Buscher, M.D.
> President, American Academy of Environmental Medicine

OPTIMAL WELLNESS

Ralph Golan, M.D.

Ballantine Books • New York

NOTICE

This book is a source of important information about optimizing health but, for more serious conditions, it cannot serve as replacement for the services of a licensed health care professional.

If you suspect you have a medical problem, you should not only seek competent medical advice, you should educate yourself about the nature of your illness and recommended treatments. Any application of the material set forth in the following pages is at the reader's discretion and sole responsibility.

Library of Congress Catalog Card Number: 92-97310

ISBN: 0-345-35874-0

Text design by Holly Johnson

Manufactured in the United States of America

First Edition: October 1995

10 9 8 7 6 5 4 3 2 1

To my parents, Maxine Rader Golan and Eugene Golan,
for the love and opportunities they have given me.

C O N T E N T S

ACKNOWLEDGMENTS

I want to thank:
- Charlyn Golan, my wife, who assisted on many stages of this work, beginning with the original 1982 self-published edition.
- Cheryl D. Woodruff, my editor, who recognized the value of this work long ago and who engineered it to completion.
- Assistant editor Leah Odze, who deserves an award for her perseverance, especially in following my road maps.
- Barbara Shor, Robert Fleming, and Sona Vogel for hand-polishing the final text.
- Bob Podrat, who was there when I needed him.
- Sharon Mehdi, who gave me the confidence to "go for it all."
- Sarabelle Prince, who encouraged me to find a publisher and provided my first introduction to Ballantine.
- Karl Mincin, B.S., N.C., and Patrick Donovan, N.D., who assisted in the preparation of the Nutritional Deficiencies chapter.
- Richard Kitaeff, M.A., N.D., C.A., Dipl. Ac. (NCCA) who contributed the Acupuncture chapter.
- David Buscher, M.D., who assisted in the preparation of the chapters on Environmental Illness, Yeast Overgrowth, and Food Allergy.
- Patrick Donovan, N.D., David Buscher, M.D., Elias Ilyia, Ph.D., Walter Crinnion, N.D., Paul Rubin, D.D.S., Sandra Denton, M.D., Russ Jaffe, M.D., Ph.D., Len Wisneski, M.D., John T. R. Ely, Ph.D., Mark Swanson, N.D., Pam Alboher-Ray, Ph.D., Eleanor Barrager, R.D., and Shelly Beckman, Ph.D., all of whom assisted in research and consultation.
- Joe Pizzorno, N.D., and Michael Murray, N.D., for their generous permission to reprint sections from their *Textbook of Natural Medicine*.
- Theron Randolph, M.D., and Ralph Moss, Ph.D., for their generous permission to reprint sections from *An Alternative Approach to Allergies*.
- Reference librarians Judy Atkinson and Chris Beahler, who tracked down many books for me.
- Patricia Huling and Mary Barton, who spent countless hours at their keyboards; and Cody Ellerd, who filled in on emergencies.
- Phyllis Kirk, who updated and compiled the sugar tables.
- My proofreading team—Maxine Golan, Charlyn Golan, Blanche Narodick, Carla Oliver, Tom Sponheim, Carolyn Anderman, Marie Fix, Tim Noah, Nancy Sanders, Charlie Gioiosa, Barbara Brainin, and Letha Hedger.
- Letha Hedger for her additional indispensable assistance and support.
- Bob Anderson, M.D., Ed Turner, Jeffrey Bland, Ph.D., Alex Schauss, Ph.D., Paul Brenner, M.D., Jonathan Wright, M.D., Alan Gaby, M.D., Kaaren Nichols, M.D., Bernard Jensen, N.D., D.C., Ph.D., Leyardia Black, N.D., Charlie Black, N.D., Steven Sandberg-Lewis, N.D., Sally Rockwell, Ph.D., Christiane Northrup, M.D., Blair Taylor, Richard Miller, Ph.D., Solveig Thomson, Ph.D., Glen Warner, M.D., Jack Schwartz, N.D., James Johnston, M.D., John Bastyr, N.D., Stephen and Ondrea Levine, Joel Levey, Davis Lamson, N.D., Ed Madison, N.D., Charlie Greene, M.D., John Thoreson, B.S., David Seaman, D.C., and many others too numerous to mention who have taught and inspired me.
- My children, Cody, Jonah, and Rose, who are my most profound teachers.
- Naturopathic medicine, the tradition that showed me a new way.
- My patients, who help me every day to become a better doctor and teacher.

INTRODUCTION

I have been a practicing physician for twenty years and have witnessed on hospital wards, in emergency rooms, and in general practice both the marvels and failures of modern medicine. The diagnostic precision of today's medical machinery, coupled with advanced surgical techniques and wonder drugs, has given us undeniable advantages in the treatment of conditions that not long ago left us feeling helpless. However, both health professionals and laypersons alike have recognized the short-sightedness and lack of effectiveness of many current high-tech medical treatments. An article in the *New England Journal of Medicine*,[1] for example, announced several years ago that despite powerful chemotherapeutic agents, radiation, and surgery (our prized "magic bullets"), we are losing the war against cancer.

Many have recognized that modern medicine cannot function as a complete health care system, one that is appropriate for all health care needs. Although obviously superb at treating some conditions, modern medicine fails miserably at and is grossly inappropriate for others. Most physicians today would agree with this assertion, but because their formal training is limited to the conventional model of crisis care and disease management based primarily on drugs, surgery, and radiation, they know of no other options to offer their patients. Thus, as competent as many physicians are in their specialties, the prejudices and limitations of their training make it difficult for some patients to receive the kind of care and education that could lead to better health. Although modern conventional medicine has finally begun to include concepts of preventive health care emphasizing nutrition, exercise, and stress management, practically speaking, current conventional medicine is a system still deeply entrenched in disease care and high technology. In what seemed to be an effort to broaden the perspectives of conventionally practicing physicians, the *Journal of the American Medical Association* published in 1991 an article on one of the world's oldest systems of holistic health care, Ayurvedic medicine.[2] However, a subsequent issue harshly criticized the article and one wonders if, in the end, physicians were only further prejudiced against alternative medicine.

After eight exciting and frustrating years of training and practicing in the modern medical system, I came to the realization that I could best serve patients (and be happiest as a physician) in my own practice of "preventive and wellness medicine," which I established in 1979 in Seattle, Washington. It is in this setting, my classes, and now in this book[3] that I offer to individuals a context of health care for which I perceive a great need.

PREVENTIVE AND WELLNESS MEDICINE

I work with people as a health consultant—a diagnostician as well as a guide and teacher. In addition to treating illness, I help my patients see what lifestyle factors may be contributing to their health problems and what actions and self-care skills they can implement to achieve and maintain a more balanced state of being. It is too easy for a physician to see a patient simply as a disease or a set of symptoms. I always strive to look at the whole person, to explore with my patients the effects of and relationships among nutrition, exercise, psychological and social factors, environmental effects, structural alignment, and personal attunement. (I examine the interplay of allergic, hormonal, digestive, and microbiologic factors as well.) To achieve optimal wellness, it is necessary to address all these elements. In addition to my formal medical education, I have been trained in clinical nutrition, orthomolecular and metabolic therapy, environmental medicine, acupuncture (auricular therapy), herbology, homeopathy, iridology, fasting and detoxification, gestalt therapy, imagery and visualization techniques, hypnosis, therapeutic touch, shiatsu, applied kinesiology, and VAS (vascular autonomic system) of pulse diagnosis.

It is my style to get to know a patient well and then choose the approaches that we both feel will be effective (and that may sometimes include prescription medications, surgery, and other conventional forms of medical therapy). By treating illness with both conventional and alternative/naturopathic approaches and emphasizing health education, self-care, and prevention, I work with my patients toward building a health reserve—achieving optimal wellness. In sharing the responsibility for their health care decisions, they develop the confidence and understanding necessary to become full participants in their health care.

This belief, that patients can be active participants in their own cure, is by no means new, but dates back to 400 B.C., when the philosophical roots of naturopathic medicine were established.

Also known as "nature cure," naturopathy traces its roots to alternative healing systems of the eighteenth and nineteenth centuries and is based on the belief that our bodies, in their "natural" state, already contain everything we need to overcome disease and restore optimal function. The physician's role is to aid the body in its healing efforts rather than to take over the functions of the body.

Naturopathy was originated in the United States by Benedict Lust, who began using the term in 1902 to describe the future of natural medicine, a future which combined the best treatments, including nutritional and exercise therapy, natural diet, herbal medicine, homeopathy, and stress reduction, among others.

As Michael Murray and Joseph Pizzorno explain in *The Encyclopedia of Natural Medicine*, naturopathic practitioners believe that "there is really but one healing force in existence and that is Nature herself, which means the inherent restorative power of the organism to overcome disease."

The naturopathic doctor, then, will always turn to the least invasive intervention possible to treat an ailment or disease, which involves such measures as eliminating unhealthy eating habits, regulating breathing and exercise, and helping the patient to attain the right mental attitude and habits.

I have much gratitude and respect for naturopathic medicine, for much of my current practice stems from the inspiration I have received from the naturopathic practitioners I have had the honor of knowing. Like any single medical approach, naturopathic medicine is not a complete health care system. However, naturopathic and modern medicine are excellent complements.

WHO WILL FIND THIS BOOK HELPFUL?

I have written this book to help you become a more knowledgeable and confident participant regarding your health. The information contained within these pages should offer insights largely unexplored by most modern medical practitioners. In a broad sense, *Optimal Wellness* is an extension of the work I do with my patients and students, most of whom fall into the following categories:

- Those who have a diagnosed illness or condition for which modern medicine offers no treatment (or treatment that is ineffective).
- Those whose medical treatments are apparently "working" but who still do not feel healthy.
- Those who are in the gray zone between health and disease, who do not feel or function very well but whose physical examinations and standard laboratory tests are usually "normal."
- Those who want to reduce or discontinue their use of medications, either because of undesirable side effects, a philosophical dislike of prescription drugs, or a preference for nonpharmaceutical or "natural" approaches.
- Those who believe that health is far more than the absence of disease and want guidelines to enhance their immune function and build a health reserve. (A health reserve may be defined as a state in which one usually functions well, in which one's many levels of being are whole and in balance. It is a state in which the strength of one level of being makes up for the deficiency of another. It is a state of increased resistance to illness or at least of adequate recuperative ability in the face of illness or injury.) Such individuals have learned to be active participants in their health care; they know or eventually recognize that what they do, in addition to what doctors offer, can greatly influence (a) how good they can feel and (b) their recovery from and avoidance of illness. These individuals do not appreciate the cloak of mystery with which many physicians shroud their interactions with patients. They will not put up with secrecy and partial or diluted information. They are devoted to learning about themselves and want to understand everything.
- Those who are healthy and want to stay that way, especially those who have a family history of major illness.
- Those health professionals and educators interested in

developing or furthering preventive, wellness, and/or naturopathic approaches in their practices and curricula.

THE COMMON DENOMINATORS OF ILLNESS

In my practice, I have observed a number of common denominators of illness—underlying causes of or significant contributors to chronic and recurring ailments. By uncovering them and implementing treatment, I have been able to help individuals build a health reserve they never thought possible while assisting many others in getting off a medical roller coaster from which they thought there was no escape.

These common denominators are:

- Dietary Hazards
- Nutritional Deficiencies
- Poor Digestion and Assimilation
- Toxic Bowel
- Sluggish Liver
- Hypoglycemia (Low Blood Sugar)
- Adrenal Exhaustion
- Yeast Overgrowth
- Food Allergies/Intolerances
- Psychoneuroimmunology (The Mind–Body Connection)

The recognition and treatment of these conditions in turn affect the competence of the immune system. This relationship is explored in Chapter Sixteen.

Many of these conditions go unrecognized by conventionally practicing doctors. Although some (for example, food allergies, hypoglycemia, and intestinal parasites) are well known, the accepted laboratory tests used to diagnose them often prove unequal to the task. Many others are not examined or given clinical emphasis in medical school or residency training programs. Some have never been described in the professional journals that conventional physicians read. In fact, some poorly designed studies and biased editorials in prestigious journals instruct their readers not to believe in such "fad" or "quack" conditions, and readers will often, without question, adopt as their own the gospel of such publications. Resistance to the recognition of these conditions, as with anything new or different in any well-established field, is basically rooted in attachment to a set of rigidly held beliefs. Regardless of the reasons cited to invalidate these conditions, I and other practitioners of similar mind see people get well so often and in such amazing ways that it is difficult for us not to continue doing what we do.

IN SEARCH OF ULTIMATE HEALTH

It is my hope that *Optimal Wellness* will assist you in regaining and/or maintaining your good health; and I do not propose that health be your ultimate goal in life. Eating natural foods, evacuating your bowels daily, and exercising regularly may not be top priorities for you. This book, however, recommends such optimal wellness measures so that with improved health you may be able to achieve your life purposes—or discover them.

HOW TO USE *OPTIMAL WELLNESS*
Part One—The Self-Care Imperative

Chapter One, "Transformation," attempts through the life stories of two of my patients to portray the wisdom and necessity of becoming your own and best health advocate. These two accounts represent, in macrocosm, the myriad conditions and aspects of health with which you may wish to become familiar.

In Chapter Two you will find the Master Symptom Survey, an abbreviated list of symptoms for most of the ten common denominators of illness listed previously. It will direct you to the underlying conditions that may be eroding your health.

Part Two—Diet and Health

Chapter Three presents the most common American dietary hazards, the illnesses they can cause, and practical choices for more healthful eating.

Chapter Four discusses dietary balance and explores the properties and energies of various foods. It also explains how you can individualize your diet based on your blood and body type. Remember, a diet suitable for one person may make another person ill, and even seasonal changes may affect dietary needs.

Finally, in Chapter Five, some "All-Star" foods are discussed, and tasty and healthful recipes are provided.

Part Three—The Ten Common Denominators of Illness

Chapters Six through Sixteen address each of the ten conditions separately. (You can use the Master Symptom Survey to pinpoint a condition and to determine the appropriate chapter.) Most of these chapters contain case histories and more detailed symptom lists to help you to identify the conditions in yourself. A number include suggested laboratory tests to help substantiate the diagnosis and treatments, many of which lend themselves to self-care and some of which require a health professional's assistance.

Chapter Sixteen offers a discussion of the immune system, the competence of which depends in large part on the recognition and treatment of these conditions.

Part Four—Common Ailments, Natural Remedies, and Preventive Approaches

Chapter Seventeen lists alphabetically over one hundred common health problems, along with suggested treatments and preventive approaches. You can also access information in this chapter through the index.

Part Five—New Age and Age-Old Approaches

In Part Five, you will find information on cleansing/detoxification/fasting, herbs, acupuncture, homeopathy, hydrotherapy, bodywork, exercise, and other alternative approaches for treatment of specific conditions listed in Parts Three and Four and for general health maintenance. Some approaches that lend themselves easily to self-care, such as cleansing/fasting and herbal medicine, are presented in detail. Services usually rendered by health professionals, such as acupuncture and bodywork, are given brief descriptions that serve primarily as an introduction or overview.

Part Six—You and the Medical Profession

Self-care implies more than what you can do for yourself directly; it also means choosing the right helping professionals when their services are necessary and using them wisely. Some guidelines for this may be found in Chapter Twenty-two.

WHAT TO EXPECT

This book does not offer a set of quick answers and simple solutions. Many illnesses are connected with deeply ingrained habits. To turn your health around, you may have to live a very different kind of life from what you are used to. You may need to relearn or readjust a lifetime of eating preferences, reward systems, habits of physical activity, and self-monitoring. The more serious your illness, the more readjusting may be required. Such changes present a potentially major stress with which to contend. If you have been struck with a life-threatening crisis, have been frightened by the prospect of dying, and cherish the possibility of productive years to come,

you will not find it so difficult to commit to a new way of life. The stress of change will likely not be insurmountable with family or other close support relationships to help you maintain your commitment. On the other hand, if your life has not been threatened, your motivation for a change in lifestyle may come from the commonsense appeal of a healthier regimen. In this case, you may encounter some difficulty.

Say, for example, you are currently eating a standard American diet, are fairly sedentary, and have never meditated before. You then decide to dive directly into a low-fat diet with no sugar, caffeine, or processed flour. You also eliminate milk products. At the same time, you decide to do a colon-cleansing regimen, and begin a schedule of enforced aerobic exercise three times weekly and skilled relaxation twice daily. You refuse to see old friends because all they do is drink, smoke, and sit around playing cards or watching television. With such abrupt and dramatic changes, you may soon feel overwhelmingly deprived, constrained, and depressed.

If you are not on the brink of physical disaster, go slowly, one step at a time. Begin in a place that is sensible and comfortable to you. Force yourself to do something healthy just one or two days a week to start. Vary your choice until you find something you truly enjoy. When you are genuinely drawn to something, you will keep coming back. A health program will work only if you stay with it, and the only way you will stay with it is if you enjoy what you are doing and begin to see tangible benefits. Experiment with different foods, different diets, different kinds of fiber or vitamin supplements, different types of exercise, different ways to relax and have fun. Find what feels right for you. It can take months, even years, to become comfortable in a new, healthier way of life.

Self-health care is an ever-changing growth process at which you will get better over time. You may begin simply by minimizing sugar in your diet. Several years later, you may find yourself having radically and comfortably changed your entire lifestyle for the better. Find the right professional guidance when needed, enlist the support of family and friends, and be prepared to encounter setbacks and discouragement along your health journey. Do not let anyone dishearten you; simply pick up where you have left off and continue on your path. Believe in yourself. Believe in your new health regime. With this deep commitment, you will succeed in achieving optimal wellness.

PART ONE

THE SELF-CARE
IMPERATIVE

CHAPTER 1

TRANSFORMATION

We begin our exploration of the self-care imperative by taking a look at two individuals, a young woman and a young man, both plagued with health problems, who find solutions that turn their lives around. Their stories demonstrate some of the glaring inadequacies of modern medicine and portray how self-care and alternative approaches to health uncover the underlying causes of their numerous symptoms. Along the way, they improve their health dramatically, and, in fact, transform their lives.

Sally's story begins our examination of optimal wellness. Limited by a host of conditions for which her doctor has her taking seven different medications, Sally feels ill most of the time, even though her examinations and laboratory tests are always normal. Her journey back to health epitomizes the core issues involved in optimal wellness and self-care—motivating yourself for change and taking responsibility for regaining wellness.

Our second story involves Steve, a young man who develops an array of disabling symptoms that lead him through a maze of specialists, none of whom are able to diagnose or treat him successfully. He is unable through lifestyle measures to turn his health around. Steve finally finds the answers and treatment he needs when he is diagnosed as having three fairly straightforward conditions, two of which mainstream medical doctors do not recognize. His experience underscores the need for some individuals to seek health professionals with a perspective broader than that of conventional medicine.

SALLY

Sally came into my office with an expression on her face that quite accurately fit her statement: "I'm a wreck, and I'm only twenty-eight years old!" She proceeded to tell me that for the last two and a half years she had been seeing a physician periodically, who gave her codeine for her headaches, diet pills for her weight problem, antidepressants for her moodiness, two different antibiotics for her acne and recurring bronchitis, vaginal cream for the yeast infections caused by the antibiotics, and water pills for her premenstrual fluid retention. He also recommended laxatives for her constipation, which had been aggravated by the codeine. It seemed, she added, that she was always using some cold or flu preparation as well and sucking on throat lozenges. Her physician never diagnosed any real disease. The examination and laboratory tests were usually "normal." He told her she was basically fine but needed to "just relax a little more" and take the medication he prescribed.

Sally related how she was sick and tired of pills. Although they sometimes gave temporary relief, she feared becoming dependent on some of them and disliked their side effects. I pointed out to Sally that most importantly, these pills were not addressing the causes of her various ailments or building up her health. She was not ill by medical standards, I explained, but she was far from healthy. In such a position, modern medicine had little to offer other than symptom-suppressing medicines. A preventive and optimal wellness approach, I encouraged her, could very well bring her out of her current impasse.

Sally also expressed fear that, like her mother, she would develop breast cancer, as well as gallbladder disease, or, like her father, end up with a heart attack and colon cancer. For years, both parents suffered numerous chronic minor conditions like Sally's that were treated similarly with a myriad of prescription drugs. They had never really felt well, but nothing ever showed up on their exams or lab tests—until their crises struck. Unfortunately, Sally's parents were of a generation that never questioned a doctor's authority or the popular belief that pills were the solution to their health problems. Even when they were diagnosed with their cancers, this attitude did not change.

I supported Sally's belief that coping with minor ailments and taking pills merely to relieve symptoms may very well have led to her parents' catastrophic diseases and surgeries. If they had gone to a doctor who sought to diagnose and treat the underlying causes of their ailments and taught them preventive and self-care measures to genuinely improve their health and well-being, they perhaps would have avoided major illness. With this speculation, Sally was onto something vital—the crux of preventive and wellness medicine.

She made another observation: through their surgeries and chemotherapy, her parents never knew or thought to do anything to promote their own recovery. Instead, they acted and lived like victims while following their doctors' treatment orders. Sally could see that years of feeling like victims, first of minor ailments, and later of major diseases, made them helpless and fearful and contributed to what she felt was a pitiful quality of life.

In grappling with the issues of her own health and not wanting to repeat her parents' patterns, Sally was deciding she was no longer going to be a victim. It was a decision made from an unshakable conviction—without even having knowledge of alternative health approaches—that there was a better way.

Sally proceeded to describe the "wreck" of her body. Over the past two years, she had become progressively fatigued and moody. Due to a host of other complaints, she said that she felt more like she was sixty-eight than twenty-eight. She said, "I am fatigued from the moment I awake in the morning. Although there are sometimes waves of energy during the day, I could fall asleep on a moment's notice if given the opportunity." She described her moodiness as frightful; the slightest confrontation with her boss at the mall supermarket or her boyfriend at home would bring on tears and either render her incapable of expressing herself or cause her to explode in a fit of irrational anger. In between such major episodes, she portrayed herself as having lost her joie de vivre. She could not remember the last time she had let out a genuine laugh.

Sally lamented over the thirty-five pounds she had gained in the previous three and a half years. She complained about her constant bouts of constipation. She read from her list of complaints: sallow complexion, acne, bad breath, recurring abdominal aches and indigestion, chronically sore throat, headaches, foggy-headed or fuzzy thinking, and poor memory. In addition, she described premenstrual symptoms of bloating, headaches, breast tenderness, and intolerable feelings of fragility and sensitivity. All of these symptoms, when combined, were severe enough to necessitate one or two sick days off from work each month. She would miss another day or two every month or so from recurrent colds that would invariably develop into bronchitis.

Her work as a supermarket checker, she related to me, was a job to which she felt ill-suited. She had nearly finished a college degree in computer science but had never completed her studies. She felt that being a supermarket checker was neither rewarding nor challenging. Sally described other undesirable aspects of her job: the alternating day and night shifts she was obligated to work kept her from establishing a consistent sleep cycle, and the fluorescent lights she stood under at her job undoubtedly aggravated her fatigue and moodiness.

She wondered if her diet was somehow connected with any of her health complaints and proceeded to describe what she ate in the course of a typical day. Breakfast was coffee and fruit. Lunch meant tuna or chicken salad, french fries, grilled cheese sandwich, or pizza. Dinner usually consisted of macaroni and cheese or fried chicken and quick rice, sometimes a small salad and french roll and canned soup. She drank two or three soft drinks and two or three cups of coffee with sugar during the day. She also had a constant sweet tooth.

In listening to Sally's story, I could see that in addition to all of the body functions that were not working properly—conditions for which I felt she was grossly overmedicated—many parts of her life were plainly out of balance: her diet, her level of physical activity, her sleep, her job, her avocation—in short, her general attitude. It was not difficult to understand how the disharmony in all of these areas interconnected and produced a downward spiral of poor health. Very little in her life was nurturing, building, harmonizing, or fun. Very little seemed to contribute to her well-being.

Although Sally was sour on nearly everything and felt as if she were hitting bottom, I could see she was a fighter. Given support, encouragement, and the right information, she would be able to pull herself up.

Sally's Recovery: From Being Sick to Living Well

The first specific area we worked on was her diet, one of the cornerstones of health. Without adequate nutritional support, the brain, as well as every other organ, gland, and system in the body, cannot function normally. Demands for vitamins, minerals, fatty acids, amino acids, and carbohydrates must be met. To function at peak efficiency, every hormone, enzyme, antibody, and neurotransmitter requires a good diet. The harmony of all these components will be disrupted not only by nutrient deficiencies, but by an overconsumption of sugar, fat, caffeine, fried and rancid foods, refined flour, and chemical food additives. Sally's diet, though normal-sounding, was excessive in all these dietary hazards and deficient in the important nutrient categories. From a basic dietary standpoint, it was no surprise that her body and mind were giving her so much trouble.

I could see that Sally's "overwhelm button" had been pushed at the prospect of having to overhaul her entire diet. It was easy for her to understand and accept the relationship between health and nutrition, but it made her visibly anxious to consider how she would make it over the hurdles of her present eating habits. I reassured Sally that making a transition to a whole-foods diet was a gradual process that she could succeed at with the right guidance. And she would not have to rely on her willpower alone. I could assist her, I explained, with the biochemical and nutrient support that would strengthen her enough to take on such changes. Such nutritional support could also minimize her cravings for and addictions to sugar and caffeine (see Chapter Three).

Correcting Low Blood Sugar

The first actual condition I examined related to Sally's carbohydrate metabolism. She displayed several indications of hypoglycemia: fatigue, irritability, shakiness, "spaciness," depression, and headaches, to name a few. She could almost predict the onset of these symptoms if she delayed her meals or snacks. However, she could have these symptoms to a lesser degree at nearly any time of the day. As is so often the case, her pancreas was overstimulated by too much sugar, which meant that her adrenal glands were likely overstressed as well. From tests we obtained subsequently, I also learned that the protein in her diet was not being adequately digested or absorbed. You may already be aware that when the brain is not being supplied with a consistent level of its most important fuel, glucose (blood sugar), hypoglycemic symptoms result. Paradoxically, one major cause of sugar deprivation to the brain is the consumption of too much refined sugar, as well as too much caffeine, not enough protein, and poor protein digestion. Making a gradual shift to a whole-foods diet, I pointed out to Sally, is the cornerstone of treatment for hypoglycemia, namely, reducing sweets and refined foods and increasing whole foods such as whole grains, legumes, and fresh vegetables. Since she was not vegetarian, I also emphasized an adequate intake of animal protein. To aid in stabilizing her blood sugar, decreasing her craving for sweets, strengthening her adrenal glands, and giving her brain a better biochemical and nutritional environment, I recommended important vitamin and mineral supplements as part of her treatment. (Chapter Three provides specific hints for overcoming sugar addiction, while

Chapter Ten lists the symptoms indicative of hypoglycemia and the corresponding dietary and vitamin recommendations. Chapter Eleven explains the concept and treatment of adrenal exhaustion.)

A New Way of Eating

Over the next six weeks and three visits—while monitoring Sally's progress, obtaining more tests, and diagnosing other conditions that would eventually require treatment—I worked with Sally primarily as a teacher, providing her with do and don't lists, even recipes, and a lot of encouragement. Although Sally had not cut out sugar completely, her diet was definitely shifting in the right direction. She was including whole-grain items (cereals, breads, crackers, and noodles) more than 50 percent of the time and using less of the refined flour counterparts. She was now occasionally preparing bean soups and other legume dishes and being sure to buy lots of fresh vegetables. She was making certain to get in some animal protein at least once a day, if not twice.

Sally was still not fully familiar with this new way of preparing food and didn't have any friends who cooked in this health-conscious manner. However, she had found some simple recipes to which she was becoming accustomed (see Chapter Five). She was also learning to shop at food co-ops and health food stores, where she could find bulk bins of whole grains, legumes, seeds and nuts, and herbal teas. Genuine whole-grain breads that had no refined and vitamin-fortified flour were also available there, as were chicken and beef not raised on hormones and antibiotics. Organic produce was frequently sold at these stores.

Many of these items, she discovered, were also available in the health food sections of some supermarkets. She was also learning to read labels and avoid so-called natural products with a lot of hidden sugars and bad oils (see Chapter Three). Sally enrolled in a natural foods cooking class in which she learned to prepare a variety of delicious, health-giving foods. She also met a woman in class who was to become a close friend and source of support on her "journey." It was at this point that she was eating sweets only three times a week and felt with the help of her program that her sweet tooth was now more a habit than a need.

Kicking the Caffeine Habit

In just the fourth week of her diet change and vitamin regimen, Sally was beginning to feel better than she had in months. She was eager to continue her recovery and rejuvenation, so we proceeded to tackle her caffeine habit. Her daily dose of caffeine had been quite high, up to three cups of coffee and three soft drinks a day, as well as chocolate and diet pills. Many of her symptoms fit the picture of caffeine intoxication (see page 67). On the first day she stopped drinking coffee all at once without tapering off. She then experienced fatigue, irritability, shakiness, and a headache so severe that she had to leave work early. Not knowing what else to do, she drank a few cups of coffee, and to her surprise her headache and other symptoms quickly subsided. She felt herself again—only to experience a slight headache, irritability, and fatigue a few hours later.

Sally quickly realized that caffeine was actually a drug to which she was addicted. When the drug was not available, her body would go through terrible withdrawal symptoms, which would subside if she drank coffee again. Her body was begging her, by means of the painful symptoms, for another "hit" of caffeine. She was hooked.

With the support that her improving diet and supplement program provided, Sally's level of energy eventually rose until she no longer felt such urgent need for a caffeine lift every morning. Her efforts to quit caffeine soon proved successful. Gradually, over two and a half weeks, she tapered the amount she was ingesting. By the time she abstained completely, she was no longer using diet pills or craving soft drinks. She cut back her coffee intake to only one cup a day. Learning about the healthful substitutes for her caffeinated beverages made things much easier during this transition. Sally discovered several herbal teas, hot and iced, that satisfied her taste and need to be drinking something continually.

Improved Digestion and Elimination

By now, with no caffeine, much less sugar, and many more whole foods in her diet, Sally realized that 60 to 70 percent of her bowel complaints were gone. This new diet, which was quite high in fiber and much lower in cheese, enabled her to have fuller and less difficult bowel movements every other day and once in a while daily (compared to every three to four days before). Her breath, she noticed, was smelling sweeter and her complexion was improving. Eventually she decided to undertake an intestinal cleansing program that I recommended. She subsequently found, to her surprise, just how much better her whole digestive system could function. (In Chapter Eight, you will find a discussion of how to assess and normalize bowel function.) But these efforts were still not enough.

Despite a pretty good diet, Sally still had a tendency to become constipated and sometimes bloated. However, she did experience much less indigestion now that she was eating a more wholesome diet, chewing her food more thoroughly, and remembering to relax at meals. She also noticed that she could avoid gas by not having fruit or anything sweet after dinner. Yet she still required

snacks between meals to avoid getting headaches and feeling spacey. My testing showed her to be deficient in both pancreatic enzymes and stomach hydrochloric acid. By supplementing her meals with pancreatic enzymes and hydrochloric acid/pepsin capsules, I solved her remaining bowel and hypoglycemic symptoms. (See Chapter Seven for suggestions on how to assess and treat digestive problems.)

Social Pressures

During the process of changing her diet and following various programs and treatments, Sally encountered a common social pitfall. Her friends ridiculed her new habits, calling her an extremist and a "health food nut," and seemed always to be inviting her to eat out at their favorite haunts. These were places where Sally was forced to exert enormous effort to resist ordering unhealthy foods while turning down the tempting morsels her "friends" dangled seductively before her on spoons. Since they did not have the health problems plaguing Sally, they did not really understand how pizza, cola, ice cream, and coffee could be bad for her. They were even less willing to understand the likely long-term effects of such a diet—cancer, heart disease, and other serious ailments with which Sally's parents were contending.

Sally occasionally surrendered to these temptations and sometimes regretted it, as her body unpredictably retaliated with the old symptoms. Her desire to maintain her new food discipline was in direct conflict with her belief that in order to be a good friend, she should participate in whatever everyone else was doing, even if it meant damaging her health. After some of her slips, she felt that precious ground had been lost.

Giving in to social pressures cost Sally a lot more than a few headaches, stomach complaints, or general malaise. It left her with feelings of self-betrayal and low self-esteem. The resulting depression would then stimulate her need to eat more sugar. If this chain of events continued long enough, it would lead her back to her previous state of physical addiction: the use of sugar and caffeine would cause symptoms—fatigue, irritability, headache—that could only be alleviated by further use of these very substances. Sally understood the dynamics of this vicious circle but felt trapped in it nonetheless.

Wisdom and Strength

Sally was able to find her way out by discovering a deeper strength and wisdom. She remembered how much she dreaded "not feeling good" and having to ride the medical roller coaster of pills and more pills. She also recalled from our discussions that her body functioned best with optimal biochemical support, so she decided to be nearly religious about taking all of her vitamin supplements. Sally knew how much better she felt when she took them regularly. She reestablished a connection with her genuine desire to be well and, as an extension of this desire, recognized the importance of being very strict in the initial stages.

Discovering Real Friends

Sally began to understand that if giving in to social pressures jeopardized her body's delicate balance and damaged her self-esteem, then something must be inherently wrong with relationships that would produce such social pressures. She began to see that a real friend would not encourage or demand her participation in anything that was destructive to her. With new resolve, she renewed her commitment to her diet and, in the process, was reminded of who her real friends were and what authentic friendship was all about. Sally was eventually able to forgive her friends when she realized that their intentions to break her resolve were motivated by their own guilt with food issues. Yet, it was some time before she decided to be with them again.

Self-Forgiveness

At some point in the course of these discoveries, I was able to teach Sally that one way out of a self-hating, sugar-eating cycle was to intervene fiercely with self-forgiveness. Only she could rescue herself, and the intervention could not be harsh, punishing, unreasonable, or unforgiving. She learned to remind herself that, although she might be having a setback or had retreated a few steps, she was still far ahead of her starting place. Her body was much healthier in many ways. She could see particularly that her attitude had improved tremendously. She had developed a genuine interest in her health; she had mustered motivation, courage, strength, and awareness. She loved seeing these qualities in herself, and when she remembered these little victories over the old Sally, she derived satisfaction and strength. Picking herself up, she would say to herself, "Well, every new and unfamiliar journey is going to have a few setbacks: getting flat tires, becoming lost, running out of gas, being unable to find a motel. Little setbacks here and there cannot ruin this wonderful trip. Let's just get up and keep going."

Big Decisions

As Sally grew healthier and stronger, her inner vision seemed to clear. She began to scrutinize what was for her the most tension-producing aspect of her current state of being, her stormy two-year relationship with her boyfriend. Although the two were lovers, she realized they were far from friends or wholesome companions

for each other. She could see how each one was using the other to fulfill genuine needs but without the compassion and love to be truly concerned about the other's welfare, growth, and development. Although some needs were being met, the most important ones were not. A relationship intended originally to be mutually supportive turned out to be mutually abusive. With the encouragement and "permission" of a counselor whom I had advised her to see and whom she came to trust, Sally was able to break away from this destructive relationship. It was a decision she had come to on her own. With some help and support, she went through with it. And she never regretted the move. Looking back, she felt that the act of taking responsibility for a major life decision was, in itself, strengthening and health-giving. From this point on, everything seemed to take a giant leap forward for the better.

A Chain Reaction of Good Events

Approximately six to seven months after Sally and I started working together, she was feeling consistently stronger, both physically and emotionally. She could now go longer between meals without hypoglycemic symptoms. She could cheat on her diet once in a while and not feel adverse effects. Eating sugar every now and then would not induce the old addiction cycle. She felt in control and could enjoy occasional indulgences without guilt. She also seemed to be able to get by on fewer vitamin and digestive supplements. Apparently, with so much less tension in her life, her body and mind felt more balanced: her adrenal glands, her metabolism of carbohydrates, her digestive system, and her nervous system all were stronger and more stable.

She quit her job at the supermarket and resourcefully used her savings and a small loan from her parents to return to school to finish her beloved computer studies. Sally then found a desirable position in her chosen field, and, through her work, seemed to grow personally as well as professionally. She started walking the two miles to and from work at least three days a week. She was rediscovering and reclaiming those aspects of her life that made her feel more complete.

Pounds Lighter

Sally experienced one unexpected benefit from her self-care journey: weight loss. Once she'd improved all the areas we addressed together, her overall health improved vastly, which was her intended goal. She had no idea, however, that she would also lose much of her extra weight. Previous "quick" weight-loss programs had not been consistently helpful; they had induced a rapid weight loss without concern for health and well-being (sometimes they'd actually drained her of energy and subjected her to mood swings). Now, controlling her weight seemed easier and much more sensible through her improved total health.

Beginnings and Endings

This is Sally's journey, or as much of it as I know. I later learned that she had married, was pregnant, and was still taking good care of herself. Her journey will continue, as all journeys do. Beginnings and endings, if there are endings at all, are all different. For Sally, the beginning was her realization that she was "hitting bottom," and her belief that there was a better way. A substantial change in her diet plus the addition of vitamin, mineral, and digestive supplements began to even her out biochemically. This helped her feel so much healthier, both physically and mentally, that she could cope much better and, in fact, enjoy life again. These very same measures were substantially lessening her risks of future illness—heart disease, cancer, osteoporosis, diabetes, stroke, and other serious diseases.

With strength and hope, she continued to work on her body, and her commitment to personal growth followed suit. Having to change her diet forced her to examine the meaning of social pressures and friendships, and later to address the issue of self-esteem. She struggled courageously. Eventually she learned to forgive and believe in herself. She realized along the way that these two factors were perhaps the most vital components to her success and happiness. She ended a destructive relationship, quit a job that held little meaning for her, and pursued a career that made genuine use of her talents. Her willingness to seek professional guidance in several areas empowered her to become more self-sufficient and whole. Her feeling of well-being eventually attained a level she had never known possible.

Inadequacies of Modern Medicine

Sally also learned to recognize something important about doctors and modern medicine. She knew her previous doctor had been doing his best all those years but later realized that the scope of his practice was insufficient for her health needs and goals. His primary concern seemed always to focus either on detecting disease or on writing a quick prescription that would make her "better" by suppressing symptoms. The structure of his practice and his concept of health did not allow for any other meaningful investigation. There was never any interest in looking for the deeper, underlying causes of all her symptoms. There was never any focus on health education or on teaching her to build her health.

While on the road to recovery, Sally tried to explain to him some of the underlying ailments from which she had been suffering for years. She shared some of the wonderful changes she had made. It was as if she were speaking a foreign language to him, however. She was somewhat surprised to learn that he did not even believe in the existence of some of these conditions, nor did he care to hear about them. His reluctance was firm despite the fact that she was feeling much better from the treatments and no longer needed most of her old prescriptions. She was, however, distinctly disappointed with his impatience, his inference that she would be better off back on his medications. His mockery of her involvement in "fringe" medicine especially annoyed her. Fortunately, Sally recognized that his opinions came from a biased and limited frame of reference. She had developed enough confidence to withstand his skepticism; she would not allow him to invalidate her own experience. Instead, she felt a mixture of anger and regret that he could not widen his perspective enough to consider another point of view.

Sally realized that modern medicine represents an incomplete system of health care and is actually more of a disease-care system. It is good for certain things, she recognized, and bad for others. She learned she should never again blindly trust a medical opinion, but rather should use it as information with which to make her own decisions. Unlike her parents, she learned that although crisis/disease-oriented medical care is important and does address a need, it cannot teach patients how to build a health reserve. Her "optimal wellness," she realized, would have to be established and maintained largely by her own attitude, learning, and efforts—which is the self-care imperative.

The Journey Continues

From the initial step of altering her diet, Sally embarked on a journey that changed her life. Over two and a half years, she developed in herself the tools and knowledge to care for her body, mind, and spirit not only to prevent disease, but to attain her full health and perhaps life potential. This is the ultimate goal of *Optimal Wellness*.

Please do not interpret this story as a "happily ever after" fairy tale, however. Sally still experiences her ups and downs, still suffers occasionally from depression, abdominal ache, and occasional bouts of constipation and weight gain if she doesn't pay attention to the factors that get her into trouble. Yet she has overcome much of the helplessness and fear experienced in dealing with her problems, after learning about self-care, after uncovering the causes of her ailments, and after determining what attitudes to hold and actions to take to pull herself up.

Sally's journey is not about evolving to a state where problems do not exist; problems will always arise. However, when problems become opportunities for learning and growth and for applying one's newfound and ever-growing knowledge and wisdom, life has been transformed.

STEVE

I could not tell if it was tears or anger that Steve was holding back as he explained to me in our first visit that he no longer had the health to be the father or husband he once knew himself to be. Employed as an engineer at a local aerospace company, Steve was currently on a medical leave of absence. Just one year before, he had enjoyed robust health, working up to fifty-five hours a week following a recent promotion that put him on a jet-set international negotiating team. However, he spent all of his free time with his wife and family. At forty-two, Steve had two sons, ages thirteen and sixteen, and a six-year-old daughter. The family played football and basketball, and spent time swimming, hiking, and camping during their free evenings and on weekends. Vacations usually meant vigorous activity. Steve had loved to work and play hard, but now his life was different.

In the previous year, he developed a progressive and overwhelming fatigue that mystified his family doctor. A complete physical examination and comprehensive laboratory tests indicated nothing abnormal. His doctor told him to take some time off, to work fewer hours, to sleep more, and to not compete so adamantly with his sixteen-year-old, who was a varsity athlete. Steve obeyed his doctor's orders. He was able, fortunately, to work half-time for one month. His employer then permitted him to take a two-week vacation, so that he had six weeks in the middle of the summer to recuperate.

To his dismay, after six weeks of taking it easy, Steve still felt no better. In fact, his condition worsened when he returned to his full work schedule. He soon experienced low-grade fevers, swollen and painful lymph nodes, a sore throat, and generalized muscle and joint aches. He felt as if he had the flu all the time. When he began losing his memory and ability to concentrate, he sought a second opinion.

The internist Steve saw proved not to be much more help than his family doctor. Using blood tests, she diagnosed chronic fatigue syndrome stemming from an Epstein-Barr virus infection, which couldn't be treated. The doctor, however, prescribed a course of antibiotics to alleviate his sore throat, fever, and swollen lymph glands. Other than that, she felt there was nothing she could offer for relief. Initially, the antibiotics seemed to help, and after two weeks on this medication Steve was encouraged. However, his symptoms returned full strength the third week. Another two-week course of medication did not help. He began to feel desperate.

He tried a complete overhaul of his diet. With his wife's help, he eliminated sugar, processed flour, fried foods, and junk foods from his meals. For six weeks, he ate fresh vegetables and fruits (nearly all organic), brown rice, and other whole grains, including homemade whole wheat bread. He also included legumes, nonfat milk products, raw seeds and nuts, and hormone- and antibiotic-free eggs and poultry. He ate minimal red meat and included fresh fish in his diet at least three times a week.

He was certain that such an obviously healthful diet would have to help, but after six weeks he had to face facts: he was making hardly any gains. He felt like giving up. He could no longer "fake it" at work. His diminishing performance was becoming evident to everyone. At home, his family hardly recognized him anymore. Once a major source of energy and enthusiasm, he was now a near invalid who would force himself out of bed every morning and drag himself home at night, with no strength to interact with anyone. He frequently went right to bed without dinner.

Over the next three months, Steve saw a series of specialists. He had developed a host of new allergies. His sinuses were frequently congested and runny. He suffered headaches from the smells of certain perfumes, exhausts, and fresh paint. He scheduled an appointment with an allergist. The scratch tests found him to be mildly allergic to mold and cats, but not enough to warrant allergy shots or to explain the severity of his fatigue and other symptoms.

When Steve asked about the possibility of a food allergy, his doctor told him flatly that foods could not be related to his illness. He next saw a neurologist, who could not find anything to explain his memory and concentration deficits or his headaches. He saw a gastroenterologist, who ordered upper and lower gastrointestinal X-rays, and even a colonoscopy, but found nothing to explain the persistent nausea and constipation. Steve declined the liver biopsy that was next on the list of tests.

By this time, Steve was anxious and depressed and needed to take a medical leave from work. He went back to his family doctor, who gave him antidepressant medication that seemed to clear his head but did not give him the strength to return to work or a normal family life.

Tracking Down the Sources of Steve's Condition

Finally, Steve ended up in my office telling me the details of his saga, one that has become extremely familiar to me. In fact, I hear similar complaints from other patients several times a day. When he was finished, I asked him if he remembered any event that occurred shortly before the onset of his fatigue, anything that might have some bearing on the deterioration of his health. Was there any injury, any emotional trauma, any unusual work stress, any paint or chemical exposure, any medication he took, anything that stood out in his mind?

Steve responded immediately that he wondered if a grueling six-day hike taken in late spring, just before the decline of his health, was connected to his current illness. He said he was tired at the start of the hike after having finished two insane workweeks. One week involved a particularly difficult and exhausting trip to Japan. He also wondered if it was important to mention that he'd drunk some river water at one of his campsites that had seemed to give him some diarrhea and mild intestinal cramps for just two days. Although his stools firmed up, he said his bowels never felt quite normal after that. He felt a sense of mild bloating, occasional nausea, and, lately, a tendency to constipation. He volunteered that three recent stool tests revealed no "bugs."

Giardia Infection

I shared with Steve that the lab testing procedure to identify parasites, especially *Giardia*, a common parasite in the waters of the Northwest where beavers live, will commonly miss the organism, sometimes even after three separate stool samples. Utilizing a lesser-known technique that can identify disintegrated *Giardia* cysts, a fecal *Giardia* antigen assay, would be far more sensitive and accurate.

Steve was not as encouraged as I by the possibility that part of his illness was due to a treatable infection. He had nearly given up hope and figured that I, like his previous doctors, would probably come up with nothing. I explained that a chronic parasite infection like giardiasis can go undetected for years, since it may simply cause minor bowel complaints that people learn to accept. However, the infection can drain the immune reserve and make an individual far more susceptible to viruses and illness, often causing generalized and even debilitating fatigue.

I obtained this test on Steve, and, indeed, he had giardiasis. With an antiparasite medication, most of his intestinal symptoms resolved. Within a few weeks, he was feeling a little stronger. His level of energy was higher, and he could exert himself more, without the usual sore throat, swollen glands, and fever that formerly developed.

Candida Onslaught

I also obtained a stool and blood test, to first determine if Steve's illness was related at all to the *Candida albicans* fungus, a yeast that is a normal inhabitant of the intestinal tract. *Candida albicans* can overgrow and cause intestinal symptoms, along with the fatigue, sore throat, achy muscles, allergies, and foggy brain that were still disabling Steve (see Chapter Twelve). It is common knowledge that antibiotics can trigger yeast overgrowth. Steve's medical history revealed that he took tetracycline for four years in high school and college for the treatment of acne. More recently was the four-week course of antibiotics he took, as well as his returning and severe sugar habit, another yeast-promoting factor. Nearly everyone with chronic giardiasis—and therefore weakened intestinal immunity—will also harbor too much intestinal yeast. So Steve had more than enough reasons to suspect a significant yeast infection. It was not surprising that his stool tests showed abundant Candida colonies, and his blood showed evidence of free-circulating Candida antigens (see Chapter Twelve).

Treating the Invaders and Allergies

After the eradication of giardiasis, and six weeks into the Candida treatment, which involved not only medication and nutritional supplements but also a very wholesome and sugar-free diet, Steve noticed significant improvement and started feeling confident that his full health would eventually return. On his first visit, I advised a weekly intravenous nutrient cocktail containing vitamins C, B complex, B-5, B-6, and B-12, and the minerals magnesium, chromium, selenium, manganese, zinc, and copper (see pages 425–426, "Chronic Fatigue Syndrome," for details). These injections would boost his energy, dissipate his fevers and lymph gland soreness, and give him a temporary sense of well-being. The effects would usually last a week or more. However, while recovering from his giardiasis and Candida infection, he found that after four shots, the injections were no longer necessary. He was gathering a reserve of strength.

Steve would get cocky occasionally and think he could go back to his three sodas a day, donuts, and candy bars, but with the prompt return of his symptoms he realized it was best to stay with the program. As he became more attuned to the effects of his diet, I encouraged him to try to eliminate some of his most repetitive foods as an experiment for ten days, replacing them with nutritionally equivalent alternatives—a self-testing procedure for food allergy/intolerance (see page 245 in Chapter Thirteen).

With the elimination of both wheat and milk products, Steve felt much sharper mentally, had clearer sinuses, less intestinal bloating, and less muscle soreness. He could reproduce these symptoms by reintroducing these foods. Thus we concluded that Steve had a significant degree of food allergy/intolerance, and decided to obtain a blood test for delayed hypersensitivity reactions to a broad panel of foods. After then having eliminated tuna, oranges, grapes, corn, aspartame, and several other items that showed up on the test, Steve experienced a new level of symptom resolution. Following four to five months of avoidance, he was able to use most of these foods regularly once again, without any apparent problems. Once his inflamed intestinal lining and "leaky gut" had healed sufficiently, he was no longer allergic (see Chapter Thirteen).

Steve was soon able to exercise without feeling worse from it. Gradually, over three to four months, he seemed to regain his full strength and health. He still had to watch his sugar intake, which meant not having dessert more than two or three times a week. But he could once again participate fully with his family and work at full capacity at his job. He was on the road to good health.

Steve may not have been diagnosed correctly. Chronic fatigue syndrome is commonly a diagnosis of exclusion, but his other physicians did not fully consider a parasite infection or a Candida-related illness or food allergy—conditions that can cause symptoms similar to chronic fatigue syndrome, but that often go unrecognized. Many physicians, in fact, are not aware of the latter two conditions, and not one of Steve's five previous specialists had even inquired about his diet.

Candida-related illness, food allergies, diet, and other areas covered in this book will someday be mainstream medical diagnoses and concerns with which all health professionals will be familiar. Giving patients suffering from chronic fatigue a trial of nutrient injections may become as common as giving patients with depression a trial of antidepressant medication. Until that time, however, individuals like Steve may have to suffer through a year of tests, six physicians, and the misspending of thousands of dollars before they find the answers they need. Steve reached an impasse with mainstream medical specialists and finally realized that he needed to find a physician with an entirely different perspective. In finding such a doctor, he found his health again.

SELF-CARE IS HEALTH CARE

From both Steve's and Sally's experiences, I hope you recognize that as sick as you might be feeling, and as little help as you might be receiving from your doctor, optimal wellness is a genuine possibility for you. From Sally's story, I hope you have recognized that optimal wellness is integrally linked to the call to self-care. It's critically important to learn what you can about all the health factors you are able to influence: your diet, exercise, stress level, relationships, self-esteem, feelings, goals, and so on. It is the call to find the right teachers, motivators, guides, and books to help you learn about yourself and your body, and to implement a health-giving way of living. It is the call to understand your weaknesses and strengths. It is also a chance to develop the measures that will return you to balance and keep you there.

As Steve's story demonstrates, the self-care imperative is also the call to find the right health professionals with the particular perspectives and approaches necessary to diagnose and treat your illnesses. Like Steve, you may have a condition draining your health reserve too severely to benefit substantially from a good diet and rest alone. You may need the right health professional to help get you over the hump so that your personal self-care measures will make a difference in the recovery and maintenance of your health. The self-care imperative is the call of Optimal Wellness—the challenge of personal empowerment. Your health is in your hands!

MASTER SYMPTOM SURVEY

The following survey is designed to help you and your doctor uncover conditions that may be responsible for your chronic or recurring health problems. Effectively addressing these conditions should put you on the road to optimal wellness.

The Master Symptom Survey is divided into twelve categories. Under each condition, you will find a list of characteristic symptoms or predisposing factors. Your responses to each section will provide important clues about which of the Ten Common Denominators of Illness may be compromising your current health.

Begin this survey by rating each symptom according to the point scale which follows, then calculate your total score. Your highest total score is a good indicator of which of the Ten Common Denominators should serve as the starting point for your self-care program.

If two or more of your total scores are close or identical, you may have several coexisting conditions. Read each of the corresponding chapters to determine where to best direct your initial effort.

Quite often, after working successfully on one condition (yeast overgrowth, for example), symptoms from other conditions you may also have, such as hypoglycemia and food allergies, may diminish or even subside. Not only does yeast overgrowth predispose to both hypoglycemia and allergies, but the treatment for the former is similar in some respects to the treatments for the latter.

If you are concerned about several conditions in particular, begin working on the one causing you the most discomfort, then see how things progress. If necessary, direct efforts at other suspects. If you lack confidence in your own assessment, especially if your complaints are not minor, or if they are persistent or worsen, you should seek the assistance of a health professional—ideally one experienced in the evaluation and treatment of these conditions.

As diet is so central to the discussion of the Ten Common Denominators of Illness, the Master Symptom Survey is followed by eleven tables of dietary excesses/hazards and their potential medical consequences. At a glance, you'll be able to tell if your diet is putting you at risk. (How to avoid dietary hazards is explained in Chapter Three.)

MASTER SYMPTOM SURVEY

HOW TO USE THE MASTER SYMPTOM SURVEY

To evaluate your current health status, complete each of the following twelve symptom surveys. Rate the occurrence of each symptom according to the scale below, then calculate your total score.

SYMPTOM RATING SCALE

0=Never
1=Seldom
2=Occasionally
3=Frequently
4=Infrequently with severe symptoms
5=Almost always

The higher your total score for any single symptom survey, the greater the likelihood that your health is being compromised by that condition. Scores in the moderate to severe range or higher indicate that you would benefit from reading the corresponding chapter(s) and noting any other conditions related to your symptoms.

Since your goal is optimal wellness, low scores may also benefit from further evaluation. If your total score for any condition falls in the mild imbalance range, or you have no total scores higher than mild imbalance in the entire Master Symptom Survey, consider reading the corresponding chapters as a preventive measure.

Note: If your symptoms persist or are severe in nature, regardless of your score, please consult your physician.

NUTRITIONAL DEFICIENCIES* (CHAPTER SIX)

Rate the occurrence of each symptom according to the scale below, then calculate your total score.

SYMPTOM RATING SCALE

0=Never   1=Seldom   2=Occasionally   3=Frequently
4=Infrequently with severe symptoms   5=Almost always

___ Hypoglycemia
___ Food allergies
___ Chemical hypersensitivity
___ Depression
___ Insomnia
___ Fatigue
___ Irritability
___ High blood pressure
___ Premenstrual symptoms
___ Recurrent colds and respiratory infections
___ Dry skin
___ Eczema
___ Seborrheic dermatitis
___ Acne
___ Diarrhea
___ Poor night vision
___ Carpal tunnel syndrome

___ Spina bifida (birth defect attributed to nutritional deficiencies in pregnant women)
___ Cervical dysplasia (abnormal Pap smear)
___ Heart rhythm disturbance (palpitations)
___ Gum disease
___ Bruising
___ High blood cholesterol
___ Arteriosclerosis
___ Phlebitis
___ Infertility
___ Arthritis
___ Excessive dietary hazards (refined carbohydrates, partially hydrogenated oils, phosphorus from soft drinks and flesh foods)

Total Score: ___

Scores in the range of 1–15 may indicate a mild imbalance.
Scores in the range of 16–25 may indicate a moderate imbalance.
Scores in the range of 26–45 may indicate a severe imbalance.
Scores in the range of 46 and over may indicate a critical imbalance.

*The general symptoms listed above represent common consequences to a range of nutritional deficiencies. For a comprehensive list of symptoms caused by specific nutritional deficiencies, see Chapter Six.

POOR DIGESTION AND ASSIMILATION (CHAPTER SEVEN)

Rate the occurrence of each symptom according to the scale below, then calculate your total score.

SYMPTOM RATING SCALE

0=Never   1=Seldom   2=Occasionally   3=Frequently
4=Infrequently with severe symptoms   5=Almost always

___ Gas
___ Bloating
___ Indigestion
___ Heartburn
___ Upper abdominal heaviness after eating
___ Nausea after eating
___ Hunger after eating
___ Feel full after eating an unusually small amount of food
___ Diarrhea
___ Constipation
___ Undigested food in stool
___ Fatigue
___ Arthritis
___ Acne
___ Food allergies
___ Iron deficiency
___ Intestinal candida
___ Intestinal parasites
___ Osteoporosis
___ Anxiety
___ Hurried meals
___ Insufficient chewing
___ Excessive fluids with meals (especially iced drinks)
___ Overeating
___ Unwise food combinations

Total Score: ___

Scores in the range of 1–15 may indicate a mild imbalance.
Scores in the range of 16–25 may indicate a moderate imbalance.
Scores in the range of 26–45 may indicate a severe imbalance.
Scores in the range of 46 and over may indicate a critical imbalance.

THE TOXIC BOWEL (CHAPTER EIGHT)

Rate the occurrence of each symptom according to the scale below, then calculate your total score.

SYMPTOM RATING SCALE

0=Never   1=Seldom   2=Occasionally   3=Frequently
4=Infrequently with severe symptoms   5=Almost always

___ Constipation (hard or difficult stools)
___ Bowel movements usually less often than
    once a day
___ Reliance on laxatives
___ Incomplete bowel elimination
___ Constipation alternating with diarrhea
___ Bad digestion
___ Excessive gas
___ Abdominal fullness, bloating
___ Hemorrhoids
___ Varicose veins
___ Hiatal hernia
___ Diverticulosis
___ Appendicitis
___ Gallbladder problems
___ Colorectal cancer
___ Diabetes
___ Heart disease

___ High blood cholesterol
___ Food allergies
___ Bad breath
___ Body odor
___ Coated tongue
___ Headache
___ Fatigue
___ Acne, boils, folliculitis
___ Eczema, psoriasis, dermatitis
___ Ulcers
___ Gum disease
___ Low back pain
___ Low-fiber diet
___ Too many refined grains
___ High-sugar diet
___ Excessive cheese
___ Insufficient fluid

Total Score: ___

Scores in the range of 1–20 may indicate a mild imbalance.
Scores in the range of 21–35 may indicate a moderate imbalance.
Scores in the range of 36–50 may indicate a severe imbalance.
Scores in the range of 51 and over may indicate a critical imbalance.

THE SLUGGISH LIVER (CHAPTER NINE)

Rate the occurrence of each symptom according to the scale below, then calculate your total score.

SYMPTOM RATING SCALE

0=Never   1=Seldom   2=Occasionally   3=Frequently
4=Infrequently with severe symptoms   5=Almost always

___ Premenstrual symptoms
___ Fibrocystic breasts
___ Food allergies
___ Chemical hypersensitivity
___ Autoimmune diseases
___ Overweight
___ Acne
___ High blood cholesterol
___ Nausea
___ Constipation or diarrhea
___ Bloating or gas
___ Greasy, fatty stools
___ Intolerance of greasy or fatty foods
___ Gallbladder problems
___ Rashes
___ Hypoglycemia tendencies
___ Achy joints and muscles

___ Itching
___ Slow wound healing
___ History of hepatitis
___ Current or past alcohol or drug abuse
___ Excessive dietary fat and protein
___ Excessive calories
___ Excessive exposure to industrial, agricultural, or garden and lawn chemicals, paints, fuels, solvents, etc.
___ Fatigue
___ Poor memory or confusion
___ Poor concentration
___ Headaches
___ Dizziness
___ Frequent urination
___ Water retention

Total Score: ___

Scores in the range of 1–15 may indicate a mild imbalance.
Scores in the range of 16–25 may indicate a moderate imbalance.
Scores in the range of 26–45 may indicate a severe imbalance.
Scores in the range of 46 and over may indicate a critical imbalance.

HYPOGLYCEMIA (CHAPTER TEN)

Rate the occurrence of each symptom according to the scale below, then calculate your total score.

SYMPTOM RATING SCALE

0=Never   1=Seldom   2=Occasionally   3=Frequently
4=Infrequently with severe symptoms   5=Almost always

Any of the following symptoms accompanying delayed or missed meals, including:

___ Fatigue   ___ Insomnia
___ Irritability   ___ Weakness
___ Headache   ___ Continual hunger
___ Depression   ___ Dizziness, light-headedness
___ Mental confusion   ___ Palpitations
___ Mood swings   ___ Excessive or unexplained sweating
___ Seizures

Symptoms not necessarily related to meals:

___ Fatigue
___ Depression
___ Nervous exhaustion
___ Craving for sweets, caffeine, alcohol
___ Difficulty coping with stress
___ Insomnia
___ Regular and/or excessive consumption of sugar, honey, maple sugar, molasses, dried fruit, fruit juice
___ Regular and/or excessive consumption of fast food, processed foods, white flour products
___ Alcoholism (active or recovering)
___ Regular consumption of alcohol
___ Excessive consumption of caffeine (coffee, black tea, soft drinks, chocolate, caffeine-containing medications)
___ Inadequate protein ingestion (especially, but not limited to, vegetarians)
___ Inadequate complex carbohydrate ingestion

Total Score: ___

Scores in the range of 1–10 may indicate a mild imbalance.
Scores in the range of 11–20 may indicate a moderate imbalance.
Scores in the range of 21–40 may indicate a severe imbalance.
Scores in the range of 41 and over may indicate a critical imbalance.

ADRENAL EXHAUSTION (CHAPTER ELEVEN)

Rate the occurrence of each symptom according to the scale below, then calculate your total score.

SYMPTOM RATING SCALE

0=Never   1=Seldom   2=Occasionally   3=Frequently
4=Infrequently with severe symptoms   5=Almost always

____ Fatigue
____ Exhaustion
____ Nervousness, irritability, anxiety
____ Depression
____ Inability to concentrate
____ Poor memory
____ Hypoglycemia (especially if resistant to normal measures or requiring persistent attention)
____ Cravings for sweets
____ Premenstrual symptoms (especially if resistant to normal measures or requiring persistent attention)
____ Always feel cold (abnormally low body temperature)
____ Less than normal perspiration
____ Food and other allergies
____ Low blood pressure
____ Light-headedness on standing up
____ Headaches
____ Difficulty overcoming infections
____ Slow recovery from any kind of stress (exercise, overwork, mental strain, inadequate sleep, emotional trauma, injury, surgery)
____ Severe or recurrent stresses

Total Score: ____

Scores in the range of 1–10 may indicate a mild imbalance.
Scores in the range of 11–20 may indicate a moderate imbalance.
Scores in the range of 21–34 may indicate a severe imbalance.
Scores in the range of 35 and over may indicate a critical imbalance.

YEAST OVERGROWTH (CHAPTER TWELVE)

Rate the occurrence of each symptom according to the scale below, then calculate your total score.

SYMPTOM RATING SCALE

0=Never   1=Seldom   2=Occasionally   3=Frequently
4=Infrequently with severe symptoms   5=Almost always

___ Gas
___ Bloating
___ Constipation and/or diarrhea
___ Spastic/irritable colon
___ Crohn's disease, colitis
___ Intestinal cramping
___ Heartburn
___ Itchy anus
___ Continual sinus problems (allergies, infections)
___ Chronic or recurring sore throat, colds, bronchitis, ear infections
___ Premenstrual symptoms
___ Menstrual cramps and other menstrual problems
___ Fatigue
___ Depression
___ Irritability
___ Inability to concentrate
___ Headaches
___ Recurrent or chronic vaginal yeast infections

___ Recurrent bladder infections or irritation
___ Infertility
___ Chronic rashes
___ Recurrent staph infections
___ Joint or muscle pain
___ Itchy ears or ringing in the ears
___ General itchiness
___ Multiple allergies
___ Weight problems
___ Craving for sweets, alcohol, bread, cheese
___ Feel drunk without having ingested alcohol
___ Chemical and fume intolerance
___ Worsening of any of the above symptoms within six to twelve months after a pregnancy
___ Multiple pregnancies
___ Antibiotic use
___ Birth control pill (oral contraceptive) use
___ Cortisone or steroid use
___ Chemotherapy or radiation

Total Score: ___

Scores in the range of 1–20 may indicate a mild imbalance.
Scores in the range of 21–35 may indicate a moderate imbalance.
Scores in the range of 36–50 may indicate a severe imbalance.
Scores in the range of 51 and over may indicate a critical imbalance.

FOOD ALLERGIES (CHAPTER THIRTEEN)

Rate the occurrence of each symptom according to the scale below, then calculate your total score.

SYMPTOM RATING SCALE

0=Never   1=Seldom   2=Occasionally   3=Frequently
4=Infrequently with severe symptoms   5=Almost always

___ Feel worse after eating
___ Flu-like symptoms that are not the flu
___ Depression
___ Fatigue
___ Total exhaustion
___ Weakness
___ Poor memory
___ Poor concentration
___ Brain fogginess, dopiness, confusion
___ Hyperactivity
___ Learning disability
___ Inappropriate rage or emotional outbursts
___ Headaches
___ Insomnia
___ Seizures
___ Delusions
___ Chronic sore throat
___ Mucus in throat, nose, or sinuses
___ Recurrent ear, sinus, or other respiratory infection
___ Canker or cold sores
___ Abdominal bloating or gas
___ Diarrhea and/or constipation

___ Spastic/irritable colon
___ Crohn's disease, colitis
___ Indigestion
___ Itchy anus
___ Arthritis
___ Muscle pains
___ Muscular weakness
___ Bed-wetting
___ Frequent urination
___ Genital itch
___ Painful or irregular menstrual periods
___ Hives, rashes, acne
___ Dark circles under eyes
___ Asthma
___ Coughing
___ High blood pressure/low blood pressure
___ Palpitations
___ Phlebitis
___ Weight problems
___ Irritated eyes
___ Anemia, low white blood cell count, or low platelet count

Total Score: ___

Scores in the range of 1–25 may indicate a mild imbalance.
Scores in the range of 26–50 may indicate a moderate imbalance.
Scores in the range of 51–85 may indicate a severe imbalance.
Scores in the range of 86 and over may indicate a critical imbalance.

CHEMICAL HYPERSENSITIVITY AND ENVIRONMENTAL ILLNESS (CHAPTER FOURTEEN)

Rate the occurrence of each symptom according to the scale below, then calculate your total score.

SYMPTOM RATING SCALE

0=Never   1=Seldom   2=Occasionally   3=Frequently
4=Infrequently with severe symptoms   5=Almost always

___ Fatigue, lethargy, exhaustion
___ General feeling of ill health
___ Flu-like symptoms that aren't the flu
___ Impaired memory and thinking
___ Headaches
___ Insomnia
___ Overeating/undereating
___ Emotional instability
___ Behavioral or personality change
___ Unwarranted depression
___ Dizziness
___ Incoordination
___ Numbness
___ Weakness
___ Tremors or seizures
___ Arthritis
___ Muscle aches and pains
___ Chest pains
___ Nausea
___ Diarrhea/constipation
___ Abdominal pain or cramps
___ Weight loss

___ Blurred or dimmed vision
___ Eye irritation
___ Loss of sense of smell
___ Hoarseness
___ Sore or irritated throat
___ Burning sensations in mouth, throat, lungs
___ Ulcerations in mouth
___ Wheezing
___ Flushing
___ Hives, rashes, acne
___ Menstrual abnormalities
___ Infertility
___ Birth defects in offspring
___ Stillbirth
___ Low body temperature
___ Thyroid disease
___ Anemia
___ Unexplained lymph swelling
___ Persistent cough
___ Parkinson's disease
___ Amyotrophic lateral sclerosis
___ Multiple sclerosis

___ Increased susceptibility to chronic fatigue syndrome, yeast overgrowth, food and inhalant allergies, autoimmune diseases
___ Symptoms occurring within several months after insertion of new dental metals
___ Symptoms generally worse after fasting, exercise, and emotional stress
___ Reactions to normal ambient levels of gas or oil heat fumes, gas range (especially if unvented), car exhaust, smoke, perfume, marker pens, glue, household or industrial cleaning agents, new synthetic carpets, fresh paint, synthetic auto and plane interiors, synthetic clothes, building materials with formaldehyde, lawn and garden chemicals, paint, paint thinner, etc.

Total Score: ___

Scores in the range of 1–30 may indicate a mild imbalance.
Scores in the range of 31–60 may indicate a moderate imbalance.
Scores in the range of 61–95 may indicate a severe imbalance.
Scores in the range of 96 and over may indicate a critical imbalance.

PSYCHONEUROIMMUNOLOGY: THE BODY–MIND CONNECTION (CHAPTER FIFTEEN)

Rate the occurrence of each symptom according to the scale below, then calculate your total score.

SYMPTOM RATING SCALE

0=Never   1=Seldom   2=Occasionally   3=Frequently
4=Infrequently with severe symptoms   5=Almost always

___ Unresolved anger, bitterness, resentment (with parents, spouse, any close relationship, or with a situation)
___ Relationships always difficult
___ Low self-esteem, inferiority complex
___ Unable to forgive yourself
___ Unable to forgive others
___ Unable to ask for what you need or want
___ Unable to confront or to say no
___ Unable to express anger, sadness, or fear
___ Feel need to be sneaky or tell "white" or blatant lies
___ Have to please others excessively
___ Always acting in ways you do not like
___ Unable to believe in your own worth
___ Unable to relax or do not allow yourself to relax
___ Unable to have fun or do not allow yourself to have fun
___ Emotions govern behavior to an excessive degree
___ Unable or unwilling to take a moral inventory of yourself
___ Out of touch with your genuine needs, feelings, desires, talents, goals
___ Unusual and insurmountable fears that limit you significantly
___ Feel you have little power or influence over your life
___ Feel like a victim
___ Addictions to alcohol, drugs, sex, work, food, etc.
___ Keep repeating negative or deleterious patterns or choices that end up harming you or others
___ Rarely touch or get touched by others
___ Lonely, isolated, lacking meaningful/fulfilling connection to another person, family, group, organization, or pet

Total Score: ___

Scores in the range of 1–15 may indicate a mild imbalance.
Scores in the range of 16–25 may indicate a moderate imbalance.
Scores in the range of 26–45 may indicate a severe imbalance.
Scores in the range of 46 and over may indicate a critical imbalance.

LOW THYROID STATUS (CHAPTER SEVENTEEN, "HYPOTHYROIDISM")

Rate the occurrence of each symptom according to the scale below, then calculate your total score.

SYMPTOM RATING SCALE

0=Never   1=Seldom   2=Occasionally   3=Frequently
4=Infrequently with severe symptoms   5=Almost always

Low thyroid status and *intestinal parasites* are also extremely common conditions. Often unrecognized, they are responsible for numerous chronic symptoms and a generally low level of health. Brief discussions can be found in Chapter Seventeen and their general symptoms are listed here.

___ Increase in weight
___ Difficulty losing weight
___ Excessive fatigue
___ Mentally sluggish
___ Always feel cold
___ Cold hands and feet
___ Constipation
___ Depression
___ Coarse, dry skin or hair
___ Headaches
___ Adult acne
___ Recurrent colds and flu
___ Frequent and lengthy colds
___ Water retention, edema

___ Lack of interest in sex
___ Premenstrual symptoms
___ Menstrual cramps
___ Periods too heavy, irregular; missed periods
___ Difficulty conceiving
___ Diminished sweating
___ Insomnia
___ Hypoglycemia
___ Diabetes
___ Anemia or low white blood cell count
___ High blood cholesterol
___ Down's syndrome
___ Lithium therapy

Total Score: ___

Scores in the range of 1–15 may indicate a mild imbalance.
Scores in the range of 16–25 may indicate a moderate imbalance.
Scores in the range of 26–45 may indicate a severe imbalance.
Scores in the range of 46 and over may indicate a critical imbalance.

INTESTINAL PARASITES (CHAPTER SEVENTEEN, "PARASITES, INTESTINAL")

Rate the occurrence of each symptom according to the scale below, then calculate your total score.

SYMPTOM RATING SCALE

0=Never   1=Seldom   2=Occasionally   3=Frequently
4=Infrequently with severe symptoms   5=Almost always

___ Gas
___ Bloating
___ Abdominal fullness
___ Nausea
___ Constipation
___ Diarrhea
___ Abdominal cramps or pain
___ Fatigue
___ Hives
___ Allergies, especially food
___ History of previous parasitic infections (even if treated)
___ History of traveler's diarrhea
___ History of family member with parasites
___ Difficulty overcoming intestinal yeast growth

Total Score: ___

Scores in the range of 1–7 may indicate a mild imbalance.
Scores in the range of 8–15 may indicate a moderate imbalance.
Scores in the range of 16–25 may indicate a severe imbalance.
Scores in the range of 26 and over may indicate a critical imbalance.

DIETARY HAZARDS AND EXCESSES

HAZARDS/EXCESSES

FAT

SOURCES

Hamburgers	Butter	Half-and-half
Hot dogs	Cheese	Cream soups and sauces
Cold cuts	Pizza	Peanut butter
Ribs	Ice cream	Cakes, pastries, and donuts
Sausage	Whole milk products	Fried foods (french fries, chips)
Margarine	Cream	Chocolate

POTENTIAL CONSEQUENCES

ATHEROSCLEROSIS	CANCER	EXCESS ESTROGEN
Heart attack	Rectum and colon	Early menstruation
Angina	Breast	Late menopause
Stroke	Prostate	Breast cancer
Claudication	Ovaries	Fibrocystic breasts
Gangrene	Testes	Premenstrual syndrome
Neuropathy	DIABETES	Ovarian cancer
Retinopathy		GALLSTONES
Dizziness		OBESITY
Senility		OSTEOPOROSIS
Impotence		
Hearing loss		

DIETARY HAZARDS AND EXCESSES

HAZARDS/EXCESSES

TRANS-FATTY ACIDS FOUND IN OVERHEATED POLYUNSATURATED OILS AND IN PARTIALLY HYDROGENATED OILS

SOURCES

Heated oils: safflower, sunflower, corn, walnut, soy, flaxseed

Partially hydrogenated oils found in:

Margarine	Pancake mixes	Many frozen foods
Mayonnaise	Baking mixes	Non-dairy creamers
Vegetable shortening	Cereals	Artificial whipped cream
Breads	Salad dressings	Candy bars
Crackers	Corn chips	Crusts
Muffins	Potato chips	Health or fiber bars
Cookies		

POTENTIAL CONSEQUENCES

ESSENTIAL FATTY ACID DEFICIENCIES AND HORMONE IMBALANCES

Arthritis	Schizophrenia	Increased susceptibility to:
Eczema and other skin conditions	Abnormal clotting and clumping of platelets	Infection
		Cancer
Premenstrual syndrome	Thrombophlebitis	Decreased fertility
Menstrual cramps	Spasm of coronary arteries	Obesity
Heavy periods	Heart attack	Prostate enlargement
Food and other allergies	High blood pressure	Diabetes
Migraine headaches	Irritable bowel syndrome	Constriction of arteries
Depression	Autoimmune disorders	Heart Attack
Irritability	Infections	Stroke

DIETARY HAZARDS AND EXCESSES

HAZARDS/EXCESSES

FREE RADICALS

SOURCES

Fats exposed to excessive heat, oxygen, and light:

Scrambled eggs	Fried foods (especially using	Grilled, broiled, charcoaled or
Dried egg products	polyunsaturated oils)	charbroiled meats
Dried milk		Poultry
Melted or crisped foods, i.e.		Fish
pizza		
nachos		
enchiladas		

POTENTIAL CONSEQUENCES

PREMATURE AGING	CANCER	GENETIC MUTATIONS
ARTHRITIS	CHRONIC DEGENERATIVE	BIRTH DEFECTS
ATHEROSCLEROSIS	DISEASES	

DIETARY HAZARDS AND EXCESSES

HAZARDS/EXCESSES

REFINED CARBOHYDRATES

SOURCES

White flour products:

Bread	Noodles	Bagels
Rolls	Cereals	Tortillas
Crackers	Cookies	White rice
	Cakes and pastries	Sugar

POTENTIAL CONSEQUENCES

CONSTIPATION	DIVERTICULOSIS	COLON AND RECTAL CANCER
BLOATING	APPENDICITIS	HIGH BLOOD CHOLESTEROL
GAS	HIATAL HERNIA	CORONARY ARTERY DISEASE
HEMORRHOIDS	GALLBLADDER DISEASE	OBESITY
VARICOSE VEINS	SPASTIC BOWEL	VITAMIN AND MINERAL
ANAL FISSURE	COLON POLYPS	DEFICIENCIES

DIETARY HAZARDS AND EXCESSES

HAZARDS/EXCESSES

SUGAR

SOURCES

Soft drinks
Candy
Cookies
Canned fruits

Sweet rolls
Ice cream
Donuts
Bread

Frozen yogurt
Sweetened cereals
Ketchup
Salad dressings

Processed foods containing: sucrose, dextrose, glucose, corn sweetener, corn syrup, high fructose, and maltose

POTENTIAL CONSEQUENCES

HYPOGLYCEMIA
DIABETES
ATHEROSCLEROSIS
   Heart attack
   Stroke
   Claudication, etc.
DEPRESSED IMMUNE
  SYSTEM

INFECTION
CANCER
NUTRITIONAL DEFICIENCIES
PREMENSTRUAL SYNDROME
OBESITY
ALLERGIES
RECURRENT RESPIRATORY
   INFECTIONS

HEADACHE
FATIGUE
ANXIETY
HYPERACTIVITY
DEPRESSION
CHRONIC YEAST
  OVERGROWTH
RECURRENT VAGINAL
  INFECTIONS

DIETARY HAZARDS AND EXCESSES

HAZARDS/EXCESSES

CAFFEINE

SOURCES

Coffee	Soft drinks	Over-the-counter and
Tea	Chocolate milk	prescription medications
Cocoa beverage	Milk chocolate	

POTENTIAL CONSEQUENCES

NERVOUSNESS	ANXIETY	MUSCLE TREMORS
IRRITABILITY	BIRTH DEFECTS	DIARRHEA
FATIGUE	PREMENSTRUAL SYNDROME	CYSTITIS
HEADACHE	INFERTILITY	BREAST CYSTS
DEPRESSION	HYPOGLYCEMIA	HEART RHYTHM
INSOMNIA	OSTEOPOROSIS	DISTURBANCES

DIETARY HAZARDS AND EXCESSES

HAZARDS/EXCESSES

FOOD ADDITIVES OR CONTAMINANTS

SOURCES

Any foods that are not "organic" or "additive/preservative free"

Artificial colorings   Artificial sweeteners   Sulfites
Artificial flavorings   Saccharin   BHT, BVO, BHA, MSG
Sodium nitrates   Sodium bisulfite   Sulfur dioxide
Propyl gallate

POTENTIAL CONSEQUENCES

HYPERACTIVITY (Artificial colorings)
CANCER (Blue No. 1, Citrus Red No. 2, Green No. 3, BHA, BHT, Propyl Gallate, Saccharin, Sodium
  Nitrite, Sodium Nitrate)
TUMORS (Blue No. 2, Red No. 3, Yellow No. 6)
ALLERGIC REACTIONS (Yellow No. 5, Yellow No. 6, MSG, Sulfur Dioxide, Sodium Bisulfite)
BEHAVIORAL DISTURBANCES (Aspartame)

DIETARY HAZARDS AND EXCESSES

HAZARDS/EXCESSES

SALT

SOURCES

Chips	Cheese	Milk shakes
Pretzels	Canned Soups	Frozen foods
Processed meats	Sardines	Fast food
Cake mixes	Herring	Prepared rice and pasta
Some breads		products

POTENTIAL CONSEQUENCES

HIGH BLOOD PRESSURE	EDEMA	HEADACHES
STROKE	PREMENSTRUAL SYNDROME	FATIGUE/WEAKNESS
HEART ATTACK	FREQUENT URINATION	

DIETARY HAZARDS AND EXCESSES

HAZARDS/EXCESSES

ASPARTAME

SOURCES

Soft drinks	Other beverages	Candy
Iced tea	Drink mixes	Gelatin desserts

POTENTIAL CONSEQUENCES

HEADACHE	DEPRESSION	ALLERGIES
FAINTING	NAUSEA	SKIN RASHES
SEIZURE	GASTROINTESTINAL	MENSTRUAL PROBLEMS
MEMORY LOSS	DISTRESS	MOOD SWINGS

HAZARDS/EXCESSES

ALUMINUM

SOURCES

Cookware	Baking Powder	Screw-on and -off bottle tops
Foil	Antacids	Deodorants

POTENTIAL CONSEQUENCES

PRESENILE DEMENTIA (ALZHEIMER'S)	OSTEOPOROSIS	BEHAVIORAL DISTURBANCES

DIETARY HAZARDS AND EXCESSES

HAZARDS/EXCESSES

HEAVY METALS (LEAD, ARSENIC, CADMIUM, ETC.) INDUSTRIAL AND AGRICULTURAL POLLUTANTS

SOURCES

Tap water (Lead)
Food from lead-soldered cans (Lead)
Food grown in soil in and around industrial areas (Lead, Cadmium, Nickel)
Fresh and salt water fish and shellfish (Mercury, Cadmium)
Grains treated with fungicides (Mercury)
Fungicides (Mercury, Cadmium)
Fertilizers (Cadmium)
Refined foods (Cadmium)
Coffee (Cadmium)
Meat—liver and kidneys (Cadmium)
Poultry (Cadmium)
Grains (Cadmium)
Insecticides (Arsenic)
Hydrogenated oils (Nickel)

POTENTIAL CONSEQUENCES

CANCER   HIGH BLOOD PRESSURE   ANEMIA
NEUROLOGICAL DISEASES

Now that you have completed the Master Symptom Survey and reviewed Dietary Hazards and Excesses, you've probably checked off enough symptoms to make you think you have every disease in this book. Well, relax, because the likelihood is you don't. When my patients complete this survey they often have the same thought. However, I point out that many of the symptoms caused by any one condition fall under several others as well. Patients frequently have only one or two conditions, and we first approach the one that's causing the most trouble through the number and severity of symptoms. This is frequently the one with the most predisposing factors as well.

Reading the relevant chapter will usually solidify your suspicions or prove them wrong. If you believe you've found the culprit, proceed with the information given. If it doesn't quite fit, read the chapter corresponding to your next most likely suspect.

One last word before you continue. If your understanding of the relationship between diet and health needs bolstering, what follows next is a comprehensive discussion of this subject. I highly recommend reading this, as the information will give you a foundation for understanding and treating the Ten Common Denominator conditions.

PART TWO

DIET AND HEALTH

DIETARY HAZARDS AND EXCESSES

In the first part of this chapter, I will review one by one the dietary health hazards so common today in the homes, restaurants, and institutions of this country. Wholesome alternatives will be offered, which together will form the basis of a whole-foods diet. Next, in Chapter Four, I will help you refine and individualize your application of whole-foods eating. No one whole-foods diet is right for everyone; no one diet will always be correct for the same individual. Seasons of the year, geography, even the time of day can dictate specific dietary requirements.

Finally, I will introduce several concepts that may help you determine a way of eating that best suits your individual and changing metabolic needs. When you begin to look at eating in a larger context, you will realize that sound nutrition involves more than establishing correct amounts of calories, protein, carbohydrates, fats, vitamins, and minerals. It is even more than whole-foods "hazard-free" eating. Ultimately, it becomes an art of individual balance.

DIETARY HAZARDS

In the last two decades, modern medicine has dramatically altered its accepted attitudes about the relationship between diet and health. Just twenty years ago when I was a medical student, the only clinically relevant nutritional information that I can remember being taught was to restrict salt for high blood pressure, restrict sugar for diabetes, and supplement with iron for anemia. Also, we were taught what the eight essential amino acids were. For the most part, however, nutrition and medicine seemed to be in two entirely different worlds. Conventional nutritional safeguards at that time, the "four food groups" and the Recommended Dietary Allowances, served to protect us primarily against diseases of blatant malnutrition. They did not and do not defend against a plethora of dietary assaults, many of them excesses, that have been linked to our most common ailments and killer diseases. From decades ago to present times, such noted physicians and scientists as Weston Price, D.D.S.,[1] Francis Pottenger, M.D.,[2] Dennis Burkitt, M.D.,[3] Nathan Pritikin, M.D.,[4] S. Boyd Eaton, M.D.,[5] C. Everett Koop, M.D., Sc.D.,[6] and Chen Junshi, M.D.,[7] have been key members of a growing list of health professionals alerting the world to the emerging health hazards of our diet.

Today, it has become nearly common knowledge that cancer, heart disease, diabetes, obesity, and high blood pressure are associated with dietary excesses of calories, fat, sugar, refined carbohydrates, salt, and food additives—the standard American fare. More than ever before, we are shunning red meat, whole milk products, eggs, sugar, white flour, additives, and other items. We are reading food labels and buying more organic produce. Many of those who do buy meat have learned to look for it free of hormones and antibiotics.

We are beginning to understand that many diseases, and the disabilities and deaths they cause, are not the inevitable result of aging. And we are now taking seriously the fact that medical treatment is inadequate for many of our common and worst diseases. We are also realizing that our doctors' attention is, for the most part, focused on finding and treating disease, not on teaching us how to avoid disease. We are wisely turning to self-care and a preventive orientation. Since diet and health have become such popular issues, there is naturally a good deal of common misinformation floating about—some of it dangerous—that I hope to straighten out in these pages.

With mistaken ideas, even the best efforts and intentions can work against us. Thus, it is hoped that the information given in this chapter will promote a keener understanding and motivation toward making dietary choices that will be sound and lasting.

DIET AND DISEASE

The known associations between the current standard American diet and disease are summarized in the following table.

COMMON DIETARY EXCESSES IN THE UNITED STATES AND ASSOCIATED EFFECTS ON HEALTH

EXCESS FATS ASSOCIATED WITH:

Cancer of the—

Colon	Prostate
Rectum	Ovaries
Breast	Testes

Arteriosclerosis and related problems:

Poor circulation	Cataracts
Coronary artery disease	Dizziness
Heart attack	Transient ischemic attacks
Angina	Stroke
Claudication	Senility
Gangrene	Hearing loss
Neuropathy	Impotence
Retinopathy	

Excess estrogen:

Early menstruation	Premenstrual syndrome
Late menopause	Fibrocystic breast disease
Breast cancer	Ovarian cancer

Also:

Obesity	Gallstones
Diabetes mellitus	Osteoporosis

EXCESS CONSUMPTION OF REFINED CARBOHYDRATES ASSOCIATED WITH:

Nutrient deficiencies of—

Magnesium	Selenium
Vitamin B-6	Manganese
Vitamin E	Zinc
Chromium	Essential fatty acids

These deficiencies and others can lead to such ailments as:

Hypertension	Birth defects
Heart attack	Weakened immune response
Stroke	leading to infections and
Arthritis	cancer
Cervical dysplasia	Depression, anxiety, and other
Premenstrual syndrome	mental disorders

Excess Carbohydrates Can Lead to Insufficient Consumption of Fiber and Such Ailments as:

Constipation	Sluggish or incomplete stool
Excessive gas	evacuation

Diarrhea	Bloating of the abdomen
Hemorrhoids	Abdominal pain or cramps
Varicose veins	Very foul-smelling stools or
Diverticulosis	gas
Anal fissures	Indigestion or heartburn
Appendicitis	Irritable bowel or spastic colon
Hiatal hernia	Gallbladder disease
Colon polyps	Coronary artery disease
Colon cancer	Elevated blood cholesterol
Rectal cancer	Heavy metal accumulation
Diabetes	(lead, cadmium, or mercury)
Stroke	Overeating tendency
Heart attack	Allergic tendencies (especially
Hypertension	to foods)
Overweight	Candida overgrowth
Hard, dry, or difficult stools	

EXCESS CONSUMPTION OF SUGAR ASSOCIATED WITH:

Hypoglycemia
Diabetes
Arteriosclerosis (heart attack, stroke, etc.)
Weakening of the immune system
Elevated uric acid/gout
Personality and behavioral aberrations (depression, fatigue, nervousness, hyperactivity, criminal behavior)
Hypertension
Nutrient deficiencies
Obesity
Yeast infections and other Candida-related ailments
Addictions
Dental caries

EXCESS CONSUMPTION OF ARTIFICIAL SWEETENERS (ASPARTAME) ASSOCIATED WITH:

Headache	Depression
Fainting	Nausea
Seizure	GI distress
Memory loss	Allergies
Mood swings	Skin rashes
Menstrual problems	

EXCESS CONSUMPTION OF CAFFEINE ASSOCIATED WITH:

Fatigue	Decreased coping ability
Headache	Gastritis and ulcers
Depression	Premenstrual syndrome
Insomnia	Fibrocystic breast disease
Anxiety	High blood pressure
Nervousness	Increased serum cholesterol
Irritability	Heart rhythm disturbances
Muscle tremors	Rectal pain and itching
Birth defects	Diuretic action
Stillbirth	Urinary loss of calcium, inositol, biotin, and other nutrients
Prematurity	
Infertility	
Hypoglycemia	Questionable association with cancers of pancreas, prostate, and bladder
Diarrhea	
Cystitis	
Prostatitis	

EXCESS CONSUMPTION OF SOFT DRINKS CREATES PROBLEMS ASSOCIATED WITH:

Excess sugar (see page 44)

Excess caffeine (see page 44)

Excess artificial sweeteners (see page 44)

Excess phosphorus: may cause calcium metabolism abnormalities leading to osteoporosis; excess vitamin D and deficient magnesium will increase this trend as well as provoke metastatic calcification (arthritis, arteriosclerosis, kidney stones, and kidney failure)

EXCESS CONSUMPTION OF SALT ASSOCIATED WITH:

Hypertension	Bloating
Stroke	Constipation
Heart attack	Craving for liquids
Edema	Frequent urination
Premenstrual syndrome	Headache
Tinnitus	Mineral imbalance
Fatigue/weakness	Osteoporosis

EXCESS CONSUMPTION OF MILK PRODUCTS ASSOCIATED WITH:

Recurrent infections:	Diarrhea
Ear	Constipation
Throat	Abdominal cramps
Sinus	Spastic colon
Bronchial	Muscle aches
Sinus congestion	Fatigue
Mucus	Heartburn
Sore throat	Indigestion
Cough	Ulcers
Colitis	Bed-wetting
Bloody stools	Thought disorders
Acne	Hyperactivity
Eczema	Poor concentration
Canker sores	Moodiness
Rashes	Irritability
Arthritis	Depression
Asthma	Schizophrenia
Headache	Delinquency
Insomnia	Antisocial behavior

EXCESS CONSUMPTION OF PEANUTS AND PEANUT BUTTER CREATE PROBLEMS ASSOCIATED WITH:

Excess fat (see above)	Increased clotting tendency
Prostaglandin hormone imbalance	Arteriosclerosis
Menstrual cramps	Liver cancer due to aflatoxin (fungal contaminant)
Thrombosis	

EXCESS CONSUMPTION OF FOOD ADDITIVES/ CONTAMINANTS CREATE PROBLEMS ASSOCIATED WITH:

Asthma	Intestinal cramps
Hives	Diarrhea
Headache	Abnormal sweating
Hyperactivity (attention deficit disorder)	Chest pain
	Palpitations
Learning disability	Osteoporosis

Epilepsy	Alzheimer's disease
Cancer	

EXCESS CONSUMPTION OF PROCESSED FOODS CREATE PROBLEMS ASSOCIATED WITH:

Excess fat (see page 44)

Insufficient fiber (see page 44)

Excess sugar (see page 44)

Caffeine (see page 44)

Salt (see above)

Food additives/contaminants (see above)

Essential fatty acid deficiencies (see page 49)

EXCESS FOOD CONSUMPTION CREATES PROBLEMS ASSOCIATED WITH:

Fatigue	Obesity:
Diminished digestion	Hypertension
Bowel and liver toxicity	Diabetes
Decreased nutrient assimilation	High blood cholesterol
	Heart attack
Bowel and other cancers	Stroke
Shorter life span	Musculoskeletal injuries and ailments
Multiple digestive complaints:	
Heartburn	
Abdominal pain	
Diarrhea	
Constipation	

The recognition of such correlations has brought about major changes in dietary recommendations from the American Heart Association, the American Cancer Society, the National Research Council Food and Nutrition Board Committee on Diet and Health, and the Office of the Surgeon General. Such changes echo the recommendations made in 1977 by the Senate Select Committee on Nutrition and Human Needs[8] and those made in 1983 by the American Holistic Medical Association in *Nutritional Guidelines*.[9]

One of the early leaders of this movement to educate the public about diet and health concerns was Weston Price, D.D.S., who in 1939 first published *Nutrition and Physical Degeneration*. Price observed that a majority of current health problems are rare in traditional cultures subsisting on basic diets. He found, however, that these cultures soon developed the same health problems when their diets were westernized. This hallmark study of traditional cultures lasted several decades and spanned three generations. Price reported the startling observation that degenerative physical changes occurred in the children of mothers who had switched to processed and refined foods. He concluded that diet can adversely influence the expression of genetic potential in as little as one generation.

The table on the next page compares the diet of traditional cultures, which remain free of most of our illnesses, with our own. It lists dietary elements as a per-

COMPARISON OF DIETARY ELEMENTS IN TRADITIONAL AND CURRENT WESTERN DIETS*

	Traditional	Western	Desired
Fat	21%	44%	20%–30%
Sugar (refined)	0	25%	10% or less
Total carbohydrates	46%–65%	25%	30%–50%
Protein	12%–33%	12%	20%–30%
Alcohol	0	7%–10%	? (consumption for optimal health highly variable: 0–1 or 2 drinks daily)
Fiber	60–150 gm	15–20 gm	30–60 gm or more
Salt	690 mg	up to 7,000 mg	1,000–3,000 mg or less
Ratio of polyunsaturated to saturated fats	1.41	.44	1.0 or more

*Adapted from The Paleolithic Prescription by S. Boyd Eaton, Melvin Konner, and Marjorie Shostak, Harper & Row, New York, 1988. Copyright © 1988 by S. Boyd Eaton, M.D., Melvin Konner, M.D., Ph.D., and Marjorie Shostak. Reprinted by permission of S.B. Eaton, M. Konner, M. Shostak, and HarperCollins Publishers, Inc.

centage of total calories. The third column notes suggested daily intakes of these elements.

From a health standpoint, both public and personal, many of our dietary habits have become hazardous. The task at hand is not simple. We need to reduce the excesses of hazardous foods to reasonable levels while replacing them with wholesome food choices. We need to learn how to make the transition, especially when food addictions seem overwhelming and old habits overpowering. And we must dispel the damaging nutritional myths that have led many of us astray.

FAT

The excessive fat content in our diet has been linked closely to some of the most serious diseases, notably heart disease, stroke, and cancer. It is a rare American these days who has not at least heard of the recommendations to decrease our intake of cholesterol and saturated fat. Many of us are making serious efforts to cut down on consumption of beef, pork, lamb, cold cuts, sausage, bacon, hot dogs, cheeses, butter, ice cream, sour cream, whole milk products, eggs, and the skin of chicken and turkey. Such foods are rich in saturated fat, the kind that has received all the bad press. Saturated fats—palmitic and stearic acid are their chemical names—are primarily of animal origin (coconut oil is a notable exception) and solidify at room temperature.

Polyunsaturated fats are derived primarily from vegetables and remain liquid at room temperature. For several decades, they have been considered the more healthful fats. We have been urged by the food industry, the media, and even our doctors to use margarine and vegetable shortening—corn, safflower, soy, and sunflower oils. We are continually reminded that they are cholesterol-free and very low in saturated fat. Yet in recent years, we have learned that even these vegetable fats and oils are linked to obesity, cancer,[10] and heart disease,[11] and that we therefore need to be far more discriminating about the kinds of vegetable oils we use, as well as to watch our total fat intake. Consequently, many health-conscious individuals have also been reducing their consumption of seeds and nuts, nut butters, avocados, chocolate, refined salad and cooking oils, mayonnaise, margarine and other foods containing partially hydrogenated oils, and sautéed, fried, and deep-fried foods.

To estimate the percentage of fat in your diet, take a look at the following table. Where do the majority of your food choices fall?

PERCENT OF FAT CALORIES IN FOODS

75% OR MORE

Avocado

Bacon

Beef—choice grade of chuck rib, sirloin, and loin untrimmed, hamburger (regular)

Coconut

Cold cuts—bologna, Braunschweiger salami

Coleslaw

Cream—heavy, light, half-and-half, sour

Cream cheese

Frankfurters

Headcheese

Nuts—walnuts, peanuts, cashews, almonds, etc.

Olives

Peanut butter

Pork—sausage, spareribs, butt, loin, and ham (untrimmed)

Salt pork

Seeds—pumpkin, sesame, sunflower

50% TO 75%

Beef—rump, corned

Cake—pound

Canadian bacon

Lake trout

Lamb chops, rib

Oysters, fried

Cheese—blue, cheddar, American, Swiss, etc.
Chicken, roasted with skin
Chocolate candy
Cream soups
Eggs
Ice cream (rich)
Perch, fried
Pork—ham, loin, and shoulder (trimmed lean cuts)
Tuna with oil
Tuna salad
Veal

40% TO 50%

Beef—T-bone (lean only), hamburger (lean)
Cake—devil's food with chocolate icing
Chicken (fried)
Ice cream (regular)
Mackerel
Milk, whole
Pumpkin pie
Rabbit, stewed
Salmon, canned
Sardines (drained)
Turkey pot pie
Yogurt (whole milk)

30% TO 40%

Beef—flank steak, chuck pot roast (lean)
Cake—yellow, white (without icing)
Chicken, roasted without skin
Cottage cheese, creamed
Fish—flounder, haddock (fried) halibut (broiled)
Granola
Ice milk
Milk, 2%
Pizza
Seafood—scallops, shrimp (breaded and fried)
Soups—bean with pork
Tuna in oil (drained)
Turkey, roasted dark meat
Yogurt (low-fat)

20% TO 30%

Beef—sirloin (lean only)
Corn muffin
Fish—cod (broiled)
Liver
Oysters, raw
Pancakes
Shake, thick
Soups, chicken noodle, tomato, vegetable
Wheat germ

LESS THAN 20%

Beans, peas, and lentils
Bread
Buttermilk
Cabbage, boiled
Cakes—angel food, sponge
Cereals, breakfast (except granola)
Cottage cheese, uncreamed
Fish—ocean perch (broiled)
Frozen yogurt
Fruits
Grains
Milk, skim and 1%
Seafood—scallops and shrimp (steamed or boiled)
Soups—split pea, bouillon, consommé
Tuna in water
Turkey, roasted white meat
Vegetables

From Jane Brody's Nutrition Book *(New York: Norton, 1981); 76–77. Reprinted from* Jane Brody's Nutrition Book *by Jane E. Brody, with the permission of W.W. Norton & Company, Inc. Copyright © 1981 by Jane E. Brody.*

According to current medical opinion, if you want to reduce the risk of fat-related illness, choose foods primarily from the last two groups (less than 30 percent of fat calories). Such a prudent diet would consist of lots of fresh fruits and vegetables, whole grains and legumes, and, if you are not vegetarian, one serving a day generally of either low-fat fish or white poultry meat, lean (or preferably, extra lean) cuts of meat, or wild game. Low-fat cottage cheese, nonfat yogurt, or nonfat (or one percent) milk would also be included.

Seeds and nuts, nut butters, and the higher-fat cheeses should be used sparingly, although vegetarians could be somewhat less strict here. Ice cream and other high-fat foods would be considered occasional treats. If you side with the Pritikin school of low-fat eating, the fat level in your diet would fall somewhere between 10 and 20 percent of total calories and thus would be even more restricted.

Not every food label will give you the percentage of fat calories so plainly, but you can calculate it quite easily with the following formula:

$$\text{Percentage of fat} = \frac{\text{the number of fat grams per serving} \times 9}{\text{the number of calories per serving}}$$

For example, look at a carton of 2 percent milk. The number of fat grams per serving is 5; multiplied by 9 this is 45. 45 divided by 120 (calories per serving) is .375. Move the decimal 2 places to the right and you have 37.5 percent.

$$\text{Percentage of fat} = \frac{5 \times 9}{120} = \frac{45}{120} = .375 = 37.5\%$$

Breaking the First Myth about Fat

What few of us realize is that heart attacks hardly occurred in this country or in England at the beginning of this century,[12] when the total fat consumption was nearly the same as in 1961[13] when death from heart attack in this country was near an all-time high. This leads us to ask more questions: Why are heart attacks and other manifestations of atherosclerosis so rare in many high-saturated-fat-consuming cultures (the Atiu-Mitario of Polynesia,[14] the Somalis and Samburus of East Africa,[15] the population around Udaipur of northern India,[16] the Swiss of the Loetschental Valley in the Valaisian Alps,[17] the Greenland Eskimos,[18] and the Masai)? Why does our Western industrialized high-fat diet seem to be associated with such a high incidence of heart attacks and other diseases while the equally high-fat diets of these other cultures—and of early America and England—are not?

"In applying [the popularized low-fat guidelines], you must recognize that not all fats are the same . . . and that the twentieth-century increase in heart disease [as well as cancer and autoimmune diseases] has *not* been accompanied by an increase in either total fat or animal fat consumption, but rather by a change in the nature of the fats consumed."[19] There is a veritable fat fear spreading across the nation—useful in some respects,

ESSENTIAL FATTY ACIDS AND PROSTAGLANDIN HORMONES

Dietary sources of essential fatty acids converted in your body to favorable prostaglandin hormones help to:

• Enhance the immune system and protect against cancer and infections.

• Protect against blood clots which cause heart attacks, strokes, and venous thromboses.

• Dilate arteries and help control high blood pressure.

• Prevent arthritis and allergies.

• Protect against autoimmune diseases.

but misleading and harmful in others. Not all fat is bad, a fact that Dr. Pritikin overlooked.[20] In fact, some kinds of fats are essential for your health.

Essential Fatty Acids

It is an unfortunate fact that much of the nutritional information generally available today fails to mention essential fatty acids. To maintain good health, we need to consume two essential fatty acids: linoleic acid (an omega-6 fatty acid) and alpha-linolenic acid (an omega-3 fatty acid). Both are polyunsaturated fatty acids and are found in many seeds and nuts, vegetable oils, and some meats. Some examples of linoleic acid–rich foods are safflower, sunflower, corn, soy, and walnut oils, and wild game, especially game birds. Domestic pigs and poultry contain lesser amounts. Flax oil is rich in alpha-linolenic acid, while pumpkin seed, soy, canola, and walnut oils contain lesser amounts. In the body, alpha-linolenic acid is converted to eicosapentaenoic acid (EPA), which is then converted to an important hormone, prostaglandin E-3 (PGE-3). EPA is found in cold-water fish, rabbit, and wild game.

There is also a third fatty acid, gamma-linolenic acid, which is not technically considered essential because the body produces it from linoleic acid. However, many factors can block this conversion, as you will soon learn. Some authors, therefore, list gamma-linolenic acid as essential. Evening primrose oil, black currant oil, and borage oil are sources of gamma-linolenic acid.

Although Americans consume plentiful quantities of polyunsaturated oils, most of the time these oils have been dangerously altered—damaged from processing and refining, and from the heating and frying to which we subject them.[21] In such an altered state, the essential fatty acids cannot perform their intended functions, and

in fact become hazardous—even more so than animal (saturated) fats.

First, let's consider this short lesson in nutritional biochemistry. Essential fatty acids are known to function as part of cellular membranes, contributing to their fluidity and electrical potentials and to oxygen transport across membranes. They are constituents of lipids in nerve tissue and affect brain development and mental state. Growth, the burning of fat, the fluidity of fat, chromosome stability, gene expression, even the absorption of sunlight in your skin are some of the functions influenced by essential fatty acids. Additionally, they are involved in adrenal stress response, muscle recovery time, vision, sperm formation, cholesterol and triglyceride transport, and all glandular functions.

Perhaps essential fatty acids are best known as building blocks for a group of highly active metabolic substances called prostaglandins,[22] a class of hormones distinct from endocrine hormones. Whereas endocrine hormones come from specific glands (estrogen from the ovaries, thyroxin from the thyroid, and cortisol from the adrenals), prostaglandin hormones are manufactured in common cells throughout the body, secreted locally, and used on the spot.

Three classes of prostaglandins and over thirty actual different prostaglandin hormones have been identified to date, which together affect the brain and nerves, blood clotting, skin, reproductive organs, joints, muscles, gastrointestinal tract, immune system, metabolic rate—essentially our whole bodies.

Some prostaglandins are considered generally protective to health and therefore "good" (PGE-1, PGE-3), while others are seen as generally destructive and therefore "bad" (PGE-2). Although all the prostaglandins are usually present to varying degrees, it is the ratio of "good" to "bad" that determines whether a diseased or healthy state exists. You can influence this prostaglandin ratio, and in effect the presence or absence of many of our most common and significant illnesses, by your choice of dietary oils and fats. By choosing the "good" oils and fats and using them wisely—knowing which ones to cook with, which ones to use unheated, which ones to refrigerate—you can make better use of the oils in your diet. "Good" oils and fats refer to those that inherently contain favorable amounts of usable essential fatty acids. The practical dos and don'ts of oil choices can be found in "The Right Oils and Fats" beginning on page 54.

If you use damaged or altered polyunsaturated oils or use "good" oils unwisely, you will be introducing into your body several toxic substances, one of which is trans-fatty acids; your body will be unable to use the essential fatty acids for needed purposes; and you will overactivate the biochemical pathways that synthesize unfavorable prostaglandin hormones. You may therefore be subjecting yourself to conditions associated with essential fatty acid deficiencies.

Good Oils/Bad Oils

If you do not want to become a premature disease or death statistic, heed the following: *avoid damaged oils*. This means primarily partially hydrogenated oil—which is what you're getting when you eat margarine. If steering clear of margarine were all you had to do, your job would be easy, but food companies use partially hydrogenated oil in more foods than you can imagine—bread, crackers, muffins, cookies, pancake or baking mixes, cereal, mayonnaise, salad dressing, potato and corn chips, frozen waffles and many other frozen foods, artificial creamer, artificial whipped cream, candy bars, even some "health food" sweet treats. In 1975, over 5.6 billion pounds of vegetable oil were hydrogenated, which comes to 28 pounds per person per year, or 34 grams a day.[23] I would guess that current figures are higher.

Nearly every item above can be found without partially hydrogenated oils; check with a local health foods

CONDITIONS ASSOCIATED WITH ESSENTIAL FATTY ACID DEFICIENCIES

Depression	Kidney failure
Irritability	Menstrual cramps
Neurosis	Premenstrual tension
Schizophrenia	Increased and prolonged menstrual bleeding
Manic Depressive Syndrome	Fibrocystic breast disease
Abnormal clotting and clumping of platelets	Insulin resistance (diabetes)
Constriction of arteries	Food and other allergies
Heart attack	Asthma
Stroke	Tinnitus (ringing in the ear)
High blood pressure	Irritable bowel syndrome
Thrombophlebitis	Alcohol intolerance and alcoholism
Arthritis	Migraine headaches
Bursitis	Autoimmune disorders (rheumatoid arthritis, multiple sclerosis, etc.)
Tendonitis	Immunosuppression (decreased T-cell lymphocyte function)
Dry, rough, or flaky skin	
Eczema	Increased susceptibility to infection
Psoriasis	Increased susceptibility to cancer
Brittle nails	Decreased fertility
Hair loss	Glaucoma
Poor wound healing	Decreased tear and saliva production
Growth retardation	Prostate enlargement
Decreased metabolic rate	Obesity

store or in the health food section of your supermarket. (Exceptions are margarine and artificial anything.) Real food, the way nature provides it, is what your body will utilize well. Butter is better than margarine, provided you do not use it in excess. Or try "better butter," a combination of butter and healthful oil that you can easily make (see recipe on page 114). For salad or cooking oils, buy only true cold-pressed and unrefined oils, as these retain their nutritional quality and leave out the hazardous agents.

Trans-fatty acids are altered forms of essential fatty acids. For example, when linoleic acid from safflower oil is exposed to the tremendous heat of the hydrogenation process during refining, trans-linoleic acid is formed. Trans-linoleic acid cannot be used constructively by the body. Even worse, it blocks the first step in the conversion of linoleic acid to the favorable prostaglandin E-1.

With too much of the unfavorable PGE-2 being produced from a diet high in flesh foods, and very little PGE-1 being made from using predominantly damaged oils, most Americans are asking for trouble. You will recall that PGE-2 suppresses the immune system, raises blood pressure, and promotes heart attacks, strokes, allergies, and other conditions. According to one recent report, "The increased intake of biologically abnormal trans-fatty acids derived from hydrogenated vegetable oils correlates better with the twentieth-century increase in heart disease and breast cancer than any other single dietary change."[24]

I would also suggest avoiding most supermarket cooking and salad oils, which are highly purified and refined by heat, solvents, bleaches, and other chemicals. They lack usable essential fatty acids and other nutrients that were originally present, notably vitamin E, and may contain trans-fatty acids.

Avoid oils that do not specify "unrefined" or "cold pressed" on labels (see p. 54 for more information on this as manufacturers use these terms rather loosely). Equally important, do not make a habit of frying, stir-frying, or baking with polyunsaturated-rich oils (corn, safflower, sunflower, soy, flax, walnut, pumpkin) even if they come from the health food store and are labeled "cold pressed," because you will inadvertently damage them. There are far more heat-stable oils to sauté and bake with (see "The Right Oils and Fats"). Fried foods, especially those that are deep-fried using polyunsaturated oils instead of lard or beef tallow, are now heralded by fast-food chains as a move toward "healthier" fried fare. Do not believe this for a second. Movie theaters promoting "healthier" popcorn (popped in soy or other polyunsaturated oil instead of coconut oil) are committing a similar error. Even health food store potato or corn chips using unrefined polyunsaturated oils are suspect, since chips are fried foods.

Figure 3-1 details the steps that essential fatty acids go through on their journey toward being converted into prostaglandin hormones. The table that follows Figure 3-1 lists food sources of essential and some nonessential fatty acids, along with their percentages. Figure 3-1 illustrates other unfavorable blockers of "good" prostaglandin synthesis: excesses of dietary saturated fat, oleic acid, alcohol, sugar, and stress; also diabetes, very high blood cholesterol, aging, copper toxicity, carcinogens, and radiation. Even in the presence of these blockers, you can see that by taking fish oil–EPA supplements, or by eating cold-water EPA-rich fish regularly, your body can still make the favorable PGE-3. And by taking GLA (gamma-linolenic) supplements (evening primrose oil, borage oil, or black currant oil) your body can still make the favorable PGE-1.

The diagram also shows that in order for essential fatty acids to be converted to "good" prostaglandins, the body also needs cofactors—nutrients that stimulate the enzymes necessary to push biochemical reactions. These cofactors include the minerals magnesium, selenium, and zinc, and vitamins C, E, B-3, and B-6. To be sure your body has sufficient amounts of these building blocks, you need to eat a whole-foods/unrefined diet. By definition, this is vitamin and mineral rich. For extra assurance, I advise most of my patients to take a multiple vitamin/mineral supplement.

SOURCES OF ESSENTIAL AND NONESSENTIAL POLYUNSATURATED FATTY ACIDS (APPROXIMATE PERCENTAGES)

LINOLEIC ACID (OMEGA-6)

Safflower seed oil (75%)	Brazil nut oil (24%)
Evening primrose oil (72%)	Pecan oil (20%)
Grape seed oil (71%)	Almond oil (17%)
Sunflower seed oil (65%)	Filbert oil (16%)
Corn oil (59%)	Flax oil (14%)
Wheat germ oil (54%)	Macadamia oil (10%)
Walnut oil (51%)	Pistachio oil (6%)
Soy oil (50%)	Chicken (20%–25%)
Sesame oil (45%)	Turkey (15%–20%)
Pumpkin oil (42%)	Egg (13%)
Rice bran oil (35%)	Pork (10%)
Canola oil (30%)	Beef (2.1%)
Peanut oil (29%)	

ALPHA-LINOLENIC ACID (OMEGA-3)

Flax oil (58%)	Walnut oil (5%)
Chia seed oil (30%)	Dark leafy greens (50%)
Poppy seed oil (30%)	Beef (0.8%)
Pumpkin seed oil (15%)	Pork (0.5%)
Soy oil (9%)	Egg (0.4%)
Canola oil (7%)	

EPA (EICOSAPENTAENOIC ACID—OMEGA-3)

Salmon	Tuna	Cod liver oil	Haddock
Mackerel	Eel	Pike	Rabbit
Sardines	Rainbow trout	Carp	Wild game
Herring			

Figure 3-1. How Polyunsaturated Oils are Converted to Prostaglandin Hormones*

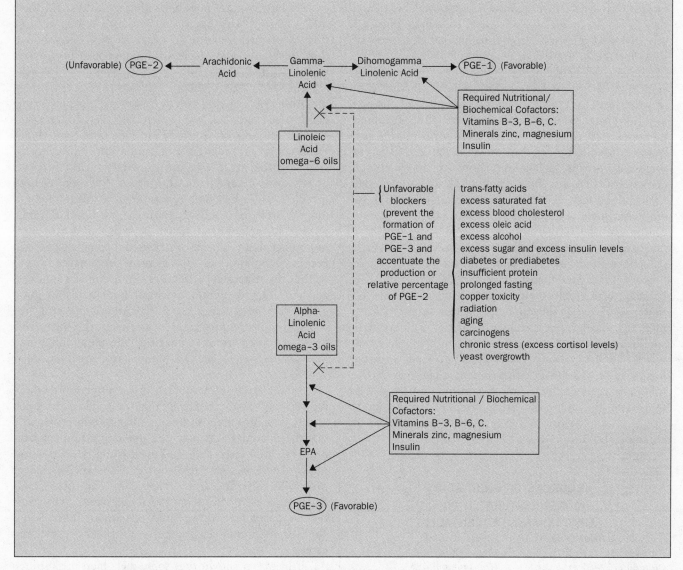

Much of the information for this figure comes from H. Sinclair, Essential Fatty Acids in Perspective, Human Nutrition, Clinical Nutrition 38-C, 1984, pp. 245–260.

GAMMA-LINOLENIC ACID (OMEGA-6)	
Evening primrose oil (10%)	Bluegreen algae (21.4%)
Black currant oil (12%)	Borage oil (up to 30%)

Sources:
1) Chicken, turkey, pork, beef: from S.B. Eaton, M. Shostak, and M. Konner, The Paleolithic Prescription (New York: Harper & Row, 1988).
2) Egg: USDA, "Composition of Foods, Dairy, and Egg Products, Raw, Processed, Prepared," Agriculture Handbook no. 8-1 (Washington, DC: USDA ARS, 1976).
3) All others are reprinted from Fats That Heal, Fats That Kill, by Udo Erasmus, Alive Books, Burnaby, British Columbia. Copyright © 1986, 1993 by Udo Erasmus. Reprinted by permission of Alive Books.

Linoleic Acid Problems

One other point should be mentioned about polyunsaturated oils. As you can see in Figure 3–1, unaltered linoleic acid (LA) can be converted to both favorable (PGE-1) and unfavorable (PGE-2) prostaglandin hormones. Too much linoleic acid can contribute to too much prostaglandin E-2, which can cause inflammation, blood clots, autoimmune problems, and other conditions. Avoid daily use of safflower and sunflower oils, which are rich in linoleic acid, or even corn oil, which is 59 percent linoleic acid. Moreover, just as linoleic acid is easily damaged by light, heat, and oxygen outside the body, it can be damaged inside the body as well—especially if your body's antioxidant defense mechanisms (see page 53) are compromised. I therefore recommend that you use only moderately linoleic acid–rich bottled oils, such as unrefined sesame, rice bran, and flax. It is also important, of course, to include omega-3 oils (flaxseed oil, cold-water fish, and other sources of EPA) for the formation of favorable PGE-3.

You've probably heard of monounsaturated (oleic acid) oils. These oils are far more stable in the presence of light, heat, and oxygen than polyunsaturated oils and are therefore preferred for cooking. One common monounsaturated oil is olive oil. Used for centuries as a staple in Mediterranean diets, olive oil has gained recent popularity because it has been shown to decrease total cholesterol, LDL or "bad" cholesterol, and triglyceride levels (blood fats related to heart disease). Olive oil lowers these lipids without also lowering HDL or "good" cholesterol and is therefore considered somewhat of a preventative for heart disease.

Other good sources of oleic acid are almond, filbert, hickory, macadamia, pistachio, and cashew nuts. Dry roasting them would subject you to minimal hazards. Of those just listed, pistachio is the highest in polyunsaturates (19 percent), but is still much safer to dry roast than sunflower seeds (65 percent polyunsaturated). In other words, for dry roasting, choose nuts and seeds with the highest oleic and lowest polyunsaturated fat content. Use this same criterion for choosing sautéing or baking oils. (See "The Right Oils and Fats" for specific suggestions.)

The table below lists percentages of oleic acid in common foods.

SOURCES OF OLEIC ACID
MONOUNSATURATED OILS
(APPROXIMATE PERCENTAGES)

High oleic sunflower seed oil (81%)	Filbert oil (54%)
Olive oil (76%–82%)	Brazil nut oil (48%)
High oleic safflower seed oil (75%)	Rice bran oil (48%)
	Peanut oil (47%–60%)
Macadamia oil (71%)	Sesame oil (42%)
Avocado oil (70%)	Walnut oil (28%)
Cashew oil (70%)	Soy oil (26%)
Hickory oil (68%)	Corn oil (24%)
Almond oil (65%–78%)	Sunflower seed oil (23%)
Pistachio oil (65%)	Flax oil (19%)
Apricot kernel oil (63%)	Grape seed (17%)
Pecan oil (63%)	Egg (48%)
Canola oil (54%–60%)	Chicken (47%)
Beech oil (54%)	Beef (40%)
	Pork (34%)

Adapted from S. B. Eaton, M. Shostak, and M. Konner, The Paleolithic Prescription (New York: Harper & Row, 1988); U. Erasmus, Fats That Heal, Fats That Kill (Burnaby, British Columbia: Alive Books, 1993); and USDA, "Composition of Foods, Dairy, and Egg Products, Raw, Processed, Prepared," Agriculture Handbook no. 8-1 (Washington, DC: USDA ARS, 1976).

The Hazards of Today's Diet

Perhaps you are now beginning to understand some of the reasons why Americans in the early years of this century seemed immune to heart attacks, even though their diets consisted of plentiful amounts of beef, pork, lard, eggs, and whole milk products. You may also have a good idea why Greenland Eskimos, Masai tribesmen, the Atiu-Mitario, and other traditional peoples rarely develop heart attacks, even when their diets contain substantial amounts of saturated fat. One important clue is the essential fatty acid/prostaglandin hormone relationship. Hydrogenated oils and trans-fatty acids, blockers of favorable prostaglandin hormones, had not yet been invented. More heat-stable, saturated fats were predominantly used for cooking. Furthermore, food refining, processing, and other nutrient-depleting measures were not widespread. Subtle nutrient deficiencies had not become common, and this, in turn, promoted and protected the nutrient cofactors that convert undamaged, unaltered dietary essential fatty acids to good prostaglandin hormones. Early Americans and traditional cultures were able to keep the favorable prostaglandin hormones ahead of the unfavorable and maintain relatively healthy immune and cardiovascular systems.

Studies have shown that nearly every culture whose members subsist on relatively high-fat foods and are relatively free of our most serious diseases subscribes to a diet that includes adequate and undamaged polyunsaturated essential fatty acids and mostly unprocessed whole foods. There is very little altered oil: no margarine or processed oils; no french fries, chips, or other foods fried in polyunsaturated "low cholesterol" vegetable oil; no partially hydrogenated oil–contaminated foods such as mayonnaise, crackers, cookies, breads, and cereals.

It has been shown that some diets high in saturated fat are commonly associated with high levels of cholesterol and the development of plaque. But the end results of plaque in the arteries—heart attacks, strokes, and peripheral vascular disease—are prevalent mostly in cultures that also consume large quantities of damaged vegetable oils and other altered/refined foods. These cultures also have a higher incidence of certain cancers and autoimmune diseases.

There are many apparent and clear advantages to reducing dietary saturated fat. But in this country we need to take even more aggressive action to protect ourselves by:

1. Using appropriate amounts of unaltered, undamaged essential fatty acids, both the omega-6 (linoleic acid) and omega-3 (alpha-linolenic acid/EPA). See "The Right Oils and Fats," page 54.

2. Avoiding damaged oils, particularly polyunsatu-

rated and partially hydrogenated vegetable oils containing trans-fatty acids.

3. Consuming a diet consisting largely of whole foods.

We also need to heed one last recommendation: minimizing free radicals.

Free Radicals and Antioxidant Mechanisms

One of the more significant and least publicized dangers of our excessive fat consumption, one that parallels the hazards of trans-fatty acids and hydrogenated vegetable oils, is rancidity, an oxidized state of fat or oil that causes direct injury to our tissues through free radicals.[25]

FREE RADICALS. A free radical is an electrically neutral molecule with an unpaired electron. Hydrogen peroxide, superoxide, hydroxyl radical, and singlet oxygen are the most studied free radicals. To satisfy their electron shortage, free radicals initiate a chain reaction of destruction on a biochemical level, causing cellular destruction and damage to proteins, enzymes, and DNA, the chromosome storehouse. They can also cause the generation of toxic compounds such as malonaldehyde that can produce similar damage.

Free radicals can injure tissues in nearly any organ or system of the body, speeding up the aging process and contributing directly to a multitude of illnesses. If the destructive process takes place in LDL cholesterol molecules or in the linings of the arteries, for example, the resulting arteriosclerotic plaque could eventually lead to coronary artery disease and heart attack. If excessive free radicals are unleashed chronically in your knee, arthritis could result. If they appear in the lining of your colon, colitis or colon cancer could develop. Free radicals have been classified as carcinogens (causing cancer), mutagens (causing genetic mutations), and teratogens (causing birth defects).

More and more scientific investigators and health professionals embrace the theory that free radicals are a common component of most of our chronic degenerative diseases, premature aging, and premature death.[26] With an understanding of the dietary contribution to the free radical process and the antioxidant mechanisms that protect us from this process, we can develop specific strategies to further defend our health. Fortunately, because you have just learned about trans-fatty acids and partially hydrogenated oils, you already know how to avoid a majority of the assaults from dietary free radicals.

Polyunsaturated fats and oils are the most susceptible to rancidity. Heat over 300° F and overexposure to air (oxygen) and especially to light will trigger the generation of free radicals. The regular consumption of foods with such damaged fats (for example, french fries cooked in polyunsaturated oil) merely invites chronic illness in years ahead.

CHOLESTEROL is a distinct entity, separate from and yet often associated with saturated fat in many foods. Unlike saturated fat, which is more resistant to oxidation, cholesterol is easily oxidized outside or inside the body. Oxidized cholesterol, not simply cholesterol, may very well be a primary cause of coronary heart disease and some forms of cancer.[27] It is for this reason that fried or scrambled eggs (or dried egg products) are significantly more dangerous to eat than soft-boiled or poached eggs or that hamburgers are far riskier than a roasted meat or a beef stew. In fact, one study showed that the consumption of fried eggs was the strongest dietary association with fatal ovarian cancer.[28] For more than a decade there has been fanfare and documentation about the excessive dietary fat/cancer link in the United States.[29] What is rarely publicized and may actually be causing the cancers are the free radicals generated from the excessive temperatures we use to cook our fat—the frying, grilling, broiling, and charcoaling of any meats (especially where charring occurs).[30] This cooking hazard also includes the melting and "crisping" of cheese for pizzas, nachos, and other foods.

How can we be practical and realistic about this free radical phenomenon without turning into dietary extremists and becoming fearful of any heated oil or fat? Well, first it may be important to know that free radicals, despite their danger, perform some essential tasks for us. They are generated by our own white cells, for instance, as they fight off infections. In addition, some free radicals kill bacteria and help to transform malignant cells and modulate the immune and inflammatory responses. Free radicals are also generated when the liver metabolizes toxic chemicals (see Chapter Nine).

ANTIOXIDANTS. Because free radicals occur naturally in our bodies and are an inherent part of certain biologic activities, we have been equipped with protective antioxidant mechanisms to safeguard our tissues. The stronger these protective mechanisms, the less likely it is that exposure to free radicals will pose a serious threat, unless the exposure is of an overwhelming nature.

Crucial to the antioxidant arsenal are dietary nutrients, such as sulfhydryl proteins/amino acids like cysteine; vitamins E and C; beta-carotene; and the minerals selenium, zinc, manganese, and copper. Other nutrients that have antioxidant capability are vitamins B-1, B-2, B-3, and B-5, dimethylglycine, glycine, glutamic acid, and factors such as coenzyme Q-10, lipoic acid, and glutathione. Several herbal agents (including pycnogenol, milk thistle, rosemary, celery seed, and myrrh) and even some naturally occurring components of our blood (such as uric acid, ceruloplasmin, and transferrin) also serve antioxidant functions.

A number of antioxidant nutrients function as cofactors in concert with free radical–deactivating

THE RIGHT OILS AND FATS

- Find the brands of polyunsaturated oils that are made using the Omegaflo® process or other processes that guarantee the exclusion of oxygen, light, and temperatures above 110° Fahrenheit. Such oils are packaged in an oxygen-free, opaque (non-see-through) container with the date of pressing and expiration.

  These oils are truly "cold pressed" and unrefined. They are usually rich in color and flavor and may be cloudy. Most important, they are undamaged (free of trans-fatty acids and free radicals), retaining their freshness and nutritional value. Supermarkets don't regularly stock these oils yet, so look in health food stores or food co-ops. Avoid purchasing large-size containers that you won't use up in two or three months, and avoid polyunsaturated oils from bulk containers that are not refrigerated or nitrogen packed.

- Keep your oils in the refrigerator or freezer in their airtight containers. If your olive oil crystallizes in the refrigerator, keep it in a dark, cool cabinet.

- I recommend using unrefined sesame, extra virgin olive, flax, walnut, hazelnut, macadamia, and rice bran oils. If available, high oleic sunflower oil (derived from a genetic hybrid sunflower seed high in oleic acid and low in polyunsaturates) is also a good oil. See recipes for salad dressings in Chapter Five.

- Do not use the following oils regularly, as they are too unsaturated: sunflower seed, corn, grape seed, and soy.

- Safflower oil has a very short history of usage (safflower seeds are not eaten, unlike other seeds). According to Andrew Weil, M.D., in *Natural Health, Natural Medicine*, ancient texts of India warn against its use in the diet.[31] It might be best to avoid regular safflower and even high oleic safflower oil.

- I usually use high oleic acid (monounsaturated) oils (such as olive or occasionally high oleic sunflower) for heating and sautéing. Canola oil is gradually becoming very popular for cooking because it is relatively high in oleic acid (54–60 percent) and very mild in flavor. However, it is still 37 percent polyunsaturated, and therefore not ideally suited for high-temperature use.

- Although food companies have jumped on the canola oil bandwagon, some authorities, such as Udo Erasmus (author of *Fats and Oils: The Complete Guide to Fats and Oils in Health and Nutrition*), strongly advise against the use of canola oil. This oil is derived from rapeseeds, a toxic component of which allegedly remains in the oil. Besides this, most canola oil is heavily refined, reason enough to avoid it.

- The only polyunsaturated oil I use for sautéing is unrefined sesame oil (41 percent polyunsaturated and 46 percent monounsaturated). You would think that 41 percent polyunsaturated is still too high for heating; however, because of antioxidants unique to sesame oil generated during heating, sesame oil is more stable in the presence of heat, light, and oxygen than other polyunsaturated omega-6 oils. I sometimes use butter or a combination of olive oil and butter, which permits me to cook at a higher temperature without burning the butter.

- Do not let these oils smoke or burn, for they will be damaged. Or use coconut oil, which is the most stable to heat. Make sautéing an occasional treat, not a regular method of food preparation. Minimize the amount of oil used by sprinkling in water or tamari sauce for a "steam-fry" effect.

THE RIGHT OILS AND FATS

- The least processed and most preferred olive oil is extra virgin. The next best is virgin; and the most processed is pure.

- Peanuts and peanut oil, along with peanut butter, have gained a bad reputation for the common fungal contaminant aflatoxin, a carcinogen. Additional medical gossip about the peanut concerns its atherogenicity,[32] the tendency to accelerate clotting of blood—not a favorable event inside an artery—and its relationship to menstrual cramps. Although peanut oil is very stable to heat and excellent for frying (and less expensive than olive oil), do not use it regularly.

- Do not cook with polyunsaturated oils such as sunflower, safflower, grape seed, corn, soy, wheat germ, walnut, and flax.

- Consult table (see page 58) to determine the fat content of various oils and other foods.

- Avoid baked or fried products containing polyunsaturated oils (safflower, sunflower, corn, soy, canola, etc.). This can prove to be virtually impossible, as most commercial cookies, cakes, crackers, breads, muffins, corn and potato chips, fresh and frozen french fries, oil-roasted nuts, snack foods, and other items contain these oils.

- How can you protect your health and still be realistic and practical? Fried foods, like chips, present the greatest hazard, because of the very high temperatures used in their preparation. So just try to avoid them, and find alternatives when you can, like baked chips made without oil.

- Commercial baked goods do not present as much of a hazard as fried foods because of the lower temperatures used in the baking process. However, since food companies rarely use unrefined or monounsaturated oils, you should include these items only occasionally in your diet. Instead, bake your own cakes and cookies using unrefined monounsaturated oil (make large batches and freeze the extra). Experiment to see which oils taste best. Try high oleic sunflower, macadamia nut, avocado, or a very mild olive oil. Sesame oil may also work. If the saturated fat content of your diet is minimal, try a little coconut oil or butter. Also check out fat-free cookies and other baked items available in health food stores and elsewhere.

- Avoid any cooked or uncooked products containing partially hydrogenated oils. Such items include margarine, mayonnaise, pancake or baking mixes, many canned soups, cereals, salad dressings, many frozen foods, artificial creamers, artificial whipped cream, cookies, cakes, crackers, chips, frozen french fries and other frozen foods, candy bars, and even carob candy.

- Avoid margarine. Use butter instead, but sparingly. Or make "better butter" (see page 114). Or, instead of a spread, use olive or flax oil.

- Store nut butters, whole-grain mixes and flours, wheat germ, bran, and bread products in airtight containers in the refrigerator (or, except for nut butters, in the freezer). Although nuts and seeds have a natural protective coating, their freshness is prolonged by refrigeration or freezing. Buy flour and flour products as fresh as possible. Grind grains yourself, if possible. Any flour you don't use for immediate purposes may be stored in airtight containers or bags and refrigerated or frozen.

- Assure dietary adequacy of alpha-linolenic acid. Unless you eat wild game, rabbit, or cold-water fish regularly (or take EPA fish or cod liver oil capsules regularly), you will likely be missing enough

THE RIGHT OILS AND FATS

of this essential fatty acid. Pumpkin, soy, canola, and walnut oils contain a small amount of alpha-linolenic acid, but these are rarely found unrefined. If you eat seeds and nuts, choose pumpkin seeds and walnuts. Flaxseeds, however, have the highest percentage of alpha-linolenic acid.

- I highly recommend that you take as a regular supplement: 1 to 2 teaspoons of expeller (cold-pressed) unrefined flax oil, nitrogen bottled in amber glass or opaque containers with dates of pressing and expiration and found refrigerated in the store. Use at least three to four times a week, mixed in cottage cheese, yogurt, hot or cold cereals, grain dishes or soups, on salads with other dressing, on bread, in juice or a blender drink, or taken straight at mealtime. Never heat it. Flax oil has a growing reputation for the treatment and prevention of cancer, cardiovascular disease, arthritis, and other diseases (See pages 106–108).

- If you have diabetes, if you use too much alcohol or have a history of alcohol abuse, if your cholesterol level is very high, or if your diet is loaded with saturated fat, you should take special nutritional supplements. Use GLA supplements (black currant seed oil, borage oil, or evening primrose oil capsules) for omega-6 sources, and EPA fish oil supplements for omega-3 needs. (Be sure EPA capsules are certified free of PCBs, other organic chemicals, heavy metals and rancidity—fish oil capsules from Carlson's Laboratories of Arlington, Illinois, have one of the best ratings.)

- Minimize charcoaling, charbroiling, grilling, and broiling—anything that chars the meat and fat. If you must use these methods, take measures to avoid charring. It is best to bake, steam, poach, boil, or stew. Slow cooking and low temperatures are least hazardous. For instance, a beef stew presents much less danger than a grilled or broiled hamburger. For eggs, poaching and soft-boiling are best. Exposing the yoke to oxygen and high temperatures of frying can damage the cholesterol, so scrambling is the least desirable method; hard-boiling will likely cause minimal damage to the fat unless, when preparing certain dishes, the yoke is exposed to air for any length of time. Avoid burning toast—or anything, for that matter.

- Do not eat broiled or high-temperature baked cheese on a regular basis. This means nachos, pizzas, omelettes with cheese, lasagna, enchiladas, and so on. Add grated cheese after the dish is out of the oven, letting the heat of the food melt it.

- If you eat out often (every day or nearly every day), find out what kind of oil is used in cooking, salad dressings, mayonnaise, etc. Chances are the food is frozen, preprepared, and contains refined, heated, and damaged polyunsaturated oils and partially hydrogenated oils. If you go to a higher-quality restaurant where the food is made from scratch, you will have better luck but may still encounter bad oils. Inquire. Conscientious chefs and owners will often respond to reasonable requests and questions.

- Choose foods that are relatively safe: baked, steamed, poached, or boiled; stews or soups, and raw vegetables and fruits. Order sauces and dressings on the side. Ask for butter or any fat or oil on the side so you can choose how much to use. Substitute olive oil and vinegar dressing. Perhaps sneak in your own healthful dressing. If you eat out only occasionally, you do not need to be as concerned; it is your daily or nearly daily habits and meals that count most. Take active, aggressive, and commonsense measures to protect your health.

THE RIGHT OILS AND FATS

- If you are a meat eater, use intact meat cuts or parts (slices, legs, chops, etc.) rather than ground meat products. In general, it is best to boil meats or poultry, a process that requires some planning. After boiling, let the water cool, refrigerate, then skim off the fat that congeals at the top. This produces a much-reduced fat content in the meat, and a low-fat, flavorful broth. You can then use the meat in a soup or stew or prepare it in other ways.

- Eat fresh fish caught from relatively uncontaminated water. Fish is generally low in saturated and total fat and highest in polyunsaturated fat of all commercially available flesh foods. Farmed fish has less optimal polyunsaturated fat (EPA) content than wild, but may be less contaminated with pollutants.

- Find butchers who sell organic or at least hormone- and antibiotic-free meats and poultry (see "Food Additives/Contaminants," page 72). Be sure to use leaner cuts of meat. For optimum fat content and ratios in meat, nothing compares with the extremely low total fat, low saturated fat, and high polyunsaturated fat percentage of wild game. Grain stuffing before slaughter is what substantially raises the overall fat and saturated fat content of commercial meats (and, from an ecologic and global perspective, may be wasting valuable resources).

- Be reasonable and practical. Occasional use of foods with damaged oils or very high fat content does not present a long-term health hazard. Eat right most of the time and protect yourself with antioxidant nutrients.

enzymes. Selenium, for example, relates to glutathione peroxidase, manganese to mitochondrial superoxide dysmutase, zinc to catalase and superoxide dysmutase, and copper to superoxide dysmutase and peroxidase.

Some nutrients, like vitamin E, work more on their own to protect cellular membranes from free radical assault. Other nutrients, such as beta-carotene, act as free radical quenchers, or trappers, by virtue of their molecular conformation. Still others serve as necessary precursors for the synthesis of elements in antioxidant systems. For example, cysteine and glutamic acid become glutathione. Several authorities now believe that all antioxidant mechanisms need to function simultaneously for effective free radical protection to take place. You can see how important a whole-foods/unrefined diet is in the fight against a free radical assault.

If your diet provides the important nutrients listed above, and you avoid excessive exposure to rancid fats and oils, you'll have an edge on free radicals. The average American, however, eats foods terribly deficient in these important nutrients, and the body's natural defenses cannot protect against diseases brought on by free radicals. Over decades, this assault contributes to a quickening of the aging process and to the development of many degenerative diseases.

The body's ability to protect itself from free radical assault can be enhanced if you make it a habit to avoid dietary sources of free radicals and prepare your meals wisely. Since your control over dietary free radicals and refined foods may not always be optimal, and in light of the increasing threat to our health from environmental pollutants, it is crucial to take supplemental antioxidant nutrients, even if only vitamins C, E, beta-carotene, B complex, and the minerals selenium, zinc, manganese, and copper. All of these are usually found in most good multiple vitamin/mineral formulas. Try to get in the following dosages every day:

Vitamin C: 500–1,000 mg two to three times
Beta-carotene: 25,000 I.U.
Vitamin E: 400–800 I.U.
Selenium: 200 mcg
Zinc: 15–30 mg
Copper: 2 mg
Manganese: 5–20 mg
Cysteine: 100–200 mg
B complex: 10–25 mg

(Chapter Six offers guidelines and precautions for many of these nutrients.) If you want more specialized anti-oxidant protection, you can use specific combination formulas including these and other antioxidants mentioned.

Rational Fat Choices

Although the consumption of excessive fat calories has been linked to many serious illnesses, it appears that the quantity ingested—or even the saturated versus un-saturated percentages—are not the only factors to be considered. In determining the balance between health and disease, the prevalence of trans-fatty acids, partial hydrogenation, and rancidity of oils is a critical issue. Once we understand essential fatty acid metabolism, the mechanisms of imbalanced prostaglandin ratios, and the associated dietary and environmental hazards that contribute to this danger, we are equipped to make safer and more rational choices about the fat in our diet.

The table below offers a comparison of fatty acid percentages in several animal sources.

REFINED CARBOHYDRATES

Why do refined carbohydrates have such a devastating effect on health? It's because refining wheat, rice, and other grains strips out most of the life-giving vitamins, minerals, oils, and fiber necessary for the optimal functioning of our minds and bodies. After years of eating white rice, white bread and rolls, white crackers, white noodles, refined cereals, pancakes and waffles, cookies, cakes, and pastries all made from white flour, subtle vitamin and mineral deficiencies can develop that sooner or later manifest as chronic ailments and disease.

Vitamins and minerals play essential roles in metabolic processes, from the production of antibodies and hormones to detoxification and the generation of energy and heat. All biochemical reactions require specific vitamins and minerals. When food sources no longer contain the rich supply of nutrients with which nature endowed them, our glands, organs, and cells may eventually be deprived of components crucial to their optimal performance. I am not referring here to gross deficiency diseases like beriberi, scurvy, kwashiorkor, or pellagra, which are now seen primarily in underdeveloped nations. However, in the context of subtle micronutrient deficiency, I'm talking about enzyme slowdown or failure and other defects that can lead to arthritis, premature senility, fatigue, depression, mental illness, adult onset diabetes, arteriosclerosis, heart attacks and strokes, impaired immunity, and defective antioxidant mechanisms that contribute to infections and cancer.

Do you think we develop all these ailments naturally, simply as part of the process of aging? No. Aging is not a disease. A more accurate explanation may be that, as a result of eating foods deficient in essential nu-

PERCENTAGE OF FAT IN COMMONLY EATEN ANIMAL FOODS AND COCONUT

| | POLYUNSATURATED | | MONOUNSATURATED | SATURATED |
	ALPHA LINOLENIC (OMEGA 3)	LINOLEIC (OMEGA 6)	OLEIC	
Chicken fat	—	22%	47%	30%
Beef fat	0.8%	2.1%	46%	51%
Lard: pork fat	0.5%	12%	47%	41%
Butter	—	4%	30%	54%
Egg	0.4%	13%	48%	30%
Coconut	—	3%	6%	91%

Sources: 1) omega 3 content for Beef and Pork and omega 6 content for Beef: S.B. Eaton, M. Shostak, M. Konner, The Paleolithic Prescription *(New York: Harper and Row, 1988), 109*
2) Egg: USDA, "Composition of Foods, Dairy and Egg Products, Raw, Processed, Prepared," Agriculture Handbook no. 8–1 (Washington, DC: USDA ARS, 1976)
3) Coconut is reprinted from Fats That Heal, Fats That Kill, *by Udo Erasmus, Alive Books, Burnaby, British Columbia. Copyright © 1986, 1993 by Udo Erasmus. Reprinted by permission of Alive Books.*
4) All others: J.B. Reeves and J.L. Weihrauch, "Composition of Foods," Agriculture Handbook no. 8–4 (Washington: US Department of Agriculture, 1979)

trients over a period of years, we gradually develop predictable ailments as these continuing deficiencies manifest in our bodies. The biochemical factories in our cells stop functioning properly when the manufacturing components and parts are unavailable. Stripping the germ and bran from a kernel of wheat, for instance, removes a significant portion of its vitamins: B-1, B-2, B-3, B-5, B-6, E, biotin, folic acid, and the minerals chromium, iron, calcium, potassium, magnesium, zinc, manganese, cobalt, molybdenum, and selenium (see the table below). Enriching flour only with vitamins B-1, B-2, B-3, and the mineral iron still leaves gaps in many of these important components.

LOSS OF NUTRIENTS IN ENRICHED WHITE BREAD

NUTRIENT	% LOST IN WHITE BREAD
Vitamin E	96
Vitamin B-6	82
Manganese	88
Fiber	78
Magnesium	78
Chromium	72
Zinc	62
Copper	58
Potassium	39

Copyright 1985, CSPI. Adapted from Nutrition Action Healthletter *(1875 Connecticut Ave., N.W., Suite 300, Washington, D.C. 20009-5728. $24.00 for ten issues).*

Begin to lessen your consumption of white flour products. Anything made from white flour, enriched, bleached, or unbleached, can be made with whole wheat flour and other whole-grain flours: buckwheat, cornmeal, brown rice, barley, millet, rye, oat, amaranth, teff, spelt, kamut, and quinoa. Brown rice can easily be used instead of white rice. None of these whole-grain products need enrichment, as nature has endowed them with enough nutrients of their own.

Using whole-grain foods, however, may require several changes in perspective and preparation. When you shop, you may need to seek out health-food stores, food co-ops, or enlightened supermarkets that offer products made from whole grains. If you want genuine whole wheat bread, be sure that the first item in the fine print on the ingredient label reads "whole wheat flour" or "wheat flour." Most breads available in supermarkets are actually made from primarily refined and enriched flour but resemble whole wheat thanks to food coloring. Very small amounts of actual whole wheat flour, if any at all, are included. The labels on such products offer an extremely long list of ingredients, the first of which is enriched flour and the last several are preservatives.

Unrefined bread contains nothing but whole wheat or other whole-grain flour, water, yeast, salt, sometimes honey, and sometimes seeds or nuts. Some bakers leave out the yeast. Whole-grain items available in the right stores include bread, rolls, buns, muffins, crackers, bagels, noodles and other pastas, pretzels, bread sticks, croissants, cereals, pancake or waffle mixes, gravy, cakes, and cookies. Many can be easily made. Even traditional foods such as chapati, pita, tortillas, and scones can be purchased or made from whole-grain flours.

If you do not spend much time in the kitchen, find the right places to buy these whole-grain items. If you already spend time cooking and baking, it's a simple matter to substitute whole-grain items for refined ingredients. Many natural food cookbooks will prove helpful as will some of the food suggestions and recipes in Chapter Five.

Many restaurants now serve whole-grain rolls, and most will at least provide whole wheat bread or toast on request. It is quite common, as well, for many to serve brown rice. Natural foods restaurants also serve whole wheat or whole-grain noodles and desserts made with whole-grain flours. Many will gladly make changes to provide what enough of their clientele request. If you eat out frequently, it is extremely important to find restaurants that support your health.

Not every meal has to contain whole, unrefined grain, especially if you are just beginning to convert from a standard white flour diet. Convert to whole-grain eating gradually, as your intestinal tract may revolt with a little distress if the change is too abrupt.

FIBER

According to Dennis Burkitt, M.D., the elimination of fiber in the refining of flour is perhaps more responsible than any other dietary factor for a good number of chronic diseases.[33] From the sizable list of conditions associated with lack of fiber (see page 45), it is quite evident that roughage serves a role beyond mere bowel regulation. Some additional functions include:

- Helping to regulate the rate of sugar entering the bloodstream.
- Helping to prevent cholesterol reabsorption and lower blood fat levels.
- Detoxifying the colon and preventing colon cancer as well as absorption into the colonic mucosa and bloodstream of bacterial and fungal metabolites.
- Preventing absorption of other toxins and heavy metals.

- Helping to control weight.
- Keeping vital, friendly intestinal bacteria happy.

Chapter Eight presents a more detailed discussion of fiber and how to monitor your transit time, one very important test of fiber adequacy and bowel health.

Whole-grain products will contribute to your fiber intake, while refined grain and refined flour products will not. If you tolerate whole grains quite well, however, it would be a mistake to attempt to derive all your fiber needs from this food category. In order to sustain a balanced diet, other fiber-rich foods should be consumed: legumes (dried beans like black, pinto, navy, soy, adzuki, garbanzo, lentils, and split peas), fresh vegetables and fruits, even seeds and nuts.

SUGAR

A refined carbohydrate that has had a devastating effect upon our health is sugar. Annual consumption of sugar by the average American in 1984 was 126.8 pounds[34]—roughly one-third of a pound per day. With table sugar alone, that's six tablespoons a day. Approximately 75 percent of the sugar we eat is hidden, added to soda, cake and cookie mixes, pie, ice cream, candy, cereals, soups, canned fruit, ketchup, salad dressings, bread, yogurt, vitamins, medications, and nearly every processed, prepackaged item on supermarket shelves. Sugar often appears as sucrose, dextrose, glucose, corn sweetener, corn syrup, high fructose corn syrup, and maltose. The closer these sugars are to the beginning of any food ingredient list, the higher the sugar content. See the following tables to get a rough idea of just how sugar-rich your diet is.

REFINED SWEETENERS (SUGAR) CONTENT OF BREAKFAST CEREALS (IN PERCENTAGE)*

Ready-to-eat Cereal	Sugar Calories as a Percentage of Total Calories
GENERAL FOODS/NABISCO	
100% Bran	35
Fruit Wheats Strawberry	28
Frosted Wheat Bites	25
Fruit Wheats Raspberry	25
Fruit Wheats Blueberry	24
Team Flakes	18
Shredded Wheat'n Bran	2
Shreded Wheat	0
Shredded Wheat Spoon Size	0
GENERAL FOODS/POST	
Golden Crisp	55
Marshmallow Alpha-Bits	47
Fruity Pebbles	44
Cocoa Pebbles	43
Raisin Bran	42
Alpha-Bits	40
Honeycomb	40
Bran'nola Raisin	36
Fruit & Fibre Dates, Raisins & Walnuts	34
Bran'nola Original	30
Fruit & Fibre Peaches, Raisins & Almonds	29
Great Grains Raisins, Dates & Pecans	25
Blueberry Morning	24
Bran Flakes	22
C.W. Post Hearty Granola	21
Grape-Nuts Flakes	20
Honey Bunches of Oats Honey Roasted Banana Nut Crunch	18
Honey Bunches of Oats with Almonds	18
Great Grains Crunchy Pecan	15
Grape-Nuts	14
Post Toasties	8
GENERAL MILLS, INC.	
Boo Berry	47
Cocoa Puffs	47
Count Chocula	47
Frankenberry	47
Total Raisin Bran	44
Wheaties Dunk-A-Balls	44
Lucky Charms	43
Sprinkle Spangles	43
Trix	42
Crispy Wheats'n Raisins	42
Apple Cinnamon Cheerios	40
S'mores Grahams	40
Golden Grahams	37
Hidden Treasures	37
Honey Nut Cheerios	37
Reese's Peanut Butter Puffs	37
Oatmeal Crisp Raisin	34
Low Fat Fruit Granola	34
Wheaties Honey Gold	33
Cinnamon Toast Crunch	31
Berry Berry Kix	30
Oatmeal Crisp Apple Cinnamon	30
Raisin Nut Bran	30
Sun Crunchers	30
Ripple Crisp Honey Bran	29
Clusters	24
Basic 4	23
100% Natural Oat Cinnamon & Raisin	23
Multi-Grain Cheerios	22
100% Natural Oat Fruit & Nut	21
Body Buddies Natural Fruit	20
Kaboom	20
Triples	20
Oatmeal Crisp Almond	19
Ripple Crisp Honey Corn	18
Total Whole Grain	18
100% Natural Oat Toasted Oats & Honey	18
Wheaties	15

Total Corn Flakes	11
Kix	10
Country Corn Flakes	7
Cheerios	4
Wheat Hearts	3
Fiber One	0
KELLOGG'S	
Smacks	58
Apple Jacks	51
Marshmallow Krispies	51
Cinnamon Mini Buns	47
Corn Pops	47
Froot Loops	47
Pop-Tarts Crunch Frosted Strawberry	47
Bran Buds	46
Double Dip Crunch	44
Cocoa Krispies	43
Frosted Flakes	43
Raisin Bran	42
Apple Cinnamon Rice Krispies	40
Frosted Bran	40
Frosted Krispies	40
Nutri-Grain Golden Wheat & Raisin	40
Pop-Tarts Crunch Frosted Brown Sugar Cinnamon	40
Fruitful Bran	38
Nut & Honey Crunch O's	37
Apple Raisin Crisp	36
Nut & Honey Crunch	33
Temptations Honey Roasted Pecan	33
Multi-Grains, Raisins, Crunchy Oat Clusters & Almonds	32
Mueslix Crispy Blend	32
Nutri-Grain Almond Raisin	32
Cracklin' Oat Bran	31
Low Fat Granola	30
Low Fat Granola with Raisin	30
Rice Krispies Treats Cereal	30
Temptations French Vanilla Almond	30
Apple Cinnamon Squares	27
Just Right Fruit & Nut	27
Raisin Squares	27
All-Bran	25
Frosted Mini-Wheats	25
Frosted Mini-Wheats Bite Size	25
Blueberry Squares	24
Complete Bran Flakes	24
Multi-Grain Flakes	24
Just Right with Crunchy Nuggets	24
Nutri-Grain Golden Wheat	24
Common Sense Oat Bran	22
Strawberry Squares	22
Mueslix Golden Crunch	21
Multi-Grain Squares	17
Crispix	15
Product 19	11
Rice Krispies	11
Special K	11
Corn Flakes	7
All-Bran with Extra Fiber	0

QUAKER OATS COMPANY	
Quaker Cocoa Blasts/Popeye Cocoa Blasts	51
Quaker Sweet Puffs	49
Quaker Marshmallow Safari	48
Quaker Fruity Ohs	44
Cap'n Crunch	43
Cap'n Crunch with Crunchberries	43
Quaker Oh's—Honey Graham	40
Quaker Low Fat 100% Natural Crispy Wholegrain Cereal with Raisin	33
Cap'n Crunch's Peanut Butter Cereal	31
Quaker Oat Cinnamon Life	30
Quaker 100% Natural Cereal—Oats, Honey & Raisins	27
Sun Country Granola—Raisin & Date	27
Quaker Cinnamon Oat Squares	24
Quaker Crunchy Bran	24
Quaker Toasted Oatmeal Cereal—Honey Nut	23
Quaker Toasted Oatmeal Cereal—Original	23
King Vitamin	22
Quaker 100% Natural Cereal—Oats & Honey	22
Quaker Life	18
Quaker Oat Bran Cereal	18
Quaker Oat Squares	18
Sun Country Granola with Almonds	17
Kretschmer Wheat Germ (Regular)	12
Quaker Unprocessed Bran	6
Kretschmer Toasted Wheat Bran	5
Quaker Puffed Wheat	1
Quaker Shredded Wheat	1
Quaker Puffed Rice	0
RALSTON PURINA	
Cookie Crisp	40
Graham Chex	32
Strawberry Muesli	27
Raspberry Muesli	25
Almond Delight	23
Multi-Bran Chex	20
Corn Chex	11
Wheat Chex	11
Rice Chex	7

*The sugar percentage for each cereal was calculated per serving and the amount of sugar per serving applied to the following formula: Sugar (in grams per serving) multiplied by 4 (calories per gram). Divide this answer by total calories per serving. Multiply this answer by 100, which gives sugar as percent of total calories. In mathematical configuration this would be:

$$\frac{Sugar\ (grams\ per\ serving)\ X\ 4}{Total\ calories\ per\ serving}\ X\ 100$$

The figures needed for this calculation were kindly provided by the cereal manufacturers. These figures can also be found in the Nutrition Facts panel on any product package. As cereal formulations may change, check this panel for current information.

AILMENTS LINKED TO SUGAR EXCESS

- Hypoglycemia, or low blood sugar, is a symptom of disordered carbohydrate metabolism. Sufferers experience fatigue, mental confusion, depression, irritability, anxiety, shakiness, dizziness, headaches, insomnia, and many other problems (see Chapter Ten).

- Diabetes mellitus is another disorder of carbohydrate metabolism. It is a chronic condition characterized by an overabundance of blood sugar (see Chapter Seventeen).

- Arteriosclerosis can be aggravated by sugar, even in a nondiabetic.[35] Excess dietary sugar can be converted by the body into saturated fat. Sugar can, therefore, raise blood fat levels (triglycerides); decrease HDL cholesterol, a blood cholesterol cleanser, in part by making linoleic acid unavailable; and increase the stickiness, or aggregation quality, of platelets. All of these contribute to either arteriosclerotic plaque formation or thrombosis, putting an individual at increased risk of heart attack, stroke, and other complications of arteriosclerosis (see "Arteriosclerosis," "Heart Attack," and "Stroke" in Chapter Seventeen).

- Sugar diminishes the strength of the immune system, partly by compromising the ability of neutrophils, or white blood cells, to engulf foreign invaders like bacteria, by diminishing lymphocyte transformation, and by other means.[36] In this way, high sugar levels increase susceptibility to infections and to cancer. Sugar consumption has been correlated with a higher incidence of breast cancer in several studies, one of which evaluated this relationship in twenty-one countries.[37]

- Sugar can raise blood levels of uric acid, causing increased susceptibility to gout.[38]

- Sugar abuse is associated with personality and behavioral aberrations, even criminal behavior.[39] Depression, fatigue, foggy-headedness, nervousness, and other mental and brain disorders have been linked to an allergy to cane sugar, corn sugar, and beet sugar (see Chapter Thirteen).

- Laboratory animal studies have confirmed the potential adverse effects of sugar on the kidneys and have linked its overuse to hypertension.[40]

- Some researchers feel that sugar leaches vitamins and minerals from the body, leading to nutritional deficiencies. Sugar certainly induces calcium loss in the urine, contributing to the possibility of developing osteoporosis as well as other calcium deficiency–related ailments (muscle cramps, menstrual cramps, insomnia, nervousness, hypertension, etc.; see Chapter Six). Sugar-induced calcium loss in the urine has also been linked to kidney stones.[41]

- The enzymes used to metabolize sugar into stored energy or fat require specific cofactor vitamins and minerals. As sugar and the refined foods rich in sugar do not replace the micronutrients used in their metabolism, deficiencies are incurred. Sugar, you see, is a metabolic freeloader. As it seems to fill a larger percentage of our diet by displacing more wholesome nutrient-rich foods, it contributes further to nutrient deficiencies.

- Sugar can lead to obesity through a number of mechanisms. By increasing blood insulin levels, fat storage is encouraged. In addition, it takes a very small quantity of sugar or sugar-rich food to deliver an alarming number of calories. Because sugar and sugar-rich foods contain little or no fiber, it is easy to consume them in large quantities before feeling full, by which time you have taken in a tremendous number of calories. Another mechanism involves the overloading of energy-producing biochemical pathways. If these pathways are overburdened with sugar molecules, they can be shunted or shifted away from energy and glycogen production toward the production of fat.

AILMENTS LINKED TO SUGAR EXCESS

- Sugar feeds *Candida albicans*, our resident yeast, and is a significant contributor to the growing yeast epidemic (see Chapter Twelve).

- Sugar can become an addiction and can therefore impair an individual on multiple levels.

- Excess dietary sugar can increase the incidence of gallstones.

SUGAR PERCENTAGE OF VARIOUS DAIRY PRODUCTS

	Serving Size	Sugar Calories as Percent of Total Calories
Frozen yogurt, whole milk	1/2 cup	62
Low-fat yogurt, fruit	1/2 cup	52
Dreyer's low-fat yogurt, vanilla	1/2 cup	56
Dreyer's fat-free yogurt, fruit	1/2 cup	70
Dreyer's fat-free yogurt, vanilla	1/2 cup	62
Vanilla ice cream	1/2 cup	40
Yogurt, flavored	1 cup	34
Chocolate milk, 2%	1 cup	24

Information provided by individual product Nutrition Fact labels and applied to the formula given at the end of the table above, Sugar Percentage of Breakfast Cereals. As product formulas may change, check labels for current information.

SUGAR PERCENTAGE OF VARIOUS DESSERTS

	Serving Size	Sugar Calories as Percent of Total Calories
Popsicle	1	100
Canned peaches, heavy syrup	1/2 cup	92
Canned applesauce	1/2 cup	58
Chocolate Jell-o instant pudding	1/2 cup	76
Hunt's snack pack pudding, chocolate	1 cup	40

Information provided by individual product Nutrition Fact labels and applied to the formula given at the end of the table above, Sugar Percentage of Breakfast Cereals. As product formulas may change, check labels for current information.

Sensible Sugar Levels in Your Diet

How much sugar is acceptable? How can you avoid excesses? How do you know if sugar is responsible for any of your health complaints? How do you know if you're addicted?

Let's begin with chronic illness. From an epidemiologic standpoint, regardless of how sugar affects you day to day, excessive use can contribute to long-term health deterioration. From one point of view, the more healthful your diet and lifestyle, the more resistant you will be to disease from sugar and many other causes. Occasional sweet treats for most of us should not pose a problem. Personally, I consider "occasional" to be definitely less than daily, perhaps more like twice weekly. But there is no way sugar use could be considered occasional if your regular daily intake contains foods with hidden sugar, such as soda, cereal, yogurt, and salad dressings.

Remember: "100 percent natural" does not mean "sugar free." You must read the list of ingredients. Trying to reduce sugar consumption by cutting out an occasional cookie or dessert might not be terribly significant if, like most Americans, you drink a sugar-sweetened soda every day or you regularly consume foods with significant amounts of hidden sugar. If you rely on convenience foods, try to find health food stores, co-ops, and enlightened supermarkets that stock sugar-free packaged, prepared, canned, and frozen foods.

Preferably you will see the wisdom of relying less on convenience foods, while making time to prepare more of your food from scratch.

For instance, take a few minutes and make oatmeal or a seven-grain cooked cereal with a small handful of raisins instead of using a sugared instant hot cereal or ready-to-eat boxed cereal. Prepare a vegetable or miso soup as opposed to a canned or packaged soup. Instead of sweetened yogurt, use plain yogurt and add some fresh fruit slices, perhaps a few raisins, and nuts.

Throw away the store-bought sweetened salad dressing, whose oil quality is usually questionable. Make your own dressing with extra virgin olive oil (the least processed and most healthful of the olive oils), or unrefined sesame or walnut oil, vinegar, and a few herbs. (Chapter Five offers several salad dressing recipes and many fairly convenient, sugar-free, make-it-from-scratch soups, cereals, and other items.)

Hard-core sugar items, such as candy bars, hard candy, soft drinks, sweet rolls, chocolate milk, cookies, doughnuts, ice cream, and chocolates, should be saved for special treats. Find more healthful alternatives.

Initially, commit to making a small percentage of your sweet needs from separate, unadulterated, natural ingredients. This way you can control the kind and amount of sweetener used. The satisfaction generated in creating something on your own—preparing it just the way you like it and the way it is good for you—is immense. And you'll find that your taste buds will grow more sensitive as you begin to cut back on sweeteners. Your own creations will be quite satisfying, while the items you previously consumed will seem oversweet.

For instance, try making a soft drink substitute (see recipe in Chapter Five) from cooled or iced herb tea. Or buy Lemon Zinger tea by Celestial Seasonings at your supermarket or health food store. Bring a cold Thermos of it to work. Have a quart or two ready to drink in your refrigerator. Make your own cookies or muffins with whole-grain flour and cut way down on the sugar. In fact, you can replace the sugar with fruit juice or concentrated fruit sweetener available now in most health food stores, or use a little honey, molasses, sucanat, or barley malt syrup (see page 65). Make your own rice pudding and other desserts (see Chapter Five) that will please yet not be overly sweet.

If you don't have the time to prepare your own treats, find bakeries and health food stores that offer relatively undersweetened items. Beware of carob and granola bars and other "health" treats that are sweetened with honey or fructose. Often these treats are as oversweetened as many sugared items and may contain bad oils as well. Many carob treats contain 48 percent sugar and have a higher saturated fat content than a Hershey's bar, with more sugar than ice cream.

Sugar and Chronic Illness

How can you know if your current chronic illness is in some way related to years of sugar excess? Quite simply, you can't. Chronic illnesses are multicausal, so pinning the blame solely on sugar would be shortsighted. From a medical nutrition standpoint, most chronic illnesses, however, would benefit from a drastic reduction in sugar intake, with similar attention paid to other dietary hazards, and the incorporation of treatments for appropriate underlying conditions (many of which will be discussed in detail in subsequent chapters). Quite often, once you make such nutritional improvements, you'll begin to feel better than you have in years.

Fatigue, nervousness, anxiety, depression, headache,

hyperactivity, recurrent respiratory infections, recurrent vaginal infections may not be recognized as symptoms of sugar addiction, but these day-to-day acute, adverse reactions are common to the syndrome. Hypoglycemic, allergic/addiction, and immune-weakening effects may all be parts of it. Most individuals I see in my practice end up tackling their sugar problem because of immediate present-day health complaints. Yes, they are concerned about their future health, but their primary desire is to feel and function their best again. A drastic reduction of sugar is one common way to achieve this.

If you are addicted to sugar, or feel that you need a lot of support in breaking the habit, consider the following suggestions.

How to Overcome the Sugar Habit

- Make sure there are adequate complex carbohydrates in your diet, particularly for meals after which you tend to crave sugar. Experiment to find the balance of complex carbohydrates that your body tolerates best. In craving sweets, your body may simply be signaling a need for carbohydrates, which you can fill with the more wholesome, unrefined variety. If your diet already contains ample whole grains, legumes, and starchy vegetables, adding more will not be helpful. It may even worsen your sugar cravings.

- Make sure your diet contains adequate protein, whether the sources are vegetarian (beans and grains, tofu, tempeh, seeds, nuts and nut butters, etc.) or animal (fish, chicken, eggs, some beef and other flesh foods, some milk products). Use the protein sources that your body assimilates and tolerates best. If you are a strict vegetarian, you may consume what seems to be an adequate amount of protein yet always feel "starved," and have a persistent sweet tooth. You may, in fact, need to increase your protein intake. If this doesn't help, some animal protein might, as contrary as that may seem to you. A small amount could possibly help you to feel more satiated and crave fewer sweets. Strict vegetarianism is not appropriate for everyone. Of course, if your diet already contains ample protein of the kind appropriate for your body, do not increase the amount. In fact, excessive protein often triggers a craving for sugar. Experiment with protein amounts and see how this affects your sweet tooth.

- Follow the dietary recommendations and supplements discussed in Chapter Ten for stabilizing your blood sugar. The regimen establishes adequate complex carbohydrates and proteins and proposes a reduction of concentrated sweets (sugar, honey, and the like). It also calls for the reduction of caffeine, alcohol, and fruit juices, but it does allow some fresh fruits (not in excessive amounts).

Supplements include vitamins B complex and C, chromium-GTF, glutamine, and biotin. Chromium, biotin, and glutamine specifically decrease sugar cravings. A strong supplement program, along with an appropriate diet, may be what you need initially to stay off sweets. If you still cannot break the sugar habit, you will nevertheless be on the way to recovery.

- Look for a chronic yeast overgrowth (Chapter Twelve). Initiation of antifungal therapy often reduces—and in many cases completely relieves—sugar craving.
- In attempting to lower your sugar intake, bear in mind that you may be allergic to the very source of your addiction. Food allergy/addiction can trigger intense withdrawal symptoms similar to drug addiction (see Chapter Thirteen). There are a number of effective ways to minimize withdrawal difficulties, as explained on page 247.

Overcoming very severe sugar addiction may require professional supervision and intravenous therapy. In addition, each of us has particular sensitivities. You may find that you can tolerate beet sugar, whereas cane or corn sugar may send you into a tailspin. Not that regular consumption of a tolerated sugar is advised. Just remember that when you do use sugar, choose wisely to avoid allergic reactions.

- Sugar may be serving an important emotional or psychological need. For this reason, it may not be wise to attempt to eliminate it from your diet until you have established adequate social and emotional support such as close friends or family, your primary other, a therapy group, individual counseling, and Overeaters Anonymous. Many sources of support are available.
- Sugar may be helping you to stay away from tobacco, alcohol, or other addictive substances from which you are recovering. Reducing your sugar consumption before you're biochemically or psychologically ready may not be a good idea. However, using sugar as a substitute addiction can create new problems that will sooner or later have to be faced and worked on.

Make a Sugar Consumption Plan

As you cultivate food consciousness and an overall understanding of health concerns, you will begin to question your desire for super bursts of sugar or even for hits of the less sweet health food treats and desserts. Later, as your metabolism becomes more balanced through dietary changes, your body will actually desire them less.

So, how much sugar should you ingest? What is a reasonable and sensible amount? You must decide that for yourself. Formulate a plan that will work for you—

and only you will know the program that can work best. Once you lessen the amount of sugar in your diet, you may find that in order not to feel deprived, you need to have a concentrated sugar once or twice a week. When you have your sugar, enjoy it thoroughly with no guilt or bad feelings. Consider the improvement and progress you have made, and be pleased that you can enjoy a little of what may once have been a problem-causing substance for you.

You may find, however, that a small indulgence of two or three times a week can keep you wanting sugar all the time, thinking often about your next opportunity to eat it. Or it may make you feel plain lousy. You may decide, then, that once a week or once every few weeks is as often as you can safely ingest it. Then again, you may consider sugar a serious addiction or be diagnosed with a serious illness and swear it off completely for six months or more, as I once needed to do. I could never eat "just a little" sugar; one cookie would turn into eight.

Know yourself and what will work for you, and establish a plan. If it doesn't work, try a different plan or seek assistance from a nutritionally oriented health professional and possibly a counselor or hypnotherapist. Eventually you will succeed.

Alternatives to Sugar

Granulated sugar, brown sugar, turbinado raw sugar, and refined fructose (such as high-fructose corn syrup) are all extremely refined products that offer relatively no vitamins, minerals, or nutritive value other than calories. The following list provides some alternatives to sugar:

Honey
Molasses
Maple syrup
Sucanat
Barley malt or rice malt syrup
Dates
Date sugar
Raisins
Fruit puree/fruit concentrate
Licorice root or anise tea
Stevia

Natural sweeteners contain simple sugars that can have adverse effects similar to those produced by table sugar (sucrose) on the blood sugar level, the pancreas, the adrenal glands, and the brain. All get converted at variable rates to the same glucose. Just because they are "natural" or generally less refined than sucrose does not mean you can use them in any amounts you wish. Yet for many individuals, these sweeteners will not trigger the same reactions as table sugar and will provide some nutritive value. Through trial and error, you may find several that in certain amounts work quite suitably for you.

There are several reasons these sweeteners are more desirable than sugar:

- The enzyme content of raw honey may have beneficial effects. Honey also contains a small amount of vitamins and minerals.
- Molasses, blackstrap and unsulfured, is a significant source of the minerals iron, calcium, phosphorus, and potassium and even contains vitamins B-1, B-2, and B-3.
- Maple syrup (100 percent), particularly grades B and C (often available in bulk in health food stores or co-ops), is less sweet and more mineral-rich (calcium and magnesium) than the more common A grade. Be careful: most supermarket maple syrup, even with "natural" on the label, is mostly sugar water and imitation maple flavor.
- Sucanat is a granulated, natural, organic sweetener evaporated from freshly squeezed sugarcane juice. Nothing is removed but the water, so it is, in effect, an unrefined, whole-foods sweetener, retaining the minerals, trace elements (even chromium), and vitamins. It contains 2.5 percent of these nutrients, whereas table sugar contains none, and brown and turbinado sugars contain only 0.5 percent. Sucanat can be substituted for table sugar teaspoon for teaspoon.
- Concentrated fruit sweetener contains fructose. Unlike the highly refined fructose usually derived from corn, it comes from pineapple, pear, grape, and other fruits and retains some of the original nutrients. You can make your own by blending chopped fresh fruit with small amounts of fruit juice. It is available commercially at most health food stores.
- Malt syrup (from barley or rice) also contains some of the nutrients from the original grains: vitamins K, B, A, C, and the mineral calcium.
- Dates and raisins both contain minerals. Try soaking some dates overnight, pitting them, and blending them in the soaking water to use as a sweetener. Try the same with raisins, or simply use a few chopped dates or a small handful of raisins to cook with a whole-grain cereal or add to a muffin batter.

Licorice root tea imparts a pleasantly sweet taste alone or when used with other herbal teas (see Chapter Nineteen for precautions). Anise may work in this regard as well. Stevia, extracted from a South American plant, is a sweetening agent used for centuries by traditional South American cultures and is popular in Japan. Two to three drops of extract can sweeten any tea or beverage quite adequately and can also be used in baking. Unfortunately, stevia is not widely available in this country, as the FDA has not yet approved it for internal use.

Artificial Sweeteners

You may be wondering about aspartame, which is available as Nutrasweet and Equal. Is it a safe alternative to sugar? According to a report in the *New England Journal of Medicine*,[42] aspartame, which is made from phenylalanine, aspartic acid (two amino acids), and methyl alcohol, can greatly imbalance levels of other amino acids and neurotransmitters in the brain. One example is a decrease in tryptophan availability and the reduction of brain serotonin levels, a prime setup for mood or sleep disturbances. This especially affects individuals exhibiting hypertension, Parkinson's disease, insomnia, hyperactivity, as well as those on such drugs as levodopa and monoamine oxidase inhibitors.

Although the average person may not feel any adverse effects from using small to moderate amounts of aspartame as a sweetener, I would hesitate to call it completely safe. Possibly because of its methyl alcohol content, large amounts of aspartame can provoke headaches, fainting, seizures, memory loss, mood swings, depression, nausea, and gastrointestinal distress. Small amounts can cause allergic or skin rashes and itching in susceptible individuals. Menstrual problems have also been linked to the use of aspartame. Heating the sweetener—in baking, for instance—creates well-known additional hazards.

FDA approval of artificial sweeteners is not always a guarantee of safety. For instance, cyclamates were used in the fifties and sixties, then banned because of their link to cancer. Saccharin is another example. Because of the controversy over its relationship to bladder cancer, the use of saccharin has not been fully deemed safe. Generally speaking, I advise my patients against the regular ingestion of artificial sweeteners and the foods and beverages containing them.

CAFFEINE

You may be unaware that caffeine is actually a drug. Approximately 400 million cups of coffee are consumed daily in the world, 16 pounds per person per year in the United States alone.[43] Abundant quantities of caffeine are found elsewhere: in black tea, soft drinks, chocolate, cocoa, and numerous prescription and over-the-counter medications.

Caffeine produces a feeling of energy, alertness, and

well-being through its direct effect on the nervous system and through stimulation of the adrenal glands. Both cortisol and adrenaline from the adrenal glands elevate blood sugar levels, which in turn stimulates the central nervous system. Because of its energizing effect, caffeine can allow an individual to continue with lifestyle habits that are causing chronic fatigue. Beneath the buzz of energy and alertness, however, the nervous system and adrenal glands continue to tire. Such use of caffeine is a time bomb. It gradually creates a need for more and more as the liver becomes conditioned to metabolizing caffeine more quickly while the body becomes increasingly tired. One or two cups of coffee may no longer deliver the same punch. Coffee drinkers may soon find themselves ingesting toxic doses of the substance to keep getting the same lift. Sooner or later, this means they will develop a number of adverse symptoms and conditions.

There has also been a suggested relationship between caffeine and cancers of the pancreas, prostate, and bladder.[44]

Some people enjoy coffee for the taste, just a cup a day or less. They never feel the need to drink more, they do not experience any of the adverse effects of caffeine use, and they do not use caffeine to boost their energy. This kind of use seems far less hazardous.

Given the possible long-term consequences of caffeine use, it might be reasonable to assume that the lower the daily dose, the less likely the incidence of long-term damage. Knowing also that coffee beans come from countries where pesticides and herbicides considered too toxic to be sold in the United States are used, one can only wonder if part of the risk of long-term damage stems from the residues of these man-made carcinogens. The same question may be raised about the decaffeinating solvents TCE (trichloroethylene, recently banned) and methylene chloride. If regular use is a must for you (unless you are pregnant or caffeine-addicted), a small daily amount might be safe, although it is best to use organic coffee or organic/water-processed decaffeinated brews.

If you feel you need to give up this habit or diminish your intake to more reasonable levels, consider the following:

- Reduce caffeine intake (coffee, black tea, soft drinks, chocolate, caffeine-containing medications). Look at all your potential sources of caffeine and see if you can gradually and steadily reduce your usage (see the tables on the next page). Some individuals prefer the "cold turkey" method of stopping abruptly. However, the withdrawal symptoms may be more intense with this method.
- Find alternatives. Instead of coffee or black tea, substitute herbal teas—there are many to choose from

SYMPTOMS OF CAFFEINE TOXICITY

Fatigue	Stillbirth
Headache	Prematurity
Depression	High blood pressure
Insomnia	Increased serum cholesterol
Decreased ability to cope	Heart attack
Anxiety	Heart rhythm disturbances
Nervousness	Hypoglycemia
Irritability	Rectal pain and itching
Muscle tremors	Diarrhea
Gastritis and ulcers	Cystitis
Fibrocystic breast disease	Prostatitis
Premenstrual syndrome	Diuretic action
Birth defects	Urinary loss of calcium, magnesium, biotin,
Infertility	inositol, and other nutrients
Osteoporosis	

(see Chapter Five); hot water with a squeeze of fresh lemon and/or slice of lemon peel; Pero, Cafix, Postum, or other roasted grain beverages; miso soup; vegetable, meat, or chicken broth. If soft drinks contribute substantially to your total caffeine use, review previous suggestions for alternatives. If you have medical conditions that require caffeine-containing drugs, consult the following ten chapters for underlying conditions that could potentially lie at the root of your symptoms. Also check Chapter Seventeen.

- Develop nutritional and dietary support. Follow the same nutrient supplement program and diet used for breaking the sugar habit and stabilizing blood sugar (see previous section and Chapter Ten). In this way, your nervous system and adrenals will be supported.
- To handle such withdrawal symptoms as headaches, irritability, anxiety, and fatigue, which may last from one day to one week, use buffered vitamin C and/or Alka-Seltzer Gold (as discussed on page 247). A gradual elimination of caffeine will lessen the severity of withdrawal. If it's more your style, going "cold turkey" is also a viable option, although a bit risky. I recommend intravenous nutrient injections for those whose withdrawal symptoms are too severe for self-help measures.

CAFFEINE CONTENT OF SEVERAL COMMON BEVERAGES AND FOODS

ITEM	MILLIGRAMS AVERAGE	CAFFEINE RANGE
Coffee (5-oz. cup)		
Brewed, drip	115	60–180
Brewed, percolator	80	40–170
Espresso, single shot (Starbucks)*	80	60–100
Instant	65	30–120
Decaffeinated, brewed	3	2–5
Decaffeinated, instant	2	1–5
Tea (5-oz. cup)		
Brewed, major U.S. brands	40	20–90
Brewed, imported brands	60	25–110
Instant	30	25–50
Iced (12-oz. glass)	70	67–76
Cocoa beverage (5-oz. cup)	4	2–20
Chocolate milk beverage (8 oz.)	5	2–7
Milk chocolate (1 oz.)	6	1–15
Dark chocolate, semi-sweet (1 oz.)	20	5–35
Baker's chocolate (1 oz.)	26	26
Chocolate-flavored syrup (1 oz.)	4	4

*Starbucks Coffee Company, Seattle, Wa.
U.S. Food and Drug Administration, Food Additive Chemistry Evaluation Branch, as reproduced in U.S. Food and Drug Administration, "The Latest Caffeine Scorecard," FDA Consumer (March 1984), 14. Based on evaluations of existing literature on caffeine levels.

CAFFEINE CONTENT OF VARIOUS SOFT DRINKS (12-OZ. SERVINGS)

BRAND	MILLIGRAMS CAFFEINE
Sugar-Free Mr. PIBB	58.8
Mountain Dew	54.0
Mello Yellow	52.8
TAB	46.8
Coca-Cola	45.6
Diet Coke	45.6
Shasta Cola	44.4
Shasta Cherry Cola	44.4
Shasta Diet Cola	44.4
Mr. PIBB	40.8
Dr Pepper	39.6
Sugar-Free Dr Pepper	39.6
Big Red	38.4
Sugar-Free Big Red	38.4
Pepsi-Cola	38.4
Aspen	36.0
Diet Pepsi	36.0
Pepsi Light	36.0
RC Cola	36.0
Diet Rite	36.0
Kick	31.2
Canada Dry Jamaica Cola	30.0
Canada Dry Diet Cola	1.2

Institute of Food Technologist (IFT) as reproduced in U.S. Food and Drug Administration, "The Latest Caffeine Scorecard," FDA Consumer (March 1984), 15. Based on data from National Soft Drink Association, Washington, DC, April 1983.

CAFFEINE CONTENT OF A FEW COMMONLY USED DRUGS

PRESCRIPTION DRUGS	MILLIGRAMS CAFFEINE
Cafergot (for migraine headache)	100
Fiorinal (for tension headache)	40
Soma Compound (for pain relief, muscle relaxant)	32
Darvon Compound (for pain relief)	32
NONPRESCRIPTION DRUGS	
Alertness tablets	
NoDoz	100
Vivarin	200
Analgesic/pain relief drugs	
Anacin, Maximum Strength Anacin	32
Excedrin	65
Midol	32
Vanquish	33
Diuretics	
Aqua Ban	100
Maximum Strength Aqua-Ban Plus	200

FDA's National Center for Drugs and Biologics, as reproduced in U.S. Food and Drug Administration, "The Latest Caffeine Scorecard," FDA Consumer (March 1984), 16.

Caffeine Withdrawal—Sam's Story

In addition to nutritional support, other factors may be quite valuable in helping to discontinue caffeine use. Consider the following case history.

Sam, a forty-one-year-old engineer, came to my office with complaints of abdominal pain, fatigue, headache, anxiety, and excess weight. He was employed by a large corporation and worked ten hours a day, six days a week.

Sam had a wife and two children, but had little energy for them during his evenings after work or on his one day off each week. Instead, he was forced to spend his free time trying to "recover." Yet when I asked him what gave him the most meaning in his life, he responded, "My family!" But he also said that he would be unable to make it through the day without coffee. He consumed over eight cups a day, and his diet included many doughnuts and fast-food sandwiches.

Sam's medical history and physical examination disclosed high blood pressure, heart palpitations, near exhaustion, a probable duodenal ulcer, and deep emotional unhappiness. This was a man under intense demands from his job. He was sacrificing not only his health, but the most important and meaningful part of his life—his relationship with his family.

When Sam first went to work for his present company, he'd been drinking only one cup of coffee a day with breakfast. However, as the demands upon him increased, his energy began to fail. That's when he began adding a cup or two of coffee during the day to give him an extra lift. On top of the caffeine, the doughnuts and convenience foods he was eating were certainly not helping his energy level, nor was his excessively sedentary lifestyle.

Sam soon found himself drinking a cup or two of coffee at home at night simply to stay awake through dinner so he could spend some time with his family. It wasn't long before Sam realized that he "needed" to drink coffee all day long. It was after a month at this level of caffeine intake that he appeared in my office. Sam was a wreck. He felt trapped in what he saw as a position necessary to obtain his goals, but one that was ruining his health and causing his life to deteriorate.

I pointed out to him the way in which coffee was contributing to his mental and physical symptoms. I explained that he would benefit by eliminating caffeine, by cleaning up the rest of his diet, and by using several "all-star foods" (see Chapter Five) and supplements. In addition, if he would begin a regular course of exercise, he'd find himself better able to deal with the stress and hours of work, while experiencing much less anxiety and fatigue. He'd still feel good enough to enjoy his family. If at that time, I continued, he found that his work still conflicted excessively with the quality of his family life, a reexamination of his work goals might be in order.

As Sam's story shows us, just as with sugar, many factors need to be considered when you're trying to eliminate coffee successfully: diet and nutrition, exercise, stress, priorities, and goals. Before eliminating a caffeine habit—or any destructive habit—you need to sit down and examine the whole picture, all the interwoven, related factors of your life that have led you step by step into an abuse of the substance. This kind of conscious, courageous, and careful planning puts you well on the road to success.

SOFT DRINKS

Haven't we incriminated this item enough for its sugar, caffeine, and aspartame content? Not quite! In addition to the hazards associated with these ingredients, you may be interested to learn that phosphates added to soft drinks, whether sugared, artificially sweetened, caffeinated, or decaffeinated, contribute to disorders in calcium metabolism.[45] When the blood phosphorus level climbs out of proportion in relation to calcium levels, homeostatic corrective mechanisms are engaged to raise the calcium level and renormalize the ratio. The parathyroid glands, which are located in the neck by the thyroid gland near the Adam's apple, control the body's calcium and phosphorus levels. They are then signaled to secrete parathormone, a hormone that causes bone to release minerals, mostly calcium, into the bloodstream.

You can see how decades of this compensatory action will contribute to a loss of bone density and strength and to the development of periodontal disease and osteoporosis. If there is a concomitant excess of vitamin D and magnesium deficiency, calcium can be deposited in undesirable areas such as blood vessels, kidneys, and joint linings. This, in turn, contributes to secondary ailments such as atherosclerosis, kidney stones, and arthritis. Not surprisingly, in Germany and other European countries where researchers are convinced of phosphoric acid's adverse effect on behavior, such additives have been outlawed.

When you are parched and want something cool to drink, have on hand your own wholesome soft drink brew. Try the delightful combination of cool lemon grass tea with a touch of apple juice and a dash of sparkling mineral water. Or have fruit-flavored unsweetened sparkling mineral water or plain spring water with a bit of fruit juice, or a squeeze of lemon or lime. When carbonation is not desired, have just the cooled herb tea plain or sweetened either with licorice root or a little fruit juice. Or have fruit juice diluted with water to diminish the sweetness—excessive fruit sugar can have some of the same effects as regular sugar. Have fresh vegetable juice or a combination of vegetable juices (especially easy if you have a juicer). Buy low-salt tomato juice or a tomato/vegetable juice combination. Health food stores carry "natural" soft drinks without phosphoric acid or other additives; however, be discriminating about these, as some are oversweetened. One of the reasons for the worldwide popularity of soft drinks is the effective hydrating qualities of the combination of water, carbonation, and sugar. Experiment to find the best-tasting and hydrating soft drink alternative.

It's not easy for a soda junkie to reform. Often, addictions to both sugar and caffeine must be overcome. As with many areas of health improvement, the first step will often be a transition phase. Follow the hints for overcoming a sugar habit (see page 64) and the treatment plan for hypoglycemia (Chapter Ten).

Soft drinks are an entirely unnecessary component of nutrition. Anyone concerned about disease prevention and health maintenance should recognize that regular use of soft drinks, which in my mind means one serving a day or even every other day, is inadvisable. Choose more healthful beverages. They are plentiful, easy to make, and pleasant tasting. By the way, for a beverage that not only quenches thirst but truly enhances your health, nothing beats a tall glass of plain, simple, pure water.

WATER

Water is unquestionably our most valuable resource.[46] All life on planet Earth depends upon water. The purity of our drinking water supply, however, has become severely endangered by industrial and agricultural pollutants. Many of these pollutants are toxic to vital organs, tissues, and contain well-known carcinogens that are often undetectable by taste, sight, or smell.

You may think your tap water is perfectly safe and wholesome, yet even the water in pristine Washington State wells were found to be contaminated with toxic organic chemicals from a local U.S. Air Force base. In California's Silicon Valley, solvents used in the manufacturing of computer chips were found to have leaked from buried storage tanks into the water supplies of several communities. Cornell University in upstate New York is studying wells on Long Island that show traces of the pesticide aldecarb, recently associated with watermelon toxicity in California. Preliminary reports indicate that the drinking water in this area may be affected for as long as 140 years. The fumigant ethylene dibromide (EDB), which causes cancer in animals, has been found in wells in Florida.

State health authorities are trying to force the cleanup of a former battery plant in Dallas, Texas, where tests reveal that soil in some areas contain 577 times the lead content considered potentially hazardous to children. Over the past few years, hundreds of Nebraska families have been drinking bottled water furnished by the Army because poisonous chemicals from a nearby ammunition plant had seeped into their well water. These are but a few of the countless examples of water whose quality has been jeopardized by contamination from human activities.

Common Water Pollutants

These fall into four categories:

1. Organic chemicals.
2. Inorganic chemicals.
3. Biological agents (bacteria, viruses, parasites, fungi).
4. Physical agents (asbestos, sediment).

Organic chemical contamination derives primarily from industrial and agricultural (herbicide and pesticide pollutants) activities.

Inorganic contaminants (heavy metals) enter the water supply through industrial pollution, through eroding water pipes, and through the leaching effect of acid rain on soil and pipes.

Chlorine and Fluoride. These inorganic pollutants are commonly added to public water supplies. Although the benefits of these two chemicals are well known, nevertheless their well-documented hazards—one of which is carcinogenesis—have been largely ignored. It is well known that the interaction between chlorine and many organic chemicals gives rise to a very toxic and potentially carcinogenic class of compounds: trihalomethane and chloramines.

It is also known that some microorganisms, especially viruses, are not adequately killed by chlorine. Conversely, we do not want chlorine killing the friendly bacteria in our intestines. Another alleged threat from chlorine, though poorly substantiated, is its association with atherosclerosis and heart attacks.[47]

Fluoride is best known for its alleged ability to reduce cavities. Tooth decay has decreased 50 to 60 percent over the last thirty years, and this improvement has largely been attributed to fluoridation of public water supplies. However, serious challenges to this assumption have shown comparable reduction of tooth decay in fluoridated and nonfluoridated areas alike.[48] It is well accepted in the scientific community that excessive fluoride can cause dental fluorosis, a condition that has symptoms ranging from mild discoloration or mottling to darkened, pitted, brittle teeth that are very sensitive to fracture. Another consequence of fluoride toxicity is skeletal fluorosis, an abnormal bone and joint condition ranging from biochemical changes in the bone to a crippling disease.

Why should we fluoridate our water when the benefits are questionable and the risks are real? Why should we fluoridate when there is a general consensus that the amounts of fluoride considered to be toxic are only a fraction higher than the "anticavity" amounts considered to be safe? With a naturally high fluoride content in the drinking water in many areas of the country, along with relaxed EPA standards allowing four parts per million fluoridation—plus an increasing amount of fluoride from other sources such as toothpastes, mouthwashes, vitamins, chewing gum, and foods—many individuals could be consuming excessive amounts of fluoride. This is especially worrisome for people who live in hotter climates and who drink far greater volumes of water.

Intensifying this controversy are the data that show unequivocal enzyme changes caused by fluoride and conflicting reports and allegations of mutagenic effects, birth defects, and cancer. Although some possible toxic effects from fluoridation have not been well proven, they have certainly not been disproven, and there is adequate reason to question its safety. It is clear that many individuals are allergic or hypersensitive to fluoride. And yet, whether or not to fluoridate has become more a political question than a medical one. I generally recommend avoiding water and vitamins that have been fluoridated.

Although chlorine is not a perfect disinfectant, and although infections, particularly viral ones, do arise, we should feel grateful that we can fill up a glass of water from the tap without worrying about contracting typhoid fever, cholera, or parasitic diseases. Yet, this issue is less important today. This is because industrial and technological advances have brought us new, far more insidious dangers that are now making clean, pure water a rarity. We just cannot continue to take for granted that our tap water is safe, even if we're using our own well or spring.

What You Can Do to Find Clean Water

Despite the fact that most of our lakes, rivers, and underground aquifers are now chemically contaminated and threaten our health, a number of measures can help us secure a pure drinking water source. One of the best is the use of a home water purification system. Such a system should satisfy the following criteria:

- Removal of organic chemicals.
- Removal of inorganic chemicals.
- Removal of biological agents (bacteria, viruses, parasites).
- Removal of such physical agents as asbestos (a common contaminant from asbestos-lined concrete pipes used in municipal water systems).
- Retention of all healthful minerals.

A good system should *not* promote growth of bacteria, require a lot of maintenance, or cost a lot of money to operate.

Methods of Water Purification

- **DISTILLATION**, heating to steam, then recondensing to water, frees water of the inorganics and physical agents. Unless the final product has been distilled two or three times, it will not be free of organic chemicals. Unfortunately, distilling water also removes all the healthful minerals, such as calcium and magnesium. This method is costly to operate, and because of the deposit of inorganic salts in the distiller, it requires a great deal of maintenance.

- **CARBON FILTRATION** effectively traps organic contaminants and any adverse tastes and odors. Unfortunately, it will not remove the inorganics, but it will let through the healthful minerals. If the charcoal filter is not changed often enough, impurities will accumulate and the system will not filter effectively—this may not be easy to determine. Any bacteria in the water will find the filter a very favorable place to breed (unless the filter is silver-impregnated).

- **REVERSE OSMOSIS** forces water through a semipermeable membrane that allows the passage only of molecules of water and some of the healthful minerals. The inorganic chemicals, most organic agents, physical agents, bacteria, and other large microorganisms, are thus separated from the final product and sent down the drain. Because this technology does not actually trap and accumulate impurities, as distillation and carbon filtration do, it is relatively maintenance free.

  Reverse osmosis technology alone satisfies all the stated criteria for excellence in water purification, provided the membrane quality is sufficient. If applied in combination with activated carbon filtration, whereby the reverse osmosis–treated water (stage 1) would then be filtered through the charcoal (stage 2), any organic pollutants remaining after stage 1 would thereby be removed. What is left is alive, tasty, clean water with some of its natural minerals. Although initial costs may be substantial for such a combination system ($300 and up), it is extremely inexpensive health insurance, one of the least expensive methods to operate, and well worth the peace of mind.

Of course, you can have spring or artesian water delivered to your home or office. Water companies usually filter and purify this water, but this ends up being far more costly per gallon than water from your own purification system—and may be, in regard to purity, less reliable. If you choose this route, request copies of water-testing results.

Testing Your Water

For a reasonable fee, you can send a sample of your drinking water to a laboratory that will test for heavy metals, organic chemicals, even minerals. Look in the Yellow Pages under "Environment" or "Water" or "Laboratories," or call your municipal water works for a referral.

If you do not find great fault with your central water supply, and the chlorine and fluoride levels are not worrisome to you, perhaps the problem rests with your plumbing pipes (lead and cadmium from old galvanized pipes, outdated lead solder from antiquated systems, and copper from copper pipes). To minimize the risk from these potential hazards, let your cold tap water run for several minutes to clear out the water that has been sitting for hours in the plumbing system. Then collect from the cold tap a large container of new water, which is fresh from the central supply. Use this container exclusively for drinking and cooking. Never drink from or cook with water from the hot tap.

One last measure you can take is to support environmental groups, state and community action groups, and legislators who will strengthen the Clean Water Act. See the following list of organizations that can provide resource information and refer you to local organizations (see also resource information in Chapter Fourteen).

Environmental Defense Fund, 257 Park Ave. South, New York, NY 10010, (212) 505-2100.
National Resources Defense Council, 40 West 20th Street, New York, NY 10011, (212) 727-4400.
Audubon Society, 8940 Jones Mill Rd., Chevy Chase, MD, (301) 652-9188.
Friends of the Earth, 1025 Vermont Ave. NW, Washington, DC, (202) 783-7400.
Sierra Club, 404 C Street NE, Washington, DC, (202) 547-1141.

FOOD ADDITIVES/CONTAMINANTS

Along with the disease-encouraging dietary habits we have adopted, we have developed methods of food processing, preserving, and packaging that call for the addition of thousands of chemicals to our foods. When these chemicals were first created, they were considered a great advance in nutritional technology, making it possible to store and ship foods, allowing people to enjoy staples and delicacies from different climates and countries, and freeing homemakers from the daily trip to the market and countless hours spent canning and drying seasonal foods. The additives made some foods cheaper and seemed to be the answer to food waste through molds, rot, and other natural decay processes. As with other contributions of industry and technology, however, what at first appeared to be a breakthrough welcomed by many has resulted in inquiries over safety issues and bannings. Although many additives have been outlawed, many more are still allowed despite reasonable suspicion of health risks. The "innocent until proven guilty" and "profit protection over health protection" creeds are putting consumers at risk, and we need to safeguard ourselves.

We use well over three thousand chemical substances foreign to our biological systems in the agricultural and food industries. Many of the substances are known toxins, known enzyme poisons, known carcinogens, known allergy- and asthma-causing and behavior-altering chemicals. There are preservatives, coloring and flavoring agents, emulsifiers, buffers, binders, bleaches, anticaking agents, flowing agents, and others. Many of these have not been adequately tested for safety. Did you know that some European countries allow only twenty additives, some allow only seven, and some allow none at all? Yet, the United States allows thousands of food chemicals—some may be safe and useful, some outright dangerous, and many more yet to be tested.

Just one example of the dangers of food additives can be seen in restaurant salad bars, where sulfite, a preservative and antibrowning agent, has come into common use. It has become evident that acute asthmatic attacks can be brought on by this additive. In fact, in many states, legislation has compelled restaurants to post a sign informing their clientele of the use of sulfite. Despite the known hazards of this preservative, food and restaurant industries adamantly lobby to maintain their right to its use.

BHA and BHT, extensively used preservatives, have known toxic effects. Adverse allergic reactions, including anaphylaxis, urticaria, and asthma, have been noted from ingestion of tartrazine, sunset yellow, ponceau red, benzoates, and other additives. You may already know that it is processed, prepared, convenience, and junk foods that generally contain harmful additives.

Buying unrefined, fresh, whole foods will not only give you more nutritional value, obviously, but will generally steer you clear of harmful additives. Read food labels. Look for the words "additive and preservative free." This is becoming far more common as food companies respond to the growing number of health-conscious consumers. There are several good references on food additives to provide you with much more detailed information.[49] The following table summarizes the dangerous, the safe, and the suspect additives.

COMMON FOOD ADDITIVES

KEY

✓ = SAFE   **?** = QUESTIONABLE   ✗ = AVOID

✓ **ALGINATE, PROPYLENE GLYCOL ALGINATE**
Thickening agents; foam stabilizer
Ice cream, cheese, candy, yogurt

Alginate, an apparently safe derivative of seaweed (kelp), maintains the desired texture in dairy products, canned frosting, and other factory-made foods. Propylene glycol alginate, a chemically modified algin, thickens acidic foods (soda pop, salad dressing) and stabilizes the foam in beer.

✓ **ALPHA TOCOPHEROL (Vitamin E)**
Antioxidant, nutrient
Vegetable oil

Vitamin E is abundant in whole wheat, rice germ, and vegetable oils. It is destroyed by the refining and bleaching of flour. Vitamin E prevents oils from going rancid.

✗ **ARTIFICIAL COLORINGS**

Most artificial colorings are synthetic chemicals that do not occur in nature. Though some are safer than others, colorings are not listed by name on labels. Because colorings are used almost solely in foods of low nutritional value (candy, soda pop, gelatin desserts, etc.), you should simply avoid all artificially colored foods. In addition to problems mentioned below, there is evidence that colorings may cause hyperactivity in some sensitive children. The use of coloring usually indicates that fruit or other natural ingredients have not been used.

✗ **BLUE No. 1**
Artificial coloring
Beverages, candy, baked goods

Inadequately tested; suggestions of a small cancer risk. Avoid.

✗ **BLUE No. 2**
Artificial coloring
Pet food, beverages, candy

The largest, most recent study suggested, but did not prove, that this dye caused brain tumors in male mice. The FDA concluded that there is "reasonable certainty of no harm."

✗ **CITRUS RED No. 2**
Artificial coloring
Skin of some Florida oranges only

Studies indicate that this additive causes cancer. The dye does not seep through the orange skin into the pulp.

✗ **GREEN No. 3**
Artificial coloring
Candy, beverages

A 1981 industry-sponsored study gave hints of bladder cancer, but FDA re-analyzed the data using other statistical tests and concluded that the dye was safe. Fortunately, this possibly carcinogenic dye is rarely used.

✗ **RED No. 3**
Artificial coloring
Cherries in fruit cocktail, candy, baked goods

The evidence that this dye causes thyroid tumors in rats is "convincing," according to a 1983 review committee report requested by FDA. FDA's recommendations that the dye be banned had been overruled by pressure from the Reagan administration.

COMMON FOOD ADDITIVES

? RED No. 40
Artificial coloring
Soda pop, candy, gelatin desserts, pastry, pet food, sausage

The most widely used food dye. While this is one of the most tested food dyes, the key mouse tests were flawed and inconclusive. An FDA review committee acknowledged problems, but said evidence of harm was not "consistent" or "substantial." Like other dyes, Red No. 40 is used mainly in junk foods.

? YELLOW No. 5
Artificial coloring
Gelatin dessert, candy, pet food, baked goods

The second most widely used coloring causes allergic reactions, primarily in aspirin-sensitive persons. This dye is the only one that must be labeled by name on food labels.

✗ YELLOW No. 6
Artificial coloring
Beverages, sausage, baked goods, candy, gelatin

Recent industry-sponsored animal tests indicate that this dye causes tumors of the adrenal gland and kidney. It may also cause occasional allergic reactions. This dye is contaminated with cancer-causing impurities.

? ARTIFICIAL FLAVORING
Flavoring
Soda pop, candy, breakfast cereals, gelatin desserts; many others

Hundreds of chemicals are used to mimic natural flavors; many may be used in a single flavoring, such as for cherry soda pop. Most flavoring chemicals also occur in nature and are probably safe, but they may cause hyperactivity in some sensitive children. Artificial flavorings are used almost exclusively in junk foods; their use indicates that the real thing (usually fruit) has been left out.

✓ ASCORBIC ACID (Vitamin C) ERYTHORBIC ACID
Antioxidant, nutrient, color stabilizer
Oily foods, cereals, soft drinks, cured meats

ASCORBIC ACID helps maintain the red color of cured meat and prevents the formation of nitrosamines (see *sodium nitrite*). It helps prevent loss of color and flavor by reacting with unwanted oxygen. It is used as a nutrient additive in drinks and breakfast cereals. SODIUM ASCORBATE is a more soluble form of ascorbic acid. ERYTHORBIC ACID (sodium erythorbate) serves the same functions as ascorbic acid but has no value as a vitamin.

? ASPARTAME
Artificial sweetener
Drink mixes, gelatin desserts, other foods

ASPARTAME, made up of two amino acids, was thought to be the perfect artificial sweetener, but questions have arisen about the quality of the cancer tests and persons have reported severe adverse behavioral effects after drinking diet soda. If you use aspartame, be careful! People with PKU need to avoid it, also.

✓ BETA CAROTENE
Coloring, nutrient
Margarine, shortening, non-dairy whiteners, butter

Used as an artificial coloring and a nutrient supplement. The body converts it to Vitamin A, which is part of the light-detection mechanism of the eye.

COMMON FOOD ADDITIVES

✗ **BROMINATED VEGETABLE OIL (BVO)**
Emulsifier, clouding agent
Soft drinks

BVO keeps flavor oils in suspension and gives a cloudy appearance to citrus-flavored soft drinks. The residues of BVO found in body fat are cause for concern. BVO should be banned; safer substitutes are available.

✗ **BUTYLATED HYDROXYANISOLE (BHA)**
Antioxidant
Cereals, chewing gum, potato chips, vegetable oil

BHA retards rancidity in fats, oils, and oil-containing foods. While most studies indicate it is safe, a 1982 Japanese study demonstrated that it caused cancer in rats. This synthetic chemical can often be replaced by safer chemicals.

✗ **BUTYLATED HYDROXYTOLUENE (BHT)**
Antioxidant
Cereals, chewing gum, potato chips, oils, etc.

BHT retards rancidity in oils. It either increased or decreased the risk of cancer in various animal studies. Residues of BHT occur in human fat. BHT is unnecessary or is easily replaced by safe substitutes. Avoid it when possible.

✗ **CAFFEINE**
Stimulant
Coffee, tea, cocoa (natural); soft drinks (additive)

Caffeine may cause miscarriages or birth defects and should be avoided by pregnant women. It also keeps many people from sleeping. New evidence indicates that caffeine may cause fibrocystic breast disease in some women.

✓ **CALCIUM (or SODIUM) PROPIONATE**
Preservative
Bread, rolls, pies, cakes

CALCIUM PROPIONATE prevents mold growth on bread and rolls. The calcium is a beneficial mineral; the propionate is safe. SODIUM PROPIONATE is used in pies and cakes, because calcium alters the action of chemical leavening agents.

✓ **CALCIUM (or SODIUM) STEAROYL LACTYLATE**
Dough conditioner, whipping agent
Bread dough, cake fillings, artificial whipped cream, processed egg whites

These additives strengthen bread dough so it can be used in bread-making machinery and lead to more uniform grain and greater volume. They act as whipping agents in dried, liquid, or frozen egg whites and artificial whipped cream. SODIUM STEAROYL FUMARATE serves the same function.

? **CARRAGEENAN**
Thickening and stabilizing agent
Ice cream, jelly, chocolate milk, infant formula

Carrageenan is obtained from seaweed. Large amounts of carrageenan have harmed test animals' colons; the small amounts in food are probably safe. Need better tests.

✓ **CASEIN, SODIUM CASEINATE**
Thickening and whitening agent
Ice cream, ice milk, sherbet, coffee creamers

Casein, the principal protein in milk, is a nutritious protein containing adequate amounts of all the essential amino acids.

COMMON FOOD ADDITIVES

✓ **CITRIC ACID, SODIUM CITRATE**
Acid, flavoring, chelating agent
Ice cream, sherbet, fruit drinks,
candy, carbonated beverages,
instant potatoes

CITRIC ACID is versatile, widely used, cheap, and safe. It is an important metabolite in virtually all living organisms; especially abundant in citrus fruits and berries. It is used as a strong acid, a tart flavoring, and an antioxidant. SODIUM CITRATE, also safe, is a buffer that controls the acidity of gelatin desserts, jam, ice cream, candy, and other foods.

? **CORN SYRUP**
Sweetener, thickener
Candy, toppings, syrups, snack
foods, imitation dairy foods

Corn syrup is a sweet, thick liquid made by treating cornstarch with acids or enzymes. It may be dried and used as CORN SYRUP SOLIDS in coffee whiteners and other dry products. Corn syrup contains no nutritional value other than calories, promotes tooth decay, and is used mainly in low-nutrition foods.

? **DEXTROSE (GLUCOSE, CORN SUGAR)**
Sweetener, coloring agent
Bread, caramel, soda pop,
cookies, many other foods

Dextrose is an important chemical in every living organism. A sugar, it is a source of sweetness in fruits and honey. Added to foods as a sweetener, it represents empty calories, and contributes to tooth decay. Dextrose turns brown when heated and contributes to the color of bread crust and toast.

✓ **EDTA**
Chelating agent
Salad dressing, margarine,
sandwich spreads, mayonnaise,
processed fruits and vegetables,
canned shellfish, soft drinks

Modern food manufacturing technology, which involves metal rollers, blenders, and containers, results in trace amounts of metal contamination in food. EDTA (ethylenediamine tetra-acetic acid) traps metal impurities, which would otherwise promote rancidity and the breakdown of artificial colors.

✓ **FERROUS GLUCONATE**
Coloring, nutrient
Black olives

Used by the olive industry to generate a uniform jet-black color and in pills as a source of iron. Safe.

✓ **FUMARIC ACID**
Tartness agent
Powdered drinks, pudding, pie
fillings, gelatin desserts

A solid at room temperature, inexpensive, highly acidic, it is the ideal source of tartness and acidity in dry food products. However, it dissolves slowly in cold water, a drawback cured by adding DIOCTYL SODIUM SULFOSUCCINATE (DSS), a poorly tested detergent-like additive.

✓ **GELATIN**
Thickening and gelling agent
Powdered dessert mix, yogurt,
ice cream, cheese spreads,
beverages

Gelatin is a protein obtained from animal bones, hoofs, and other parts. It has little nutritional value because it contains little or none of several essential amino acids.

✓ **GLYCERIN (GLYCEROL)**
Maintains water content
Marshmallow, candy, fudge,
baked goods

Glycerin forms the backbone of fat and oil molecules and is quite safe. The body uses it as a source of energy or as a starting material in making more complex molecules.

COMMON FOOD ADDITIVES

✓ **GUMS: Guar, Locust Bean, Arabic, Furcelleran, Ghatti, Karaya, Tragacanth**
Thickening agents, stabilizers
Beverages, ice cream, frozen pudding, salad dressing, dough, cottage cheese, candy, drink mixes

Gums derive from natural sources (bushes, trees, or seaweed) and are poorly tested. They are used to thicken foods, prevent sugar crystals from forming in candy, stabilize beer foam (arabic), form a gel in pudding (furcelleran), encapsulate flavor oils in powdered drink mixes, or keep oil and water mixed together in salad dressings. Tragacanth has caused occasional severe allergic reactions.

? **HEPTYL PARABEN**
Preservative
Beer, noncarbonated soft drinks

Heptyl paraben—short for the heptyl ester of para-hydroxybenzoic acid—is a preservative. Studies suggest this chemical is safe, but it, like other additives in alcoholic beverages, has never been tested in the presence of alcohol.

? **HYDROGENATED VEGETABLE OIL**
Source of oil or fat
Margarine, many processed foods

Vegetable oil, usually a liquid, can be made into a semi-solid by treating with hydrogen. Hydrogenation reduces the levels of polyunsaturated oils. We eat too much oil and fat of all kinds, whether natural or hydrogenated. High-fat diets promote heart disease, obesity, and probably cancer.

✓ **HYDROLYZED VEGETABLE PROTEIN (HVP)**
Flavor enhancer
Instant soups, frankfurters, sauce mixes, beef stew

HVP consists of vegetable (usually soybean) protein that has been chemically broken down to the amino acids of which it is composed. HVP is used to bring out the natural flavor of food (and, perhaps, to use less real food).

? **INVERT SUGAR**
Sweetener
Candy, soft drinks, many other foods

Invert sugar, a 50–50 mixture of two sugars, dextrose and fructose, is sweeter and more soluble than sucrose (table sugar). Invert sugar forms when sucrose is split in two by an enzyme or acid. It represents "empty calories," contributes to tooth decay, and should be avoided.

✓ **LACTIC ACID**
Acidity regulator
Spanish olives, cheese, frozen desserts, carbonated beverages

This safe acid occurs in almost all living organisms. It inhibits spoilage in Spanish-type olives, balances the acidity in cheese-making, and adds tartness to frozen desserts, carbonated fruit-flavored drinks, and other foods.

✓ **LACTOSE**
Sweetener
Whipped topping mix, breakfast pastry

Lactose, a carbohydrate found only in milk, is Nature's way of delivering calories to infant mammals. One-sixth as sweet as table sugar, it is added to food as a slightly sweet source of carbohydrate. Milk turns sour when bacteria convert lactose to lactic acid. Many non-Caucasians have trouble digesting lactose.

✓ **LECITHIN**
Emulsifier, antioxidant
Baked goods, margarine, chocolate, ice cream

A common constituent of animal and plant tissues, it is a source of the nutrient choline. It keeps oil and water from separating out, retards rancidity, reduces spattering in a frying pan, and leads to fluffier cakes. Major sources are egg yolk and soybeans.

COMMON FOOD ADDITIVES

✓ **MANNITOL**
Sweetener, other uses
Chewing gum, low-calorie foods

Not quite as sweet as sugar and poorly absorbed by the body, it contributes only half as many calories as sugar. Used as the "dust" on chewing gum, it prevents gum from absorbing moisture and becoming sticky. Safe.

✓ **MONO- and DIGLYCERIDES**
Emulsifier
Baked goods, margarine, candy, peanut butter

Makes bread softer and prevents staling, improves the stability of margarine, makes caramels less sticky, and prevents the oil in peanut butter from separating out. Mono- and diglycerides are safe, though most foods they are used in are high in refined flour, sugar, or fat.

? **MONOSODIUM GLUTAMATE (MSG)**
Flavor enhancer
Soup, seafood, poultry, cheese, sauces, stews; many others

This amino acid brings out the flavor of protein-containing foods. Large amounts of MSG fed to infant mice destroyed nerve cells in the brain. Public pressure forced baby food companies to stop using MSG. MSG causes "Chinese Restaurant Syndrome" (burning sensation in the back of neck and forearms, tightness of the chest, headache) in some sensitive adults.

? **PHOSPHORIC ACID; PHOSPHATES**
Acidulant, chelating agent, buffer, emulsifier, nutrient, discoloration inhibitor
Baked goods, cheese, powdered foods, cured meat, soda pop, breakfast cereals, dehydrated potatoes

PHOSPHORIC ACID acidifies and flavors cola beverages. Phosphate salts serve many purposes. CALCIUM and IRON PHOSPHATES act as mineral supplements. SODIUM ALUMINUM PHOSPHATE is a leavening agent. CALCIUM and AMMONIUM PHOSPHATES serve as food for yeast in bread. SODIUM ACID PYROPHOSPHATE prevents discoloration in potatoes and sugar syrups. Phosphates are not toxic, but their widespread use has led to dietary imbalances that contribute to osteoporosis.

✓ **POLYSORBATE 60**
Emulsifier
Baked goods, frozen desserts, imitation dairy products

POLYSORBATE 60 is short for polyoxyethylene–(20)–sorbitan monostearate. It and its close relatives, POLYSORBATE 65 and 80, work the same way as mono- and diglycerides, but smaller amounts are needed. They keep baked goods from going stale, keep dill oil dissolved in bottled dill pickles, help coffee whiteners dissolve in coffee, and prevent oil from separating out of artificial whipped cream.

✗ **PROPYL GALLATE**
Antioxidant
Vegetable oil, meat products, potato sticks, chicken soup base, chewing gum

Retards the spoilage of fats and oils and is often used with BHA and BHT, because of the synergistic effects these additives have. The best long-term feeding study was peppered with suggestions (but not proof) of cancer. Avoid.

✗ **QUININE**
Flavoring
Tonic water, quinine water, bitter lemon

This drug can cure malaria and is used as a bitter flavoring in a few soft drinks. There is a slight chance that quinine may cause birth defects, so pregnant women should avoid quinine-containing beverages and drugs. Very poorly tested.

COMMON FOOD ADDITIVES

✗ SACCHARIN
Synthetic sweetener
"Diet" products

Saccharin is 350 times sweeter than sugar. Studies have not shown that saccharin helps people lose weight. In 1977, the FDA proposed that saccharin be banned, because of repeated evidence that it causes cancer. It is gradually being replaced by aspartame (NutraSweet).

✗ SALT (SODIUM CHLORIDE)
Flavoring
Most processed foods: soup, potato chips, crackers

Salt is used liberally in many processed foods. Other additives contribute additional sodium. A diet high in sodium may cause high blood pressure, which increases the risk of heart attack and stroke. Everyone should eat less salt: avoid salty processed foods, use salt sparingly, enjoy other seasonings.

✓ SODIUM BENZOATE
Preservative
Fruit juice, carbonated drinks, pickles, preserves

Manufacturers have used sodium benzoate for over 70 years to prevent the growth of microorganisms in acidic foods.

✓ SODIUM CARBOXYMETHYLCELLULOSE (CMC)
Thickening and stabilizing agent; prevents sugar from crystallizing
Ice cream, beer, pie fillings, icings, diet foods, candy

CMC is made by reacting cellulose with a derivative of acetic acid. Studies indicate it is safe.

✗ SODIUM NITRITE, SODIUM NITRATE
Preservative, coloring, flavoring
Bacon, ham, frankfurters, luncheon meats, smoked fish, corned beef

NITRITE can lead to the formation of small amounts of potent cancer-causing chemicals (nitrosamines), particularly in fried bacon. Nitrite is tolerated in foods because it can prevent the growth of bacteria that cause botulism poisoning. Nitrite also stabilizes the red color in cured meat and gives a characteristic flavor. SODIUM NITRATE is used in dry cured meat, because it slowly breaks down into nitrite.

✓ SORBIC ACID, POTASSIUM SORBATE
Prevents growth of mold
Cheese, syrup, jelly, cake, wine, dry fruits

SORBIC ACID occurs naturally in many plants. These additives are safe under normal circumstances.

✓ SORBITAN MONOSTEARATE
Emulsifier
Cakes, candy, frozen pudding, icing

Like mono- and diglycerides and polysorbates, this additive keeps oil and water mixed together. In chocolate candy, it prevents the discoloration that normally occurs when the candy is warmed up and then cooled down.

COMMON FOOD ADDITIVES

✓ **SORBITOL**
Sweetener, thickening agent, maintains moisture
Dietetic drinks and foods; candy, shredded coconut, chewing gum

Sorbitol occurs naturally in fruits and berries and is a close relative of the sugars. It is half as sweet as sugar. It is used in noncarinogenic chewing gum because oral bacteria do not metabolize it well. Large amounts of sorbitol (2 oz. for adults) have a laxative effect, but otherwise it is safe. Diabetics use sorbitol, because it is absorbed slowly and does not cause blood sugar to increase rapidly.

✓ **STARCH, MODIFIED STARCH**
Thickening agent
Soup, gravy, baby foods

Starch, the major component of flour, potatoes, and corn, is used as a thickening agent. However, it does not dissolve in cold water. Chemists have solved this problem by reacting starch with various chemicals. These modified starches are added to some foods to improve their consistency and keep the solids suspended. Starch and modified starches oftentimes replace more nutritious ingredients.

✗ **SUGAR (SUCROSE)**
Sweetener
Table sugar, sweetened foods

Sucrose, ordinary table sugar, occurs naturally in fruit, sugarcane, and sugar beets. Americans consume about 65 pounds of sucrose per year. Sugar, corn syrup, and other refined sweeteners make up about one-eighth of the average diet, but provide no vitamins, minerals, or protein. Sugar and sweetened foods may taste good and supply energy, but most people eat too much of them. Unless you enjoy large dentist bills and a large waistline, you should eat much less sugar.

✗ **SULFUR DIOXIDE, SODIUM BISULFITE**
Preservative, bleach
Dried fruit, wine, processed potatoes

Sulfiting agents prevent discoloration (dried fruit, some "fresh" shrimp, and some dried, fried, and frozen potatoes) and bacterial growth (wine). They also destroy vitamin B-1 and can cause severe reactions, especially in asthmatics. Avoid all forms of this additive, since it has caused at least seven deaths.

✓ **VANILLIN, ETHYL VANILLIN**
Substitute for vanilla
Ice cream, baked goods, beverages, chocolate, candy, gelatin desserts

Vanilla flavoring is derived from a bean, but VANILLIN, the major flavor component of vanilla, is cheaper to produce in a factory. A derivative, ETHYL VANILLIN, comes closer to matching the taste of real vanilla. Both chemicals are safe.

In addition to food additives, toxic residues from insecticides and herbicides contaminate much of our food and water, exposing us to other significant dangers. To offer a few examples (adapted from *An Alternative Approach to Allergies* by Theron Randolph, M.D., and Ralph Moss, Ph.D.):

- Fruit orchards are sprayed with pesticides ten to fifteen times a season from the blossom stage to just a few weeks before harvest. Apples, cherries, and peaches are apparently the more contaminated fruits.
- Cabbage, broccoli, and cauliflower are sprayed regularly, making them some of the most contaminated items among vegetables.
- Dates and dried fruit are treated with methyl bromide.
- Corn is soaked in sulfur dioxide, which prevents its fermentation. This chemical residue finds its way into virtually hundreds of corn-based foods, including corn syrup, corn sweetener (dextrose), cornstarch, cornmeal and flour, and corn oil.
- In restaurants, french fries, potato chips, even fresh-cut apple and peach slices are soaked in sulfur dioxide to prevent browning.
- Fruit is commonly dusted with sulfur. Ethylene gas is used to ripen bananas. Fungicides are used on crates of citrus and other fruits and produce shipped in railway cars.
- Phenol, or carbolic acid, is used to line tin cans in order to prevent the metal from bleaching the food contents. This contaminant can cause headaches, depression, asthma, and other ailments.
- Paraffin, a petrochemical, is used to polish green peppers, apples, and cucumbers.

Animal Food Contaminants

The way animals are fed and raised and the methods used to process and butcher meat are equally hazardous. Most commercial meat and poultry contain residues of several toxic substances. Animals are often fed antibiotics to increase their weight for sale, one consequence of which has been the transference to humans of bacterial infections (salmonella) resistant to antibiotics.[50] (Because of such infections, even deaths, there has been a movement to restrict the use of growth antibiotics in slaughter animals.)

Commercial meat and poultry products also contain significant quantities of hormones and growth promoters such as resorcylic acid lactones and other metabolites with estrogenlike activity derived from zearalenone, a known carcinogen, and teratogen, which is derived from a mold. The content of this toxin in commercial animal products may partly explain the observed association between the consumption of these animal products and the incidence of colorectal and breast cancers. Cattle feed is often sprayed directly with pesticides and fungicides (cell and enzyme poisons), which we inevitably end up ingesting. Of course, nitrates are used as preservatives, flavoring, and coloring agents in cured beef and pork products like bacon, hot dogs, salami, sausage, bologna, corned beef, pastrami, pepperoni, and practically all luncheon meats. You may know that, once in our bodies, nitrates can be converted to nitrosamines, a class of potent carcinogens.

As if all this weren't horrifying enough, a number of industrial and agricultural toxins (PCB and dioxin, to name just two) manage to find their way into domestic beef cattle, pork, lamb, and chickens and are concentrated in the meat and milk up to *four hundred* times the levels found in the plant foods and water that the animals eat and drink. The higher up on the food chain we eat, the more concentrated the toxins are—an additional reason for choosing vegetarianism.

Total System Assault

Food additives and agricultural contaminants, along with the toxic industrial pollutants and petrochemicals in the air, soil, and water, provide a potential cumulative assault on our immune systems and can render us susceptible to disease. I know this all may seem quite discouraging, and you may feel that it is useless to attempt a way out of this chemical mess. Again, our best protection is to be informed and alert. Read food labels carefully. Try to avoid foods processed and packaged by food companies that use additives and preservatives. Additive-free items are becoming quite popular and more available due to an increasingly informed and demanding public. Find sources of organic and chemical-free foods in health food stores, food co-ops, and, where possible, public markets.

A few local butchers and a food co-op in Seattle, where I live, stock chemical- and hormone-free beef, lamb, pork, chicken, turkey, and rabbit. Though not completely organic, these products are far "cleaner" than their regular commercial counterparts. In fact, one unique local supermarket chain has introduced organic produce and meats.

The mainstream food industry is slowly coming to terms with the situation, making it possible for us to purchase wholesome, nutritious foods with greater ease. From a realistic, practical standpoint, however, it still is just not possible to eat chemical- and additive-free food all the time, and organic produce is not always available, reasonably priced, or good looking. I take comfort in the likelihood that my whole-foods diet and nutritional supplements provide the nutrients necessary for my liver to detoxify whatever chemicals my sometimes-impure diet contains.

SALT

Salt has received a great deal of bad press over the years, which has informed the public of its many hazards: high blood pressure, stroke, heart attack, fluid retention, edema, premenstrual syndrome, and so on. On the one hand, salt is a necessary part of the diet for health maintenance; on the other, its excess can maim. However, the hazards of salt intake may not derive simply from its excess, but also from the techniques used to process and refine the product itself.

Despite the known correlation between excessive salt intake and some killer diseases, the food industry continues to oversalt our foods. If we do not add salt directly, many processed and prepackaged household food items cause us inadvertently to consume far too much salt. At the bottom of the page is a list of common overly salty foods that often find their way into our diets.

The following table lists the salt content of various common foods:

SODIUM CONTENT OF SOME COMMON FOODS

FOODS	AMOUNT	SODIUM (MG)
Vegetables		
Fresh (most varieties)	½ cup	0–40
Frozen	½ cup	0–40
Canned	½ cup	230–460
Tomato juice (S&W or V-8)	163 ml.	380–430
Celery, beets	½ cup	75

SALT-RICH FOODS

Instant flavored hot cereals
Some breads
Cake mixes
Prepared rice and pasta products
Smoked and pickled products
Ham
Bacon
Sausage
Luncheon meats
Fast-food hamburgers
Fast-food chicken
Milk shakes
Dried meats
Frankfurters
Corned beef
Canned fish
Herring
Sardines
Canned meat
Pork sausage
TV dinners
Canned soups
Prepared meat extenders
Fruit products containing
  sodium
Tomato juice (canned)
Vegetable juice (canned)

Sauerkraut
Pickles and olives
Relish
Packaged vegetables in seasoned sauces
Buttermilk
Processed cheeses
Processed cheese foods
Salty cheeses (Parmesan, blue, feta, edam,
  Romano, provolone, cottage cheese, gouda)
Frozen pizza
Salted nuts
Corn chips
Potato chips
Salted popcorn
Salted crackers
Pretzels
Some brands of mineral water
Garlic salt
Onion salt
Soy sauce
Baking soda
Baking powder
Monosodium glutamate
  (MSG—in Chinese food)
Any additive or preservative with the word
  "sodium" in it

Fruits

Fresh or canned	½ cup	0
Fruit juice (most varieties)	½ cup	0

Grains

Rice, macaroni, noodles	½ cup	0
Hot cereals (examples)		
Instant	1 oz.	0
Instant flavored	1 oz.	200
Quick	1 oz.	80
Ready to Eat cereals (examples)		
Shredded Wheat (Nabisco)	2 biscuits	0
All-Bran (Kellogg's)	½ cup	80
Corn Flakes (Kellogg's)	1 cup	330
Cheerios (General Mills)	1 cup	280
Grape Nuts (Post)	½ cup	350

The figures are approximations based on data in U.S. Department of Agriculture, Sodium Content of Foods, *Handbook 456 (Washington DC: U. S. Government Printing Office, 1985). Tomato juice, V-8, and cereal data obtained from Nutrition Facts panel on product packages.*

LOW-SODIUM MEATS

MEATS	AMOUNT	SODIUM (MG)
Beef, lamb, pork	1 oz.	20–30
Chicken, turkey, veal	1 oz.	20–30
Hamburger	3 oz.	46
Bacon, crisp	1 strip	80

HIGH-SODIUM MEATS

MEATS	AMOUNT	SODIUM (MG)
Ham	1 oz.	288
Pork sausage	1 oz.	276
Hot dog	1	460
Bacon, Canadian	1 oz.	690

From Eat for Health *by William Manahan, M.D. Copyright © 1988 by William Manahan, M.D. Reprinted by permission of HJ Kramer Inc., P.O. Box 1082, Tiburon, CA. All rights reserved.*

COMMON HIGH-SODIUM LUNCH AND DINNER FOODS

FOODS	AMOUNT	SODIUM (MG)
LUNCH		
Tuna salad sandwich	1	400–600
Tossed salad, dressing, croutons	1	400–600
Luncheon meat sandwich	1	570–670
Macaroni and cheese	1 cup	746
Campbell's canned soup	1 cup	800–930
Spaghetti with meat	1 cup	730–1,100
Chef Boyardee Beefaroni	1 cup	950
DINNER		
Potpie	8 oz.	900–1,670
TV dinner (with meat)	12 oz.	850–1,775
Pizza, frozen or mix (14")	½	1,200–1,800
Marie Callender's Turkey with gravy and dressing	1	2,030
Sloppy joe mix (dry, no meat)	1½ oz.	3,565

From Eat for Health *by William Manahan, M.D. Copyright © 1988 by William Manahan, M.D. Reprinted by permission of HJ Kramer Inc., P.O. Box 1082, Tiburon, CA. All rights reserved.*

SODIUM TOTALS FOR COMMON FAST-FOOD MEALS

FOOD	AMOUNT	SODIUM (MG)
Whopper (Burger King)	1	1,000
Hot ham and cheese sandwich (Arby's)	1	1,400
Chicken breast sandwich (Arby's)	1	958
Kentucky Fried Chicken	3 pieces	1,439

From M. Franz, Fast Food Facts: Nutrition and Exchange Values for Fast Food Restaurants *(Minneapolis: International Diabetes Center, 1994).*

SODIUM CONTENT OF A TYPICAL MEAL AT McDONALD'S

FOOD	AMOUNT	SODIUM (MG)
Big Mac	1	890
French fries	20	110
Chocolate low-fat milk shake	1	240
Apple danish	1	370

From M. Franz, Fast Food Facts: Nutrition and Exchange Values for Fast Food Restaurants *(Minneapolis: International Diabetes Center, 1994).*

SODIUM-CONTAINING COMPOUNDS

COMPOUND	USE
Baking soda (sodium bicarbonate or bicarbonate of soda)	For leavening in the preparation of breads and cakes; sometimes added to vegetable cookery; as an alkalizer for indigestion
Baking powder	In the preparation of breads and cakes
Brine (salt and water solution)	In the processing of foods and in canning, freezing, and pickling
Disodium phosphate	In some quick-cooking cereals and processed cheeses
Monosodium glutamate (MSG)	As a seasoning in home and restaurant cooking and in many packaged, canned, and processed frozen foods

Sodium acetate	For pH control
Sodium alginate	For smooth texture in chocolate milks and ice creams
Sodium aluminum sulfate	For leavening
Sodium benzoate	As a preservative in condiments
Sodium calcium alginate	For smooth texture or thickening
Sodium citrate	For pH control
Sodium diacetate	As a preservative
Sodium erythorbate	As a preservative
Sodium hydroxide	In the processing of some fruits and vegetables, hominy, and ripe olives
Sodium nitrate	As a preservative
Sodium propionate	As a preservative
Sodium sorbate	As a preservative
Sodium stearyl fumarate	As a maturing and bleaching agent or dough conditioner
Sodium sulfite	As a bleach for some fresh fruits and as a preservative in some dried fruits

Salt and Hypertension

It is evident that much packaged, precooked, and processed food contains excessive quantities of salt. The National Academy of Sciences has estimated that a daily intake of 1,100 to 3,300 milligrams of sodium is safe and adequate for the general public.[51] Some studies indicate that we generally consume 5,600 to 7,600 milligrams daily,[52] 75 percent of which is added to foods by the food industry. Here we see the importance of preparing food from scratch or at least finding low-sodium prepared products. You may need to do a little investigating to secure the information you need, but beware: Food package labels may not always disclose all ingredients.

Perhaps a moderate amount of salt would not be damaging, particularly if we consumed adequate quantities of potassium, magnesium, and/or calcium. Research indicates that perhaps only 30 percent of the population are salt sensitive—and would develop high blood pressure from sodium overload.[53] For the majority of us, however, it would take an accompanying deficiency of any of the above minerals to tip the balance. Adequate potassium may protect many of us from hypertension even without sodium restriction.[54]

Vegetarians tend not to develop high blood pressure, probably because of the generous amounts of potassium inherent in their diets—whole grains, legumes, fresh vegetables and fruits, sea vegetables like kelp and dulse, and unsalted seeds and nuts. And even with sodium restriction, many hypertensive individuals fail to normalize their blood pressure. This seems to indicate that sodium is not solely responsible for the condition.

Other evidence indicates that deficiencies in magnesium and calcium also contribute to hypertension.[55] Deficient magnesium stores will trigger a host of ailments and conditions, one of which is chronically tense smooth muscle tissue, the very muscles in your arteries. Adequate magnesium will displace calcium, help relax these muscles, dilate the arteries, and lower blood pressure.

Both potassium and magnesium are primarily intracellular minerals; consequently common blood tests for these minerals may be quite normal when, in fact, the body's intracellular stores are low. Other studies have shown that it's the chloride part of salt more than the sodium that may determine high blood pressure.[56]

Other Problems with Salt

Salt excess has been linked to such problems as edema and swollen tissues—including feet and ankles; headaches; premenstrual complaints such as bloating and tender breasts; excessive liquid cravings and frequent urination; constipation, which can occur if the high salt concentration in the bloodstream forces fluid from the intestines to dilute it; and fatigue, weakness, and tinnitis (ringing in the ear).

The quantity of salt consumed by many Americans may certainly explain these problems. However, the fact that the salt we purchase in supermarkets (and ingest courtesy of the food and restaurant industries) is a highly processed food may contribute to these problems as well. The refining of salt results in both an altered form that cannot effectively accomplish its relatively unknown purposes and a loss of vital minerals and trace elements.

Sea Salt

If mineral-rich, unprocessed sea salt were used, some salt-related health problems could likely be prevented. Celtic salt is a prime example—a heavy, slightly sticky, rough-textured, gray salt, hand-harvested from the coast of Brittany from natural clay beds and purified through a process of ionization. Celtic salt contains eighty-two trace minerals in addition to sodium chloride. Regular salt, even most sea salt sold in health food stores, contains for the most part only sodium chloride.

COMPARISON OF CELTIC NATURAL GRAY SEA SALT TO BOILED MEXICAN SALT

MINERAL	CELTIC (%)	BOILED MEXICAN (%)
Magnesium	1.00	0.1
Manganese	0.01	0.0001
Boron	0.001	0.0001
Copper	0.001	0.0001
Silicon	0.01	0.001
Iron	0.1	0.01
Nickel	0.0001	0.0001
Moisture % by weight	5.79	0.31

J. de Langre, Sea Salt's Hidden Powers: How to Tell Its Integrity and Use It Correctly, 1985; published by the Grain and Salt Society, P.O. Box DD, Magalia, CA 95954.

Jacques de Langre, in *Sea Salt's Hidden Powers*,[57] reports that moderate amounts of unprocessed sea salt will not bring on thirst, water retention, or edema, nor will it contribute to high blood pressure, as does the heat-processed, refined, purified, smooth, white, free-flowing, and mineral-depleted salt we are most accustomed to using. According to de Langre, the heat processing used to make common salt removes the majority of the magnesium and other minerals.

Unrefined sea salt, de Langre continues, can help normalize the excessive acidity created by the standard American diet. It can help promote hydrochloric acid production and improve digestion and absorption. Moreover, it provides trace nutrients needed for triggering bioelectric impulses crucial to cellular metabolic efficiency, maintenance, and renewal. And it's cleaner—it contains no anticaking agents, bleaches, or conditioners. Did you know that many brands of salt on supermarket shelves contain sugar and aluminum?

Of course, you should avoid excess ingestion even of unrefined salt, but such an event is not likely to occur if you're the one controlling the amount of salt in your food. Natural Celtic sea salt is available through the Grain and Salt Society, 14351 Wycliff Way, P.O. Box DD, Magalia, CA 95954, (916) 873-0294.

Salt Alternatives

Should you wish, you may also choose from among the many salt alternatives available. Several varieties of salt substitutes are made from ground dried vegetables and herbs or a premixed combination of herbs alone. These substitutes may be found in many health food stores and some supermarkets. Granulated sea vegetables, such as kelp and dulse, provide a somewhat salty flavor, as do other sea vegetables—wakame, kombu, arame, and hijiki—all good soup additions. They also contain abundant quantities of potassium, calcium, iodine, and other trace minerals important for health. Miso, a fermented, pastelike substance made from soybeans, barley, and other grains, is commonly used in soup for its salt effect, unique flavor, and myriad health benefits (see Chapter Five).

MILK

Much controversy exists as to whether cow's milk is as wholesome a food as Americans think. At one extreme, some authors contend that cow's milk is fit only for calves. Others propose that we drink several glasses a day. However, few of us are aware of the startling relationship between milk products and a host of symptoms and conditions.

Even thought disorders, hyperactivity, poor concentration, moodiness, irritability, depression, schizophrenia, delinquency, antisocial behavior, and diabetes have been related to the consumption of milk.[58] Although many of these problems are triggered by food allergies (see Chapter Thirteen), other mechanisms are responsible as well.

What exactly in milk is allergy-producing? It appears that milk protein such as casein, lactalbumin, and lactoglobulin is the most usual culprit. Many milk-allergic individuals, who react unfavorably to milk, cheese, and yogurt, can tolerate butter and full cream, which have no milk protein. Others, however, are allergic even to butter. On rare occasions, I have seen a patient react to pasteurized milk products but have absolutely no problem with raw milk products. And others who react inconsistently to raw milk products may actually be responding to the food source of the cow, such as grains. When the animal is primarily pasture fed, the milk is tolerated without distress. Finally, many individuals do not produce enough of the enzyme lactase to digest lactose, milk sugar. This condition gives rise to a condition known as lactose intolerance (technically not an allergy), which causes gastrointestinal distress (see page 243). So you see, milk reactions can occur from a variety of mechanisms.

THE PREVALENCE OF LACTASE DEFICIENCY IN HEALTHY ADULTS

POPULATION GROUP	% WITH DEFICIENCY
Filipinos	90
Japanese	85
Taiwanese	85
Thais	90
Indians	50

Peruvians	70
Greenland Eskimos	80
American blacks	70
Bantus	90
Greek Cypriots	85
Arabs	78
Israelis	58
Finns	18
Danes	2
Swiss	7
American whites	8

Reprinted from Don't Drink Your Milk, © *1983 by Frank A. Oski. Published by Teach Services, Inc., RR1, Box 182, Brushton, NY 12916-9738.*

THE LACTOSE CONTENT OF DAIRY PRODUCTS

	AMOUNT	LACTOSE (GM)	% LACTOSE
Milk, whole	½ cup	6.0	30
Milk, 2%	½ cup	6.5	41
Milk, skim	½ cup	5.7	57
Yogurt, lowfat	½ cup	8.0	46
Cheese, cheddar	1 oz.	0.5	2

From Eat For Health *by William Manahan, M.D. © 1988 by William Manahan. Reprinted by permission of H.J. Kramer, Inc., P.O. Box 1082, Tiburon, CA 94920. All rights reserved.*

Fats in Milk Products

Because some milk products contain a significant quantity of fat, they can contribute to the problems listed previously for excessive fat intake: elevated blood cholesterol, heart disease, and cancer.

FAT CONTENT OF MILK

TYPE OF MILK	FAT CONTENT (% OF TOTAL CALORIES)
Whole	48
2%	31
1%	15
Skim	2–8

From Eat for Health *by William Manahan, M.D. Copyright © 1988 by William Manahan, M.D. Reprinted by permission of HJ Kramer Inc., P.O. Box 1082, Tiburon, CA. All rights reserved.*

As you can see from the above table, 2 percent milk is not extremely lowfat; 31 percent of its calories are fat calories (it is less fatty, however, than the 48 percent of whole milk). How does the milk industry get away with calling a 31 percent fat milk "2 percent"? Well, the fat content in a glass of this milk is 2 percent of its total weight! True, but deceiving. If you use milk products regularly and are trying to significantly reduce your fat intake, it is best to use skim (nonfat) or at most 1 percent milk products.

Homogenization

Research suggests that homogenization of milk can indirectly damage the arteries, predisposing milk drinkers to arteriosclerosis and heart attacks.[59] Apparently, homogenization enables the milk's xanthine oxidase into

SOME SYMPTOMS RELATED TO THE CONSUMPTION OF MILK PRODUCTS

Recurrent respiratory infections: ear, throat, sinus, and bronchial infections
Sinus congestion
Excess mucus
Sore throat
Cough
Asthma
Headaches
Insomnia
Diarrhea
Constipation
Abdominal cramps
Spastic colon

Colitis
Bloody stools
Microscopic blood or protein in the urine
Acne or eczema
Canker sores and other skin disorders
Arthritis
Muscle aches
Fatigue
Heartburn
Indigestion
Stomach and duodenal ulcers
Bed-wetting

the bloodstream. This enzyme injures the arterial wall by destroying plasmologen. Once injured, the arterial wall is predisposed to the development of plaque formation. ("Arteriosclerosis," in Chapter Seventeen, explains how a process of free radical pathology is involved in this damage.) In unhomogenized milk, active xanthine oxidase will not absorb into the bloodstream.

The 1 and 2 percent and nonfat homogenized milks commonly sold in supermarkets—and purported to diminish arteriosclerotic risk by lessening the fat content—are processed, altered foods that may actually contribute to the risk of heart disease and stroke. Take, for example, the parallel situations in Finland and France. Both countries consume much dairy. The Finns use homogenized milk products. The French, who use primarily cheese and butter, do not. The result is that the French have half the incidence of heart attack that the Finns experience. In the United States, heart attacks were rare before the introduction of homogenization. True, homogenization is only one variable among many, and although medical opinion does not support the relationship between homogenized milk products and heart disease,[60] I still feel this potential danger is worth mentioning. Whole milk products would bypass this issue, but everyday usage of substantial amounts could add up to excessive fat.

Calcium

Some people feel that milk products are a necessary part of the diet because they alone ensure adequate quantities of calcium. This is a fallacy. A large percentage of the world's population is lactose intolerant and does not consume milk products at all. They take in perhaps half the calcium that we do, yet generally do not develop osteoporosis or other calcium-deficiency ailments. In fact, the incidence of osteoporosis is highest in countries that consume the most milk.[61] This disorder may have far more to do with excesses of dietary protein inherent in milk products and flesh foods and other elements that stimulate calcium loss through the urine rather than any outright dietary deficiency of calcium.

Those opposed to milk products also declare that the bioavailability of, or capacity of the body to utilize, milk calcium makes it a relatively ineffective source of calcium. I have yet to see hard data on this point. It is irrefutable, however, that milk products can deliver one of the highest absolute amounts of calcium per serving of food (see the following table).

CALCIUM IN DAIRY PRODUCTS

ITEM	SERVING SIZE	CALCIUM (MG)
Low-fat yogurt, plain fortified	1 cup	415
Part-skim ricotta cheese	½ cup	335
Low-fat milk (2%)	1 cup	300
Whole milk	1 cup	290
Buttermilk	1 cup	285
Vanilla soft-serve ice milk	½ cup	275
Swiss cheese	1 oz.	270
Cheddar cheese	1 oz.	210
American cheese	1 oz.	175
Vanilla soft-serve ice cream	½ cup	170
Cottage cheese	1 cup	112
Vanilla ice cream	½ cup	100
Cream cheese	2 tbsp	20
Coffee cream	1 tbsp	15

Source for cottage cheese: E. Ilyias, DiagnosTechs Clinical and Research Laboratory, Seattle, WA.

Many nondairy foods are abundant sources of calcium. The following table provides a spectrum of both high- and low-calcium content.

CALCIUM CONTENT OF SOME NONDAIRY FOODS

ITEM	SERVING SIZE	CALCIUM (MG)
Sesame seeds, unhulled*	3½ oz.	1,160–1,200
Canned sardines with bones	3½ oz.	300–437
Sesame seeds, hulled	3½ oz.	204–308
Almonds**	3½ oz.	254
Soybeans, dried	3½ oz.	226
Filberts**	3½ oz.	200
Canned salmon, with bones	3½ oz.	200–250
Parsley	3½ oz.	203
Oysters	¾ cup	170
Collard greens, boiled, drained	3½ oz.	188
Brazil nuts	3½ oz.	188
Dandelion greens, boiled, drained	3½ oz.	187
Kale, boiled, drained	3½ oz.	187
Turnip greens, boiled, drained	3½ oz.	184
Watercress	3½ oz.	151
Chickpeas (garbanzos), dried	3½ oz.	150
White beans, dried	3½ oz.	144
Mustard greens	3½ oz.	138
Pinto beans, dried	3½ oz.	135
Broccoli, cooked or raw	3½ oz.	130
Sunflower seeds	3½ oz.	120
Beet greens	3½ oz.	118
Mung beans, dried	3½ oz.	118
Tofu	4 oz.	113
Spinach, cooked**	½ cup	106
Shrimp, canned	3 oz.	100
Corn muffins	2 medium	90
Chili with beans	1 cup	90
Walnuts, roasted	3½ oz.	83
Okra, cooked	3½ oz.	82

Peanuts, roasted	3½ oz.	74
Chard, cooked**	3½ oz.	73
Baked beans	½ cup	70
Raisins	3½ oz.	62
Parsnips, cooked	3½ oz.	57
Rutabaga, cooked	3½ oz.	55
Orange	1 medium	55
Kidney beans, cooked	3½ oz.	40
Egg	1 large	30
Green beans, cooked	½ cup	30
Whole wheat bread	1 slice	20
Peanut butter	2 tbsp.	20
Lettuce	⅙ head	15
Spaghetti, cooked	1 cup	15
Orange juice	4 oz.	10
Apple	1 medium	10
Hamburger patty	3 oz.	10
Chicken	3 oz.	10
Rice, cooked	½ cup	10
Tuna	3 oz.	5
Seaweeds		
Agar	3½ oz. (100 gm)	567
Dulse	3½ oz. (100 gm)	296
Hijiki	3½ oz. (100 gm)	1,400
Kelp	3½ oz. (100 gm)	1,093
Kombu	3½ oz. (100 gm)	800
Wakame	3½ oz. (100 gm)	1,300

Although sesame seeds appear to be a superior source of calcium, most of the calcium is in the hull, along with oxalic acid, which is thought to interfere with calcium absorption. Hulled sesame seeds contain only 17.5 to 26.6 percent of the original calcium (and approximately 5 percent of the original oxalic acid), which makes it still a fairly good and absorbable source of calcium.

**The calcium in these foods is less available due to the relatively high oxalic acid content.*

From U. S. Department of Agriculture, Composition of Foods: Raw, Processed, Prepared (Washington, D.C., USDA Agriculture Handbook No. 8–11, 1984; No. 12, 1984; and No. 16, 1986); M. Kushi, The Book of Macrobiotics: The Universal Way of Health and Happiness (Tokyo, Elmsford, NY: Japan Publications, 1977); N. Clark, "Calcium Content of Some Commonly Eaten Foods," Physician and Sports Medicine 12 (1984), 143; and Ford Heritage, Composition and Facts about Food and Their Relationship to the Human Body (Mokelumne Hill, CA: Health Research, 1971).

In order for these milk-free sources of calcium to satisfy your calcium requirements, you will need to make a drastic departure from the high-protein, high-fat, high-salt, high-sugar, high-caffeine habits that can demineralize your body. If you cannot change your eating patterns yet still want to eliminate milk products, you might consider adding mineral supplements (see "Osteoporosis" in Chapter Seventeen, and "Calcium" in Chapter Six).

Chemical and Hormone Contamination

Just as chemicals become concentrated in meats, so residues of pesticides and herbicides find their way into milk. Dairy products also contain residues of the antibiotics and hormones given to cows. The newest potential assault is synthetic bovine somatotropin, a genetically engineered growth hormone, given to most dairy cows.[62] This hormone results in abnormal increases in milk production and higher rates of udder infections and subsequent antibiotic use. To avoid the known and unknown consequences of this type of contamination, it is best to minimize the commercial dairy products containing this hormone. Find out from your supermarket manager or milkman if there are brands free of this drug. Remember, the FDA does not require labeling of milk products that contain this hormone.

Melted Cheese

The melted-cheese craze (pizza, tuna melts, nachos, enchiladas, lasagna, etc.) presents another hazard, that of heat-damaged fat. If you prefer your cheese melted, add it just after the rest of the ingredients are done cooking and out of the oven. Let the heat of the food melt the cheese. This can be done quite easily with omelets, frittatas, and casseroles. If you must cook cheese, avoid broiling, and be sure to use the lowest temperature possible.

Testing for Milk Allergy

To test yourself for milk allergy/intolerance, cut out all milk products for two to four weeks, particularly if you experience any of the milk-related symptoms previously listed. (See the list of both obvious and hidden sources of milk on pages 251–252.) If you are milk allergic or intolerant, you may be surprised to notice a reduction in or even the disappearance of one or more symptoms that you have had for years. Following this period of abstinence, begin to reintroduce a large portion of your previous dairy food(s). You may then encounter a dramatic return of the symptoms anywhere from several hours to three days after reintroduction. You may be surprised to learn that individuals with type O blood usually have milk allergies (see Chapter Four).

Cultured Milk Products

It is generally agreed that the cultured, fermented forms of milk products, such as yogurt, buttermilk, and kefir, are preferable to plain milk, cheese, and other milk products. In addition to the beneficial bacteria they provide in the colon, there are innumerable other benefits (see Chapter Five, "Cultured Milk Products," and Chapter Eight for discussion). Health food stores offer yogurt made from whole (nonhomogenized) milk and nonfat yogurt made from organic milk.

Goat, Soy, Rice, and Nut Milks

Goat's milk products are often good nutritional substitutes in the event of an allergy to cow's milk. (If used as a primary staple for an infant, however, folic acid must be added.)

Many nutritionally oriented physicians, such as Bernard Jensen, D.C., N.D., Ph.D., consider goat's milk to be a superior food source. However, occasionally, cross-reactions will occur, in which case goat's milk products will trigger allergic symptoms as well. As with cow's milk products, a goat's milk lactose intolerance may be relieved with the use of lactase products.

Various soy milk products are also available in health food stores and food co-ops. They come regular or 1 percent fat, plain (with a distinct soy taste), or mildly and pleasantly sweetened and naturally flavored. I avoid the brands that use sugar as a sweetener and vegetable oil as an additional ingredient. Soy milk works exceptionally well in cereals and for cooking. Or you might try other milk substitutes: rice-based "Rice Dream," or the almond-based "White Almond Beverage" (1 or 2 percent), available in most health food stores. Seed and nut milks can be made quite easily in a blender (see recipes in Chapter Five).

The Risks of Milk and Milk Products

As you can see, there are some problems with milk products: allergies, lactose intolerance, excessive fat, damaged fat, excessive protein, homogenization/ xanthine oxidase, and chemical and hormone contamination. If milk products are not a large part of your diet, you don't need to overly concern yourself with these potential hazards. However, if they are central to your diet it will be to your advantage to minimize the obvious and proven risks.

The one risk that is still uncertain is homogenization/xanthine oxidase. Should you give up eating your daily low-fat cottage cheese or nonfat yogurt because of the potential risk? I can't make a definite recommendation in this regard. But I can certainly suggest that you look for organic milk products where available, and whenever feasible use soy, rice, and nut milks.

PEANUTS AND OTHER NUTS AND SEEDS

Peanuts are felt to be a potentially hazardous food source, for several reasons. An aspect of peanut meal is known to inhibit a clot-dissolving enzyme, fibrinolysin. Because of this and certain traits of peanut oil, peanuts can be considered atherogenic (causing arteriosclerotic plaque formation).[63] Eating peanuts or peanut butter or using peanut oil exposes one to this risk. Peanut oil, primarily oleic acid, can, in excess, inhibit the metabolism of essential fatty acids and cause menstrual cramps and other conditions. I always ask women who complain of menstrual cramps if peanut butter is a common item in their diet, and, if so, I suggest they omit it for a month or two. It often makes a difference.

Consumer Reports published the extraordinary finding that all brands of peanut butter they tested (natural and supermarket varieties alike) contained a liver carcinogen, aflatoxin, the product of a fungal infestation resulting from the storage of peanuts.[64] I use peanut butter, but only occasionally, and try to find brands that certify on the label "aflatoxin free." I am also sure to use brands free of partially hydrogenated oil and sugar.

Instead of peanuts, you can use almonds, sunflower seeds, pumpkin seeds, pecans, walnuts, filberts, cashews, pine nuts, brazil nuts, chestnuts, beechnuts, sesame seeds, pistachios, and many others. Seed or nut butters are available in health food stores (common are sesame, almond, cashew, macadamia, pistachio, sunflower, and filbert butters) and can be made at home with a blender. Seeds, nuts, and nut butters are generally very high in fat and calories, so they should be used modestly. Most of these seeds and nuts are rich in oleic acid and have low polyunsaturated oil content (sunflower is an exception), making them relatively resistant to damage from heat. Dry roasting them would be acceptable.

Buy seeds and nuts raw and ideally in the shell. Especially if shelled, keep them in the refrigerator (or freezer) in airtight containers. Commercial dry-roasted nuts and seeds may be okay, but you can't know for sure if the oils have been damaged in the roasting. I prefer to light-roast my own, plain, without oil, at 250° F until slightly browned. If you make your own nut butter, use raw seeds and nuts, adding some roasted for the flavor.

For those who want to go the extra mile to obtain maximum digestibility, soak raw seeds and nuts overnight, then strain, dry, and store in the refrigerator. Do not store too many at once—moisture makes them more susceptible to mold. The soaking greatly enhances their digestibility, as it initiates the sprouting process and eliminates a digestion-inhibiting factor (a trypsin inhibitor) present in the unsoaked nuts. Not every seed or nut lends itself well to soaking—try almonds, sunflower seeds, and filberts for a start. Soaked seeds and nuts also make an excellent base for blender drinks (see recipes in Chapter Five).

BREAD

Bread, the "staff of life," has been the subject of much controversy in the health literature. Many authors and practitioners—Ann Wigmore, N.D.,[65] Hazel Richards-Griffen,[66] Bernard Jensen, N.D., D.C., Ph.D.,[67] Victoras Kulvinskas,[68] Pierre Pannitier, N.D., Dr. Randolph Stone, John Ray, N.D., and others—have linked bread with chronic illness. They consider it a "dead" food lacking enzymes and warn us of the dangers of all common baked flour products.

As for Drs. Wigmore and Jensen, whom I know, they have kept themselves well and vital into old age by practicing what they preach, part of which is usually to keep bread off their tables. Their concepts are appealing to me, but their somewhat strict approaches, though important for ill individuals, may not have to be applied so rigorously to those who are generally well. But I would still recommend that well individuals adhere to these principles much of the time.

A definite part of the problem with bread and other baked flour products is their frequent use. Think of how often most of us ingest wheat: in bread, rolls, crackers, bagels, croissants, scones, sweet rolls, muffins, noodles, cookies, pretzels, tortillas, chapatis, pancakes. This overuse is what can lead to the "catarrhal accumulation" that Drs. Jensen and Wigmore feel causes ill health. From my own experience, I know that such frequent inclusion of wheat products often leads to wheat allergy/intolerance, which can produce a multitude of symptoms and conditions (see Chapter Thirteen). Food allergy aside, wheat can be an intestinal irritant for many individuals.

If you enjoy bread and are not wheat sensitive, there are several good types from which to choose. Most of the breads available today are raised predominantly with baker's yeast. Jacques de Langre, author of the forthcoming *Bread's Biological Transmutation*,[69] cites research studies from the Lima Institute in Latem-St. Marten, Belgium, where much work has been done on phytic acid. When bread is leavened naturally, as it was by our ancestors, the fermentation inherent in the process removes approximately 90 percent of the phytic acid (a naturally occurring element in many grains). Today's yeasted breads (and "Essene" bread as well, which is available primarily in health food stores) undergo very little fermentation. Therefore, the phytic acid remains intact and binds some of the grains' vital minerals, such as zinc, iron, and magnesium. Any whole wheat bread made with yeast is phytic acid–rich and cannot, states de Langre, deliver these nutrients effectively. They remain trapped in the bran and cannot be absorbed very well.

The natural fermentation process, however, breaks down the bran and releases the essential minerals, in addition to enhancing the wheat's amino acid profile. Because of the nature of the fermentation process, the bread can be stored simply by wrapping it in a cloth. After several days, it has undergone minimal loss of moisture. In fact, it is even more nutritious and tastier. By contrast, yeast breads become less nutritious and get stale rather quickly. Over time, the lack of mineral absorption from using regular yeast-raised bread is compounded as we ingest this dietary staple. This may lead to a mineral-deficient condition that could very well be related to the high level of susceptibility to chronic illness in this country, according to de Langre.

Bread made from the traditional sourdough leavening natural fermentation method makes the most health sense to me and feels the most satisfying to my body. I highly recommend that you try it. The usual commercially available sourdough bread or roll, incidentally, is far from the real thing; it is basically yeasted bread with a little sourdough starter added. (You can obtain a recipe for naturally fermented sourdough bread by writing the Grain and Salt Society, P.O. Box DD, Magalia, CA 95954, (916) 873-0294.)

If you use standard, yeast-raised bread, I recommend the varieties containing nothing other than whole wheat, water, salt, yeast, and perhaps a small amount of natural sweetener. Other whole-grain flours, seeds, and nuts may sometimes be incorporated as well. Steer clear of varieties that have enriched flour as their main ingredient (enriched with vitamins and minerals that do not begin to make up for what is refined out). Most breads that appear to be whole wheat use primarily enriched flour. Buy the real thing! The brands with chemical additives and preservatives, which should be avoided, are usually the ones with enriched flour. Oil is not really a necessary ingredient, and if it is partially hydrogenated, it is a hazard.

In your overall diet, try to avoid ingesting wheat so frequently. Instead, incorporate a variety of whole grains (millet, buckwheat, brown rice, barley, rye, corn, oats, quinoa, amaranth, spelt, kamut, and teff) as side dishes, cereals, noodles, in casseroles or soups, or as rice cakes and tortillas. Health food stores and co-ops have abundant choices. (See Chapter Five for recipes.) In this way, you will not overindulge in wheat, one of the more potential allergy/intolerance-inducing grains. When you do have some, you will appreciate it.

ALUMINUM

Aluminum is a relatively inexpensive and lightweight metal used in cookware and kitchen utensils. It is also used in antacids, antiperspirants, cans, bottle tops, baking powder, baking soda, commercial toothpastes, cigarette filters, and processed cheese. And thanks to the ever-increasing presence of acid rain, elevated levels of aluminum are now turning up in our drinking water. Aluminum can become toxic to our tissues, particularly to the brain.[70] It has been related to presenile dementia, Alzheimer's disease, and osteoporosis (the latter from an induced hyperparathyroidism). To slow the accumulation of this potentially toxic metal, you need to take preventive measures:

1. Use nonaluminum cookware and utensils—Pyrex, enamel, earthenware, stainless steel, or cast iron—and avoid aluminum foil. (Anodized aluminum cookware may be acceptable.)

2. Use aluminum-free baking powder and mixes.

3. Avoid drinking directly from bottles that have aluminum tops. Aluminum residue is left on the bottle threads every time the cap is screwed on and off.

4. Use a filter to purify tap water.

5. If you depend on antacids to relieve heartburn or indigestion, try aluminum-free products such as calcium carbonate or aloe vera juice or other herbal digestive aids instead (see Chapter Seven).

6. Use aluminum-free alternatives to deodorants and other products.

7. Support legislative measures to reduce acid rain.

PROCESSED FOODS—ALTERATIONS, ADDITIONS, AND NUTRIENT LOSS

By now, you're aware of the many dangers of processed food. You're also aware of the significant nutrient loss that occurs when the bran and germ of a grain are stripped from a kernel of wheat in the making of white flour.

One more point about nutrient loss: Micronutrients, or vitamins and minerals, are delicate, fragile, and fleeting parts of any food, easily broken down, easily lost to the air, and especially susceptible to heat. As soon as a fruit is harvested, a vegetable picked, or an animal slaughtered, a loss of micronutrients begins. Most fruits and vegetables are picked prematurely, long before they have wholly ripened and developed their full nutritive value. The longer the time between harvest and consumption, the more significant the nutrient loss. Then there is also blanching, boiling, freezing, pickling, smoking, canning, drying, prebaking, prebroiling, and preserving.

Once it comes time to prepare a meal, a food's nutritive properties may have already been significantly compromised, and if it is a processed food, seriously depleted. The trout caught, lightly cooked, and eaten by the riverside is best. The ripe apple picked and eaten is the best. The tomatoes, basil, swiss chard, beet greens, and corn on the cob picked from the backyard garden and prepared for dinner are best. Not all of us have op-

portunities every day to eat such fresh, vital food. But the alfalfa sprouts and produce you buy in the supermarket or the brown rice or seven-grain cereal you take the time to cook will certainly be superior in micronutrient content and life energy than the canned vegetables, TV dinner, or reheated frozen pizza you would normally eat.

Alternatives to Processed Foods— What You Can Do

Find the least adulterated and damaged foods in any of the food groups. You will be ahead by minimizing the prepackaged and prepared items. Whatever you use, read labels and choose judiciously. Try to make a good portion of most of your meals from scratch, particularly when cooking vegetables. If you think it impossible, start with just one meal a week. You may be able to find more time for cooking like this than you think.

Search for homegrown or locally grown produce in farmers' markets. In terms of nutrient content, freshly picked produce wins hands down to that picked days before and shipped from out of state, even if it's been organically grown.[71] If you depend on the fresh produce section of your supermarket, you will still be getting nutritious and "live" food. Learn how to sprout and grow your own indoor greens year round (see Chapter Five). Consider planting a vegetable garden in your yard. Even a small patch of zucchini or tomatoes will be enough to get you started. If you don't have a yard, garden in planting containers on a porch, doorstep, window box, even your roof. Plant a fruit or nut tree. You'll come to value it. Take any or all of these measures to maximize your micronutrient intake. You may lose a few minutes, but you'll gain a reserve of health.

OVEREATING

Food gives us the physical and mental energy to accomplish our goals. Yet it can also work against us—even an organic whole-foods diet. How can good food, which we all know builds health, be bad for us?

One of the more energy-demanding metabolic processes in our body is the manufacturing of hydrochloric acid in the stomach, a secretion necessary for the initial step of protein digestion as well as eventual mineral absorption. If the stomach cells that manufacture hydrochloric acid are under constant or excessive demand to perform their function, they will be forced to draw from energy reserves. This energy drain can extend over long periods of time and result in the accumulation of a debt. Then you will feel tired—not just immediately after a meal, but throughout the day and on a regular basis. It is that simple. When one part of the body is forced to do extra work, it will steal energy from wherever it can find it. In this way, overeating can sap vitality.

Eventually, the functioning of your overworked digestive system will deteriorate, which will lead to both diminished nutrient assimilation and bowel and liver toxicity. You have already begun to learn of the far-reaching effects of nutrient deficiencies, and Chapters Eight and Nine will emphasize the seriousness of a bowel/liver toxic condition. In addition, excessive calories have been linked to several cancers, notably of the bowel, and to a generally shortened life span.[72] Obesity is certainly not the least consequence of excessive calories. You should consider, as well, the resultant risks of high blood pressure, diabetes, elevated cholesterol levels, heart attack, stroke, cancers, and numerous musculo-skeletal difficulties.

Alternatives to Overeating—What You Can Do

By establishing a whole-foods and therefore nutrient-rich diet, you might eliminate one of the more common causes of overeating: the impulse itself. Your body's need for nutrients will be fully satisfied, while the fiber in whole foods will force you to chew thoroughly, eat more slowly, and thus become satiated with fewer calories. Fiber-rich foods will feel more filling, besides.

You may need to improve your digestive and assimilative processes before a whole-foods diet can exert the maximum effect on your overinflated appetite. Concentrate on chewing your food completely. Avoid excessive fluids or very cold or hot fluids with meals. Pay attention to food combinations, and apply the other measures to improve digestion outlined in Chapter Seven. You may need to do a bowel- and liver-cleansing regime, even a series of fasts (see Chapter Eighteen), to reverse the damage to your digestive system. Frequently, candidiasis and food allergies stimulate cravings and overeating, so treating these conditions (Chapters Twelve and Thirteen, respectively) can often normalize appetite.

Overeating is commonly triggered by dietary imbalances other than those involving nutrient quantities. A diet that is too acidic or too alkaline, too expansive or too contractive can bring on maddening cravings. You will learn in the next chapter how to balance these and other food opposites.

How many of us eat because we are bored, angry, depressed, lonely, excited, nervous, or anxious? Many of us would do well to sit quietly and reflect several minutes before our meals. By doing this, we may bring to the surface the thoughts, feelings, and anxieties that can often unconsciously trigger us to overeat. Food, as you know, is a powerful tranquilizer and sedative. Some individuals find that conquering their overeating requires a major effort in the areas of psychoemotional balance and personal growth (see Chapter Fifteen).

YOUR DOCTOR—ANOTHER NUTRITIONAL HAZARD?

Depending on your doctor for sound and complete nutritional advice may pose an unexpected hazard. As mentioned earlier, clinical nutrition is not a required course in most medical schools or residency programs. You may very likely know as much as or more than your doctor about nutrition. Doctors are generally concerned with making a correct diagnosis and treating disease. Once they are confident in their diagnosis and management of your problem, they consider their primary job completed. They often eschew the role of teacher.

Your doctor's nutritional knowledge may not extend far beyond such basic information as increasing fiber and reducing fats, sugar, salt, and calories. If you suffer from coronary artery disease, diabetes, or high blood pressure or are terribly constipated or overweight, your doctor will most likely make one or more of these nutritional recommendations. However, it's unlikely that he or she will touch on any of the finer nutritional points that can help you reduce your medication and even overcome your condition. Most physicians feel that many ailments are permanent and must simply be "managed" with medications. Worse than that, your doctor may encourage you to use the very items that contribute to today's killer diseases: margarine and polyunsaturated oils. Some pertinent nutritional knowledge and common sense can protect you from this white-coated hazard.

EATING BETTER MEANS FEELING BETTER

Although the dietary obstacles to good health are substantial, they are by no means overwhelming, and I hope by now, from all the options offered in this chapter, you're feeling encouraged and empowered. Improving your diet can make a dramatic difference in how you feel today, and it can help prevent a catastrophic illness tomorrow.

But, as I have cautioned, make your changes gradually. Do what feels comfortable at any given time. Don't attempt to overhaul your entire diet in a few weeks, or even in a month. Every few weeks, or once a month, implement a new change and get comfortable with it before moving on. Changing too much too quickly can backfire on you.

Working toward a hazard-free whole-foods diet is a laudable goal; however, we are all individuals. Some of us will grow healthier as vegetarians; others will not. Some will thrive on milk products; others will get ill. In the next chapter, I will present some information to help you adjust your diet to your personal needs.

SUGGESTED READING

Airola, Paavo, N.D. *Are You Confused?* Phoenix, AZ: Health Plus, 1971.

Budwig, Johanna, M.D. *Flax Oil as a True Aid Against Arthritis, Heart Infarction, Cancer and Other Diseases.* Vancouver: Apple, 1992.

Carper, Jean. *The Food Pharmacy: Dramatic New Evidence That Food Is Your Best Medicine.* New York: Bantam, 1988.

Colbin, Annemarie. *Food and Healing: How What You Eat Determines Your Health, Your Well-Being, and the Quality of Your Life.* New York: Ballantine, 1986.

Diamond, Harvey and Marilyn. *Fit for Life.* New York: Warner Books, 1985.

Eaton, S. B., Shostak, M., and Konner, M. *The Paleolithic Prescription: A Program of Diet and a Design for Living.* New York: Harper & Row, 1988.

Erasmus, Udo. *Fats That Heal, Fats That Kill.* Burnaby, British Columbia: Alive Books, 1993. To order: (800) 661-0303.

Gittleman, Ann Louise. *Beyond Pritikin: A Total Nutrition Program That Goes Beyond the Pritikin Principles by Adding Essential Fats for Rapid Weight Loss, Longevity, and Good Health.* New York: Bantam, 1988.

Hausman, Patricia, and Hurley, Judith Benn. *The Healing Foods: The Ultimate Authority on the Curative Power of Nutrition.* New York: Dell, 1989.

Jacobsen, Michael, Ph.D. *The Complete Eater's Digest and Nutrition Scoreboard.* New York: Doubleday, 1986.

Kilham, Christopher S. *The Bread and Circus Whole Food Bible: How to Select and Prepare Safe and Healthful Foods Without Pesticides or Chemical Additives.* Reading, MA: Addison Wesley, 1991.

Lappé, Frances Moore, and Collins, Joseph. *Food First: Beyond the Myth of Scarcity.* New York: Ballantine, 1978.

Manahan, William, M.D. *Eat for Health: A Do-It-Yourself Nutrition Guide for Solving Common Medical Problems.* Tiburon, CA: H.J. Kramer, 1988.

McDougall, John A., M.D. *The McDougall Program: 12 Days to Dynamic Health.* New York: Plume, 1990.

McDougall, John A., M.D., and Mary A. *The McDougall Plan.* Hampton, NJ: New Win Publishers, 1983.

Nutrition Action Healthletter. Center for Science in the Public Interest (1501 16th Street NW, Washington, DC 20036).

Nutrition Search, Inc. *Nutrition Almanac.* New York: McGraw-Hill, 1979.

Pitchford, Paul. *Healing with Whole Foods: Oriental Traditions and Modern Nutrition.* Berkeley: North Atlantic Books, 1993.

Robbins, John. *Diet for a New America: How Food Choices Affect Your Health, Happiness, and the Future of the Earth.* Wallpole, NH: Stillpoint, 1987.

Schmid, Ronald. *Traditional Foods Are Your Best Medicine.* New York: Ocean View/Random House, 1989.

Smith, Lendon, M.D. *Feed Your Kids Right.* New York: McGraw Hill, 1979.

———. *Feed Yourself Right.* New York: McGraw Hill, 1983.

Wigmore, Ann, N.D. *The Hippocrates Diet and Health Program.* Wayne, NJ: Avery, 1984.

CHAPTER 4

FINDING YOUR OPTIMAL DIET

We have considered the typical American diet and learned how to safeguard ourselves from its hazards. We have spoken in detail about specific elements of a whole-foods diet, which will be summarized subsequently. We will now attempt to clarify the issues of balance and polar opposites to refine your understanding of food properties and energies. Using this information, as well as concepts relating blood type and body type to diet, we will then examine ways to individualize whole-foods eating. Much of the information in this section is adapted from *Food and Healing* by Annemarie Colbin (Ballantine, 1986).

WHOLE-FOODS DIET

By now, I am sure you are aware that whole foods are not strange specialty items with bizarre flavors and textures, used exclusively by extremists or food faddists. They're natural foods, simply what nature provides for us: whole grains, legumes, fresh vegetables, sea vegetables, fresh fruits, seeds and nuts, eggs, meat, fish, poultry, and milk products—all obtained as fresh as possible, in season, and preferably grown or obtained locally. (And, of course, "natural foods" also include unrefined oils, natural sweeteners, and condiments such as unrefined sea salt, soy sauce, unpasteurized miso, herbs, and spices.)

Your foods should closely resemble the forms in which they are found in nature (unrefined, unbleached, unprocessed, with the least amount of chemicals and additives, and organic, if possible). It is best if meats are from animals raised without hormones and antibiotics. Meals should be prepared with care to retain as much

nutritional content as possible, without creating or adding substances hazardous to health.

Consult the following suggestions for initial guidelines on amounts and portions. However, realize that you may need to make further individualized adjustments and refinements.

1. COMPLEX CARBOHYDRATES GROUP: 2 to 3 servings a day from either of the following two groups:
- Whole grains (whole wheat, oats, barley, rye, corn, brown or wild rice, millet, buckwheat, amaranth, quinoa, spelt, kamut, teff): two to three servings a day. (See Chapter Five for some examples of how to use grains.)
- Winter squash (butternut, buttercup, acorn, blue hubbard, etc.) or other starchy vegetables, such as potatoes, sweet potatoes, and yams: one to two servings a day.

2. PROTEIN GROUP: At least two servings a day from any of the following four groups:
- Fish, fowl, eggs, meat: up to seven servings a week, depending on vegetarian or carnivorous preferences.
- Legumes (split peas, lentils, black beans, adzuki beans, etc): three to nine servings a week, depending on vegetarian or carnivorous preferences.
- Milk products: one to two servings a day, depending on the use of other protein sources and any potential allergies/intolerance to milk products.
- Seeds, nuts, and nut butters, although protein rich, are even more fat rich. Use sparingly unless

the remainder of your diet is lacking in protein and fat.

3. MODERATELY LOW-STARCH ROOT VEGETABLES (turnips, parsnips, rutabaga, carrots): one to two servings a day.

4. GENERAL VEGETABLES (zucchini, broccoli, cauliflower, cabbage, celery, onions, scallions, radishes, tomatoes, green, red, yellow, and other sweet peppers, eggplant, etc.): one to two servings a day.

5. GREENS (lettuce, spinach, kale, chard, collard, bok choy, beet greens, sunflower greens, buckwheat greens, etc.): at least one serving a day.

6. SEA VEGETABLES such as dulse, kelp, nori, hijiki, kombu, wakame: two to five servings a week.

7. RAW FRUIT: one to two servings a day, more often in the warmer seasons; cooked (stewed, etc.) and less often in the colder seasons.

8. FERMENTED FOODS containing bacteria favorable to the intestinal tract: one serving a day from any one of the following:

- Unpasteurized sauerkraut (see Chapter Five).
- Unpasteurized miso.
- Tamari/shoyu.
- Tempeh.
- Pickled vegetables.
- Yogurt, buttermilk, or kefir, if dairy is being consumed.

SEVEN-DAY MEAL PLAN

The following suggested week's meal plan offers some practical hints on how to implement the previous suggestions. Although each day's meals or any one particular meal may not conform exactly to the macronutrient percentages (fat, 20 to 30 percent; protein, 20 to 30 percent; carbohydrates, 40 to 60 percent) suggested for good health, taken as a whole, the overall plan should conform. Mild "excesses" on one day are balanced by appropriate "shortages" on another, or different meals in one day may offset imbalances. Feel free to make appropriate substitutions, additions, and/or deletions to conform with your tastes and individualized needs. Recipes for many items can be found in Chapter Five, although I recommend you have on hand several whole-foods cookbooks to enrich your options. (See "Recommended Cookbooks" at the end of Chapter Five.)

DAY 1

Breakfast: Fresh fruit, whole-grain cereal, herbal tea.
Lunch: Minestrone soup (see recipe, page 109), corn bread (see recipe, page 114) or whole-grain bread, salad.

Dinner: Baked or poached fish, steamed vegetables, including greens such as chard and kale, brown rice, salad, herb tea, whole-grain cookies.

DAY 2

Breakfast: Sliced fruits with seeds or nuts (soaked or lightly roasted) and yogurt (optional), whole-grain toast.
Lunch: Soft-boiled or poached eggs, sliced raw vegetables (tomatoes, cucumbers, green pepper, etc.), whole-grain crackers/tortilla or whole-grain bread.
Dinner: Baked squash (see recipe, page 112) and black bean (or adzuki bean) dish, salad, corn bread, raw sauerkraut condiment (see recipe, page 109).

DAY 3

Breakfast: Fruit and nut blender drink (see recipes, page 107), or whole-grain cereal.
Lunch: Mixed vegetable-and-greens salad with baked potato and avocado, whole-grain roll, herbal tea.
Dinner: Chicken noodle soup (see recipe, page 109), salad, corn on the cob or whole-grain roll, rice pudding (see recipe, page 114), herbal tea.

DAY 4

Breakfast: Soft-boiled, poached, or "steam fried" eggs Mexican style, served with corn tortilla and black beans with taco sauce, or soft-boiled egg, fresh fruit salad, bread or warmed tortilla or chapati.
Lunch: Baba ghanoush (eggplant dip) or hummus (see recipe, page 111), with raw vegetables or served as a sandwich in whole-grain pita pocket.
Dinner: Miso soup (see recipe, page 108) with a sea vegetable, vegetable/millet/almond medley (see recipe, page 112), salad, bancha tea, strawberry cream pie (see recipe, page 114).

DAY 5

Breakfast: Miso soup, whole-grain bread or mochi (a dense, chewy, and slightly sweet toast alternative made from rice—available in health food store freezer).

Lunch: Vegetable salad (red leaf lettuce, parsley, to-
             matoes, cucumbers, green onions, green
             or red peppers, mushrooms, avocado,
             etc.), diced cooked yam or potato,
             lemon tahini dressing (see recipe, page
             111), whole-wheat or corn tortilla or
             chapati.
Dinner: Hummus or baba ghanoush with raw vege-
             tables, steamed or lightly broiled tofu
             or tempeh and vegetables over brown
             rice with a cashew ginger sauce (see
             recipe, page 111), sauerkraut condi-
             ment, herbal tea.

DAY 6

Breakfast: Fresh fruit salad with nuts and yogurt, or
             whole-grain cereal and fruit.
Lunch: Vegetarian chili (see recipe, page 112) with
             grated cheese (optional), whole-grain
             bread or roll, salad.
Dinner: Miso soup, soy-bulgur casserole (see recipe,
             page 113), lettuce/tomato/red onion/
             avocado salad (see recipe, page 110)
             with sliced roasted almonds, herbal tea,
             raw sauerkraut condiment.

DAY 7

Brunch: Fresh fruit, pancakes, eggs, or oatmeal, veg-
             etable omelette, toast. Go ahead, have
             a cup of coffee.
Dinner: Vegetarian refried bean taco salad (see rec-
             ipe, page 114), herbal tea, apple-
             almond cream (see recipe, page 114) or
             whole-grain cookies.

There are many ways to combine the different elements of a whole-foods diet, some of which will not be
right for any one individual all the time. Although we all
require a certain amount of protein, carbohydrates, and
fats, as well as vitamins and minerals, our differences in
health, metabolism, personal taste, and body type/
genetics influence our choices in diet—one person's
needs may not be the same as those of another. The following accounts demonstrate the necessity for individuality of diet selection.

TO EACH HIS OR HER OWN DIET

Consider Jack, a thirty-three-year-old patient who had
adopted a strict vegetarian diet. He had previously been
in generally robust health on a fairly heavy meat-based
diet but decided he could maintain his health at an even

higher level on vegetarian fare. For three to four
months, Jack did seem to feel better. However, with the
onset of fall and winter, he came into my office with various complaints. He'd grown a little pale and had dark
circles under his eyes. He would awaken every morning
a bit tired, despite adequate sleep. He was also craving
sweets.

Jack was over six feet tall and had a powerful frame,
square shoulders, and a prominent brow. He was confident, assertive, and outgoing—the independent type. He
looked like a fierce physical competitor, one endowed
with a very strong constitution.

An examination and lab tests revealed no evidence
of any disease. My feeling was that his present diet, with
lots of fruit, vegetables, and an apparently adequate
amount of whole grains, legumes, seeds, and nuts, was
not quite right for him. I recommended that he modify
his vegetarian diet and reintroduce animal protein at
least three times a week. He had eaten meat almost
seven days a week before his switch to vegetarianism. I
also suggested that because it was winter, he have less
raw vegetables and fruit and more hearty soups and
stews with beans and meat or poultry.

When Jack returned for a follow-up visit in three
weeks, he was nearly back to his previous vim and vigor.
Although he was attached to the idea of minimizing animal sources of protein, he finally agreed that meat was
beneficial and perhaps essential for him. (He had type O
blood, the significance of which will be discussed
shortly.) He decided to see how infrequently he could include meat in his diet, varying the amount with the season, and still retain his strength and stamina.

We also agreed that low-fat, omega-3 fatty acid-rich
flesh foods such as fish, rabbit, and game meat would be
preferable to red meat (and even to poultry), but that he
would need to choose the animal protein that felt most
satisfying to his taste and his body. Naturally, he would
try to find chemical- and hormone-free sources and, if
possible, grass/range-fed beef or other low-fat meats. Finally, we agreed that longer periods, more than a few
days, of strict vegetarianism or cleansing diets would be
restricted to the warmer seasons.

Eventually Jack found red meat was by far the most
strengthening animal source of protein for him and that
eating it twice a week seemed to keep him functioning at
his best. Moreover, he discovered he felt healthier if he
had his main protein meal of the day at dinner. He had
tried for a while to eat "breakfast like a king, lunch like
a prince, and dinner like a pauper," but his body never
felt quite satisfied with the arrangement. Thus he
learned to gauge the appropriateness of his diet through
several key indicators:

• Physical energy and stamina
• Mental clarity, quickness, and stamina

- Mood
- Digestion and elimination
- Body temperature comfort
- Facial features (pallor, acne, dark circles under the eyes, swollen tissues)
- Oral features (coated or sticky tongue, bad breath)
- Weight and fat distribution
- Skin texture and nails

When his body had been denied meat for a period of several months, Jack would slow down physically and mentally, become somewhat irritable, grow pale and develop dark circles under his eyes, and lose weight even with abundant calories from other sources. He would also tend to feel cold. Jack found that he could improve his condition somewhat with fish and poultry, but red meat a few times a week was undeniably the most effective cure.

On the other hand, with too much meat and other animal proteins, he would again begin to slow down physically and mentally. He would feel heavy and food would sit longer in his stomach. He would get a little constipated. His appetite would no longer be keen, and his face would look a little swollen. His tongue would become slightly coated, his breath strong. He would also crave salt and sometimes sweets.

Blood Type and Diet

Some fascinating information on diet and blood type has been presented in recent years by Peter D'Adamo, N.D., of Greenwich, Connecticut.[1] The first human inhabitants on Earth had type O blood. These early people were hunter/gatherers. In other words, their diets consisted of what they could kill, pick, or dig (flesh foods, eggs, berries or other wild fruit, greens, seeds, nuts, and root vegetables). Evolutionarily speaking, this is the diet to which their systems were best suited. They did not consume grains, legumes, or milk products. These foods did not become available until the agrarian age, when blood type A evolved.

Individuals today with type O blood, therefore, may have fewer diet-related health problems if they generally stick to the hunter/gatherer diet by choosing low-fat flesh foods at least several days a week, or more. Their preferable starch/carbohydrate sources should be root vegetables, such as potato and yam, and winter squash such as acorn, buttercup, and butternut. Grains and legumes should not be as abundant foods in their diet, but more than anything else, the regular use of milk products should be avoided.

Individuals with type O blood do not generally make good vegetarians, at least not for extended periods of time. However, those with type A blood generally do. Type A's seem to be able to handle cultured milk products (like yogurt) better than noncultured dairy (milk, ice cream, etc.). They also do well generally on grains and legumes. Those with type B blood should minimize lecithin-rich foods (corn, chicken, buckwheat are examples). Blood type O individuals have the most clearly delineated food group dietary boundaries. Types B and AB (which has only been in existence for eight hundred years) are more mixed. Dr. D'Adamo has developed a blood test involving blood typing that can help individualize your diet. It can serve not only to prevent disease and optimize health but, if you are seriously ill, assist your body back to health. It is a test your physician can obtain for you.[2]

Body Type and Diet

The subject of body types/personalities and appropriate diet will be touched upon only briefly here. The system that has, I believe, the longest history in this type of diet individualization is Ayurvedic medicine, a form of natural medicine practiced in India for several thousand years. This system recognizes three main constitutional types, each with a specifically recommended diet. Excessive departures from your particular recommended diet will usually result in predictable ailments. Dr. Vasant Lad's *Ayurveda: The Science of Self-Healing* (Lotus Press, 1984) is an easy-to-use and thorough guide to identifying your type and corresponding diet. Also, see Dr. Deepak Chopra's *Perfect Health: The Complete Mind-Body Guide* (Harmony, 1990).

In 1983, Elliot Abravanel, M.D., first published *Dr. Abravanel's Body Type Diet and Lifetime Nutrition Plan.* In this and his more current books, he categorizes people by their dominant endocrine gland (thyroid, pituitary, adrenal, or gonad) through questionnaires and photographs, then lays out specific breakfasts, lunches, and dinners that are quite different for each type.

One of the more comprehensive works I have seen on individualizing diet according to body type, personality, and other factors has been done by T. Glynn Braddy of Sydney, Australia. (A forthcoming book, entitled *The Four Foods System,* may be available through T. Glynn Braddy and Associates, P.O. Box 766, Manley, NSW 2095, Australia, who also sponsors Braddy's international seminars.)

EXPERIMENTING WITH DIETARY OPPOSITES

You may need to experiment to find the diet that is best for you—even in a whole-foods context and even with the guidance of a health professional. He or she may have an idea of the foods that would be best, but in the end your body rules this decision with its ultimate wisdom. Follow how you feel and function while trying out different diets and foods.

Try eating differently if your doctor does not know why you have not been feeling well and you feel the problem may be diet related. If your main meal has been at dinner, try having it at breakfast or lunch. If you have included a number of milk products on a regular basis, try going without them for a few weeks. If you have been vegetarian and have taken in very little animal protein, try adding a portion of meat three or four times a week. If you have had abundant raw foods, try more cooked foods. If your diet is largely cooked, try more raw food dishes. If you have been a heavy meat eater, try more vegetarian fare for a while. If you have been an overeater, try being an undereater. If you consume too much bread, pasta, and other grains, substitute potatoes, yams, and winter squash.

We tend to imbalance our bodies with extremes. Too much of even a good thing can become harmful. Try the opposite, or at least somewhat opposite, of what you've become used to. You may be pleased by how well you do. But after a while, you may need to modify your initial counterstrategy as your body approaches a state of balance. The following discussion may help clarify this concept:

The Law of Opposites

Building/Cleansing When we look at health as a state of dynamic balance—for example, the balance between tissues in our bodies wearing down as they normally do (catabolism) and tissues being replaced and rebuilt (anabolism)—we can see how elements in our diet parallel these metabolic activities. For worn body cells to be "washed" away most effectively, cleansing and elimination foods are required. For tissues to be rebuilt and replaced, building foods are needed.

BUILDING/CLEANSING FOODS

BUILDING	CLEANSING/ELIMINATION
Proteins:	Low-starch vegetables:
meats, poultry, fish,	greens, cucumbers,
dairy, eggs	tomatoes, celery,
Complex carbohydrates:	broccoli, cauliflower,
whole grains, legumes,	zucchini, summer squash,
potatoes, yams,	cabbage, asparagus,
winter squash	string beans, etc.
Fats:	Fruit
seeds and nuts,	
oils	

Adapted by permission of Ballantine Books, a division of Random House, Inc., from Food and Healing *by Annemarie Colbin. Copyright © 1986 by Annemarie Colbin.*

The standard American diet offers an excess of building foods and not enough cleansing foods. This results in ailments of excess: obesity, cancer, hypertension, heart disease, diabetes, and bowel and liver toxicity. On the other hand, individuals who are always on some kind of purifying or cleansing diet or fast, whether it be vegetables and fruits or simply juices, usually come to my office complaining of fatigue, poor concentration, spaciness, lack of motivation, poor wound healing, pallor, low blood sugar, low adrenal symptoms, and a general lack of vitality. To someone with conditions stemming from excessive building foods, I might recommend initially a diet of mostly vegetables and fruits such as the purifying diet on pages 180–181. To those who have overdone the cleansing diets, I would strongly suggest adding the building foods that would be well tolerated.

Acidic/Alkaline The body's enzyme systems work best in a fairly small range of acidic/alkaline balance: a pH between 7.35 and 7.45, to be exact. Within the body, both metabolic and respiratory mechanisms compensate for abnormalities. For instance, physical exercise (muscle metabolism) produces an acidic state that is quickly eliminated in the form of carbon dioxide, by quicker and deeper respiration.

ACIDIC/ALKALINE FOODS

ACIDIC FOODS	BUFFERS (NEUTRAL)	ALKALINE-FORMING FOODS
Meat, fish,	Butter	Most vegetables
poultry, etc.	Raw milk products:	Most fruits
Most grains:	milk, ice cream,	Salt
wheat, rice, etc.	yogurt, cheeses	Soybeans
Most nuts and	Tofu	Miso
seeds		Tamari/soy sauce
Sugar and honey		Sea vegetables
Most legumes		Almonds and Brazil
Decaffeinated coffee		nuts
Pasteurized milk		Millet and buckwheat
products		
Raw tomatoes		
Cranberries, plums,		
and prunes		

Adapted by permission of Ballantine Books, a division of Random House, Inc., from Food and Healing *by Annemarie Colbin. Copyright © 1986 by Annemarie Colbin.*

The standard American diet tends to emphasize acidic foods, creating an imbalance often characterized by a sticky, sour taste in the mouth. If alkalinizing dietary minerals are insufficient, chronic acidity will contribute to the demineralization of your body's tissues, teeth, and bones. Your cells (including bone cells) will relinquish their minerals at any expense to keep the blood pH in normal range—one of the more powerful metabolic priorities.

Consequently, as minerals leave the nervous system, you can develop nervous and emotional disorders. As they leave the jaw, periodontal disease results. As they leave the nail beds, broken or weak nails develop. As they leave bones, osteoporosis may set in. Osteoporosis is a disease of excess and acidity rather than a simple deficiency of dietary calcium (see, in Chapter Seventeen, "Osteoporosis").

Cravings may be evidence of innate body wisdom, alerting us to dietary imbalance. If, for example, a diet contains excessive amounts of vegetables and fruits, which is too alkalinizing, and not enough grains, beans, or animal protein, which is acidic, one will often crave sugar for its acid effect. Conversely, eating a lot of meat (acidic) will often cause a craving for salt (alkaline). Some nutritionally oriented health practitioners assess the acidic/alkaline balance by testing urine and/or saliva pH. The most sophisticated use of acid/alkaline balance that I have seen comes from the work of Emanuel Revici, M.D., of the Institute of Applied Biology in New York City, who in 1961 self-published *Research in Physiopathology as a Basis of Guided Chemotherapy with Special Application to Cancer.*

Warming/Cooling Chinese medicine classifies many diseases as "cold" or "hot." Cold ailments include arthritis, colic, and diarrhea, for which warm foods are indicated. Hot ailments include headaches, abnormal sweating, and circulatory problems, for which cooling foods are indicated. Chinese theory gets far more interesting when you learn that each of the main organs correlates to both an element (earth, water, air, fire, or metal) and a season of the year, and that specific seasonal measures, guided by the associated organ and element, will help you preserve your health.[3]

Too many of us experience health problems because we tend to ignore the seasons of the year and eat in the winter as we do in the summer. Hot oatmeal for breakfast is far more fitting in the wintertime than fresh fruit or dry cereal. A hearty soup or stew is far more protective from the cold than a seafood salad. Generally, the building foods are also warming, and the cleansing foods cooling.

COOLING/WARMING FOODS

COOLING FOODS	WARMING FOODS
Raw fruits	Cooked and dried fruits
Raw vegetables	Cooked vegetables
Cucumbers	Cabbage
Summer squash	Winter squash
Citrus fruit	Coconut
Raw tomatoes	Tomato sauce
Papaya	Avocado
Leafy vegetables	Root vegetables
Soybeans	Tempeh
Tofu	Lentils
Mung beans	Kidney beans
Sea vegetables	Potatoes
Bulgur	Yams
Corn on the cob	Oats
Rice (brown or white)	Kasha
Ice cream	Barley
Yogurt	Cornmeal
Milk	Butter
Sprouts	Cream
Egg white	Eggs
Clams	Cheese
Lobster	Nuts and seeds
Crabs	Egg yolk
Sashimi (raw fish)	Fish (cooked, fried)
Pork	Poultry, beef, organ meats
Coffee	Chocolate
	Kuzu (a thickening agent)

HERBS, SPICES, FLAVORINGS	
Cooling Herbs	Warming Herbs
Curry	Garlic
Turmeric	Ginger
Dill	Cumin
Parsley	Caraway
Hot peppers	Basil
Coriander	Thyme
Pickles	Oregano
Tamari	Bay leaf
Shoyu	Black pepper
White sugar	Coriander seed
Salt	Cinnamon
	Cloves
	Vanilla
	Miso
	Brown sugar
	Salt

COOKING TECHNIQUES	
Cooling	Warming
Steaming	Boiling
Stir-frying	Sautéing
Pickling	Frying
	Baking
	Dry roasting

Adapted by permission of Ballantine Books, a division of Random House, Inc., from Food and Healing *by Annemarie Colbin. Copyright © 1986 by Annemarie Colbin.*

Expansive/Contractive The expansive/contractive polarity, known also as yin/yang, derives from an age-old Asian conceptualization and understanding of life. The macrobiotic tradition, acupuncture, and Oriental medicine have introduced Westerners to this concept, which describes the energetic qualities in nearly all aspects of life, not merely diet.[4] Macrobiotics, as you may know, is based on a philosophy of living in harmony with nature, with others, and with oneself. (See Chapter Twenty-one for a further explanation of the yin/yang principle.) Disease can be categorized as expansive or contractive in association with the excesses of associated expansive and contractive foods. The following table lists foods that range from the expansive to contractive in nature.

EXPANSIVE/CONTRACTIVE FOODS

EXPANSIVE

Drugs
  Alcohol
    Fruit juices
      Aromatic herb teas
        Vegetable juices
          Tea/coffee
            Sugar
              Spices
                Fats and oils
                  Tropical fruits
                    Temperate fruits
                      Sprouts/lettuce
                        Fast-growing vegetables
                          Tubers
                            Bitter greens
                              Sea vegetables
                                Winter squashes
                                  Roots
                                    Nuts
                                      Beans
                                        Grains
                                          Fish
                                            Fowl
                                              Beef
                                                Eggs
                                                  Tamari
                                                    Miso
                                                      Salt

CONTRACTIVE

Adapted by permission of Ballantine Books, a division of Random House, Inc., from Food and Healing *by Annemarie Colbin. Copyright © 1986 by Annemarie Colbin.*

Excesses of expandng foods and deficiencies of contracting foods may lead to expanding ailments: mental confusion, spaciness, difficulty in concentrating, hyperactivity, disjointed motion, hypoglycemia, cysts, and mucus discharges. Excesses of contracting foods may lead to contractive ailments: hypertension, arteriosclerosis, arthritis, and physical and mental rigidity. Of all the polarities listed here, this one is more far reaching. However, the acidic/alkaline swing, according to Annemarie Colbin, is most responsible for our body's out-of-balance cravings.

Raw Foods/Cooked Foods One last set of polar opposites is raw versus cooked food. Raw food, such as a vegetable, contains maximum amounts of vitamins, minerals, enzymes, and life energy, particularly if picked ripe and eaten within the day. The live enzymes in such food assist in its digestion and put less strain on the enzyme-producing cells of the pancreas and small intestine. For these reasons, raw food enthusiasts endorse eating anything uncooked that you can eat that way: fruits, vegetables, seeds, nuts, sprouted seeds and legumes, sprouted grains, milk products, and fish (sushi or sashimi).

Fermented foods and sprouts greatly aid in the process of digestion and assimilation, and for this reason are often included in raw food and strict vegetarian diets. These include yogurt, unpasteurized miso, unpasteurized sauerkraut, unpasteurized tamari/shoyu, pickled vegetables, sprouts, and traditionally fermented sourdough bread. Generally speaking, fermented and sprouted foods are an important addition to the diets of strict vegetarians. (For helpful books on vegetarianism, see the titles by Rudolph Ballantine, M.D., John McDougall, M.D., Ann Wigmore, M.D., and Frances Moore Lappé listed under Suggested Reading, page 101.) Advocates of a raw foods diet contend that cooking kills the food: it destroys enzymes, causes the loss of many nutrients, and creates the potential for heat-induced damage (trans-fatty acids, free radical pathology, and so on).

On the other hand, cooking softens cellulose and other substances difficult for the digestive system to metabolize. Cooking, in effect, predigests food. Granted, enzymes and some nutrients are lost in the cooking, but if you choose fresh, whole foods and use healthful cooking methods, much nutrient value remains after the cooking, while your digestive processes are spared having to work on cellulose.

Life energy is characterized by far more than enzyme content. Energy exists on many levels. For example, according to Colbin, cooking does not necessarily destroy the electromagnetic energy in foods. In addition, cooking allows for tastes and textures not offered by many raw foods, which for most of us creates a more satisfying meal. Cooked food is generally warming, both physically and emotionally. Raw food is much less so.

As mentioned previously, a raw foods diet may be

extremely valuable as a therapy. It is excessively expanding, cleansing, alkalinizing, and cooling. Such a diet is useful for conditions and symptoms that arise from a diet that is excessively contracting, building, acidifying, and warming (the typical American diet). I recommend periodic raw food cleansing diets for many of my patients (see "Liver Flush and Purifying Diet," pages 180–181, and Chapter Eighteen).

Like anything else, raw foods need to be used in a balanced manner. The uniqueness of your digestive system, the climate in which you live, the season of the year, and your personal preferences will determine how much raw food/cooked food is suitable for the maintenance of your health.

THERAPEUTIC DIETS

Many diets have been proposed expressly to help undo the excesses of the standard American diet. Their successes can be explained with an understanding of the law of opposites. Many of these regimes—the Pritikin diet,[5] for example, and Wigmore's Hippocrates Health Institute Raw Foods Diet[6]—have worked marvelously for many individuals, helping reverse such conditions as angina, arteriosclerosis, hypertension, hypercholesterolemia, diabetes, obesity, and arthritis. However, these diets operate under the principle of extremes—they need to be modified once they have performed their rescue missions and brought an individual back to a state of balance and health.

Although often used therapeutically, the macrobiotic diet is designed to maintain balance indefinitely. This diet restricts the intake of raw foods, and is low in flesh foods, primarily allowing for the consumption of fish. It does not include milk products. Often, however, this diet seems too rigid, even to many vegetarians.

Without being a strict follower of macrobiotics, one can still benefit greatly from its general principles of balance and some of its key ingredients, such as sea vegetables, miso soup, fermented vegetables, high complex carbohydrate content, and low animal protein content. Similarly, while many meat eaters benefit by adopting some habits of vegetarianism, other individuals can benefit equally by adopting macrobiotic principles.

LIVING THE GOLDEN MEAN

For any diet to be successful, it must be balanced and satisfying, both in the way it tastes and in how your body feels and responds to it. The more excesses you indulge in, the more extreme your compensation will need to be. After years of these severe swings, your mental/physical balance and health may well be rather precari-ous. Find the most even and satisfying diet for yourself so that your body/mind will not crave excesses. Use the information given here, read some of the books and articles I've mentioned about individualizing your diet. Trust your preferences and experiment. Your body is your best teacher.

Remember to allow yourself occasional indulgences without guilt. Food can be a central part of social gatherings and celebrations. It's not what you do once in a while—a major festive event, an evening on the town, a party or other occasion—that will have a substantial impact on your long-term health. It's what you eat and how you live every day.

SUGGESTED READING

Abravanel, Elliot D., and King, Elizabeth A. *Anti-Craving Weight Loss Diet*. New York: Bantam, 1990.

———. *Dr. Abravanel's Body Type Program for Health, Fitness & Nutrition*. New York: Bantam, 1986.

———. *Dr. Abravanel's Body Type Diet and Lifetime Nutrition Plan*. New York: Bantam, 1986.

Aihara, Herman. *Basic Macrobiotics*. Tokyo: Japan Publications, 1988.

Ballantine, Rudolph, M.D. *Transition to Vegetarianism*. Honesdale, PA: Himalayan Press, 1987.

Chopra, Deepak. *Perfect Health: The Complete Mind-Body Guide*. New York: Crown, 1991.

Colbin, Annemarie. *Food and Healing: How What You Eat Determines Your Health, Your Well-Being, and the Quality of Your Life*. New York: Ballantine, 1986.

Diamond, Harvey and Marilyn. *Fit for Life*. New York: Warner Books, 1985.

Kushi, Michio. *The Book of Macrobiotics*. Elmsford, NY: Japan Publications, 1977.

Lad, Vasant. *Ayurveda: The Science of Self-Healing*. Wilmot, WI: Lotus Press, 1984.

Lappé, Frances Moore. *Diet for a Small Planet*, 10th ed. New York: Ballantine, 1986.

Lappé, Frances Moore, and Collins, Joseph. *Food First: Beyond the Myth of Scarcity*. New York: Ballantine, 1978.

McDougall, John A., M.D. *The McDougall Program: 12 Days to Dynamic Health*. New York: Plume, 1990.

McDougall, John A., M.D., and Mary A. *The McDougall Plan*. Hampton, NJ: New Win Publishers, 1983.

Pitchford, Paul. *Healing with Whole Foods, Oriental Tradition and Modern Nutrition*. Berkeley: North Atlantic Books, 1993.

Pritikin, Nathan, with Leonard, J. and Hofer, J. L. *Live Longer Now: The First 100 Years of Your Life.* New York: Grosset & Dunlap, 1974.

Pritikin, Nathan, and McGrady, P. M. *The Pritikin Program for Diet and Exercise.* New York: Grosset & Dunlap, 1979.

Richards-Griffen, Hazel S. *Ninety-two Years: Perfect Health in an Unpolluted Body.* Available from Sur-

vival Ministries, 4415 Semoran Farms Road, Kissimmee, FL 34744 or 10249 Coachilla Canals Road, Niland, CA 92257.

Wigmore, Ann, N.D. *The Hippocrates Diet and Health Program.* Wayne, NJ: Avery, 1984.

Wiley, Rudolf A., Ph.D. *Biobalance: The Acid/Alkaline Solution to the Food Mood Health Puzzle.* Tacoma, WA: Life Sciences Press, 1989.

CHAPTER FIVE

ALL-STAR FOODS

FRESHLY MADE VEGETABLE AND FRUIT JUICES

Fresh juices contain abundant enzymes, vitamins, and minerals that require minimal digestion and thus can be assimilated quite readily. They are used therapeutically for fasting and as natural cures for numerous ailments, including cancer. Whole fruits and vegetables, the benefits of which include fiber as well as vitamins, minerals, and enzymes, are certainly important, if not crucial, for health maintenance. Fresh juices, however, provide a superior vehicle by which unusually high quantities and concentrations of the food's life force can be consumed.

The difference between commercially sold juices and those you prepare yourself is vast. Commercial juices may contain sugar, preservatives, and other undesirables, while your own prepared juices are clearly "cleaner," fresher, and higher in nutrients as well as enzymes. If you consume the juice within fifteen minutes of making it, you will get the benefit of the enzymes—the "alive" quality of the juice—which is so heralded by nature cure physicians.

In the world of juicing, the carrot is superior. Carrot juice is sweet and often used alone, although it is commonly added to flavor blander juices and to sweeten the less palatable or bitter green juices. The green juice is considered most cleansing and nutritive, particularly because of its chlorophyll content (see pages 448–449).

Try one or more of the following greens with just enough carrot juice to taste: parsley, watercress, collard, chard, beet greens, mustard greens, kale, celery, or broccoli leaves. You can make a gourmet drink from carrot, celery, spinach, parsley, cucumber, and a little beet. To get a slight kick, add a radish, a garlic clove, or a bit of onion or slice of ginger root. This is a genuine treat that you and your body will treasure. Also try juicing your watermelon—if it's organic, juice the rind as well.

In Chapter Eighteen, you'll read about fasting. A day on fresh juices alone will be like no other. But begin, perhaps along with your regular diet, with a glass a day. Drinking a glass of juice ten to thirty minutes before breakfast is good, but any time will do. Even vegetable-phobic children will often drink carrot juice!

A juicer is an essential piece of kitchen equipment. Talk to people who have one to get an owner's assessment of the strengths and weaknesses of the different types available, or rent or borrow one. One important quality is how well the juice is extracted: Is the residue pulp fairly dry, or do you need to run a wet residue through and juice a second time to get more out? Good juicers do it sufficiently on the first try. Then there are juicers that include the fiber pulp as well. Although pulp-containing juices are not generally used in nature cure programs, they are still certainly nutritious and "alive."

Even with an ordinary blender, you can make fresh green juice. Cut up one or more greens, blend together with water and enough carrot or apple juice to sweeten, strain and serve. For a wonderful-tasting green juice treat, try blending celery tops and parsley with pineapple juice/water. You can also blend green juice with tomato juice (add fresh basil if available). For a second "harvest," combine the strained pulp with new water/juice and start over. For more tips, see *Juicing for Life, A Guide to the Health Benefits of Fresh Fruit and Vegetable Juicing*, by Cherie Calbom, M.S., C.N., and Maureen Keane, M.S., C.N. (Avery, 1992).

SPROUTS

A sprout is the embodiment of life and growth; it is life awakened. As a seed germinates, its vitamin and mineral content may double or even triple. Moreover, sprouting changes the carbohydrate and protein in the seed to much more readily digestible substances. Some of the complex carbohydrate changes to simple sugars, some of the protein to amino acids. In other words, sprouting begins the digestion process of its own macronutrients. The most common seeds used for sprouting are alfalfa, mung beans, red clover, and sunflower, although radish, Chinese cabbage, grains, and legumes can also be used. Most health food stores and many supermarkets carry sprouts, and you can grow them easily yourself.

Basic Sprouting Guidelines

To grow sprouts, you need:
a quart or ½-gallon jar
plastic or cloth mesh
a rubber band

Or you can buy special sprouting kits.

Soak small seeds (e.g., alfalfa) three to five hours, large seeds (e.g., lentil and sunflower) twelve hours. After soaking, drain off water. Put seeds in jar (1 tbsp. per quart for small seeds; ¼ cup per quart for large seeds). Cover with mesh, secure tightly with rubber band. Place jar upside down at a 45° angle to drain. Cover with a towel. Rinse the seeds every twelve hours or more often in hot weather, turning the jar upside down each time to drain off the water. Repeat the rinsing/draining/covering process until sprouts are done. (Small seeds will sprout in four to five days.) On day 3, expose to sunlight to develop the chlorophyll in leaves. When ready to harvest, place sprouts in a pan of water; the hulls will float to the surface, and you can skim off and remove them. Return sprouts to jar, drain well, and transfer to plastic bags or jar and refrigerate. Be sure to drain well before storing, and perhaps put a paper towel inside the bag to absorb excess water. Rinse every two or three days to maintain freshness. Drain well after rinsing, because excess water will cause sprouts to rot.

Larger seeds are usually ready when the root is nearly as long as the seed. They can be eaten raw or cooked. *The New Laurel's Kitchen* has sprouting instructions, as do the books by Ann Wigmore (see Recommended Cookbooks and Suggested Reading lists on p. 115).

Growing Buckwheat and Sunflower Greens (Also Wheat, Barley, Rye, and Oat Grass)

You can grow fresh greens year round, even indoors in the winter. Obtain a large baking or plastic tray or make a tray from plywood, approximately 2 feet by 3 feet by 2 to 3 inches deep. A nursery flat will do if you line the bottom with a piece of plastic. Fill with 1 to 2 inches of garden soil, composted soil, potting soil, or any good dirt from your yard. Soak sunflower seeds and buckwheat groats with hulls in separate jars for about fifteen hours. Empty the water and let seeds sit lightly covered in the jar for four to six hours. Then spread the sunflower seeds over half the moistened dirt, the buckwheat groats over the other half. Completely cover the dirt with a carpet of seeds one layer thick.

Cover with five sheets or so of moistened newspaper and a sheet of dark plastic. Let sit in a warm room, or at least one that isn't too cool, for four to five days, making sure the newspaper remains moist. When the growth has begun to lift the newspaper, remove and expose to light. It is normal for mold to develop on the dirt and seeds from the darkness and dampness. Do not let that deter you. Find a good window for the tray, or use a growing light. Water only enough to keep dirt from drying. Greens are ready for harvest when 4 to 8 inches high. Eat the leaves and the stems; they are extremely tasty and delicate. Reuse the dirt once—just turn it over in the tray and start again with new soaked seeds. After this second batch, return it to your yard or compost pile. Use new dirt.

If you are growing one of the grain grasses, you'll need a special juicer to extract the potent juices. See your health food store for such a device, or refer to the books by Ann Wigmore and Hazel Richards-Griffen in Recommended Cookbooks at the end of this chapter.

SEA VEGETABLES

Sea vegetables contain abundant minerals, particularly trace minerals that are not usually available in appreciable amounts in commercially grown foods. In addition to trace elements, some sea vegetables are extremely high in calcium (hijiki and arame, for example), and nori is rich in protein. Kelp and dulse are rich in calcium, potassium, and iodine. Dulse and kelp powders can be used in place of salt and added to almost anything. Dulse leaves can be soaked, then added to salads, grain dishes, and soups. Kombu and wakame can be added to soups; so can nori. The latter can also be used for making rice balls (see recipe section of this chapter). Nori is the dark leafy seaweed used to wrap sushi. It can also be cut into small pieces and added to salads, cereals, rice, or casseroles. Hijiki and arame should be soaked, then sautéed and simmered briefly. They can be used in grain or vegetable dishes and salads.

Most of these sea vegetables are available in health

food stores and Asian markets, especially Japanese grocery stores. They often come with recipes on their package labels. It is beneficial to regularly include a variety of sea vegetables in your diet. Evidence suggests that some algin-containing sea vegetables, like kelp, help protect against heavy metals and ionizing radiation.

MISO

This traditional Japanese staple is an aged, fermented food made from a variety of grains or from soybeans. Barley (mugi) miso is one of the milder and more popular kinds. Its flavor is unique and delicate, and it is used primarily in soups. Miso soup can be a very pleasant way to begin the day and is a regular breakfast item in Japan and for many Americans following a macrobiotic diet. It can also be used to flavor bean and vegetable soups and served for lunch or dinner. Because of the natural fermentation process, miso is in a sense predigested and rich in friendly bacteria and enzymes. It is therefore very easily digested, and its nutrients are assimilated readily. It is soothing, ideally suited to those with acute or chronic stomach and digestive disturbances, and extremely nutritious (some varieties are over 70 percent protein). Miso must not be boiled (the enzymes and bacteria are heat sensitive). Instead, add it to a soup bowl at the table or to the soup pot after the cooking is completed. Those who suffer from hypertension and are salt sensitive should monitor their blood pressure if using miso regularly. Incidentally, there have been anecdotal reports of its successful use in treating individuals injured by nuclear radiation at Hiroshima and Nagasaki. (See the miso soup recipe in the All-Star Recipes section of this chapter.)

CULTURED MILK PRODUCTS

Chapter Eight explains how necessary friendly intestinal bacteria are for good health. Cultured milk products, such as yogurt, buttermilk, and kefir, are useful sources of these organisms. Even some milk-allergic individuals can tolerate cultured milk products. Be sure the yogurt you purchase contains live cultures. Many popular supermarket brands do not contain live cultures and are oversweetened. Buy a health food brand without sweetener and add sliced fresh fruit.

RAW SAUERKRAUT

Raw sauerkraut, as opposed to the regular commercial variety, which is cooked or pasteurized, contains not only the nutrients of fermented cabbage, but also the enzymes and friendly bacteria that assist in the digestive process and in intestinal health. (For a further discussion, see pages 100 and 152.) It takes only a few bites of raw sauerkraut to serve these healthful purposes.

Raw sauerkraut is available in the refrigerated section of many health food stores and co-ops, or you may want to make it yourself and witness the fermentation process. I have successfully used the sauerkraut recipe in the All-Star Recipes in the next section of this chapter.

BREWER'S YEAST

Brewer's yeast is a source of many nutrients: amino acids, B-complex vitamins, choline and inositol, and important minerals such as chromium (the glucose tolerance factor necessary for the proper functioning of insulin and control of blood sugar levels). Manganese, zinc, and other minerals are present as well. Yeast is recommended for general use as a food supplement and specifically for such conditions as hypoglycemia and fatigue. You may need to experiment until you find the brand that is most palatable to you. Tablets are also available.

Nutritional yeast may taste a little better but often lacks GTF chromium, which you should insist upon if you suffer from blood sugar problems. However, if taste dictates whether you will use the yeast or not, go with whichever variety you tolerate best. If GTF is not present, the amino acids and the B-complex vitamins will still be very useful. Have it in diluted fruit juice or vegetable juice, blender drinks, on salads, in grain dishes, in soups, or on popcorn. Begin with a ½ teaspoon once or twice a day. Gradually, over several weeks, work up the dose to 1 tablespoon a few times a day. Allergy to yeast is common, especially if you have a candida overgrowth. If, after using yeast, you experience bowel or other symptoms that do not subside within a week or two, discontinue use. If you are prone to food allergies and find yeast helpful, take it only every three to four days. Daily or repetitive use may cause you to develop an allergy.

GARLIC AND ONIONS

Garlic and onions have numerous medicinal uses, as discussed in detail in Chapter Nineteen.

ALOE VERA

A common succulent plant from which juice and gel can

be extracted, aloe vera has many medicinal uses, as discussed in Chapter Nineteen.

MICROALGAE (SPIRULINA, BLUE-GREEN ALGAE, CHLORELLA)

Microalgae are rich sources of amino acids, minerals (particularly iron and potassium), vitamins (especially the Bs), trace elements, essential fatty acids, enzymes, and chlorophyll. They contain an abundant supply of beta- and other carotenes, as well as essential fatty acids, germanium, boron, selenium, and magnesium. Microalgae are concentrated sources of protein (particularly suited to vegetarians), but their usefulness as a source of vitamin B-12 is debatable. They're also beneficial in weight-management programs since they suppress appetite while providing low-calorie, high-quality nutrition. For this reason, microalgae are also included in fasting and detoxification programs.

Some brands of microalgae come in tablet form, although I prefer powdered, which I blend with water (and fruit juice to taste). Other ingredients can be added according to your taste (see page 107). I recommend Pure Synergy (from the Synergy Company of Moab, Utah), a combination of the three microalgae listed above in addition to wheat and barley grass, herbs, Chinese mushrooms, royal jelly, and other "superfoods" with known health-enhancing effects. Whole Life Food Concentrate (from Bernard Jensen International of Escondido, CA) is a chlorella/superfood concentrate also worth trying.

Microalgae can be preserved for many years and thus serve as an efficient nutritional source in times of food shortage. Because of quality-control issues, use microalgae products that are either U.S. or Japanese grown.

HERBS

Herbs are not only used to season food and beverages, they also provide us with minerals, and offer medicinal uses. Why not drink herbal teas (hot or cold) and use seasonings that not only taste good, but also nourish and heal? See Chapter Nineteen for a discussion of herbs and their medicinal benefits.

BEE POLLEN

Honeybee pollen is an exceptional source of concentrated nutrients. Because pollen consists of the germinal components of the plant from which it comes, it contains the vital forces required to reproduce that plant and is a life-giving food. Its vitamins, minerals, amino acids, enzymes, carbohydrates, and fatty acids supply us with elements that may be missing in other food sources, catalysts that regulate and stimulate our metabolism.

Bee pollen can serve as a valuable food supplement to assist in the maintenance of health. It is also believed to contain a small amount of antibiotic and antifungal activity, potentially increasing one's resistance to infection. Although I have not used it in treating infections, I have used it successfully to lessen pollen allergies and to support weight-management programs.

Begin with just a few granules a day and increase the regular dose gradually over several weeks up to 1 to 3 teaspoons a day. Eat it by itself, mix it in juices or blender drinks, or sprinkle it on top of yogurt, fruit salad, cereals, and other foods. Raw, relatively undried pollen, which must be stored in the freezer, is the most potent; however, this form is not widely obtainable. In most cases, dried pollen will do.

FLAXSEED OIL AND FLAXSEEDS

Flaxseed is an important oil to include in your diet because of its exceptionally high alpha-linolenic acid content. It can help prevent essential fatty acid deficiencies, and has been cited for its use in the treatment of chronic degenerative diseases.[1] Look for expeller- and/or cold-pressed (processed under 96° F) varieties, and be sure it is bottled in an opaque oxygen-free or amber glass container with the date of pressing and expiration marked. Keep it refrigerated. Use it raw, unheated, approximately one to two teaspoons a day with salad dressings and soups, in blender drinks or on cereal, cottage cheese, and yogurt. Never cook with it. Dr. Johanna Budwig recommends using flaxseed oil emulsified with protein (blended with low-fat cottage cheese or yogurt. See recipe on page 108). Flaxseeds can be ground fresh and mixed in blender drinks, hot or cold cereals, yogurt, ice cream, and soups. Use one to three tablespoons a day.

ALL-STAR RECIPES

Because the scope of this book does not allow for a lengthy recipe section, and because there are numerous other sources available with this information (see the list of Recommended Cookbooks at the end of this chapter), I will restrict my selections to a few specialty recipes, many of which have therapeutic uses and are mentioned elsewhere in the text. I have also included several others simply because they're great!

BEVERAGES AND BLENDER DRINKS

Lemon Water

1 whole lemon (organic preferred) very thinly sliced, soaked overnight in 1 to 2 quarts water. May be warmed up.

Iced or Cooled Herbal Tea

Make lemon grass tea. Let it cool, then add a splash of apple juice or mineral water and a squeeze of lemon. Make a quart or two and keep in the refrigerator. A perfect soft drink substitute. Or try lemon grass and licorice root teas brewed together and cooled. Experiment with other blends. Try Celestial Seasonings Lemon Zinger or Red Zinger, cooled.

Seed or Nut Milk

(Adapted from Hazel Richards-Griffen's *Ninety-two Years: Perfect Health in an Unpolluted Body*; see Recommended Cookbooks.)

You can use almonds, sesame or sunflower seeds, filberts, cashews, or any other raw seeds or nuts.

1. Soak seeds or nuts overnight in water. Dry and store leftovers in the refrigerator for a future drink or a chewy snack.

2. Soak several pitted dates or a small handful of raisins overnight to use as a sweetener, if desired.

3. Use ¼ to ½ cup of the soaked seeds or nuts. Grind in a blender with the soaking water (add additional water if needed to achieve desired consistency); discard the soaking water used for almonds. Add just enough dates or raisins to mildly sweeten. (You can also use fruit juice.)

4. Optional: Add ⅛ to ¼ teaspoon kelp or dulse powder.

5. Blend ingredients. Serve over cereal or as a beverage.

Fortified Health Drink

1. Blend 2 to 3 teaspoons flaxseeds into powder or use a preground health food store brand that is made with the Omegaflo™ method.

2. Add 2 to 4 tablespoons soaked seed or nut of your choice, or substitute yogurt.

3. Blend in 2 to 3 cups of water to desired consistency.

4. Then add the following optional ingredients:
   2 tablespoons plain nonfat yogurt (you can add more if not using the seed or nut base)
   ¼ to ½ teaspoon powdered kelp or dulse
   1 to 2 teaspoons rice polish or rice bran
   ¼ to 1 teaspoon rice bran syrup (if not using rice polish or rice bran)
   1 sliced apple or other fresh fruit and 1 banana (fresh or frozen)
   Berries, fresh or frozen, to taste
   1 teaspoon powdered microalgae (spirulina, blue-green algae, chlorella) or 1 to 2 tablespoons liquid chlorophyll
   1 to 3 teaspoons bee pollen
   1 to 2 teaspoons brewer's or nutritional yeast
   1 teaspoon flaxseed oil
   If more sweetness is desired, add 2 or 3 soaked, pitted dates, a small handful of soaked raisins, some fruit juice of your choice, or even a little raw honey.

5. Blend and serve.

Banana, flaxseeds, and other fiber powders will all thicken the drink, especially if you let the mixture sit a while. Use less of the nut base, more fruit, and more liquid to make the drink lighter. Experiment with lessening or deleting some items and adding more of others to suit your taste. Rice bran syrup, spirulina, and yeast all have very strong flavors and small amounts can easily alter the overall taste. Reduce their portions or leave one or more out if the taste is too strong. Try even a little bit of vanilla extract or cinnamon. Create your own favorite combination of ingredients.

Morning Tea

(Can be found commercially in health food stores as Umeshoban by Mitoku of Tokyo.)

1. Mix together 1 teaspoon kuzu powder and 1 teaspoon cold water. Mash in ⅓ of umeboshi plum (avail-

able in health food stores), then add ½ teaspoon soy sauce (tamari/shoyu) and ¼ teaspoon ginger juice.

2. Obtain ginger juice by grating washed ginger root, including skin, then squeezing grated ginger in cheese cloth. Stir well again.

3. Add hot bancha twig tea (3 to 4 ounces) until mixture starts to look clear. Stir well. Drink slowly. This beverage can often stimulate and invigorate (without caffeine).

Yogi Tea

Can be purchased premixed in health food stores. If unavailable, try the following:

1. Mix together ⅛ cup Ceylon cinnamon, ⅛ cup ginger root, 1 tablespoon whole black peppercorns, ⅛ cup green cardamom, and 1 tablespoon cloves.

2. Bring 3 cups water to a rapid boil. Add 1 tablespoon tea mixture. Let this low-boil for twenty minutes. Add 1 cup milk and return to low heat for a few minutes. Remove from heat, strain immediately, and serve with honey.

Yogi tea is said to be of great benefit during the first weeks after childbirth to help stop bleeding. It is also an energizing, tasty, and healthful drink.

SNACKS
Avocado Apple Garlic Spread

Spread mashed avocado onto a rye cracker, squeezing a little lemon on it to preserve color and enhance flavor. Sprinkle on a little salt. Add a few thin slices of garlic, then thin apple slices. Crumble a little feta cheese on top.

Rice Ball

Add lightly roasted sesame seeds to cooked rice or millet (soy sauce or tamari optional). Shape mixture into a ball or roll and pack firmly. Wrap ball in a strip of nori (available in most health food stores). Pass the nori lightly over a stove flame or electric burner before using it. The ball can be refrigerated or kept at room temperature for a good part of the day. Eat a few when you're craving a snack of some sort.

CEREALS
Rice Cream

Very nutritious and easy to digest and assimilate, this cereal is recommended for those with sensitive or recovering stomachs and intestines.

Toast (lightly brown) 1 cup brown rice in a skillet (use no oil). Grind or blend rice into a powder. Mix 5 tablespoons roasted ground rice powder with 4 cups water. Boil, add a pinch of sea salt or some kelp or dulse powder. Cover and simmer thirty minutes, stirring occasionally. Store remaining rice powder in refrigerator. Good as a breakfast cereal or at any meal; also good with vegetable soup.

Flaxseed, Fruit, and Cottage Cheese Blend

(Adapted from William L. Fischer's *How to Fight Cancer and Win*; see Suggested Reading.)

1. Layer in a bowl the following:
   2 to 3 tablespoons freshly ground flaxseeds
   1 or 2 fresh seasonal fruits, sliced or diced, and/or fresh fruit juice, to taste
   1 to 2 teaspoons of freshly ground almonds or other seeds or nuts (optional)
2. In blender, add 3 to 4 ounces cottage cheese, 1 to 2 tablespoons flaxseed oil, 1 teaspoon raw honey, 3 tablespoons nonfat milk or juice (try lemon or orange) or a combination. Blend together, adding more liquid if necessary. Try adding a banana, vanilla, cinnamon, or other ingredients for variety.
3. Add blended mixture to the ingredients in the bowl, and serve.

SOUPS
Miso Soup

Place soup pot over medium heat and add 1 teaspoon high oleic oil (olive or high oleic sunflower) or unrefined sesame oil. When oil is hot, add 1 sliced onion; stir for two to five minutes until onion is slightly transparent. Add a handful of carrot slivers. Add 5 cups of water and a pinch of sea salt, and bring to a boil. Reduce heat and simmer, covered, for twenty minutes. Remove from heat; dilute ¼ cup white or yellow miso or barley miso with about ¼ cup soup broth and stir into soup. Cover pot and allow to steep for about five minutes before serving. Miso should not be boiled, as this destroys its valuable digestion-aiding enzymes and microorganisms.

This soup is good for breakfast or with lunch or dinner. Use your choice of vegetables along with the onions, or make wakame-miso soup by adding a handful of soaked and chopped wakame seaweed instead of the carrot slivers, or substitute leeks for the onions. Shortly before serving, you can also add some chunks of tofu.

Chicken Noodle Soup

1 chemical-free cut-up chicken
8 cups water
1 bay leaf
1 to 1½ teaspoons sea salt
⅛ to ¼ teaspoon pepper (or 6 peppercorns)
½ teaspoon sage
½ teaspoon thyme
¼ cup dried parsley
Cut-up vegetables: celery, carrots, onions
1¾ cups uncooked noodles of your choice (I like
    Eden's garlic/parsley durham ribbons)

Bring chicken to a boil in medium pot with bay leaf, salt, and pepper. Simmer, covered, for thirty to forty minutes or until chicken is tender. Remove chicken from broth and refrigerate. Skim fat that forms on top of broth by cooling overnight in refrigerator or by putting in freezer compartment for one to two hours. Skin chicken and discard the skin. Remove chicken from bones and cut into bite-sized pieces. Return broth to medium heat, add cut-up vegetables, sage, and thyme, and continue cooking until vegetables are slightly tender. Then add diced chicken, parsley, and the uncooked noodles, and cook ten more minutes or until noodles are done. Season to taste.

Minestrone Soup

(From *The New Laurel's Kitchen*. Copyright © 1976, 1988 by The Blue Mountain Center of Meditation, Inc. Reprinted by permission of Ten Speed Press, Berkeley, CA; see Recommended Cookbooks.)

1 onion, finely chopped
1 to 2 cloves garlic
1½ cups chopped celery
1½ tablespoons olive oil
4 cups chopped tomatoes with juice or 1 six-ounce
    can tomato paste and 3 cups vegetable stock
2 bay leaves
1 teaspoon oregano
2 teaspoons basil
Pinch fennel seed
2 cups or more chopped carrot, zucchini, potato,
    broccoli, green beans, green pepper, cabbage,
    peas, corn, sautéed mushrooms
1 cup cooked beans: lima, kidney, pinto, black, or
    garbanzo
A handful of raw or cooked whole wheat pasta
Tender greens, cut up and ½ cup chopped parsley
Salt to taste and plenty of pepper

A richly flavored tomato-based soup that welcomes infinite variations. Begin with the tomato soup base and include any of the suggested beans and vegetables.

Sauté onion, garlic, and celery in oil until soft. Crush garlic. Add tomatoes or tomato paste, stock, and herbs. Simmer the soup gently while you prepare whatever vegetables, beans, or grains you wish to add.

At least thirty minutes before serving soup, add beans and noodles. Minestrone welcomes leftover steamed vegetables, but if you are cooking them fresh, I suggest steaming or simmering them before adding to the soup because vegetables cooked with tomato will lose their color. Incorporate the vegetable cooking water into the soup. Parsley and tender greens will keep their color and not be overcooked if you add them just a few minutes before serving. Don't count them as part of the 2 cups vegetables.

After combining all the ingredients, bring the soup to a boil, simmer briefly, and correct the seasonings. If you like, garnish each bowl with a spoonful of Parmesan cheese.

Makes about 10 cups—all to the good, because it's even better the next day. Serves six generously.

Vegetable (High-Potassium Mineral) Broth

Excellent for fasting or when solid food is not digesting well. Replenishes electrolytes. Very nutritious.

2 carrots with tops
2 beets with tops
1 onion
1 bunch parsley
2 stalks celery with leaves
Some spinach
Half bunch of watercress or any edible greens

Chop all ingredients and add to 2 quarts water. Bring to a boil, reduce heat to simmer, and cook until vegetables are soft. Use only the broth. May refrigerate for future use. Serve hot or cold.

CONDIMENTS

Raw Sauerkraut

A bushel of white and red cabbages
2 ounces juniper berries
5-gallon glazed earthenware crock with heavy lid or
    plate that fits inside the crock
1 or 2 well-washed heavy stones

Wash cabbage leaves, then thinly slice or grate them. Place the first layer at the bottom of the well-washed crock and crush the cabbage with a heavy unbreakable bottle until the juice runs out and a froth forms. This and each of the successive layers should be pressed down so that the cabbage will be saturated with its own juice. After each layer, sprinkle on some juniper berries.

Repeat these steps until the container is full. Add a few whole cabbage leaves on top. Place plate or lid within crock, on top of the layer of leaves, and weight it down with one or two heavy stones or other clean heavy weights. Store crock in a warm place (70° to 80° F), so that the fermentation process will begin. Cover with a clean cloth to protect from dust. Remember, fermenting food can emit a very strong odor, so choose the location of your processing accordingly.

Every two or three days, scoop off the scum that forms and wash the plate and stones. When the scum no longer rises, the fermentation process is finished (allow two to four weeks). Store the sauerkraut in glass jars and keep in refrigerator. Your efforts will produce many jars of this special food, which will keep for many, many months. You can experiment with the flavor by adding various layers of sliced beets, carrots, cauliflower, wakame, onions, bell peppers, and cucumbers.

SALADS

Late Summer Tomatoes with Balsamic Vinegar and Basil

(From *The Greens Cookbook* by Deborah Madison and Edward Espe Brown. Copyright © 1987 by Edward Espe Brown and Deborah Madison. Used by permission of Bantam Books, a division of Bantam Doubleday Dell Publishing Group, Inc.; see Recommended Cookbooks.)

1½ pounds juicy, vine-ripened tomatoes
4 to 5 tablespoons extra virgin olive oil
2 to 3 tablespoons fresh basil or other herbs, chopped
Salt and pepper to taste
Balsamic vinegar (or wine vinegar) to taste

Use a serrated knife to slice a plateful of tomatoes. Pour the olive oil over the tomatoes, scattering basil, and sprinkle on salt and pepper. Add vinegar to taste. If the tomatoes are going to sit for some time before serving, wait to add the salt until the last minute, as the salt will draw the juice out of the tomatoes, diminishing their flavor and texture. Serves four to six.

Lettuce/Tomato/Red Onion/Avocado Salad

Place sliced tomatoes on top of red or green leaf lettuce leaves. Thinly slice a Bermuda onion, separating the rings, and put them on top of the tomatoes.

Next, arrange slices of ripened avocado among the tomatoes and onions. Sprinkle on crumbled feta cheese and a flavorful vinaigrette dressing. (See "Salad Dressings" below.)

Apple Walnut Salad with Orange Dressing

1 large head butter or Boston lettuce, washed and carefully dried and torn into bite-sized pieces
1 large tart red apple
¾ cup broken-up walnut pieces
1 to 2 stalks celery, sliced thinly

Combine all ingredients and toss together.

Orange Dressing: In a blender, mix 1 organic orange cut up with 1 tablespoon chopped zest (peel), 2 tablespoons unrefined oil (sesame or rice bran is good), 1 tablespoon white wine vinegar, ¼ teaspoon salt, and 2 teaspoons honey. (Or try Black Swan Cygne d'Or Original Orange Dressing from Black Swan Inc. of Redmond, Washington.)

SALAD DRESSINGS

Charlyn's Honey Mustard Salad Dressing

1 teaspoon honey mustard, or use a Dijon-style mustard
2 tablespoons mayonnaise (without partially hydrogenated oil)
2 teaspoons nonfat plain yogurt
1 teaspoon balsamic vinegar
1 teaspoon rice vinegar (optional)

Combine all ingredients and mix well. Excellent for salads, dips, sandwiches (you can always use less mayonnaise and increase the yogurt to lower the fat content).

Olive Oil/Balsamic Vinegar

For 1 to 2 large servings:

2 to 3 teaspoons olive oil (extra virgin)
1 to 2 tablespoons balsamic vinegar
¼ to ½ teaspoon minced fresh or dried basil (optional)

Sesame Oil/Rice Vinegar

For 1 to 2 large servings:

2 to 3 teaspoons toasted (or plain) unrefined sesame oil
1 to 2 tablespoons rice vinegar

Tarragon Dressing

2 cloves garlic minced in garlic press
½ teaspoon dried basil
1 teaspoon tarragon
½ teaspoon dried dill
Sea salt and paprika to taste
1 tablespoon Dijon-style mustard
1 tablespoon raw honey (optional)
3 tablespoons spring water
½ cup high oleic unrefined sunflower oil, unrefined canola oil, or sesame oil
½ cup olive oil (extra virgin)
2 tablespoons apple cider vinegar
Juice of 2 lemons

Mix garlic, herbs, seasoning, mustard, honey, and water in blender for several seconds. Add oils, lemon, and vinegar and blend for a few minutes more. If a blender is not available, combine minced garlic and herbs. Mix mustard and honey in water and pour in the herbal mixture and seasonings. Slowly add the oils, stirring constantly. Add lemon and vinegar. Pour mixture into a bottle and shake vigorously. Refrigerate. Shake well before each use.

Lemon Tahini Dressing

½ cup unrefined sesame oil
3 tablespoons tahini (or sesame butter)
1 teaspoon tamari
Juice of 1 lemon
1 to 3 tablespoons water
2 tablespoons minced fresh parsley
½ cup finely chopped celery
½ cup finely chopped green pepper
¼ cup finely chopped onion
Pinch of cayenne

Combine all ingredients and blend well. Shake before using.

DIPS AND SAUCES

Tahini Mustard Miso Dip

Mix equal parts white miso and tahini, and 1 tablespoon mustard (preferably Dijon). Blend well, adding a little unrefined sesame oil and water to the desired consistency. (You can thin it more and use it as a salad dressing.) Barley (mugi) miso is fine, but use less, since the taste is very strong. Try this dip with artichokes. It's an extraordinary replacement for melted butter.

Cashew Ginger Sauce

2 cups plain, unsalted cashews that have been toasted slightly in the oven
3 cups water
2 teaspoons freshly grated gingerroot
2 teaspoons tamari/shoyu
½ teaspoon salt

Place all ingredients in blender and puree until smooth. You may need to adjust the amount of water to obtain desired consistency. Heat slowly and gently, stirring occasionally. This sauce is wonderful over steamed vegetables and rice.

Baba Ghanoush

(Use as a side dish, spread, or dip.)

3 medium eggplants
⅓ cup tahini or sesame butter
Small pinch of cayenne
½ teaspoon cumin, or more to taste
2 teaspoons finely chopped garlic
1 tablespoon olive oil
½ cup finely chopped parsley

Prick eggplants in several places with fork. Roast on rack in oven (about forty-five minutes) or until they are sagging, wrinkled, crumpled, and totally soft. Remove them carefully from the oven, wait until they're cool enough to handle. Scoop out the insides and mash well, or whir in a blender a little at a time. Combine mashed eggplant with all other ingredients, except the olive oil. Chill the Baba Ghanoush completely. Just before serving, drizzle the olive oil over the top.

Hummus

(Use as a side dish, spread, or dip.)
To 6 to 7 cups water add 2½ cups garbanzo beans. Soak overnight, then simmer two to three hours, checking occasionally to see if you need to add more water. Cook garbanzos until very soft. Measure out 4 cups beans (use leftovers in salads).
Mix in:

½ cup tahini
Juice from 1 lemon
¼ cup finely chopped green onions
12 cloves garlic mashed in a garlic press
A little olive oil
Add 1 to 2 teaspoons cumin
Sea salt to taste

Mix well or puree all ingredients together in food processor. You might need to add a little water to puree. Use sesame butter rather than tahini if you can find it.

ENTRÉES

Stuffed Acorn Squash

(From *The New Laurel's Kitchen*. Copyright © 1976, 1986 by The Blue Mountain Center of Meditation, Inc. Reprinted by permission of Ten Speed Press, Berkeley, CA; see Recommended Cookbooks.)

3 small winter squashes (acorn, delicata, or any
    other small variety of winter squash)
3 green onions, chopped
2 tablespoons oil
1 cup diced celery
1 bunch spinach, coarsely chopped
½ to 1 cup whole wheat bread crumbs tossed with
    ½ teaspoon of salt

Preheat oven to 350°. Halve and clean seeds from squash. Place cavity face down in a greased baking dish and bake for twenty-five to forty-five minutes, until tender to a fork. The time will depend on which squash you choose.

Meantime, sauté onions in oil until soft. Add chopped celery. Cover and simmer over medium heat until just tender. Add spinach; stir to wilt.

Stuff squashes with vegetable mixture. Sprinkle with salted bread crumbs. Return to oven for ten to fifteen minutes. Serves four to six, depending on size of squash.

Vegetable Almond Medley

(From *Moosewood Cookbook*. Copyright © 1977, 1992 by Mollie Katzen. Reprinted by permission of Ten Speed Press, Berkeley, CA; see Recommended Cookbooks.)

3 pounds (4 to 5 cups chopped) mixed vegetables—
    your favorites
1 cup chopped onion
2 medium cloves minced garlic
1 cup chopped almonds
2 cups water
2 tablespoons butter
1 teaspoon prepared horseradish
Dash or two of Tabasco
½ teaspoon dry mustard
1 tablespoon tamari
Topping: additional ½ cup chopped, toasted
    almonds

Steam-sauté onions and garlic in 1 tablespoon butter and a little water (about five to seven minutes), then add longer-cooking vegetables like celery to the pan, then the shorter-cooking vegetables such as zucchini, peppers, and mushrooms. They should all be tender crisp.

Toast 1 cup chopped almonds. Place in blender with water. Puree until smooth. This is "almond milk." Add seasonings and 1 tablespoon melted butter.

Combine vegetables and almond sauce and pour into oiled or buttered casserole. Sprinkle top with additional chopped almonds. Bake uncovered, at 400° for fifteen minutes.

Barbara's Three-Bean Vegetarian Chili ("Best Chili East of the West")

(From Barbara Shor, a transplanted Southwesterner in New York.)

The amounts given are for a party-sized batch—ten to twenty people—depending on how ravenous they are or how many other dishes you're adding to the board of fare. To serve six to eight, simply cut the amounts in half. However, since you're making the chili anyhow, why not make the whole amount and freeze what you don't eat in meal-sized amounts. Chili only gets better as it ages.

Beans
In a large, heavy pot add:

1 cup dry chickpeas
1 cup dry black beans
1 cup small red kidney beans
1 medium onion, peeled and quartered
5 to 6 cloves of garlic, peeled and halved
1 teaspoon salt

Add cold water at least 2 to 3 inches above the level of the beans, onion, garlic, and salt. Bring to a brisk boil. Cover, turn off the heat, and let the beans soak overnight, or at least four to six hours. After soaking, cook just until black beans are tender, as the chickpeas and kidney beans will be fairly soft after the soaking period. Check the water level from time to time to see if you need to add more. Drain after all the beans are done. Beans must be thoroughly cooked before adding to the chili mixture, because they won't get any softer in the tomato-chili sauce.

If you're in a hurry, of course, you can use two 12-ounce cans each of drained chickpeas, kidney beans, and black beans. But try the home-cooked beans at least once—the flavor will spoil you for the canned variety.

Chili
In a large heavy skillet add:

1 to 2 tablespoons of extra virgin olive oil, enough to film the bottom of the pan

1 teaspoon cumin seeds, let pop in the warming oil

Add:

2 very large or 4 medium-sized onions, coarsely chopped

6 ribs celery, coarsely chopped

6 to 8 medium carrots, scrubbed and coarsely chopped

When onions, carrots, and celery begin to soften, add:

6 medium zucchini or summer squash, scrubbed and cut into bite-sized pieces

1 pound medium mushrooms, rinsed, quartered, stems sliced

6 to 8 large cloves garlic, minced

When vegetables begin to cook but are still crisp, add:

1 2-pound, 3-ounce can of Italian peeled plum tomatoes with basil

1 2-pound can of crushed tomatoes

1 6-ounce can tomato paste

Bring to a simmer, stirring to get in all the sautéed bits. Add in the chili seasonings. Remember that once you add the beans, they will soak up a great deal of the flavor as well as the heat. The chili mixture needs to be seasoned strongly enough to withstand the beans.

Seasonings

1 cup Mecca Coffee Company Chili Mix (THE secret ingredient of this chili. It can be ordered in 1-pound bags from the Mecca Coffee Co., Inc., 1143 East 33rd Place, Tulsa, OK 74105.)

Or ¼ cup any very good, mild chili spice mix. Add more if needed. The end goal is rich flavor, not searing heat. That can be added later.

4 or more tablespoons fresh ground cumin, to taste

6 or more good shakes Tabasco sauce, to taste

1 or more small dried hot pepper, crumbled—more to taste or ½ teaspoon dried chile pequins. The smaller amounts of the chiles make a medium-hot chili; it will be mild for those who prefer flamethrowers.

2 to 4 tablespoons good soy or tamari sauce, or Worcestershire sauce, and/or 1 teaspoon tamarind sauce

Add *no salt* until you have added all the ingredients at the end of the cooking period, because the soy products to be added at the end of the cooking period are very salty.

Transfer the chili mixture to a large stew pot, big enough to hold both the vegetable mixture and the beans. An electric stewpot or crockpot is very useful for this. Add the drained beans to the chili. From time to time, check the flavor level of the seasonings to see if any more are needed. Remember, no salt until the end. Let the entire mixture simmer for another thirty minutes. Without meat, chili cooks faster, and you don't want soggy vegetables. Nevertheless, because chili improves on aging it's best to make it the day before you plan to serve it. This way all the flavors have time to meld.

After cooking is done, but before serving the chili, add:

¼ cup mild white barley miso, or a smaller amount of red soy bean miso, which will make the mixture even richer

1 pound firm tofu, cut in bite-sized pieces

Don't allow mixture to cook after adding miso or tofu. If serving the next day or freezing, do not add miso or tofu until after reheating and just before serving the chili.

Now is the time to take a final taste test of the seasonings. After you have added the miso and tofu, check to see if any additional salt is needed, or any other flavorings.

Serving Suggestions

Serve with bowls of freshly grated cheddar and finely chopped red onions.

Excellent when accompanied by hot corn bread or tortillas, as the corn and the beans form a complete protein. The miso is also very high in protein.

Soybean Bulgur Casserole

Soak ¾ cup raw soybeans in a large amount of water for at least 4 hours. Soak 1 cup raw bulgur in boiling water for fifteen minutes. (If you are avoiding wheat, use cooked millet or brown rice instead.)

2 medium green peppers, chopped

4 medium fresh tomatoes, chopped

1½ cups onion, chopped

¼ cup freshly chopped parsley

3 tablespoons tomato paste

1½ cups crumbled feta cheese

2 cloves crushed garlic

Ground cumin (to taste)

1 teaspoon basil

Dash of cayenne pepper and a dash of sea salt

Place soaked soybeans in blender with 1½ cups of water, puree. Combine pureed soybeans with soaked bulgur, or cooked rice or millet.

Steam-sauté onions and garlic in a little butter with a tablespoon or two of water. When soft, add peppers. Cook five minutes.

Combine all ingredients except feta cheese. Place in

a large buttered casserole. Bake one hour at 375° (covered, first forty-five minutes, uncovered last fifteen).

Vegetarian Taco Salad

2 3-ounce cans vegetarian refried black or pinto beans
Baked tortilla chips (no oil)
1 head leaf lettuce, torn into bite-sized pieces
1 ounce can sliced black olives
2 tomatoes, diced
3 to 4 green onions, chopped
1 avocado, cut into bite-sized pieces
½ cup shredded medium cheddar cheese
Juice of ½ lemon
Jar of salsa
Low-fat sour cream, or nonfat quark

While refried beans are heating, assemble the rest of the ingredients.

On a large platter or individual plates arrange a border of tortilla chips. Add the lettuce, olives, tomato, green onions, and avocado to form a ring inside the chips. Sprinkle with lemon juice. In the center of the salad ring, heap in the heated refried beans and sprinkle the shredded cheddar cheese on top. Serve with salsa and sour cream.

DESSERTS

Apple-Almond Cream

4 apples
2 tablespoons apple juice
1 banana
1 tablespoon honey
2 tablespoons almond meal (almonds blended into a powder)
2 tablespoons plain yogurt
¼ to ½ teaspoon almond extract

Combine peeled apples, juice, banana, and honey in blender. When smooth, add almond meal, yogurt, and extract and blend again for a few seconds. Pour into sherbet glasses and chill. Serves four.

Strawberry Cream Pie

(Adapted from Hazel Richards-Griffen's *Ninety-two Years: Perfect Health in an Unpolluted Body*; see Recommended Cookbooks.)

1. In a blender, grind into a powder the following: ⅓ to ½ cup whole oats (oat groats), ½ cup sesame seeds, ¼ cup almonds or cashews. You will need to grind each of these separately.

2. Mix the ground ingredients in a bowl. Add 1 teaspoon kelp or dulse powder or unrefined sea salt, 1 to 2 tablespoons unrefined sesame or olive oil, a few blended soaked dates or 2 tablespoons date sugar, raw honey, or pure maple syrup. Add a little water (1 to 3 tablespoons) for desired consistency.

3. Press crust into oiled glass pie plate and bake at 350° until slightly browned. When crust is cool, add freshly whipped raw cream or any whipping cream, then fresh strawberries (or frozen and thawed). Or try other seasonal fruits. Refrigerate until ready to serve.

Rice Pudding

Cook 1½ cups short-grain brown rice in 5 cups water with ⅓ cup raisins for approximately forty minutes. Mix ¼ to ⅓ cup tahini with ½ cup warm water. Mix into rice. Add 1 or 2 beaten egg yolks (optional), 1 to 2 teaspoons vanilla, ¼ teaspoon sea salt, 1 teaspoon cinnamon. Put in a casserole dish, sprinkle top with a little nutmeg if you like. For sweetness, add 2 to 3 tablespoons pure maple syrup or raw honey to the rice when you are adding the egg yolks. Bake twenty minutes at 300°.

Corn Bread

In a bowl, add ½ cup coarsely ground cornmeal, ½ to ¾ cup corn germ, ½ cup buckwheat flour, ¼ teaspoon dulse or kelp powder or salt, a little cinnamon and nutmeg (optional). Mix to blend dry ingredients. Add ¼ to ½ cup sunflower seeds (optional), ½ teaspoon vanilla extract or ⅛ teaspoon almond extract, ½ cup soaked dates or raisins, 1 beaten egg (optional), 1 to 1½ cups water, and 2 to 3 tablespoons pure maple syrup, raw honey, sucarat, date crystals (optional). Or sweeten instead with fruit concentrate and/or fruit juice in place of some of the water.

Put mixture in oiled baking pan (best not to use aluminum) and bake at 300° to 350° for thirty to forty-five minutes.

A BETTER BUTTER

Better Butter

(Adapted from *The New Laurel's Kitchen*, Laurel Robertson, Carol Flinders, and Brian Ruppenthal.)

2 cubes sweet cream butter (raw is best) softened to room temperature with wrapper on (to avoid excessive exposure to oxygen). Then remove wrapper and blend or beat butter with approximately 1 cup unrefined ex-

peller pressed oil (high oleic sunflower, unrefined sesame, extra virgin or virgin olive, rice bran, or canola). Rice bran and canola oils work the best as their tastes are very mild (and therefore allow the butter taste to prevail). However, rice bran oil is difficult to find "unrefined." Put mixture in an old margarine tub or other container that has a tight-fitting lid and always keep covered and refrigerated when not in use.

Optional additions to the recipe are:
- ¼ teaspoon lecithin
- 2 tablespoons water
- 2 tablespoons dry skim milk powder
- ½ teaspoon sea salt (omit salt if your butter is already salted)

RECOMMENDED COOKBOOKS

Colbin, Annemarie. *The Book of Whole Meals: A Seasonal Guide to Assembling Balanced Vegetarian Breakfasts, Lunches, and Dinners.* New York: Ballantine, 1983.

Diamond, Marilyn. *The American Vegetarian Cookbook from the Fit for Life Kitchen.* New York: Warner Books, 1990.

Esko, Edward and Wendy. *Macrobiotic Cooking for Everyone.* New York: Japan Publications, 1980.

Gerras, Charles, ed. *Rodale's Basic Natural Foods Cookbook.* New York: Fireside/Simon & Schuster, 1984.

Hurd, Frank, and Hurd, Rosalie. *Ten Talents Cookbook.* Available from Box 86A, Route 1, Chisholm, MN 55719.

Jensen, Bernard. *Vital Foods for Total Health.* Available from 24360 Old Wagon Road, Escondido, CA 92027.

Katzen, Mollie. *Moosewood Cookbook.* Berkeley, CA: Ten Speed Press, 1977.

——. *The Enchanted Broccoli Forest.* Berkeley, CA: Ten Speed Press, 1982.

——. *Still Life with Menu Cookbook.* Berkeley, CA: Ten Speed Press, 1988.

Kilham, Christopher S. *The Bread and Circus Whole Food Bible: How to Select and Prepare Safe and Healthful Foods Without Pesticides or Chemical Additives.* Reading, MA: Addison Wesley, 1991.

Lappé, Frances Moore. *Diet for a Small Planet*, 10th ed. New York: Ballantine, 1986.

Madison, Deborah, and Brown, Edward Espe. *The Greens Cookbook.* New York: Bantam, 1987.

Ornish, Dean, M.D. *Eat More, Weigh Less.* New York: HarperCollins, 1993.

Richards-Griffen, Hazel S. *Ninety-two Years: Perfect Health in an Unpolluted Body.* Available from Survival Ministries, 4415 Semoran Farms Road, Kissimmee, Florida 34744 or 10249 Coachilla Canals Road, Niland, CA 92257.

Robertson, Laurel, Flinders, Carol, and Ruppenthal, Brian. *The New Laurel's Kitchen.* Berkeley, CA: Ten Speed Press, 1986.

Stone, Sally and Martin. *The Brilliant Bean.* New York: Bantam, 1988.

Thorpe, Susan, N.D., D.O. *Four Seasons Vegetarian Cook Book.* New York: Thorsons, 1986.

Wigmore, Ann, N.D. *Recipes for Life.* Available from Hippocrates Institute, 25 Exeter Street, Boston, MA 92116.

——. *The Hippocrates Diet and Health Program.* Wayne, NJ: Avery, 1984.

SUGGESTED READING

Brown, Royden. *The World's Perfect Food.* Prescott, AZ: Hohm Press, 1993.

Budwig, Johanna, M.D. *Flax Oil as a True Aid Against Arthritis, Heart Infection, Cancer, and Other Diseases.* Vancouver: Apple, 1992.

Fischer, William, L. *How to Fight Cancer and Win.* Burnaby, B.C., Canada: Alive Books, 1987.

PART THREE

THE TEN COMMON DENOMINATORS OF ILLNESS

NUTRITIONAL DEFICIENCIES

OVERFED, UNDERNOURISHED: THE WISDOM OF SUPPLEMENTATION

Nutritional deficiencies are extraordinarily prevalent in the current American diet.[1] Despite consuming a sufficient amount of proteins, carbohydrates, and fats, individuals often develop vitamin and mineral deficiencies that trigger a host of ailments and diseases. In Chapter Three, I discussed nutrient loss from food refining and processing. In addition to this concern, some health practitioners and investigators maintain that even whole foods grown in this country's soils cannot supply all the micronutrients we need to stay healthy. There's little question in their minds about the importance and necessity of adding nutritional supplements to our diet. The issue is no longer whether, but how best, to supplement.

JEREMY

Jeremy, a forty-eight-year-old philosophy professor, suffered from recurrent muscle spasms in his upper back, high blood pressure, a heart rhythm disturbance, high blood cholesterol, and mild insomnia. His doctor prescribed various muscle relaxers periodically, blood pressure medication twice a day, an antiarrhythmic drug, and sleeping pills. Jeremy didn't take the sleeping pills because they made him too groggy in the morning. The antiarrhythmic medication left him depressed and constipated, and the blood pressure drug robbed him of his libido. Jeremy's main request was to be freed of all these medications.

In reviewing his diet, I realized that Jeremy, like most Americans, consumed inadequate amounts of magnesium. He was marginal in many other nutrients as

well, but his ailments fit perfectly the picture of magnesium deficiency. Magnesium is a natural calcium channel blocker; it prevents an excessive muscle-contracting action of calcium, whether the muscles are in the back, the bronchioles (air passages in the lungs), the coronary arteries, or the heart. For Jeremy's condition, I recommended a daily intake of 800 milligrams of a very absorbable form of magnesium.

Over a period of six weeks Jeremy was able to taper both his blood pressure and antiarrhythmic medications. And with the calcium supplement I eventually suggested, he seemed to experience fewer back spasms, and his insomnia problem even began to lessen.

DETERMINING YOUR SUPPLEMENT NEEDS

There are a number of preventive nutritional measures you can undertake beyond establishing a whole-foods diet. Food supplementation is perhaps the most common and the most diverse. It covers the following four categories: (1) general preventive, (2) symptom- or ailment-directed, (3) susceptibility-directed, and (4) laboratory-directed.

A general preventive/maintenance approach usually employs a broad-spectrum multiple vitamin/mineral formula, which is used to cover suspected nutritional deficiencies resulting from poor food quality and poor eating patterns.

By matching your symptoms and ailments with the associated nutrients in the Symptom Survey for Nutritional Deficiencies (see page 122), you may be able to determine specific nutrient needs. In some cases, these associations may not strictly designate a deficiency. The recommended nutrient may act instead as a therapeutic

REASONS FOR USING SUPPLEMENTS

1. *Nutritional deficiencies in the U.S. food supply*: Suboptimal food quality begins with the agricultural practices that have been compromising soil health and depleting its minerals for decades. Nutrients lacking in the soil cannot possibly be present in the food. There has been a documented steady decline in the mineral content of both soils and whole foods over the last half century.[2] Other factors include premature harvesting, extended storage and shipping, food additives, and less-than-ideal storage and preparation by consumers.[3]

2. *Environmental stress*: We are deluged with environmental pollutants—herbicides, pesticides, exhaust fumes and particulates, industrial chemicals and wastes, household and office chemicals, formaldehyde, hydrocarbon-based synthetics, recirculating air systems, microwave radiation and other electromagnetic disturbances, and noise! All of these environmental stresses place heavy demands on our bodies' nutrient reserves, antioxidant arsenals, and detoxification systems. Our nutrient needs are greatly increased by such common exposures.

3. *The inadequacy of the RDAs*: The Recommended Dietary Allowance (RDA) established by the federal government for most nutrient needs of people today were initially set in the 1940s. For the limited nutrients that are considered, the intention was, and still is, to prevent a disease due to a deficiency of a corresponding nutrient. Although the standards have been revised in recent years and have an alleged margin of safety for many nutrient levels, the RDAs are set only to prevent gross deficiency diseases like scurvy, beriberi, or pellagra—which are rare. RDAs are not established to help prevent cancer, heart disease, or many of our most common serious illnesses. The standards, in general, are set too low. In addition, they do not compensate adequately for nutrient-depleting agricultural and food-handling practices, current environmental stressors, or biochemical individuality.[4]

One aspect of the latter pertains to nutrient absorption. It is an established medical fact, for example, that 50 percent of individuals over fifty years old consistently show a marked decline in stomach hydrochloric acid secretion.[5] This deficiency causes not only protein maldigestion but diminished absorption of many essential minerals, such as iron, calcium, and manganese. With each advancing decade the percentage of hydrocholoric acid deficiency rises, increasing nutrient malabsorption. Some RDA nutrient levels cannot begin to meet the needs of the elderly.

agent for the respective symptom/ailment. For example, recurrent bouts of colds and flu may not indicate a vitamin C deficiency. However, extra vitamin C, as a therapeutic agent, may help prevent colds and flu. Many of the listed symptoms and ailments also benefit from other therapeutic modalities. One last qualifier about matching nutrient needs to symptoms: Simply treating the symptoms with a vitamin may not necessarily be the wisest course of action; in the long run it may prove more beneficial to look for an underlying cause.

Once you understand the limitations and qualifications of such a symptom survey, you can use it in context. Read on for a discussion of the recommended nutrient doses for specific ailments. Chapter Seventeen

provides more in-depth discussion and a reference guide for your particular ailments. The Master Symptom Survey in Chapter Two can lead you to underlying conditions discussed in greater detail in Part Three. The index at the end of the book can also guide you.

By knowing what ailments and diseases you are susceptible to, you can plan a logical preventive program using nutrients. For instance, if you are interested in preventing osteoporosis, you will learn in Chapter Seventeen that you should ensure an adequate intake of calcium, magnesium, zinc, copper, manganese, boron, vitamin K, and silicon. If you are concerned about heart disease or stroke, you will learn, again in Chapter Seventeen, that you should monitor your intake of vitamins

C, E, B-6, magnesium, essential fatty acids, chromium, and selenium. In your efforts to establish any preventive program, I advise that you enlist the help of a nutritionally oriented health professional.

If your medical conditions necessitate more objective documentation, you can obtain a laboratory diagnosis of nutrient deficiencies. I often order a few select tests specific to a patient's complaints but do not routinely arrange for comprehensive nutritional profiles—they are expensive and sometimes rather involved. Instead, I evaluate an individual's nutritional intake and digestive capacity, as well as symptoms and susceptibilities, and recommend the foods and supplements that are indicated.

The following table lists several nutrients and the methods of laboratory diagnosis that best assess their status. As some of these methods are not available through standard laboratories, I have listed several labs that your doctor can contact.

SUGGESTED LABORATORY TESTS OF NUTRIENT STATUS

NUTRIENT	TEST
Vitamin A	Serum level, also dark adaptation test
Beta-carotene	Serum level
Vitamin B-1	Erythrocyte (red blood cell) transketolase; lymphocyte growth response
Vitamin B-2	Erythrocyte glutathione reductase; lymphocyte growth response
Vitamin B-3	Urinary 1 N-methyl nictotinamide; lymphocyte growth response
Vitamin B-5	Lymphocyte growth response
Vitamin B-6	Erythrocyte glutamic oxalo-acetic transaminase; lymphocyte growth response
Vitamin B-12	Methylmalonic acid assay; elevated mean corpuscular volume; lymphocyte growth response; serum level unreliable unless the result is abnormally low: successful therapeutic trial (resolution of symptoms by an intramuscular injection of the nutrient)
Folic acid	Neutrophilic segmentation index; serum level reliable only if low; RBC folate may be most accurate
Vitamin C	Urinary concentration
Vitamin D	Serum level
Vitamin E	Serum level
Vitamin K	Whole blood or red blood cell content; prothrombin time
Calcium	Lymphocyte growth response; sublingual cell smears; white blood cell content (lymphocytes, leukocytes, platelets), as well as plasma and urine; hair analysis
Magnesium	White or red blood cell content; magnesium retention test; lymphocyte growth response; sublingual cell smears; serum is unreliable unless abnormally low
Potassium	Whole blood, sublingual cell smears; serum is unreliable unless level is abnormally low
Zinc	White blood cell content; lymphocyte growth response; zinc sulfate 7 hydrate taste test; hair analysis only if results are abnormally low
Copper	Red blood cell level, ceruloplasm
Chromium	Hair analysis
Manganese	Whole blood, lymphocyte content
Iron	Serum ferritin level
Selenium	Glutathione peroxidase functional assay
Molybdenum	Urinary sulfates/sulfites
Essential fatty acids	Red blood cell membrane
Essential amino acids	Urine or plasma
Protein	Serum prealbumin, retinol binding protein

For more information on nutritional laboratory tests, contact:

Doctor's Data, Inc., P.O. Box 111, 30 W. 101 Roosevelt Rd., West Chicago, IL 60185, (800) 323-2784

IntraCellular Diagnostics Inc., 533 Pilgrim Drive, Suite B, Commerce Park, Foster City, CA 94404, (415) 349-5233 (sublingual cell smears)

Liberty Testing Laboratory, 1176 Liberty St., Brooklyn, NY, (718) 647-7080

Meridian Valley Clinical Laboratory, 24030 132nd Ave., S.E., Kent, WA 98042, (800) 234-6825

Metametrix Medical Research Laboratory, 3000 Northwoods Pkwy., Suite 150, Norcross, GA 30071, (404) 446-5483

Monroe Medical Research Laboratory, Route 17, P.O. Box I, Southfields, NY 10975, (914) 351-5134

Omegatech, P.O. Box 1, Troutdale, VA 24378, (800) 437-8888

Physicians Clinical Laboratories, 15613 Bellevue Redmond Rd., Bellevue, WA 98008, (206) 881-2446

Spectra Cell Laboratories, 515 Post Oak Blvd., Suite 80, Houston, TX 77027, (800) 227-5227 (lymphocyte growth response)

Wholesale Nutrition, Box 3345, Saratoga, CA 95070, (800) 325-2664 (vitamin C strips)

SYMPTOM SURVEY FOR NUTRITIONAL DEFICIENCIES

Many of the symptoms and conditions listed here are related directly to a deficiency of the specific nutrient and will improve with nutrient supplementation. Some, however, may not strictly be a result of the deficiency, but rather, associated with it. For example, I have listed low stomach acid under vitamin B-12 because it commonly coexists with B-12 deficiency. However, B-12 deficiency does not cause low stomach acid, nor will B-12 supplementation ameliorate the condition. But if you learn that you have either one of these conditions, this table will alert you to consider the possibility of also having the other.

VITAMIN A/BETA-CAROTENE

Bumps on the backs of arms and elsewhere	Diminished salivation
Pimple-like red spots at the base of hair follicles on thighs	Dry, hard skin
	Headaches
Night blindness/poor night vision	Dull, lusterless hair
	Rigid nails that peel easily
Recurrent colds and infections	Low white blood cell count
Sinus problems	Diminished fertility in women
Acne	Loss of sense of smell
	Loss of appetite

Achy, tired, burning, itchy eyes	Epithelial cancers (skin, lungs, gastrointestinal, genitourinary)
Dry eyes	
Inflamed eyelids	
Eyeball pain	Drugs associated with deficiency: cholestyramine, mineral oil, neomycin, oral contraceptives, colchicine
Vitamin E deficiency	
Hypothyroidism	
Diabetes	

B-COMPLEX VITAMINS IN GENERAL

Fatigue	Nausea
Depression	Tongue changes (reddened, stippled, coated, cracked, scalloped, glossy)
Nervousness	
Sleep disturbance	
Loss of appetite	

B-1 (THIAMINE)

Depression	Indigestion
Insomnia	Diarrhea or constipation
Numbness or burning in feet or hands	
	Poor appetite
Apathy	Oversensitivity to pain
Confusion	Low blood pressure
Emotional instability	Fatigue
Irritability	Alcoholism
Weight loss	Drugs associated with deficiency: oral contraceptives
Oversensitivity to noise	
Headache	

B-2 (RIBOFLAVIN)

Trembling	Bloodshot, watery eyes
Dizziness	Oily, scaly skin
Insomnia	Scaling around nose, mouth, forehead, ears
Mental sluggishness	
Purplish/magenta tongue	Whiteheads
Cracks in corners of mouth and lips	Prominence of surface blood vessels
Chapped lips	Sensitivity to light
Progressively smaller upper lip	Hair loss
	Loss of eyebrows
Watery eyes	Alcoholism
Eyelids crusted	

B-3 (NIACIN/NIACINAMIDE/ NICOTINIC ACID)

Pellagra	Abdominal pain
Diarrhea	Constipation
Dermatitis (skin changes: initially dry, scaly, coarse, and wrinkled; becoming red, itchy, and burning, then tense, swollen, atrophied, and brown)	Tongue changes: tip reddened (engorged with blood), taste buds enlarged, tongue appears stippled; becoming white-coated, with deep midline crevices and cracks, then red and swollen with scalloped margins; taste buds atrophied
Dementia (apprehensions, fears, delusions, hallucinations)	
General and mental fatigue	
Irritability	Sore mouth, swollen and painful gums

Feelings of anxiety, anger, gloom
Depression
Insomnia
Loss of appetite
Inability to concentrate
Headaches
Loss of strength, muscle weakness
Burning sensations over body
Nausea and vomiting
Dizziness
Migraines
Acne

Low hydrochloric acid secretion: poor nutrient absorption, gas, and foul-smelling stools
Osteoarthritis
High blood cholesterol
Coronary artery disease
Peripheral vascular disease
Menière's disease
High blood pressure
Drugs associated with deficiency: isoniazid, tetracycline

B-5 (PANTOTHENIC ACID)

Fatigue
Insomnia
Sullenness
Depression
Adrenal exhaustion
Low blood pressure
Teeth grinding

Frequent respiratory infections
Loss of appetite
Constipation
Burning sensation in feet
Allergies

B-6 (PYRIDOXINE)

Nervousness
Mood swings
Depression
Insomnia
Hypoglycemia
Water retention
Dandruff
Oily scales at the scalp, eyebrows, around nose and ears
Seborrhea
Numbness
Cramping in arms and legs
Mouth and tongue cracked and sore
Morning nausea
Iron-resistant anemia
Premenstrual syndrome
Morning sickness with pregnancy
Fatigue
Arteriosclerosis

Arthritis
Osteoarthritis, especially with nodules on distal joints of fingers
Eczema
Kidney stones
Acne
Fibrocystic breast disease
Autism
Neuritis
Asthma
Diabetes
Muscle twitches
Carpal tunnel syndrome
Learning disorders
Drugs associated with deficiency: estrogen, hydrazines, hydralazine, oral contraceptives, cycloserine, L-Dopa, isoniazid, d-penicillamine

B-12 (COBALAMIN)

Fatigue
Apathy
Nervousness
Mood swings
Depression
Paranoia
Hallucinations
Difficulty concentrating
Difficulty learning

Confusion
Tongue changes: reddened tip but smooth and without bumps on tips or sides; shiny red
Mean corpuscular volume (a red blood cell parameter) 95 or higher

Megaloblastic anemia
Bursitis
Calcific tendonitis
Poor memory
Asthma (especially exertional)
Low stomach acid
Plantar spurs
Sciatica
Alcoholism

Drugs associated with deficiency: cholestyramine, clofibrate, chloramphenicol, colchicine, cycloserine, para-amino salicylic acid, potassium chloride, phenytoin/dilantin, triamterene, trimethoprim, neomycin, oral contraceptives

FOLIC ACID/FOLICIN/FOLATE

Fatigue
Depression
Disorientation
Confusion
Poor memory
Apathy
Withdrawal
Irritability
Slowing of mental processes
Decreased stomach acid
Decreased integrity of intestinal mucosa
Malabsorption
Diarrhea
Scaling of lips
Anemia
Low white blood cell count

Tongue sore and cracked
Cracks in corners of mouth
Decreased resistance to disease
Cervical dysplasia
Colon cancer prevention in those with colitis
Alcoholism
Drugs associated with deficiency: phenytoin, dilantin, mysoline, estrogen, oral contraceptives, tetracycline, triamterene, trimethoprim, methotrexate, aspirin, cholestyramine, cycloserine, pyrimethamine, sulfasalazine

VITAMIN C (ASCORBIC ACID)

Frequent colds
Fatigue
Listlessness
Lassitude
Confusion
Depression
Anxiety
Haggard, frowning, pained expression
Easy bruising
Bleeding gums or spongy, puffy congested gums
Petechiae (tiny skin hemorrhages)
Nosebleeds
Varicose veins
Aneurysms
Arteriosclerosis
Loss of appetite
Breathlessness
Anemia
Fleeting joint and limb pains
Loose teeth
Poor wound healing
High blood cholesterol
Hepatitis

Mononucleosis
Pneumonia
Malignant and benign tumors
Heavy metal toxicity
Drug toxicity
Drug, alcohol, tobacco, and sugar withdrawal
Food allergy/addiction withdrawal
Spinal disk problems
Back problems
Fractures
Schizophrenia
Substances and conditions that increase one's need for vitamin C: cigarette smoking, air pollution, chronic stress
Drugs associated with deficiency: oral contraceptives, estrogen, aspirin, steroids
Treatments whose outcomes are ameliorated by and side effects tenuated with vitamin C: radiation, chemotherapy

BIOFLAVONOIDS

Easy bleeding (cuts, nosebleeds, gums)
Easy bruising
Habitual and threatened miscarriages
Heavy and prolonged menstrual bleeding
Hemorrhoids
Varicose veins
Allergies
Eczema
Asthma
Arteriosclerosis

VITAMIN D

Poor absorption of calcium and phosphorus
Poor bone and tooth formation
Soft bones (osteomalacia) and teeth
Bone pain
Muscle weakness
Symptoms of calcium deficiency (see page 133)
Drugs associated with deficiency: cholestyramine, glutethimide, mineral oil, neomycin, dilantin

VITAMIN E (TOCOPHEROLS)

Infertility
Miscarriages
Menopausal symptoms (hot flashes, atrophic vaginitis)
Fibrocystic breast disease
Fatigue
Nervousness
Insomnia
Shortness of breath
Heart palpitations
Elevated serum cholesterol
Heart attack
Arteriosclerosis
Peripheral vascular disease/ claudication
Thrombophlebitis
Thrombosis
Pulmonary embolism
Anemia
Tendonitis
Muscle cramps
Accelerated aging
Burns, scarring, scar contracture
Intestinal malabsorption (celiac sprue, cystic fibrosis, chronic diarrhea)
Skin ulcers
Gangrene
Air pollution
Drugs associated with vitamin E deficiency: oral contraceptives
Treatment side effects lessened by vitamin E: radiation and chemotherapy
Substances that increase one's needs for vitamin E: air pollution, cigarette smoke, polyunsaturated oils, and ultraviolet light
Drugs associated with deficiency: cholestyramine, mineral oil, neomycin

VITAMIN K

Easy bleeding and bruising
Bleeding disorders
Nausea during pregnancy
Osteoporosis
Drugs associated with deficiency: antibiotics, anticoagulants, cholestyramine, mineral oil

CALCIUM

Muscle twitching
Muscle cramps, especially calves and back
Lower backaches
Depression
Irritability
Nervousness
Anxiety
Osteoporosis
Menstrual cramps
Brittle nails
Periodontitis
Dental caries
Arthritis

Drugs associated with deficiency: cholestyramine, neomycin, dilantin/phenytoin, tetracycline
Memory impairment
Insomnia
High blood pressure

MAGNESIUM

Twitching
Tremors
Increased sensitivity to noise
Fatigue
Depression
Grouchiness
Nervousness
Tension
Insomnia
Premenstrual syndrome, especially depression
Hyperactivity
Convulsions
Kidney stones
High blood pressure
Diabetes mellitus
Rapid or irregular heartbeat
Failing or weak heart
Diminished metabolic efficiency of the heart
Coronary artery spasm
Angina
Heart attack
Increased platelet adhesiveness
Esophageal spasms
Skeletal muscle spasms from injury or trauma
Menstrual cramps
Gangrene
Eclampsia of pregnancy
Lead toxicity
Alcoholism
Drugs associated with deficiency: cycloserine, furosemide, thiazide, hydrochlorothiazide, other diuretics, tetracycline, oral contraceptives

ZINC

Dwarfism, small stature
Mental retardation
Stretch marks on skin
Dark, excessively pigmented skin
White spots on nails
Poor growth of hair and nails
Hair splits and breaks easily
Cracks in skin of fingertips or behind the ears
Slow or poor wound healing
Delayed menstruation
Irregular menses
Male impotence
Underdeveloped or delay in development of sexual organs
Growing pains
Disturbed sense of taste/smell
Diminished immune status
Chemical hypersensitivity
Allergic swelling of nasal and eustachian tubes
Oily skin
Hair loss
Lack of appetite
Lethargy
Acne
Eczema
Prostatic hypertrophy
Night blindness unresponsive to vitamin A
Low thyroid status
Diabetes
Schizophrenia
Alcoholism
Drugs associated with deficiency: steroids, furosemide, oral contraceptives

COPPER

Iron-resistant anemia
Reduced childhood growth
Pathologic fracture in infants
Decreased immune status
Mental symptoms/decreased levels of neurotransmitters
Failure in myelination
High blood cholesterol
Reduced pigment in hair and skin
Cardiac and connective tissue defects
Arteriosclerosis
Cardiac arrhythmias
Abnormal glucose tolerance, especially diabetes

CHROMIUM

Diabetes
Hypoglycemia
High blood cholesterol
and triglycerides

Aneurysms
Arteriosclerosis
Craving for sweets

MANGANESE

Frequent injuries of
cartilage, ligaments, tendons in joints, back, neck
Slow healing of above
Arthritis

Persistent or recurring back or
neck problems
Diabetes
Tardive dyskinesia
Osteoporosis

IRON

Anemia
Fatigue
Crankiness
Behavioral problems
Inattention
Learning problems
Poor school performance
Depression
Dizziness
Diarrhea
Brittle, lusterless, flat-
tened, or spoon-shaped
nails

Vertical ridges on nails
Swollen ankles
Abnormal hair loss
Increased susceptibility to
infections
Heavy, prolonged, or frequent
menstruation
Pregnancy
Drugs associated with defi-
ciency: cholestyramine,
clofibrate, neomycin,
sulfasalazine, tetracycline

POTASSIUM

Muscle weakness, fatigue
Cardiac fatigue
Weak, slow pulse
Heart rhythm abnormalities
Constipation
Muscle cramps
Poor appetite

Mental apathy
Drugs associated with deficiency: aldactone, colchicine, steroids, furosemide,
and other diuretics, penicil-
lin

SELENIUM

Cardiomyopathy,
weakness and failure of
heart muscle
Heart attack
Free radical injury

Diminished immune
status
Osgood Schlatter's disease
Increased susceptibility
to chemical hypersensitivity

ESSENTIAL FATTY ACIDS

Heart attack
Stroke
Cancer
Arthritis
High blood pressure
Depression
Schizophrenia

Dry skin
Eczema
Brittle nails
Decreased fertility
Premenstrual and other men-
strual disorders

ESSENTIAL AMINO ACIDS IN GENERAL

Fatigue
Lethargy
Apathy
Weakness
Depression
Hypoglycemic tendency
Poor or slow healing

Edema (water retention)
Skin lesions
Weight loss (muscle and
fat)
Liver damage
Depigmentation of hair

VITAMINS AND MINERALS FOR GENERAL PREVENTIVE PURPOSES

If you have no specific ailments or susceptibilities but want to feel better generally or simply take supplements for preventive measures, consider the following multiple vitamin-mineral formula:

Vitamin A: up to 10,000 I.U.
Beta-carotene: up to 15,000 I.U.
B-1: up to 100 milligrams
B-2: up to 50 milligrams
B-3 (niacin/niacinamide): up to 150 milligrams
B-5 (pantothenic acid): up to 500 milligrams
B-6: up to 50 milligrams
B-12: up to 500 micrograms
Folic acid: up to 800 micrograms
Biotin: up to 400 micrograms
Choline: up to 100 milligrams
Inositol: up to 100 milligrams
PABA (para-aminobenzoic acid): up to 100 milli-
grams
Vitamin C: up to 1,200 milligrams
Bioflavonoids: up to 500 milligrams
Vitamin D: 50–200 I.U.
Vitamin E: up to 400 I.U.
Calcium: up to 500 milligrams
Magnesium: up to 500 milligrams
Potassium: up to 100 milligrams
Copper: up to 3 milligrams
Manganese: up to 20 milligrams
Zinc: up to 30 milligrams
Iodine: up to 150 micrograms
Chromium: up to 200 micrograms
Selenium: up to 250 micrograms
Molybdenum: up to 500 micrograms
Vanadium: up to 200 micrograms
Boron: up to 3 milligrams

Up to 18 milligrams of iron is included in most multiple vitamin/mineral formulas, which is a mistake. Generally speaking, iron should be taken only by those
adults who have documented low iron stores, or a sus-

ceptibility to such, and by pregnant, lactating, or menstruating women. If you do not fit these categories, you should probably not take any supplemental iron, either in a multiple or separately (see discussion of iron, page 137). If you have a documented copper excess, find a copper-free multiple. Some multiples will also include herbs, sea vegetation, spirulina (or other algae), bee pollen, barley grass, and other high-nutrient elements, which I feel are useful if no allergy to them exists.

The amounts above are considered megadoses by conservative standards—at least several of the nutrients (mostly B vitamins) are fifty times the RDA. These doses are potent, but not excessive. Such formulas are offered in capsule or tablet form, one or two taken three times a day. By comparison, a standard multiple vitamin with recommended RDA levels would be taken once a day and would feature drastically scaled-down amounts for the B vitamins (1 or 2 milligrams each) and most of the minerals. Many of the generic supplements available in drugstores and supermarkets do not contain even half of the minerals listed above.

Which Potency Is Right for You?

When I feel that an individual is fairly depleted nutritionally, I suggest a high-dose multiple. If significant improvement occurs, I recommend staying at the same dose for several months. After this, I usually suggest a multiple with 20 to 50 milligrams a day of B-complex vitamins. If there is a letdown, I suggest staying at the higher dose a while longer, then tapering again.

High-dose supplement therapy, however, is not meant to be more than a temporary measure—up to a year, if necessary. Once treatments of underlying disorders and dietary and lifestyle changes have raised the level of health sufficiently, such megadoses are often unnecessary. I believe in the long-term preventive value of vitamin/mineral supplements, and I suggest using a multiple similar to the formula above, but with low to moderate potency B vitamins (20 to 50 milligrams a day). If you do not believe in taking vitamins, then be sure to maintain a whole-foods, balanced diet (see Chapters Three and Four) and frequently include "All Star" foods and foods that are especially high in nutrients (see Chapter Five). For city dwellers or anyone exposed to significant car exhaust fumes and other pollutants, I suggest at least an antioxidant formula (see page 58).

Most vitamins are water soluble, and quantities more than the body can use will be excreted, usually harmlessly, in the urine. Is it therefore pointless to take more than the body needs? According to the thinking of orthomolecular medicine, to give the body sufficient nutrients many individuals need saturation levels, which inevitably lead to some "spill-over."

Vitamins A, D, E, and K are fat soluble and are stored in the body. They can reach toxic levels if taken in excessive quantities, but the amounts in multiple vitamin/mineral preparations are generally safe when taken according to label recommendations. (One exception may be vitamin D; see discussion on page 135.)

Some Adverse Effects

Although natural to the body, high and concentrated doses of water-soluble vitamins may cause some problems. For example, 1,500 to 3,000 milligrams a day of vitamin B-3 (nicotinic acid, niacin, or niacinamide) for several months can cause temporary inflammation of the liver in a small percentage of individuals.[6] It's advisable to have your physician monitor your liver function. Be on the lookout for such liver symptoms as nausea, poor appetite, fatigue/malaise, abdominal discomfort, very dark urine, and yellowing of the skin. Discontinuing the B-3 will reverse the inflammation and the symptoms.

Niacinamide is used to treat anxiety, depression, and osteoarthritis; niacin to lower cholesterol levels and to treat anxiety and some forms of schizophrenia.

Niacin can cause temporary diffuse itching, heat sensation, and redness of the skin. This is a harmless reaction attributed to the dilation of small arterioles, a desired effect, which can occur at low doses (25 to 50 milligrams) if you have never supplemented with this vitamin before. It may require much higher doses (up to 1,000 milligrams) if you have. Although timed-release niacin preparations produce less "flush," some reports have implicated them in cases of serious liver inflammation and have suggested that they be avoided.[7] Preparations utilizing niacin esters (inositol hexaniacinate) do not cause the flush and appear to be safe.

Another example of adverse reactions to megadoses is vitamin B-6, which may induce temporary and reversible peripheral nerve symptoms of tingling and numbness.[8] This finding has been reported usually when B-6 is taken in very large doses (over 500 milligrams a day) for many months, and without other B vitamins. Such side effects rarely occur in daily doses of 100 milligrams or less along with the whole B complex.

Many individuals find that B-complex vitamins boost their energy while calming their nerves and improving sleep. In some rare cases, they can cause sleep difficulties. If this happens to you, take your Bs earlier in the day. In a very small percentage of cases, high doses of B-complex vitamins can cause severe restlessness and agitation at any time, whether taken in the morning or at night. However, with a little common sense, B-complex vitamins can be used safely.

Unless you have been diagnosed with a vitamin dependency, megadoses of B-complex vitamins (100 milligrams or more) for extended periods of time are probably not necessary. By paying attention to your diet and lifestyle and by treating any hidden ailments you may have, you should be able to reduce your B-complex to low (10 to 25 milligrams) or moderate (25 to 50 milligrams) daily doses. If you cannot function well on less than 100 milligrams a day of B-complex vitamins, and there are no underlying conditions to explain such a need, staying on such a dose is unlikely to cause any problems.

Some individuals with mental or behavioral disorders require extremely large doses of vitamins to control or manage their symptoms. For example, because of metabolic defects, autistic children and adults seem to require high doses of vitamin B-6 (500 to 1,000 milligrams a day).[9] If these doses are discontinued, mental and behavioral deterioration will occur within days. Most of us, however, can benefit from reducing vitamin doses. Though high doses under certain circumstances can be helpful and sometimes even necessary, incessant and unnecessary overloading may not be wise.

Periodic Discontinuance

It might be a good idea periodically to discontinue or at least reduce the dosage of your vitamin and mineral supplements for one or two days a week when you have fewer demands and responsibilities, and perhaps for one or more weeks every three to four months, especially when you're on a vacation or in a quieter, cleaner, less stressful environment. This is not indicated if you have an ailment, susceptibility, or lifestyle that demands continual use of certain high-dose supplements.

If you have never experimented with periodic discontinuance or reduced dosage, give it a try and see if you continue to feel healthy. In the past, I have grown enamored of certain supplements because of the initial benefit they brought me and continued to take them zealously. When, inadvertently, I discontinued them, I often found that I felt just as healthy without them—in some cases, even better. What works well at one period of your life may not be appropriate on a sustained, long-term basis; in fact, prolonged use may even create an imbalance. After a condition or ailment has stabilized or improved with the help of megadose supplements, you may no longer require the same high doses to maintain your health.

If you are being treated by a nutritionally oriented health professional, have a discussion about this particular issue. Your body, however, will usually let you know what is best for you. If you intend to discontinue megadoses, it is best, for vitamin C at least, to taper off gradually. For example, if you regularly take 10 grams of vitamin C a day, it is wise to decrease the dose by 1 or 2 grams every few days. Tapering is generally unnecessary for nutrients if you are on more moderate doses.

Synthetic/Natural/Whole-Food Concentrates

Most vitamins are synthetic even if their labels say "natural." A small percentage of the actual natural vitamin might be included. However, the bulk will usually be synthetic, especially with B-complex and C vitamins. The size and cost of "all-natural" 50- or 100-milligram B-complex tablets or 1,000-milligram vitamin C tablets would be prohibitive. For example, according to Dr. Michael Colgin, in *Your Personal Vitamin Profile*, a 1,000-milligram tablet of vitamin C made entirely of rose hips would weigh nine pounds. A year's supply of vitamin C tablets made entirely of acerola would cost $1,380. A 200-milligram niacin (vitamin B-3) tablet made entirely from yeast would, according to Colgin, weigh one pound.[10]

The body recognizes and uses molecules of most synthetic vitamins, so do not be excessively purist about this distinction. One notable exception is vitamin E. Synthetic vitamin E, the dl form, has very little vitamin E activity. Avoid it. Use the d form only (see discussion on page 131). (D and dl refer to molecular conformations.)

On the other hand, there are low-dose multiples, B-complex supplements, and innumerable combinations of nutrients made entirely from natural sources and whole-food concentrates that, unlike synthetic forms, contain some unknown nutritional factors and synergists that act in concert with known nutrients. Such concentrates provide a balanced support to the body rarely achieved by synthetic ingredients. Some examples are wheat grass tablets or powder, barley grass powder, alfalfa tablets, algae/plankton (spirulina, blue-green algae, chlorella), bee pollen, royal jelly, and herbal concentrates.

Whole-food concentrates, brewer's or nutritional yeast, sea vegetation tablets, and synthetic vitamins all have their appropriate places in supporting your wellbeing. Until my health stabilized, I relied on high-potency multiple vitamin/mineral supplements. Now I lean toward whole-food or herb concentrates. Yet, I still often use a low potentcy multiple vitamin/mineral preparation. And as extra antioxidant fortification I'm careful to get in 2,000 milligrams a day of vitamin C, 25,000 I.U. of beta-carotene, and 400 I.U. of vitamin E.

Additives and Allergens

One caution applies to any vitamin, however: *Beware of additives and food allergens*. Some supplements contain sugar, artificial food coloring and flavoring, chlorine, phenol, shellac, talc, and other chemicals that are unwarranted and sometimes hazardous. Read labels carefully; avoid these brands. Some supplements contain products from corn, wheat, soy, milk, and yeast—foods to which you may be allergic or sensitive. If you are especially allergic to beef or pork, you should know that the gelatin capsules are usually beef- or pork-derived. If you wish, you can open the capsules and just use the powdered contents. In addition, for those sensitive to corn, all vitamin C is made from corn unless otherwise stated on the label.

If the vitamins you begin to take make you feel worse, it may be that they (or their doses) are incorrect for you. It is also possible, however, that you are reacting to additives or allergens in the supplements. For those with a yeast overgrowth and yeast allergy, yeast-based supplements should be initially avoided. One advantage to synthetic vitamins is that some brands are entirely free of the major allergenic foods.

Other Important Aspects of Supplements

Chelated Minerals   Minerals are best absorbed from the digestive tract into your circulation in their chelated form (in which they are "bound" to amino acids or other substances). There are many chelation vehicles on the market with a wide variation in absorption. How do you know whether to buy calcium carbonate or calcium malate; magnesium oxide or magnesium fumarate? The answer is to buy the ones with the highest absorption efficiencies: malate, ethanolamine phosphate, ascorbate, citrate, fumarate, peptonate, succinate, lysinate, glycinate, picolinate, and acetate. Moderately high efficiency absorption vehicles are: amino acid chelate, aspartate, chloride, sulfate, gluconate, and phosphate. The lowest absorption efficiency vehicles (and the least-expensive) are carbonate and oxide.

Some companies chelate a mineral with several carriers. For example, the calcium label might read "calcium from malate, lysinate, citrate, ascorbate, and carbonate." If carbonate, being the last listed, is the least abundant, this combination would be highly absorbable and therefore a good choice.

Timed-release Formulas   Unfortunately, timed-release or sustained-release formulas may not dissolve adequately and therefore fail to release their nutrients in time to be absorbed. There are specific places throughout the intestinal tract designed for the absorption of specific nutrients. As hard-coated tablets (and they do not necessarily have to be timed-release) travel through the intestinal tract, certain nutrients may miss their stops while still bound to an undissolved tablet and fail to be absorbed. This is a waste of good intentions and hard-earned money.

Encapsulated timed-release supplements may be somewhat less unpredictable. Buy supplements that will have the best chance of dissolving on time and getting absorbed. As mentioned earlier, there are potential dangers of some timed-release niacins. I am not aware of any similar hazards for any other timed-release nutrients.

Maximum Absorption   Look for nutritional supplements that are absorbed quickly. Nutrients bound up in hard-coated tablets may never make their way into the bloodstream. Loose powder, which can be mixed in fluid, or capsules, soft-gel, or quickly dissolving tablets are fast-acting forms that permit optimal absorption. If you are attached to a particular formula that comes only in hard-coated tablets, it is best to cut them up into several small pieces or to chew them somewhat before swallowing.

If you happen to be taking digestive supplements, do not chew hydrochloric acid tablets, as the acid can harm tooth enamel, and do not chew enzymes, as they may begin "digesting" your tongue. If you require these digestive supplements, find HCl in capsules and use enzymes with an enteric coating or those that are acid stable to protect the enzymes from the stomach's acidity.

Two processes, emulsification and micellization, reduce the size of oil droplets of such fat-soluble nutrients as vitamin E, vitamin A, and gamma-linolenic acid and greatly enhance their absorption. This is especially important when nutrient absorption is impaired by liver/gallbladder disease, pancreatic enzyme insufficiency, and other conditions discussed in Chapter Seven. Emulsified and particularly micellized vitamins become nearly as absorbable as water-soluble vitamins.

One final point concerning absorption: The general consensus is that vitamin supplements tend to absorb better when taken with a meal. The interaction of solid food and vitamin supplements, along with digestive secretions, enhances vitamin supplement assimilation. However, there appears to be some controversy about whether or not to take mineral supplements with or separate from meals. Some reports suggest that mineral supplements are best taken a half hour or more before or several hours after meals to achieve the best absorption. Other reports suggest that when minerals are taken with meals their absorption is enhanced.[11] Since life is complicated enough, keep things simple and take supplements with meals (except for those that specifically require other times).

Zinc/Copper Ratio   Zinc and copper antagonize each other. If you supplement with extra zinc, over time you may develop a copper deficiency. To maintain good health, keep the ratio between zinc and copper at 8 to 1 or 15 to 1. For example, using the 15 to 1 ratio, if you take 30 milligrams of zinc, take at least 2 milligrams of copper. You should also take a copper-free multiple if copper excess has been documented.

Some forms of chronic anemia as well as high blood

cholesterol levels, arteriosclerosis, low white blood cell count, and osteoporosis can be caused by a copper deficiency. Copper is an essential mineral (the RDA is 2 milligrams), but an excess amount in relationship to zinc is undesirable. Common sources of copper toxicity are copper plumbing that contaminates drinking water and mineral supplements with too much copper and not enough zinc.

Multiple Vitamin/Mineral Formulas The multiple vitamin/mineral supplement may be the most convenient and economical way of including extra nutrients in your diet. It would be worth your while to find one that takes into account the factors I have discussed above. You may not find every aspect optimal in any one multiple, but if most fit the criteria I have outlined, be satisfied. Do some homework on this, but try not to drive yourself crazy. If you're sold on your one-a-day multiple, at least break it in half and take half in the morning, say, and the other eight hours later, so that you can get the benefit of these nutrients over a twenty-four-hour stretch.

Certain long-term medications can prevent absorption or utilization of nutrients.[12] If you must be on a drug for longer than a month or two, be certain to get detailed information from your doctor or the drug company. Ask how the medication can interfere with nutrient absorption and/or utilization. You may need to take an extra dose of a specific vitamin or mineral to compensate for the drug's effect.

Health is not found solely in a vitamin pill. Since it's so easy and convenient to take vitamins and minerals, many people tend to overdo them and neglect other aspects of health maintenance. It would be a mistake to think that supplements make up for a junk-food diet or to imagine that the detrimental effects of sugar, bad oils, soft drinks, coffee, food additives, or fast foods will be offset by taking a multivitamin. Do not think that your supplements can take the place of clean air, of getting adequate sleep and exercise, or of learning how to love and accept yourself or cope with daily stresses. Nutritional supplements can certainly help compensate for a less-than-optimal environment, diet, lifestyle, and mental state, but they are not replacements. They are merely adjuncts to an appropriate self-care health program.

SELECTED VITAMINS AND MINERALS
Vitamin C

Vitamin C plays an important role in the maintenance of health and the treatment of disease.[13]

Among its many activities, vitamin C:

- Helps in the formation of collagen, giving strength to cartilage, bone, connective tissue, and dentine.
- Aids the integrity of blood vessels, and thus helps prevent arteriosclerosis, aneurysms, varicose veins, nosebleeds, easy bruising, and bleeding gums.
- Gives strength to all supporting tissues, including those surrounding tumors, and thus can help prevent or delay the spread of tumors.
- Stimulates white blood cell migration, and thus can inhibit viruses and bacteria and bring about rapid recovery from colds, flus, and more serious infections like hepatitis, mononucleosis, and viral pneumonia.
- Is important for wound healing.
- Detoxifies and helps remove from the body heavy metals such as lead, cadmium, arsenic, and mercury.
- Can help reduce drug toxicity, including that caused by chemotherapy.
- Can decrease toxicity from radiation therapy.
- Can be used in the treatment and prevention of cancer, partially by stimulating the production of lymphocytes, decreasing tumor metabolism of glucose, and providing cellular antioxidant defense.
- Can elevate levels of HDL cholesterol and reduce the dangerous atherosclerosis-promoting effects of LDL cholesterol by inhibiting oxidation of LDL.
- Has potent antihistamine properties and can be used to control and prevent allergies.
- Is instrumental in recycling vitamin E, helping to convert it to its active form after being used in fighting free radicals.
- Is one of the body's more important water-soluble antioxidants, helping to slow cellular aging/destruction and delaying chronic degenerative disease.
- Has a protective effect on the lungs and can reduce the cancer-causing, damaging effects of cigarette smoke.
- Plays an important role in adrenal function.
- Improves iron absorption.
- Protects sperm from DNA (genetic) damage that can cause inherited disease or cancer in a man's children.

Vitamin C usually works better in the presence of bioflavonoids, plant-derived substances with a broad spectrum of actions. Hesperidin, naringin, quercetin, and other flavonoids are almost always present in the foods in which vitamin C is found. Some practitioners recommend daily supplemental intake (up to 500 milligrams) of a bioflavonoid complex that is commonly included in some vitamin C preparations. Bioflavonoids can also be taken separately in higher doses for specific treatments. (See pages 392, 406, and 423 for discussion.)

Food sources of vitamin C include primarily raw vegetables and fruits and their juices—especially fresh ones. Richest sources include acerola berries, rose hips, strawberries and other berries, guava, black currant, red and other sweet bell peppers, broccoli, and brussels sprouts. Cabbage, cauliflower, mustard greens, beet greens, spinach, watercress, parsley, and most citrus fruits contain a substantial amount of vitamin C. And asparagus, lima beans, potatoes, turnips, tomatoes, melons, grapefruits, and limes have a fair amount as well. Of course, some of these items are best eaten cooked, which will cause the loss of some of their vitamin C content.

Our need for vitamin C increases with exposure to cigarette smoke, air pollution, chemotherapy, radiation, free radicals of any kind, oral contraceptives, infections, stress, and overworked adrenal glands.

Too much vitamin C can cause intestinal gas and diarrhea. The amount the bowel can tolerate is called the bowel tolerance level. During an infection such as flu, hepatitis, or mononucleosis, the bowel tolerance level may rise from perhaps 7 grams a day to 100 grams, enabling absorption of vitamin C megadoses so helpful in combating these infections.

An excess of ascorbic acid can also cause an irritated or "acid" stomach. Using an ascorbate vitamin C (buffered with calcium, potassium, or magnesium) can alleviate this problem; sodium ascorbate is also available, but if you must restrict your intake of sodium, stick with the other ascorbates.

The RDA for vitamin C is 60 milligrams. I feel that most adults should take from 1,000 to 1,500 milligrams twice a day. Researchers such as the late Dr. Linus Pauling recommend taking 10 grams of vitamin C a day, even when you're in good health, while others suggest a dosage well below that amount. So you see, there are many opinions. A good way to test for adequate vitamin C intake is to measure urinary output using a disposable test strip that measures the concentration of ascorbate in the urine. You want to maintain a concentration of 100 milligrams per deciliter of urine or greater. The test strips can be purchased from Wholesale Nutrition, Box 3345, Saratoga, CA 95070, (800) 325-2664.

Of concern to those individuals with elevated levels of oxalate in the urine and a propensity for forming calcium oxalate kidney stones is the possibility that supplemental vitamin C will raise urinary oxalate levels and therefore contribute to the formation of these stones. Although one study has suggested this association, most of the medical literature does not, even in studies using 6,000 milligrams of vitamin C daily. Some authors have suggested that those who have a history of calcium oxalate stones need not avoid vitamin C. Instead, they should adjust their diet and take vitamin B-6 (approximately 50 milligrams a day) and magnesium (up to 500 milligrams a day). This can lower urinary oxalate excretion and reduce the risk of stone formation.[14] (See Chapter Seventeen, "Kidney Stones.")

Taking vitamin C in doses greater than 2 grams a day may also promote copper loss. Although this finding has not been generally recognized, if you feel you need much larger doses of vitamin C regularly and do not take a multiple with copper, it would be useful to have your serum and red blood cell copper levels checked periodically. Vitamin C can falsely lower blood and urine glucose measurements, particularly if the device or test strips utilize Fehlings Reagent. Those utilizing hexose oxidase are less susceptible to alteration by vitamin C, and those using glucose oxidase are the least susceptible to alteration and are the preferred method.

Ascorbyl palmitate is a fat-soluble form of vitamin C that provides additional intramembrane antioxidant activity. You will see it with regular vitamin C (its more common water-soluble partner) in some antioxidant formulas and in some multiple vitamin/mineral formulas emphasizing antioxidant protection. (It is also available separately, and doses recommended are generally low—up to 300 milligrams a day.) A topical vitamin C (Derma C Cream from Interplexus of Kent, Washington) can be applied to muscles and joints that have been strained, sprained, overused—any musculoskeletal condition where there is inflammation or free radical damage (arthritis). Applying it to wrinkles—for its collagen-enhancing effect—may, according to anecdotal reports, have cosmetic benefit. It may also decrease sunburn and sun allergy.

Vitamin E

Vitamin E is a potent fat-soluble antioxidant that can protect cell membranes from environmental pollutants and radiation and from dietary and metabolic free radicals. In so doing, it prevents the oxidation of polyunsaturated fatty acids and cholesterol.[15]

Vitamin E:

- In its capacity as an antioxidant, protects against a host of chronic degenerative diseases.
- Can decrease LDL cholesterol and plaque deposits on the walls of arteries. It thus can be considered one of the most important nutrients in reducing susceptibility to angina, heart attack, stroke, peripheral vascular disease, and any manifestation of atherosclerosis.
- Is especially important for diabetics, who are six times more prone to arteriosclerosis and its complications than nondiabetic individuals. Vitamin E has been shown to reverse diabetic gangrene and prevent amputations.
- Helps keep the blood from clotting abnormally by decreasing platelet aggregation, which reduces the chances of thrombosis (heart attack, stroke, pulmonary embolism, or thrombophlebitis). It can be used as well in the acute treatment of these conditions.

- Protects red blood cells from rupture by enzymes that break down the fatty acids and cell membranes.
- Has vasodilating properties, can stimulate collateral circulation, can increase the oxygen-carrying capacity of blood, and can help chronic skin ulcers heal.
- Is used to diminish, prevent, or reduce the risk of tendonitis, muscle cramps, cardiovascular disease, and such autoimmune inflammatory diseases as polymyositis, vasculitis, scleroderma, Raynaud's phenomenon, and lupus. It is also useful in combatting neurological degenerative diseases, cancers—especially lung, oral, breast, stomach, and pancreatic cancers, as well as cancer of the colon and urinary tract—fibrocystic breast disease, atrophic vaginitis in postmenopausal women, cataracts, and tissue damage from traumatic injuries to various organs and tissues.
- Is used topically to reduce scar formation and to help burns and wounds heal.
- Helps protect against environmental pollutants such as toxic metals and chemicals (benzene compounds, carbon tetrachloride, and other chemical oxidants), oxidizing radiation (free radicals), and radiation therapy.
- Helps protect against and may reduce the toxic effects of drugs used in chemotherapy, particularly Adriamycin, Mitomycin C, and 5-Fluorouraril (5-FU).
- May help protect against the cancer-causing damage of cigarette smoke.

Adequate levels of vitamin E enhance antibody response and improve white blood cell activity, phagocytosis, and host resistance. These positive immune-enhancing effects are related to the vitamin's basic antioxidant function, which protects the fatty membranes of immune cells. In the process of killing bacteria, macrophages and neutrophils produce free radicals for which adequate antioxidants, including vitamin E, are necessary to protect these cells from autodestruction.

Food sources of vitamin E include expeller-pressed unrefined vegetable and seed oils, raw seeds and nuts, dates, organ meats, raw wheat germ, green leafy vegetables, millet, oats, barley, wheat and other whole grains, soybeans, avocado, alfalfa, asparagus, and cabbage.

Substances that increase the body's demand for vitamin E include rancid fats and oils, polyunsaturated fats and oils, oral contraceptives, refined flours, iron, lead, and copper.

The RDA for vitamin E is 30 I.U. daily. I usually recommend a preventive dose of 400 to 800 I.U. daily. Excess vitamin E can cause high blood pressure in a small percentage of individuals.

If you have high blood pressure, diabetes mellitus, valvular damage from rheumatic heart disease or other causes, heart damage from a previous heart attack or other cause, and are not currently taking vitamin E,

carefully adhere to the following. Begin vitamin E supplementation with 30 I.U. daily and increase the daily dose every week by 30 I.U. until at the desired dose level. Have your doctor monitor you. (Carlson's Laboratories of Arlington, Illinois, carries 30-I.U. vitamin E capsules.) If you take coumadin or any other blood thinner or have a bleeding disorder, consult your doctor about vitamin E supplementation.

Although the d-alpha tocopherol fraction (tocopherol is the biochemical name for vitamin E) has been found to be the most active component, the other tocopherols (beta, gamma, and delta) occurring naturally with the alpha form also have antioxidant activity and may possibly act as synergists. Some practitioners will therefore recommend d-alpha that contains some of these other tocopherols. I do not find them necessary. I recommend the esterified forms (d-alpha tocopheryl succinate or acetate), which have improved stability over and longer shelf life than the unesterified d-alpha tocopherol form. However, if fat digestion is impaired due to having no gallbladder, pancreatic enzyme deficiency, liver/gallbladder disease, or cystic fibrosis, the water-soluble (emulsified or micellized) d-alpha tocopherol form is preferred. D-alpha tocopherol is best for topical applications, but the tocopheryl forms will do. Be certain to avoid any dl-alpha tocopherol or dl-alpha tocopheryl, the synthetic form (with minimal vitamin E activity). Find the d-alpha forms (D and dl refer to molecular conformation).

Vitamin A

Vitamin A, a fat-soluble nutrient, is necessary for cellular growth.[16] It is especially important for the mucosal cells lining the respiratory, gastrointestinal, and genitourinary tracts, the eye membranes, and the ducts of secretory glands. Vitamin A acts somewhat like a hormone, stimulating these cells and triggering their vital secretions including mucus, enzymes, and other substances, one of which is the secretory component for a crucial antibody, secretory IgA. This antibody safeguards mucous membranes throughout our bodies from invasion by infectious and allergic assaults. In addition to its role in maintaining mucous membrane health, vitamin A helps preserve the integrity of red blood cell membranes and the skin.

It is known that people with lung cancer generally have very low vitamin A levels in their blood. Vitamin A has important preventive properties for this as well as cervical cancer and any epithelial cancers. It is used therapeutically to stimulate the thymus and increase the number of circulating cancer-fighting lymphocytes. Vitamin A also plays a role in the prevention of colds and flus, partially as a result of its immunostimulatory function but also because of its secretory IgA contribution.

Carotenes

There are about five hundred carotenes occurring in the plant kingdom. Some have vitamin A activity and some do not. Of the ones with vitamin A activity, beta-carotene, a precursor of vitamin A, is the most active and well studied.[17] A portion of the beta-carotene in the foods we eat will normally be converted by the body into vitamin A. What is said about vitamin A, therefore, applies to beta-carotene.

Beta-carotene has some properties unique to itself as well. It is a potent scavenger of toxic oxygen radicals, especially those produced by chemicals in the air and those generated by our own metabolism. It has stronger immune-stimulating and thymic supportive activity than vitamin A. It confers protection from lung cancer and the damages of cigarette smoking on the lungs and from ultraviolet-induced skin cancers. Beta-carotene is also an essential nutrient for normal ovarian function (ovulation, regular menstrual cycles, hormonal output). Other carotenes thought not to be as effective precursors to vitamin A formation have more potent free radical and cancer-protecting functions than beta-carotene. It is therefore preferable to find a mixed carotene supplement, a concentrate of what you are getting in so-called beta-carotene-rich vegetables. Scientific Botanicals of Seattle, Washington, makes such a supplement, called Beta Plex.

Together, vitamin A and beta-carotene are important in the prevention of night blindness, burning and itching of the eyes, drying up of the cornea and tear ducts, drying up of the salivary glands and respiratory tract membranes, loss of smell and appetite, allergies (food and respiratory), drying and hardening of the skin, dry hair, blemishes, kidney stones and urinary tract infections, bone growth retardation, and soft tooth enamel.

Food sources of vitamin A include fish oil, beef liver, white fish, eggs, and butter. Sources of carotenes are any green, orange, or yellow vegetables and any orange or yellow fruits, including broccoli, kale, chard, carrots, sweet potatoes, yams, winter squash, apricots, and cantaloupe. Green algae (chlorella, blue-green algae and spirulina) are also rich sources of carotenes.

Substances that antagonize or increase the body's demand for vitamin A include alcohol, coffee, excessive iron, mineral oil, and cortisone, not having a gallbladder and pancreatic enzyme deficiency.

The RDA for vitamin A is 5,000 I.U. daily for adults. I usually recommend both vitamin A and beta-carotene supplementation, between 10,000 and 15,000 I.U. daily of vitamin A and 10,000 to 50,000 I.U. of beta-carotene supplement (preferably containing other carotenes as well).

Vitamin A is one of the few vitamins discussed here that has the potential of toxicity. Toxic symptoms arising from excessive vitamin A include persistent headache; dry mouth; dry, rough, itchy skin; dizziness; irritability; loss of appetite, nausea and vomiting; bone and joint pain; hair loss; and liver inflammation/jaundice. There is no toxicity to beta-carotene except for an orange coloring of the skin. This in itself is harmless, although it does indicate tissue saturation levels, and doses should be lessened somewhat.

Vitamin B-6

Vitamin B-6 (pyridoxine) is one of the more important vitamins, as it acts as a cofactor in several hundred different biochemical reactions in the brain, liver, skin, joints, muscles, arteries, and nearly every other part of the body.[18] Because it is one of the vitamins most easily lost in food processing and cooking, many Americans, not surprisingly, are lacking even RDA amounts of this vitamin. Vitamin B-6 is important for energy production, for the proper functioning of the brain, for the formation of hemoglobin, and for optimal immune function. It facilitates glycogen removal from the liver and absorption of amino acids through the intestinal walls. In some cases, B-6 deficiency can lead to arterial damage, resulting in plaque formation. B-6 is useful in the treatment and prevention of arthritis, allergies, anemia, eczema, oxalate kidney stones, seborrheic dermatitis, neuritis, asthma, hair loss, diabetes, carpal tunnel syndrome, depression, learning disorders, autism, and premenstrual syndrome. For more information, see *The Doctor's Guide to Vitamin B-6* by Alan Gaby, M.D. (Rodale Press, 1984).

Food sources of vitamin B-6 include meats, organ meats, grains, brewer's yeast, bananas, blackstrap molasses, legumes, wheat germ, green leafy vegetables, prunes, peas, corn, brown rice, nuts, and fish.

Substances and factors that antagonize or increase the body's need for vitamin B-6 include alcohol, coffee, cigarette smoke, pregnancy, aging, radiation, air pollution, certain drugs (oral contraceptives, hydralazine, penicillamine, isoniazid, antibiotics, and some anticonvulsants), oxidation, ultraviolet light, heat, stress, high protein intake, and exercise.

The RDA for B-6 is 2 milligrams. I usually recommend a preventive dose between 25 and 50 milligrams a day. A dose of approximately 10 to 20 milligrams of pyridoxal-5 phosphate (the active form of B-6) may be equivalent. B-6/pyridoxal-5 phosphate should be taken in combination with the entire B-complex spectrum. For premenstrual syndrome, up to ten times the above doses of B-6 are frequently needed, but only during the premenstrual phase (see Chapter Seventeen, "Premenstrual Syndrome").

The toxicity of vitamin B-6 is minimal and reversible. Peripheral neuropathy, numbness or tingling in hands or feet, has been practically the only symptom identified, and happens very rarely when B-6 is taken according to the recommendations listed above.

Calcium

Calcium is essential for building and maintaining strong bones and teeth.[19] It acts as a nerve nutrient involved in electrical transmissions of the heart and of the skeletal muscles and assists in normal blood clotting. Calcium deficiency can result in muscle cramps, especially in the legs and back, menstrual cramps, brittle nails, insomnia, nervousness, osteoporosis, dental caries and periodontitis, arthritis, heart rhythm disturbances, high blood pressure, and colorectal cancer.

The RDA for calcium is 800 to 1,200 milligrams a day, up to 1,500 milligrams during pregnancy/lactation and menopause. It is interesting to note that in some cultures daily calcium intake does not exceed 300 milligrams, yet diseases like osteoporosis that we attribute to calcium deficiency are rare. In these cultures, a healthy diet and lifestyle prevent the excessive urinary calcium loss and abnormal calcium utilization common in many individuals in Western cultures.

Substances and factors that antagonize or increase the need for calcium include excess dietary phosphorus (flesh foods—beef, lamb, poultry, fish, etc.—and phosphoric acid containing soft drinks); excess dietary fat and protein; excess sugar, salt, and caffeine; nicotine; stress; lack of exercise; vitamin D deficiency or excess; and inadequate hydrochloric acid production (see Chapter Seven). Excess dietary phytates, like wheat bran fiber, may also be a factor. In order to compensate for our dietary excesses and a sedentary lifestyle, we are told to take what some sources consider to be excessive (1,500 milligrams) amounts of supplemental calcium. Rather than going to that extreme, it makes far more sense to clean up the diet and start exercising, although it is considered by many to be generally safe to consume that much supplemental calcium.

Because the RDA of calcium covers total calcium from foods and supplements, it is important to know the dairy and nondairy sources of the mineral (see tables on pages 87 and 88). For nonvegetarians who do not incorporate milk products into their diet, I recommend 500 to 1,000 milligrams a day of supplemental calcium. If meat products (flesh foods) are eaten every day, the high end of that range is appropriate; if meat is not part of the daily diet and lifestyle habits are not antagonistic to calcium, the low end is preferable. I suggest less supplemental calcium for vegetarians (300 to 500 milligrams a day), more for individuals with conditions such as acute insomnia and muscle and menstrual cramps. Professional advice about calcium supplementation is needed for those with a history of calcium oxalate kidney stones.

Although there is a tendency to restrict calcium supplementation in diseases that promote abnormal calcification (arthritis and atherosclerosis, for example), such a practice may not be warranted, as it is a normal body response to heal inflammation/injury with calcium. An individual with coronary artery disease still requires calcium and should be given it, although attention to enough magnesium and avoidance of excessive vitamin D is crucial here (see following sections). In such cases, it is best to direct efforts toward eliminating or reducing the cause of the inflammation/injury and therefore avoid the abnormal calcifications.

The most absorbable forms of calcium are citrate, malate, and ascorbate, which do not depend on the interaction with stomach acid. Calcium glycinate and calcium from microcrystalline hydroxyapatite are also gaining recognition. The carbonate and oyster shell forms require for their absorption adequate hydrochloric acid production from the stomach, which many adults over fifty do not have. Even with good stomach acid, absorption of these forms is relatively poor. Furthermore, the carbonate form functions as an antacid, which counters the stomach's digestive process. If used continually for acid indigestion, it does not address the underlying cause of digestive symptoms (see Chapter Seven). It also can overalkalinize the gastrointestinal system, giving rise to candida overgrowth (see Chapter Twelve) and, in large doses, overalkalinize the urine and contribute to stone formation. I do not recommend using the carbonate form as the only source of calcium. At least three-fourths supplemental calcium should be from more absorbable forms. Absorbed calcium has many known benefits, one of which is to decrease parathyroid hormone and therefore decrease the chances of colon and rectal polyps and cancer. However, unabsorbed calcium, which stays in the intestines, binds bile acids and carcinogens, forming "soaps" with fat. This also diminishes chances of colon cancer and may lower cholesterol levels.

Many companies now offer calcium supplements that include calcium from several absorbable sources in addition to a little carbonate. Avoid bone meal and dolomite, which may contain significant quantities of lead. In some individuals, calcium is constipating, an effect that can often be offset by magnesium.

Because magnesium assists in calcium uptake, many calcium supplements come with magnesium in amounts half that of the calcium. Some controversy exists over the calcium/magnesium ratio, and a few sources recommend equal amounts of calcium and magnesium or even twice as much magnesium as calcium. I have often recommended twice as much calcium as magnesium, but I currently prefer using equal amounts of both. I recommend up to twice as much magnesium as calcium for treating atherosclerosis, coronary heart disease, heart rhythm disturbances, spastic colon, nervous irritability, high blood pressure, and dry skin not helped by essential fatty acids or improved fat absorption.

Magnesium

Magnesium is a cofactor for over one hundred enzyme reactions occurring in the body. This means it is important for protein formation, DNA production, and nerve conduction.[20] Among its many activities, it helps maintain normal intracellular potassium levels, blocks the entry of excessive calcium, slows the release of both adrenaline and noradrenaline, increases the metabolic efficiency of the heart, decreases insulin resistance in diabetics, and increases pancreatic islet beta cell response and insulin action.

What this all means is that magnesium can be used to treat high blood pressure and prevent heart attacks from coronary artery spasms and diminished cardiac metabolic efficiency. It is useful in treating angina and is often the key therapeutic agent that normalizes heart rhythm disturbances. In fact, when given immediately after a heart attack and for the following four weeks, magnesium has been shown to significantly reduce the occurrence of dangerous arrhythmias and aid in recovery. Magnesium can also inhibit excessive platelet stickiness and raise HDL cholesterol levels, both useful for decreasing chances of heart attack and stroke.

Magnesium is beneficial for asthma, esophageal spasm, Raynaud's disease, skeletal muscle spasm from injury or trauma, menstrual cramps, gangrene, eclampsia of pregnancy, diabetes, kidney stones, epilepsy, and lead toxicity. Magnesium helps to prevent the cardiovascular, musculoskeletal, and renal complications associated with excess vitamin D and phosphorus, and is given as a supplement in diuretic therapy. As mentioned above, magnesium is also useful for treating spastic colon, nervous irritability, and dry skin not helped by essential fatty acids or improved fat absorption.

Cardiac crises and other serious problems almost always require intravenous injections to quickly raise magnesium stores to therapeutic levels. For less urgent needs and following acute crises, intramuscular injections and/or oral supplementation may suffice.

The most common laboratory test used to assess magnesium status is the serum magnesium level. You can believe the result only if it is low because magnesium is an intracellular mineral, and normal serum levels may exist when there is an intracellular shortage. White or red blood cell magnesium levels are far more sensitive. The magnesium load/retention test is the most sensitive.

The RDA for magnesium is 350 milligrams. I recommend at least that amount as a daily preventive dose and twice as much or more therapeutically. Unless you have chronic kidney disease, these amounts are safe. If your oral magnesium causes diarrhea, you must lower the dose or try a different brand. The most absorbable forms of magnesium are malate, ethanolamine phosphate, citrate, ascorbate, glycinate, and fumarate. Magnesium oxide, though inexpensive, is very poorly absorbed.

Magnesium-rich foods include dark leafy greens (kale, collard, chard, parsley, dandelion, beet, mustard, sorrel, chickweed, watercress, and the like), whole grains, legumes, nuts, seeds, fruits, potatoes, seafood, chicken, and blackstrap molasses.

Factors that interfere with and increase the need for magnesium are calcium supplementation, phosphorus supplementation or dietary phosphorus excess, vitamin D excess, alcohol, caffeine, sugar, excess fat, phytic acid (in grain fiber), oxalic acid (found in some vegetables and nuts), low stomach acid, and rapid intestinal transit time (caused by stress, allergies, and other factors). Drugs that interfere with magnesium include diuretics, anticonvulsants, antibiotics, digitalis, and lithium.

Selenium

Selenium is another antioxidant nutrient, a mineral that works synergistically with vitamin E to prevent or at least slow down aging and deterioration of tissues through free radical oxidation.[21] Among its many benefits, it:

- Helps protect against the effects of chemical pollution and hypersensitivity.
- Is crucial for the maintenance of healthy heart muscle and in the prevention of heart attack.
- Increases antibody response to a variety of foreign agents.
- Enhances the ability of phagocytes to destroy bacteria and increases the capacity of macrophages and related cells to attack tumor cells.
- Helps fight cancer by protecting against carcinogens (through its basic antioxidant function of protecting cell membranes from lipid peroxidation).
- May help to counteract the immunosuppressive effects of corticosteroids while at the same time aiding their anti-inflammatory effects.
- Can help protect against lead intoxication and poisoning.

Food sources include smelt, brewer's yeast, wheat germ, Brazil nuts, garlic, scallops, barley, whole wheat, lobster, swiss chard, oats, brown rice, molasses, mushrooms, radishes, carrots, and cabbage—if grown on selenium-rich soils.

The RDA for selenium is 225 micrograms a day. Since many soils are deficient in selenium, and since we face many environmental assaults from toxic chemicals, it is important to take a selenium supplement, whether in the form of a multiple vitamin/mineral, selenium-rich brewer's yeast, or separate selenium dose. Note that toxic doses of selenium are not much higher than the recommended dose. For example, only 500 micrograms can result in immunosuppression as well as dry hair, loss of hair, loss of nails, streaked nails, irritability, dizziness, fatigue, and dermatitis.

Zinc

Zinc takes part in approximately ninety enzymatic reactions, including those involved in carbohydrate metabolism; protein synthesis; activities of the immune system; membrane stability; liver detoxification; activities of the prostate, thymus, thyroid, and adrenal glands; and neurotransmitter metabolism.[22] Deficiencies of zinc may contribute to loss of taste, slow growth, brittle hair, acne, eczema, hypothyroidism, delayed sexual development, poor wound healing, chronic infections, prostatic hypertrophy, menstrual dysfunction, dyslexia, abnormal behavior, anorexia nervosa and bulimia, and chemical hypersensitivity. Zinc is an extremely important immune enhancer used in combating cancer, specifically promoting T-cell activity, the central core of the cell-mediated branch of the immune system. It also protects against the accumulation and toxic effects of lead, cadmium, and copper.

Food sources include oysters, gingerroot, lamb, pecans, split peas, Brazil nuts, beef liver, egg yolks, whole wheat, rye, oats, peanuts, lecithin, almonds, walnuts, sardines, chicken, buckwheat, and hazelnuts.

The RDA for zinc is 15 milligrams a day. A 50-milligram daily dosage is safe for most adults. With zinc citrate or picolinate, two of the more absorbable forms, 15 to 30 milligrams a day will suffice. Sometimes higher doses are recommended therapeutically. However, excessive doses can suppress the immune function. Excess zinc can also cause digestive disturbances such as nausea, vomiting, diarrhea, and abdominal pain. Zinc supplementation can suppress copper levels. Thus, taking zinc and copper in the proper ratios (15 milligrams zinc to 1 to 2 milligrams copper) is important.

Factors that increase the need for zinc include cadmium exposure, burns, surgery, chronic infections, chronic inflammatory disease, alcoholism, diabetes, kidney and pancreatic disease, psoriasis, thalassemia, sickle cell disease, anorexia nervosa, antibiotics, diuretics, oral contraceptives, penicillamine, anticancer drugs, anticonvulsants, and corticosteroids.

Copper

Copper's role in cardiovascular health is discussed in Chapter Seventeen, and its role in antioxidant defenses is presented in Chapter Three. It has numerous other functions. When complexed with salicylate or sebecate, it has potent anti-inflammatory, anti-free radical, and wound-healing effects, making it a therapeutic agent for arthritis, ulcers, and other ailments.[23]

Vitamin D

Vitamin D is more a hormone, actually, than a vitamin. It is made (like many hormones) from cholesterol. It is needed for calcium and phosphorus absorption and utilization. Vitamin D is important for growth, especially of bones and teeth, and is used in the treatment of rickets, osteoporosis, and hypocalcemia. Recently it has been linked to the prevention of polyps and cancer of the colon and rectum.[24]

Probably the healthiest and safest way to procure an adequate supply of vitamin D is through limited exposure to sunlight. According to a recent Tufts University study, approximately fifteen minutes a day of midday sunlight supplies an adequate amount of vitamin D for the average adult.[25]

The RDA for vitamin D is 400 I.U. daily. In excessive amounts, vitamin D is toxic, having a narrower margin of safety than any other vitamin. Studies have shown as little as 1,200 I.U. of vitamin D (dietary and supplement sources combined) to be correlated with increased incidence of elevated blood cholesterol levels, heart attack, and kidney stones. That dose is only three times the RDA. Excess vitamin D's cardiovascular complications are attributed, in part, to its ability to decrease intramyocardial (heart muscle) magnesium, rendering the heart less metabolically efficient and more susceptible to rhythm disturbances and heart attack. In addition, excess vitamin D can be directly angiotoxic (injurious to arteries).

In extreme excess (over 25,000 I.U. daily), it can cause severe acute illness consisting of loss of appetite, nausea, vomiting, abdominal pain, excessive urination, excessive thirst, headache, and weight loss. Some of these symptoms are attributed to the high blood levels of calcium that excess vitamin D produces. Ironically, excess vitamin D pulls calcium out of bone—an invitation to osteoporosis—which can then be deposited in joints, arteries, and kidneys. It thus can lead to arteriosclerosis, arthritis, kidney stones, and kidney failure.

Most Americans receive too much vitamin D, as the food industry fortifies milk (100 I.U. per quart), other milk products, cereals, and grain products. Add to this the extra amounts in poultry, eggs, and meat from vitamin D–fortified animal feed as well as naturally high vitamin D foods: liver, cod liver oil, and fatty fish such as sardines, mackerel, salmon, and tuna. There is also the 400 I.U. of vitamin D in most multiple vitamin formulas, not to mention the vitamin D commonly added to calcium supplements.

Just ten years ago, the average daily intake for an adult was about 2,300 I.U., nearly six times the RDA and easily into the range of increased heart attack risk. I generally recommend diminishing the intake of vitamin D–fortified foods. If you use a multiple vitamin formula, find one with reduced amounts of vitamin D (50 to 200 I.U. per daily dose). Natural vitamin D-3 (cholecalciferol) is preferable to synthetic D-2 (ergocalciferol).

The ability to manufacture vitamin D from sunlight decreases with age. An eighty-year-old manufactures only half the amount that a twenty-year-old does, so the elderly, especially if they are not regularly exposed to sun, should maintain a daily intake of 400 to 800 I.U. Any younger adult who does not spend at least fifteen minutes in the midday sun several times a week and does not regularly consume vitamin D–fortified foods should have a total daily dose of 400 I.U. Those individuals who regularly consume vitamin D–fortified foods should avoid supplemental vitamin D and should diminish their consumption of fortified foods and find whole-food alternatives when possible.

Drugs that increase the need for vitamin D are anticonvulsants, sedatives, corticosteroids, blood cholesterol–lowering agents, antibiotics for tuberculosis, antacids, mineral oil, other cathartics, and laxatives. Certain conditions causing maldigestion/malabsorption of fats (and therefore of fat-soluble nutrients) will increase the need for diet/supplement-dependent vitamin D: pancreatic enzyme deficiency, gallbladder disease (or if you have no gallbladder), cystic fibrosis, and small bowel disease. In these cases, up to 1,000 I.U. daily may be advised under professional supervision. Still, other conditions and medicines can lead to vitamin D overdose: Addison's disease, cancer, hyperthyroidism, osteoporosis from being bedridden, sarcoidosis, parathyroid hormone–producing tumors, diazide diuretics, and vitamin A overdose.

Chromium

Chromium is a trace mineral essential for the proper utilization of glucose (blood sugar).[26] Through its potentiating effect on insulin at the cellular level, chromium helps glucose enter cells, thus preventing both diabetic and hypoglycemic tendencies. It also has the observed effect of diminishing sugar craving. The insulin-chromium interaction plays a key role in protein synthesis and amino acid transport. Chromium helps maintain cardiovascular health by lowering total serum cholesterol and triglycerides and by preventing atherosclerotic plaque formation.

According to many nutritionally oriented physicians and scientists, nearly everyone in this country is deficient in chromium. As with selenium and many other trace elements, the chromium content of the American diet is rapidly diminishing through soil depletion, food processing, and poor eating patterns. More than 90 percent of hair analyses (one method of assessing chromium status) show very low or nearly nondetectable levels. Anyone with blood sugar–related problems, sugar craving, coronary or other atherosclerotic involvement, and/or cholesterol and triglyceride elevations should consider supplementing chromium.

Elemental, inorganic chromium salts, such as those that plate the bumper on your car, cannot be used by the body. Only the organic complex form of chromium—glucose tolerance factor (GTF), which contains cofactors of niacin and glutamic acid—is biologically active. This preformed GTF, which occurs in food concentrate extracts such as brewer's yeast, can be used directly, although humans have a varying ability to make their own GTF from organic chromium. One tablespoon of various brands of brewer's yeast can provide from 20 to 60 micrograms of chromium.

Valuable chromium supplements other than brewer's yeast (and easier to use) include trivalent chromium-amino acid complex, chromium polynicotinate, Chromemate™, chromium picolinate, and Ultrachrome™.

Although considered an essential element by the Committee on Dietary Allowances, chromium is often overlooked in dietary recommendations because such minute amounts are required. A tentative level of 50 to 200 micrograms was established in the 1980 Recommended Dietary Allowance for adults, and 200 micrograms daily is considered a substantial maintenance level. Up to 1,000 micrograms daily is used therapeutically. One of the few adverse reactions I have seen from inadvertent high-dose supplementation (3,000 micrograms daily) was headache, which promptly subsided upon discontinuation. Since insulin requirements in the diabetic may lessen with chromium supplementation, blood sugar levels should be monitored carefully. Additionally, some people have been known to have allergic reactions to chromium, especially if it is derived from a yeast source.

Populations particularly susceptible to deficiency include the elderly, pregnant women, and malnourished children. Those who subsist predominantly on refined foods, who suffer from diabetes, hypoglycemia, or coronary heart disease, or are on long-term intravenous therapy—especially with dextrose-containing liquids or hyperalimentation without chromium—may also be deficient.

Foods with the highest amounts of chromium include brewer's yeast, beer, oysters, potatoes with skins, nuts, and liver. Foods with a medium level are whole grains, seafoods, chicken, cheese, fresh vegetables and fruit, and bran. Refining whole wheat removes most of the chromium, since it is largely contained in the germ and bran. Refining sugar results in a total loss of chromium.

Coenzyme Q-10

Coenzyme Q-10 (CoQ-10), also known as ubiquinone, is a naturally occurring fat-soluble molecule similar in structure to vitamin K. As a cofactor in the electron transport chain, the biochemical pathway at the heart of cellular functioning from which metabolic energy is derived, CoQ-10 is essential for the health of all tissues and organs.[27]

Although CoQ-10 is manufactured in the body, deficiencies have been reported in a wide range of clinical conditions, including cardiovascular disease (angina, congestive heart failure, hypertension), periodontal disease, diabetes, gastric ulcer, muscular dystrophy, AIDS and HIV-positive conditions, and age-related deterioration of the immune system. CoQ-10 can be used therapeutically for all of the above. Deficiencies have been documented by testing a CoQ-10-dependent enzyme system known as succinate dehydrogenase–CoQ-10 reductase. If there is adequate CoQ-10 in the body, then the addition of supplemental CoQ-10 will not boost enzyme activity. More recently, serum levels of CoQ-10 have been used to detect deficiencies.

A need for supplemental CoQ-10 could arise from impaired biosynthesis due to nutritional deficiencies, a genetic or acquired defect in CoQ-10 synthesis, or increased tissue needs resulting from a particular health condition or from some medications. Such cholesterol-lowering agents as lovastatin, pravastatin, or simvastatin block the synthesis of CoQ-10. Because of the central role CoQ-10 plays in cellular metabolism, a deficiency may manifest itself in many different conditions. In a study of HIV-infected individuals representing various stages of clinical disease, from asymptomatic to full-blown AIDS, the deficiency of CoQ-10 increased with the severity of the disease. When these individuals were treated with CoQ-10, there was marked improvement in their ability to fight opportunistic infections.[28]

CoQ-10 appears to be nontoxic at the usual dosage of 30 milligrams a day. In cases of severe cardiac disease, up to 100 milligrams has been used with no adverse effects. Some individuals may have allergic reactions to CoQ-10, and its safety has not been evaluated during pregnancy and lactation. Reports are preliminary, and further testing will need to be done before it becomes widely used.

For chronic conditions, I recommend up to 60 milligrams a day (and up to 120 milligrams for more severe conditions) over a trial period of at least two months. It is expensive, but you may find it well worthwhile. If it brings significant benefit, find the lowest dosage that produces the desired effect. CoQ-10 is found in such foods as sardines, spinach, beef, and peanuts.

Iron

Iron is the most abundant of the essential trace elements in the body. It is the central figure in hemoglobin, which transports oxygen throughout the body's tissues. Functioning in numerous enzyme systems, iron is involved in electron transport, peroxide metabolism, DNA synthesis, and adrenaline metabolism.[29] The body stores iron in the form of myoglobin, a compound similar to hemoglobin, found in muscle fibers. Absorption of iron requires adequate stomach acidity and healthy mucosa in the small bowel. Hypochlorhydria (see Chapter Seven) and inflammatory bowel disease can give rise to malabsorption-induced iron deficiency.

The risk of iron deficiency is greatest during pregnancy and lactation, infancy, rapid growth phases, and excessive menstruation. Repetitive and excessive physical exertion can also predispose. Left unchecked, depleted iron stores can lead to iron-deficiency anemia, symptoms of which include extreme fatigue and/or weakness, shortness of breath, cold extremities, rapid or fluttering heartbeat, and cravings for ice, dirt, or clay.

Children with iron deficiency may show learning and behavioral problems. Deficient levels of iron can adversely affect the immune system. It may cause lymphoid tissue to atrophy and reduce the number of T and B cells in the blood. Because of the oxygen deprivation, all immune cells may be affected. Anemia from chronic disease or from occult blood loss may have similar and other symptoms.

A simple blood count is most often used to diagnose iron-deficiency anemia. However, you could be iron deficient and exhibit symptoms from it even with a normal hematocrit or hemoglobin count. A serum ferritin is a far more sensitive indicator of bodily stores of iron. If your ferritin is low, consult your doctor first to discount occult or obvious blood loss or chronic illness. If this is not a factor, the problem may stem from insufficient dietary iron or insufficient absorption of dietary iron.

The two dietary forms of iron are heme, the most readily absorbable, found exclusively in flesh food, and nonheme, found in plant foods and supplements. In addition to adequate stomach acid, the absorption of nonheme iron can be favorably influenced by ascorbic acid (vitamin C). Because of the dangers associated with iron excess, it is a good idea to get your normal maintenance iron from food. Whole grains, wheat germ, nuts, seeds, seafoods, liver, vegetables, blackstrap molasses, brewer's yeast, and flesh foods all contain significant amounts of iron. Chlorophyll-rich foods also build blood.

If you have symptoms of iron deficiency (see page 125) and your blood tests verify it, or if you are in high-risk categories for deficiency and want to prevent an imbalance, take some supplemental iron. Of the three main forms of supplemental iron (ferrous, ferric, and reduced iron), ferrous is the most readily absorbed and widely available. In terms of absorption, there is little difference among the fumarate, sulphate, gluconate, peptonate, lactate, succinate, glycinesulphate, glycinate, and glutamate forms (the fumarate, succinate, and glycinate forms, however, seem to cause fewer gastrointestinal complaints). Some of the most gentle iron preparations are botanically (herbally) based liquids, available in some health food or herb stores or from herb distributors.

The RDA for iron is 18 milligrams. For therapeutic supplementation, 60 milligrams or more of elemental iron may be prescribed. Frequent accompanying symptoms of such high supplementation may include constipation and black, tarry-looking stools.

Conflicting drug interactions include antibiotics such as tetracycline, chloramphenicol, and neomycin; antacids containing carbonates and any calcium carbonate supplements; cholestyramine, indomethacin, and dactinomycin. Iron and vitamin E conflict with each other as well.

Iron is a double-edged sword: an excess can cause a number of adverse effects, including oxidative damage to cells and organs. Iron may be the most commonly misused supplement, the toxicity for which may be difficult to track.

Excessive amounts in the body may be manifested in a variety of ways. Iron is a catalyzer of lipid peroxidation and free radical pathology, which among other things can increase the likelihood of cellular deterioration, accelerated aging, arterial damage, coronary artery disease, and cancer. Some forms of diabetes mellitus are related to excess iron (and can be reversed using an iron-chelating drug). Adults (other than anemics or menstruating, pregnant, or lactating females) should avoid supplemental iron; this includes most vitamin/mineral preparations (find one that is iron-free). Also avoid iron-fortified foods—refined bread, noodles, crackers, and cereals. If your serum ferritin is high or even near high normal, and especially if you have a susceptibility or strong family history of coronary artery disease, consider donating blood to a blood bank several times a year to lower your iron stores. (But as elevated ferritin may also represent inflammation and not necessarily excess iron, check with your doctor first.)

Predisposing red blood cell diseases that cause iron overload to tissues include sideroblastic anemia, thalassemia, and sickle cell or other hemolytic anemias. The liver and heart are most susceptible to damage by iron overload, termed hemochromatosis/iron storage disease.

Although excess iron eventually damages the liver, pre-existing liver damage from alcohol, fat, or chemicals greatly increases the risk of iron toxicity.

Symptoms of toxicity are usually not clear until the condition has progressed. The symptoms may include fatigue, abdominal or joint pain, bronze coloring of the skin, weight loss, and diabetic symptoms such as excessive urination, thirst, and hunger. Examination may reveal an enlarged spleen, damaged joints or heart, and reduced size of testicles. Early detection is extremely important for recovery. Serum ferritin levels are helpful. Immune system effects of excessive iron include the reduction of macrophage phagocytosis and increased susceptibility to infection. Iron supplementation during an acute infection may reduce host resistance. Unless iron deficiency is present, iron supplementation should be avoided in any kind of malignancy, as it favors tumor growth.

Essential Fatty Acids

For a discussion on the benefits of essential fatty acids, as well as recommended sources and amounts, see pages 48–51.

Amino Acids[30]

Amino acids, the building blocks of protein, support the growth, repair, and maintenance of every system of your body. Amino acids serve multiple roles as constituents of antibodies, hormones, neurotransmitters, enzymes, skin, muscle, bone, blood, connective tissue, hair, nails . . . everything. Although there are over forty amino acids and 1,600 different types of proteins in the body, there are eight essential amino acids that you must consume. From these eight your body can synthesize the rest. They are leucine, isoleucine, valine, threonine, lysine, tryptophan, phenylalanine, and methionine.

You may have heard the term "complete protein." This refers to the amount and balance of the essential amino acids in any one food source or combination of food sources. For example, many animal-derived foods (meat or eggs) are fairly complete, but vegetable-derived proteins are incomplete and need to be combined in specific ways to provide completeness (amino acid complementarity). This subject has been thoroughly addressed in other publications: *Diet for a Small Planet* by Frances Moore Lappé (Random House, 1982), *The McDougall Plan* by John McDougall, M.D., and Mary McDougall (New Wind, 1983), and *Transition to Vegetarianism* by Rudolph Ballantine, M.D. (Himalayan Press, 1987).

Specific amino acids can be used therapeutically, like vitamins and minerals, for a broad range of conditions and symptoms. An amino acid analysis (blood or urine testing for up to forty amino acids) can certainly help refine treatment choices. The following discussion is but a brief example of the vast extent to which amino acid therapy can be utilized.

Phenylalanine, an essential amino acid, is metabolized, with the help of vitamins C and B-6, into a brain neurotransmitter (norepinephrine) that is partially responsible for mood, clarity of thought, and alertness. It also helps stimulate the release of growth hormone from the pituitary gland. Supplemental phenylalanine (100 to 1,000 milligrams on an empty stomach at least one hour before meals) may be recommended for premenstrual syndrome, as well as those exhibiting depression, wavering concentration, anxiety, faulty memory, cloudy or foggy thinking, or difficulty with linear thought and evaluative judgment.

Because phenylalanine stimulates the release of cholecystokinin, a hormone from the cerebral cortex that acts on the hypothalamus to suppress appetite, it can be used to treat those who are overweight or for whom overeating is a problem. For those with chronic pain of any kind, the dl form of phenylalanine (approximately 350 to 1,000 milligrams one to three times a day on an empty stomach) may be helpful.

Tyrosine is a nonessential amino acid formed as an intermediary in the conversion of phenylalanine to norepinephrine. It is also a precursor to the neurotransmitters epinephrine and dopamine and stimulates the production of phenylethylamine in the cerebellum. Tyrosine has been used to treat narcolepsy, but its main therapeutic use is in the treatment of depression. Some forms of depression are due to insufficient amounts of these neurotransmitters in the brain, which is sometimes the result of an impaired ability to convert phenylalanine to tyrosine. Taking tyrosine, therefore, can be beneficial (100 to 500 milligrams a day and, under a physician's supervision, up to perhaps several thousand milligrams daily). Tyrosine is also an essential nutrient in the formation of thyroid hormone (see Chapter Seventeen, "Hypothyroidism").

Tryptophan, an essential amino acid (present in milk and turkey), is necessary for the production of the neurotransmitter serotonin. A deficiency of serotonin may be responsible for insomnia and depression. Tryptophan has been shown to ease these symptoms as well as impaired memory, concentration, and evaluative judgment. It has also been used successfully in treating some cases of premenstrual syndrome and pain syndromes.

In 1989, however, the Centers for Disease Control reported evidence linking tryptophan supplements to a blood disorder called eosinophilic myalgic syndrome. The Food and Drug Administration then recalled all products containing tryptophan. There has since been ample evidence demonstrating that the illness was caused by a contaminant from one particular manufacturer, and it is hoped that the FDA will soon allow this valuable therapeutic amino acid to be sold again. If so, tryptophan, like any of the amino acids discussed in this section, should be taken at least one and a half hours before or after any protein foods; otherwise the amino acids in protein will compete with the tryptophan to cross the blood-brain barrier, and some of the tryptophan will be left behind.

To facilitate entry into the brain, take it with juice or other carbohydrates. Use 500 to 1,000 milligrams near bedtime. Formulas combining tryptophan with niacinamide, vitamin B-6, and other synergists of neurotransmitter metabolism will also hopefully be available again. They have sometimes produced better results than tryptophan alone, depending upon the individual. Until the FDA reverses its decision, your doctor can prescribe a metabolite of tryptophan, 5-hydroxy tryptophan, an even more effective—and more expensive—way of increasing serotonin levels. Use 100 to 400 milligrams once or twice daily.

Glutamine, the amide form of the nonessential amino acid glutamic acid, is an important source of fuel for the brain. Its most important therapeutic use is in the treatment of alcoholism. Glutamine reduces alcohol craving and can prevent the mental deterioration seen in alcoholics. Alcoholics may have a biochemical lesion preventing the conversion of glutamic acid to glutamine and/or preventing the entry of glutamic acid into the brain. Paradoxically, alcohol tends to increase the transport of glutamic acid into the brain, a potential biochemical cause of alcohol craving. Doses of 1,500 to 3,000 milligrams a day (higher amounts under the supervision of a physician) have proven helpful.

Glutamine has also been used in the treatment of hypoglycemia. In providing an alternate fuel to the brain, it may lessen the consequences of a fall in blood sugar level and even diminish sugar craving. Glutamine has also been used in the treatment of some forms of schizophrenia, to help increase the intelligence quotients in children, and as a preferred substrate for mucosal cells of the small intestine, in food allergies and "leaky gut" syndrome (see page 242).

Cysteine is an extremely versatile sulfur-containing amino acid.[31] N-acetyl cysteine, a derivative of cysteine, is becoming the preferred form because of its superior absorption qualities. Cysteine/N-acetyl cysteine pulls from tissues mercury, gold, silver, and possibly arsenic and other metals, which are then combined with glutathione and excreted in the bile. Cysteine/N-acetyl cysteine increases glutathione synthesis, which not only helps in the excretion of heavy metals and toxic chemicals but serves in two crucial antioxidant enzyme systems: glutathione peroxidase and glutathione reductase.

Noteworthy is cysteine/N-acetyl cysteine's contribution to the deactivation of acetaldehyde, a toxic waste product from the liver's metabolism of alcohol (and is also present in smog and cigarette smoke), acetaminophen, and carbon tetrachloride. These substances are potent free radical generators. In excess, without antioxidant mechanisms that cysteine/N-acetyl cysteine support, they could cause massive cellular damage, particularly in the liver, and death. Cysteine/N-acetyl cysteine protects us from some mutagens and carcinogens as well as from the free radicals liberated by cancer chemotherapy. Doses of 500 milligrams three or four times a day for a limited period of treatment are suggested, although smaller amounts (300 to 1,000 milligrams a day) can be used safely over a long period of time for bolstering antioxidant capability. Cysteine/N-acetyl cysteine can leach such essential minerals as zinc and copper from the body. Sustained use of this amino acid requires supplementation with these minerals (15 to 30 milligrams daily of zinc and 2 to 3 milligrams daily of copper).

N-acetyl cysteine thins mucus and allows it to run more freely, which is extremely helpful in treating such respiratory problems as asthma, sinusitis, bronchitis, otitis media, and pneumonia. It can be taken for acute infections in high doses for one to three days (up to 500 milligrams four to five times a day). Patients with recurrent respiratory infections or chronic bronchitis can be administered a long-term dose of 200 to 500 milligrams twice a day.

N-acetyl cysteine has potent immune-enhancing effects. You may recall that free radicals are released when white blood cells attack infectious organisms or cancer cells. Because of its antioxidant function, N-acetyl cysteine protects cells of the immune system (neutrophils, macrophages, and lymphocytes) from destruction by their own free radical release. Thus it is appropriate to incorporate N-acetyl cysteine in any treatment of chronic infections and cancer. It has also been used in the treatment of AIDS and ARC to enhance T-cell counts and inhibit HIV replication.

Finally, cysteine/N-acetyl cysteine has been used successfully to lower serum cholesterol levels in the treatment and prevention of atherosclerosis. Specifically, N-acetyl cysteine has been used to lower apolipoprotein (a), the fraction associated with LDL cholesterol. It does so quite dramatically and safely as long as supplementation continues. One study published in the medical journal *Lancet* showed that the most significant lipid-lowering effect was based on a daily dose of 4 grams, although a 2-gram dose also had beneficial effects.[32]

Most of the studies documenting the effects of cysteine have been done with N-acetyl cysteine. I recommend this form. If you use cysteine, take vitamin C in at least equal or double the amounts of cysteine to prevent its conversion to cystine—another amino acid with entirely different functions. Vitamins B-1 and C work synergistically with cysteine.

Methionine is another sulfur-containing amino acid and, like cysteine, can be very useful in detoxifying harmful agents like lead, mercury, arsenic, and cadmium. It is also essential for protein synthesis, RNA/DNA formation, and the metabolism of vitamins and fats. In combination with inositol and choline, it is used in the treatment of disorders arising from a sluggish liver (premenstrual syndrome, fibrocystic breast disease, high blood cholesterol levels, poor digestion, and obesity; see Chapter Nine). Doses up to 1,000 milligrams a day have been administered.

Lysine is an essential amino acid needed for proper growth, enzyme production, and tissue repair. In particular, it has been found useful in the treatment of herpes type I and type II infections both orally and in topical preparations. Lysine is antagonistic to herpes virus replication and in doses of 500 milligrams a day can help prevent recurrences (see Chapter Seventeen, "Herpes"). It is given in doses up to 1,000 milligrams three times a day for acute recurrences. It has been used as well in similar doses for chronic Epstein-Barr virus infections (another virus in the herpes family).

THE VITAL ROLE OF VITAMINS AND MINERALS

Vitamins and minerals are essential to maintaining health and fighting disease. Without these micronutrients, the body could not function properly. You may now understand that a seemingly healthy diet may not be providing you with sufficient amounts of vitamins and minerals.

Food processing/refining and soil nutrient depletion make it all too easy to incur vitamin/mineral deficiencies and the myriad symptoms and illnesses associated with them. Age, illness, stress, pollution, activity level, and other factors may increase your need for micronutrients well beyond the RDA levels. Eating whole foods and supplementing your diet with vitamins and minerals can safeguard your health. But, as you will learn in the next chapter, it is not necessarily what you eat that determines your state of health, but what you can and cannot digest and assimilate.

SUGGESTED READING

Grant, Anne, and DeHoog, Susan. *Nutritional Assessment and Support*, 3rd ed. Self-published, 1985.

Hamilton, Kirk. *Clinical Pearls in Nutrition and Preventive Medicine*. Sacramento, CA: IT Services, 1992, 1993, 1994.

Hausman, Patricia. *The Right Dose: How to Take Vitamins and Minerals Safely.* Emmaus, PA: Rodale Press, 1987.

Lesser, Michael. *Nutrition and Vitamin Therapy.* New York: Grove Press, 1980.

Kraus, Marie, and Mahen, Kathleen. *Food, Nutrition and Diet Therapy: A Textbook of Nutritional Care,* 7th ed. Philadelphia: W. B. Saunders, 1984.

Kutsky, Roman. *Handbook of Vitamins, Minerals and Hormones,* 2nd ed. New York: Van Nostrand Reinhold, 1981.

Nestle, Marion. *Nutrition in Clinical Practice.* Greenbrae, CA: Jones Medical Pub., 1985.

Passwater, Richard, and Cranton, Elmer. *Trace Elements, Hair Analysis and Nutrition.* New Canaan, CT: Keats, 1983.

Pfieffer, Carl. *Mental and Elemental Nutrients: A Physician's Guide to Nutritional Health Care.* New Canaan, CT: Keats, 1975.

Werbach, Melvyn. *Nutritional Influences on Illness: A Sourcebook for Clinical Research.* Tarzana, CA: Third Line Press, 1987.

Wright, Jonathan, M.D. *Dr. Wright's Book of Nutritional Therapy.* Emmaus, PA: Rodale Press, 1979.

——— *Dr. Wright's Guide to Healing with Nutrition.* Emmaus, PA: Rodale Press, 1984.

CHAPTER 7

POOR DIGESTION AND ASSIMILATION

You've probably heard the dictum "You are what you eat." It's only partially true. Stated more accurately, you are what you digest and assimilate. Regardless of how wholesome the food you're eating may be, you must absorb it in order to derive any nutritional benefit. And to absorb it, your digestive organs need to be doing their proper job. In this chapter, we will begin with a case history, followed by a review of the process of digestion and methods for testing its different phases. Throughout, I will offer steps you can take to restore and maintain this system.

KIRBY

Kirby is a thirty-five-year-old landscape architect whose wife, Anne, knew there was something definitely wrong with his digestive system. Kirby was six foot five inches and weighed only 165 pounds. He could never gain any weight in spite of eating huge amounts of food every two hours. In fact, he had to overeat to keep from losing weight. And the quantities he consumed, his wife felt, had to be contributing to his recurring heartburn and unsettled stomach. His bowel movements were always too loose and had an unusually foul odor, and he had excessive gas, as well.

Eating every two hours would prevent the onset of "shakes," a difficulty he had with thinking clearly, and intense irritability. If he did not eat on schedule, he would also want to fall asleep. Kirby's complexion was always pasty, even when he went skiing. He was subject to acne and to strange rashes on his legs. And his tongue was always coated and his breath odor very strong.

Anne had read books on nutrition and, thinking Kirby was hypoglycemic, had drastically reduced the amount of sugar in his diet. This did not help much, unfortunately, nor did a mostly vegetarian diet with an emphasis on whole grains and legumes, as well as fruits, seeds, and nuts. She wondered if, in fact, this healthy food could be making him a little worse, but they liked being vegetarians so had maintained this diet for several years.

When Kirby told me about his history of travel and use of antibiotics, I suspected that some of his symptoms were due to intestinal pathogens and yeast overgrowth. His tests, in fact, showed *Dientameoba fragilis*—an intestinal parasite; *Helicobacter pylori*—a bacteria that can infect the stomach and duodenum; and a yeast overgrowth in the colon. It was comforting for both Kirby and Anne to find such tangible and treatable causes of his problems, and over the next month he diligently followed the medical and nutritional treatment I prescribed.

On the next visit, however, I learned that in spite of taking all the medications and supplements and following the diet, not much had changed. Although Kirby reported having much less heartburn and a more settled stomach, nothing else had improved. I suggested then that we test his digestive function directly—his pancreatic enzyme output and his stomach hydrochloric acid level.

We discovered that Kirby's fecal chymotrypsin test was nearly zero—meaning his pancreas was secreting extremely low levels of the enzymes necessary to digest his dietary proteins, carbohydrates, and fats. Supplementing his meals with a tablet of digestive enzymes proved to be the single most beneficial measure I or any previous physicians had suggested to him. Within four to six weeks his excessive gas and bloating was gone; he no longer had loose stools; he could comfortably make it through the day eating only three meals—he no longer needed to snack or eat huge quantities—and he had gained five pounds!

Anne was most pleased that he was no longer preoccupied with food. His acne and leg rash had also cleared, and his pasty complexion had improved. I had also suggested he add some low-fat flesh foods to his diet (often helpful for hypoglycemia), use less grains and legumes (which had been an excessive percentage of his daily intake), and add more starchy vegetables.

Kirby finally consented to the testing of his stomach acid when, after four months, his treatment had not yet improved his foul-smelling stools, his coated tongue, or his bad breath. The test demonstrated obvious low acid levels. After three to four weeks of taking hydrochloric acid/pepsin supplements, these residual complaints finally cleared to both his and his wife's satisfaction. As an additional bonus, within a year he gained fifteen welcome pounds.

YOU ARE WHAT YOU DIGEST

Digestion refers to the mechanical and chemical process of breaking down food, from large molecules to small ones. Assimilation (or absorption) refers to the transport of nutrients across membranes of the gastrointestinal tract into the bloodstream and lymph system, where eventually they are carried into cells throughout the body for utilization.

The gastrointestinal tract has been marvelously designed with glands and organs that on demand secrete specialized fluids and perform intricate churning actions, which, in turn, transform food into a state that the highly specialized intestinal lining can absorb. The whole digestive tract is lined with millions of goblet cells that produce mucus to lubricate things and protect the mucosa from mechanical and chemical injury. However, injury, imbalance, and malfunction seem inevitable for many Americans.

The digestive tract is one of the more abused systems of our bodies. A multimillion-dollar industry has evolved to treat such digestive disorders as indigestion, heartburn, burping, bloating, gas, abdominal cramps, constipation, diarrhea, coated tongue, bad breath, and body odor. These nuisance ailments, as uncomfortable as they may be, are minor in comparison with other conditions that may arise in part from poor absorption: fatigue, hypoglycemia, anemia, arthritis, osteoporosis, atherosclerosis, hypertension, and states of lowered immune competence, which render the body more susceptible to infections and cancer. Knowing that the stakes are so high, you can appreciate the importance of maintaining your digestive and assimilative capacities. Figure 7-1 gives an overview of the digestive system.

THE PROCESS OF DIGESTION

The first phase of digestion, the cephalic phase, actually begins before you take your first bite of food. Intricate neurological and hormonal communications occur between the brain and the digestive system. These signals, triggered by the odors of food, the anticipation of eating, and the sensation of hunger, prepare the digestive organs for the work in which they will be engaged.

As a general rule, eating when you are hungry, relaxed, and able to enjoy your food allows these hormonal communications to set the digestive mechanisms in action. Anxiety, tension, frustration, unresolved anger, or even overexcitement at the time of a meal can inhibit neurohormonal reflexes and interfere with digestion. Such emotions also trigger the release of adrenaline, which decreases all digestive functions by shunting blood circulation away from the gastrointestinal tract. If you feel your digestive disorders may be due to stress, I suggest you try a premeal relaxation exercise (see Chapter Fifteen for a discussion on stress). If conditions do not allow you to relax sufficiently, at least thank your food and generate a momentary feeling of gratitude. Plan not to make your meal very large.

Chewing

Chewing is the next stage in the digestive process. If food is not thoroughly broken down by the mechanical act of chewing, often only the outer surfaces of the large food morsels will be exposed to your digestive secretions. In such a condition, you might feel satiated, but the food in your belly does not necessarily mean that nutrients are reaching your cells. To make matters worse, the undigested remnants reaching your colon will trigger a state of toxicity.

Chewing thoroughly is a major factor in good digestion and assimilation. Ideally, you should eat slowly and take small bites, making sure to chew food thoroughly before swallowing. It should be nearly liquefied before swallowing. If chewing is difficult, you may need to use a blender to make foods more easily digestible.

Besides readying your food for assimilation, thorough chewing further enhances the digestive process by stimulating, through the sense of taste, the hormonal signals that prepare the stomach, gallbladder, and pancreas for their work and by enhancing the salivary gland's secretion of ptyalin, a carbohydrate-digesting enzyme. Under the influence of ptyalin, long chains of starch molecules begin to break down right in the mouth. This could be an important step for carbohydrate digestion in someone whose pancreatic enzymes are compromised. Although the action of ptyalin may not substitute for pancreatic amylase,

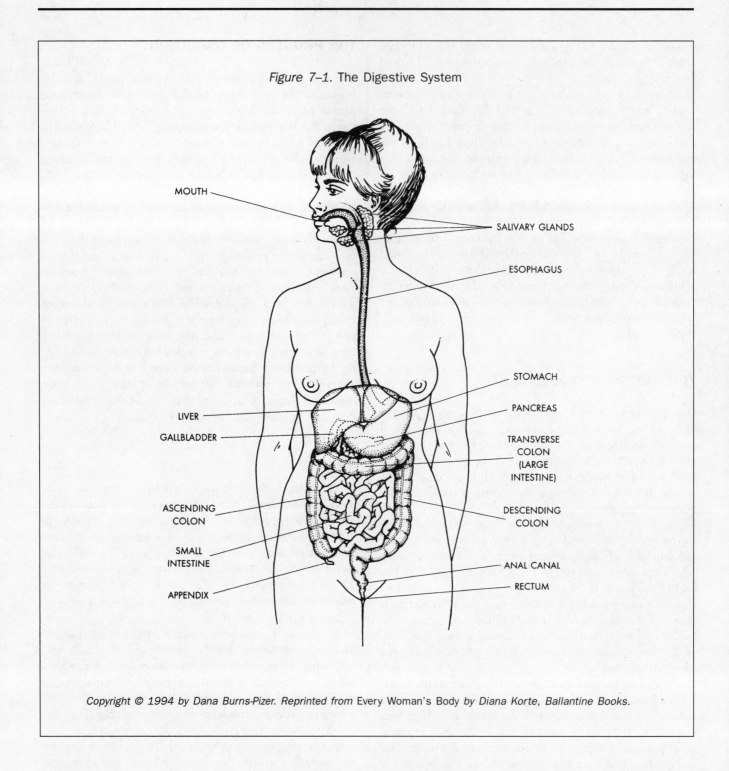

Figure 7–1. The Digestive System

MOUTH

SALIVARY GLANDS

ESOPHAGUS

STOMACH

PANCREAS

LIVER

GALLBLADDER

TRANSVERSE
COLON
(LARGE
INTESTINE)

ASCENDING
COLON

DESCENDING
COLON

SMALL
INTESTINE

ANAL CANAL

APPENDIX

RECTUM

the body's primary starch-digesting enzyme, it certainly can help.

Finally, by chewing your food thoroughly, some nutrients can pass through the mucus membranes of the mouth and enter the bloodstream directly. This absorption occurs, as with certain medications, through the rich venous network under the tongue. Although only a small fraction of food nutrients enters the bloodstream in this manner, every little bit can help. I encourage my patients who make their own fresh vegetable and fruit juices to swish these juices in their mouth before swallowing.

Fluids

Many people drink too much fluid with meals, weakening or diluting digestive secretions and impairing nutrient absorption. Ideally, most of your daily fluids should be taken thirty to forty-five minutes or more before—or at least two to three hours after—main meals. With meals, a cup of herbal tea or a small glass of water is fine. Neither very hot nor ice-cold beverages should be taken with meals since these can slow down or arrest digestive secretions and action.

A reasonable amount of wine with dinner on occasion may be fine if you are in good health. Some reports even attest to the digestion-aiding capacities of wine.[1] However, do not interpret this as free license to use alcohol inappropriately.

Portions

Overeating is another common cause of poor digestion and assimilation. A man of average strength can lift 100 pounds, but if you burden him with 250 pounds, he's not likely to be able to lift the weight at all. Eating more at one meal than the digestive system can adequately handle, and eating in this manner routinely, will overburden the acid-, enzyme-, and bile-secreting capabilities of the digestive system and the eliminative function of the colon.

Continual snacking between meals and late-night meals may also cause system burnout. Your energy is lowest at night. Sleep is for recharging your batteries, not digesting a recent meal. Your gastrointestinal tract needs an opportunity for rest and rejuvenation. Eating appropriate amounts at mealtimes and minimizing snacks will enable your digestive system to function at its best. Yet some individuals find that full meals make their digestive systems work too hard. Grazing—having five or six small, frequent meals throughout the day—is often an effective solution.

Food Combinations

Poor food combinations may partially contribute to inadequate digestion and assimilation. Several books and nutritional philosophies adhere to strict food-combining principles, some of which make good sense, while others seem rather restrictive and perhaps extreme.[2] The rationale of these principles is a bit difficult to document in the scientific literature.

I have known many individuals in my medical practice, however, who were unable to handle proteins and starches together yet could eat them separately without apparent difficulty. I have also known individuals who could handle grains and milk products separately, but not together at the same meal. The exact reason for this is unclear, but we can assume that with the more settled feeling in their stomachs from "correct" combinations, the patients' digestion and nutrient assimilation are more complete. I have also known patients whose difficulties with overweight were best managed using food-

combining principles. Although these principles may not be relevant for everyone, experiment with them. See if the combinations suggested in the diagram that follows ("Food-Combining Principles") improve how food feels in your stomach.

You may want to experiment to see how you can make your digestion more comfortable. Perhaps you don't need to be ultra strict. You may be interested in the books referenced in this section. They base their very strict food-combining principles not only on what will help your digestion, but on your overall health and well-being.

Physical Activity

Avoid excessive physical exertion immediately before or after a main meal. Your digestive system needs a lot of energy around food time, especially a main meal. Excessive muscular activity will shift your body's focus and circulation away from your digestive system toward your muscles, leaving the digestive system on hold and unable to do its job well. A short walk, however, soon after eating can actually enhance the digestive process.

Bowel Function

Having full, regular bowel evacuations is a requirement of health and well-being. If the lower end of the gastrointestinal tract becomes sluggish (constipation), the digestive functions farther up become impaired. You may have a sluggish colon and yet have one or more bowel movements every day. Test your transit time (see instructions on page 160) to see whether or not you are constipated. If so, take appropriate measures to correct this condition, as it may be a primary cause of your digestive symptoms. Realize, however, that diminished hydrochloric acid secretion from your stomach is also a cause of constipation.

Hydrochloric Acid

Even before you eat, just being hungry and thinking about food initiates neural reflexes that trigger the release of the hormone gastrin that stimulates stomach cells. Chewing food continues this process. Protein digestion begins as the stomach's parietal cells secrete hydrochloric acid and the chief cells secrete pepsin. It is the enzyme pepsin that acts on protein, breaking it down into polypeptides, or chains of amino acids.

This enzymatic action, however, requires a very low pH (acidic environment) and will therefore occur only under the influence of adequate hydrochloric acid production. Pepsinogen is the actual substance secreted by the chief cells; it becomes pepsin only by the action of the acid. Hydrochloric acid also acts to kill ingested bacteria and parasites, and may itself, by its denaturing

FOOD-COMBINING PRINCIPLES

Avoid mixing fruits with other foods, especially proteins.

Mixing more than one protein at a meal is hard on the digestive system. Milk does not combine well with other foods. Dairy products go best with grains or the green, less starchy, vegetables.

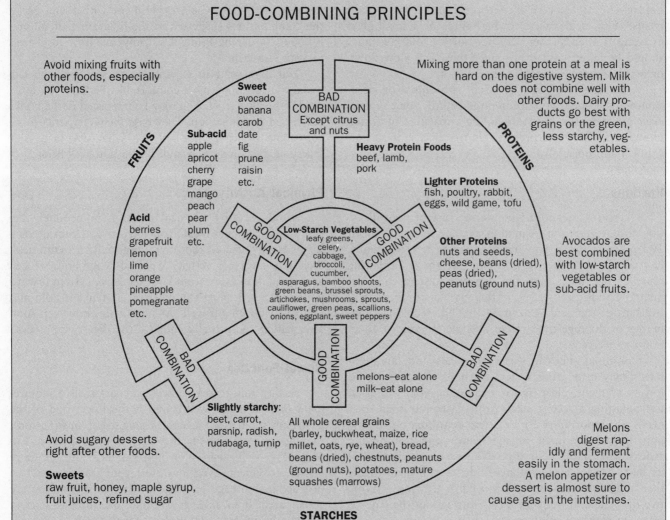

FRUITS

Sweet
avocado
banana
carob
date
fig
prune
raisin
etc.

Sub-acid
apple
apricot
cherry
grape
mango
peach
pear
plum
etc.

Acid
berries
grapefruit
lemon
lime
orange
pineapple
pomegranate
etc.

PROTEINS

BAD COMBINATION
Except citrus and nuts

Heavy Protein Foods
beef, lamb, pork

Lighter Proteins
fish, poultry, rabbit, eggs, wild game, tofu

GOOD COMBINATION

Low-Starch Vegetables
leafy greens, celery, cabbage, broccoli, cucumber, asparagus, bamboo shoots, green beans, brussel sprouts, artichokes, mushrooms, sprouts, cauliflower, green peas, scallions, onions, eggplant, sweet peppers

GOOD COMBINATION

Other Proteins
nuts and seeds, cheese, beans (dried), peas (dried), peanuts (ground nuts)

Avocados are best combined with low-starch vegetables or sub-acid fruits.

BAD COMBINATION

GOOD COMBINATION

melons–eat alone
milk–eat alone

BAD COMBINATION

Slightly starchy:
beet, carrot, parsnip, radish, rudabaga, turnip

All whole cereal grains (barley, buckwheat, maize, rice millet, oats, rye, wheat), bread, beans (dried), chestnuts, peanuts (ground nuts), potatoes, mature squashes (marrows)

STARCHES

Avoid sugary desserts right after other foods.

Sweets
raw fruit, honey, maple syrup, fruit juices, refined sugar

Melons digest rapidly and ferment easily in the stomach. A melon appetizer or dessert is almost sure to cause gas in the intestines.

Adapted from Staying Healthy with the Seasons, © *1981 by Elson M. Haas, M.D. Reprinted by permission of Celestial Arts, Berkeley, CA.*

- Do not combine in the same meal heavy or lighter protein foods with starchy foods, such as beef with bread. Being less strict, you might try a grain like brown rice with the lighter proteins, or bread with eggs. Experiment to see what will work.

- Do not combine heavy or lighter protein foods with milk or milk products or have a dairy dessert right after these proteins.

- Do not combine raw fruit or fruit juices with slightly starchy vegetables or with any nonfruit meal. Your digestive system may need to wait at least a half hour between them. Better to have them at separate meals. Lemon juice may be an exception.

- Do not have sweets of any kind with protein foods or immediately after a protein meal. This includes fruit, honey, maple syrup, and table sugar. Fresh pineapple and papaya are exceptions. They can be eaten with or immediately after protein. Wait at least thirty minutes for dessert.

FOOD-COMBINING PRINCIPLES

The following combination recommendations may be helpful:

- Combine any protein foods with leafy or low-starch vegetables.

- Combine starchy foods with leafy or low-starch vegetables.

- Have milk alone or experiment to see if it works with grain foods like cereals.

- Experiment to see if cheese works well with either fruit or vegetables, or try it with grain products or egg dishes.

- Papaya and pineapple, which contain abundant digestive enzymes, may combine well with any of the food groups, especially proteins.

- Experiment to see how nuts or seeds and unrefined oils combine with any of the food groups.

- Depending on your digestive system, fruits may or may not be combined with seeds and nuts, grains, or milk products.

ability, help slightly in breaking down protein. Although protein theoretically has another good opportunity to be digested by pancreatic enzymes, many practitioners suggest that the stomach's action is a prerequisite for optimal digestion and assimilation to occur. Such conditions as anemia and osteoporosis can result in part from insufficient amounts of hydrochloric acid, even with iron- and calcium-rich diets.[3]

A surprisingly large percentage of adults, particularly those over fifty years of age, have hypochlorhydria.[4] Even some children with asthma have been found to be deficient in hydrochloric acid.[5] Hypochlorhydria is a common digestive deficiency. Individuals with pernicious anemia and resultant vitamin B-12 deficiency often have no stomach acid (achlorhydria), a condition that can be inherited.

Theories abound as to why a deficiency of hydrochloric acid occurs in adults:

- Some practitioners have suggested that hypochlorhydria is a manifestation of autoimmune disease. Antiparietal cell antibodies can be measured in the blood and may play a role in diminishing stomach function.

- In the last several years it has been shown that a bacterial infection, helicobacter pylori (formerly named campylobacter pylori), suppresses hydrochloric acid production. It also digests the mucin—the stomach's protective layer—and denudes the mucosa, allowing the small amount of hydrochloric acid that is present to burn and cause pain, even ulcers. It has been estimated that over 90 percent of duodenal ulcer patients, 70 to 80 percent of gastric ulcer patients, and 50 percent of patients with nonulcer gastritis/indigestion/heartburn have a helicobacter pylori infection.[6] This infection may eventually turn out to be a commonly recognized cause of hypochlorhydria, and its treatment may be necessary for a return to normal acidity. (To test for helicobacter pylori, I usually obtain a blood test, helicobacter pylori IgG antibody. Far more costly and invasive is gastroscopic biopsy and culture.)

- Some practitioners have suggested that low stomach acid may result from years of eating devitalized food, therefore depriving stomach cells of nutrients required to produce hydrochloric acid and pepsin.

- Excessive dietary fat and sugar may inhibit hydrochloric acid and pepsin secretion.[7]

- Overeating may be another cause of low stomach acid. In order to make 1 liter of gastric juice, stomach cells have to expend 1,500 calories of energy and concentrate hydrogen ion four million times the amount found in arterial blood. Knowing this, you can begin to appreciate how overstimulation and overwork (from overeating) may lead to depletion.

- Weakened adrenal function (see Chapter Eleven) and hypothyroidism (see "Hypothyroidism," in Chapter Seventeen) can also cause a deficiency of hydrochloric acid.

SYMPTOMS OF INSUFFICIENT HYDROCHLORIC ACID

Symptoms of hydrochloric acid insufficiency (otherwise known as hypochlorhydria) include:

Heartburn/indigestion   Gas and bloating
Upper abdominal fullness or heaviness   Chronic constipation
The feeling of food not moving along;   Undigested food in stools
   "it just sits there"   Coated tongue
Feeling hungrier after eating   Bad breath

Insufficient hydrochloric acid may result in problems outside the digestive tract. I have seen other diffuse and chronic symptoms in association with low stomach acid:

Arthritis (osteoarthritis)   Weak, peeling, and cracked fingernails
Muscle cramps   Adult acne
Fatigue   Iron deficiency anemia
Multiple food allergies   Chronic intestinal parasites
Itchy anus   Chronic intestinal candida overgrowth
Dilated capillaries in the cheeks and nose   Toxic colon
   (in nonalcoholics)   Osteoporosis

Although not necessarily a direct cause, low stomach acid is seen in numerous diseases:

Addison's disease   Lupus erythematosus
Asthma   Myasthenia gravis
Chronic autoimmune disorders   Osteoporosis
Celiac disease   Pernicious anemia
Dermatitis herpetiformis   Psoriasis
Diabetes mellitus   Rheumatoid arthritis
Eczema   Rosacea
Gallbladder disease   Sjögren's syndrome
Graves' disease   Hyper- and hypothyroidism
Hepatitis   Vitiligo
Chronic hives

Source: "Heidelberg Gastric Analysis" from A Textbook of Natural Medicine *by J.E. Pizzorno, M.T. Murray, S.A. Barrie (eds.), Bastyr University Publications, 1994, Section II: Heidel 1–4. Reprinted by permission of Bastyr University Publications, 144 N.E. 54th Street, Seattle, WA 98105.*

- Stress can correlate directly to hypochlorhydria by inhibiting neurohormonal mechanisms necessary for hydrochloric acid and pepsin secretion, and indirectly through weakened adrenal function.
- A salt-restricted diet may contribute to hydrochloric acid insufficiency.
- Some practitioners believe that the body will strive at all costs to maintain an acid/alkaline balance. (Alkaline is the opposite of acid.) If your body runs too much on the alkalotic side, it will be very selfish about donating hydrogen ions to make hydrochloric acid when it may need these acid-forming ions to fight a metabolic alkalosis.

Tests to Diagnose Hypochlorhydria   The gastro test is a simple and inexpensive method to determine adequacy of stomach acidity.[8] After an overnight fast, the gastro capsule is swallowed. This special weighted capsule has a string protruding from one end, which is held while the capsule is swallowed. The capsule carries the remaining string to the stomach, where the capsule melts and the highly absorbent cotton string soaks up gastric juices. Within fifteen minutes, the string is gently pulled out and tested for its pH by a colorimetric reading. If there is insufficient acid, the test is over and hypochlorhydria can be diagnosed. If there appears to be normal acidity, 3 teaspoons of a saturated solution of baking soda are taken orally to see if the stomach can reacidify. The test is repeated in forty minutes. Upon retesting, if the reading shows low acidity, a diagnosis of hypochlorhydria can then be made. Two or more baking soda challenges may be necessary to determine if the stomach does not adequately reacidify. If after the final challenge, however, a normal acid level still shows, the stomach most likely produces sufficient acid.

A more expensive and somewhat better method is the Heidelberg gastrogram, which electronically measures hydrochloric acid levels.[9] A capsule containing a microtransmitter is swallowed, and the stomach acid level is measured. As the patient drinks challenging doses of the baking soda solution, the transmitter measures the drop in acidity and subsequent acid rebound or lack of response, all of which is recorded on a graph. The Heidelberg test clearly demonstrates the speed and gradation of reacidification.

Another method of assessing stomach acid is a twenty-four-hour comprehensive urinalysis. The urinary pH and chloride excretion are read together, along with other data, to determine the acid/alkaline balance. Finding a high pH and low chloride level is usually indicative of alkalosis or insufficient acid, but several other variations are indicative of this condition as well. A positive urinary indican (Obermeyer) test is also indirectly suggestive of hypochlorhydria (see page 160).

Many physicians do not seem aware of the importance of assessing stomach acid sufficiency and are therefore unfamiliar with these tests. Years later, they end up diagnosing and treating the end-stage conditions and illnesses that result from low stomach acid which could be avoided with early preventive-oriented tests and intervention.

In terms of stomach acidity, most physicians' concern is usually with excess acidity and ulcers. They are quick to prescribe antacids or acid-antagonists, which usually help the symptoms of heartburn and indigestion, but bypass the underlying cause and invite ulcer recurrences. Furthermore, not testing and compensating for low stomach acidity will inevitably lead to future health deterioration.

It is interesting to note that many cases of heartburn and indigestion thought to be a result of too much acid, are successfully treated with supplemental hydrochloric acid. This paradox can be explained by the fact that the stomach's exit valve, the pylorus, needs a certain amount of acid to open and release food into the duodenum. If the stomach does not secrete enough acid, the pylorus will not open effectively, the stomach contents will sit, and the small amount of acid you do make will pool and cause discomfort.

Once a diagnosis of hypochlorhydria has been made, or at least strongly suspected, it can be treated or helped in several ways:

1. Commonsense measures: Make sure you are relaxed and hungry before meals. Chew your food thoroughly. Avoid excessive fluids and amounts of food. Avoid excessively hot or cold fluids with meals. Pay attention to food combinations. Avoid excessive fat and sugar. Take a short walk after eating. Avoid constipation.

2. Look for underlying thyroid or adrenal insufficiency, autoimmune disease, or helicobacter pylori infection.

3. Supplement with bitters that stimulate hydrochloric acid secretion.

4. Supplement with hydrochloric acid.

As a preliminary step, follow the commonsense measures above. They can make a major difference in your digestion. Incidentally, a brief walk after a meal will stimulate the production of acid through muscle metabolism. This, in turn, may convince your stomach's parietal cells that they do not have to conserve acidity.

Have your doctor check you for a helicobacter pylori infection and, if indicated, the other conditions listed in step 2 above.

Bitters, such as gentian and goldenseal (hydrastis), seven parts to one part in a tincture form, are often recommended by naturopathic physicians to stimulate hydrochloric acid production, as well as pancreatic and biliary secretions. Fifteen to twenty drops or about one teaspoonful in a few ounces of warm water sipped twenty minutes before mealtime may do the trick. (Try Bitters Formula, available from Herb Pharm of Williams, Oregon.) If alcohol is not contraindicated, an aperitif, such as Campari or Angostura bitters, may work in the same manner.

Although anyone can purchase proteases and other plant and aspergillus-derived enzymes from a health food store, it is unlikely that this alone will successfully balance pH levels and restore full stomach function. Additionally, you should seek the supervision of a doctor skilled in the use of comprehensive urinalysis and the various enzyme formulations designed for metabolic balancing.

If your doctor has found that your system is too alkaline, you may need a more acidifying diet (see Chapter Four) or a systemic acidifier such as ammonium chloride. This can increase the stomach's ability to produce adequate amounts of hydrochloric acid.

For many individuals these measures may be ineffective, in which case hydrochloric acid itself can be supplemented: either betaine hydrochloride with pepsin (10-grain capsules) or glutamic acid hydrochloride with pepsin (7.5-grain capsules). Most physicians familiar with this therapy will recommend starting with one capsule at the beginning of each main meal. If, after using supplements in this manner for three days, you have not experienced any stomach pain, burning, queasiness, abdominal or lower chest discomfort, the dose may be increased to two capsules per main meal.

Again, after two to three days without the appearance of these particular symptoms, you may increase the dose to three per meal or however many your health practitioner has advised. If any one particular dose does trigger these symptoms, reduce by one capsule or use the next lower dose at which you experienced none of the symptoms. For smaller meals that will not require as much digestive assistance, reduce the dose appropriately. If your stomach has gone years without sufficient hydrochloric acid, introducing even just one capsule—a dose far below what you may need—may cause burning and other discomfort. It is important to work with a knowledgeable physician who can help your stomach acclimate to the supplement. Otherwise, you may mistakenly interpret the burning as a signal that your stomach already has sufficient acidity.

To treat any acute symptoms from an excess of acid supplement, use yogurt or milk (if not milk allergic), baking soda, Alka-Seltzer Gold (does not contain aspirin), or any alkalinizing agent you can tolerate.

One significant risk with using hydrochloric acid supplements is the very rare instance of *not* having any symptoms indicating an excessive dose, which could lead to a silent ulcer and a life-threatening hemorrhage or perforation. The onset of black tarry-appearing stools would signify upper gastrointestinal bleeding. If this occurs, immediately discontinue the supplements and notify your doctor (see "Ulcers," Chapter Seventeen). You may want to decide with your doctor what dose to use with each meal and test your stool periodically for blood. In this way, you can detect very early signs of bleeding and prevent further complications.

Using aspirin, ibuprofen, and other nonsteroidal anti-inflammatory drugs (as well as steroids) will pose additional risk for ulcers, particularly with acid supplements. It is best to discontinue the hydrochloric acid if you need to be on a prolonged course of these medicines.

If taking hydrochloric acid tablets relieves your digestive disturbances, chances are you have hydrochloric acid deficiency. Your stomach also may not be producing enough intrinsic factor either, a substance necessary for the assimilation of vitamin B-12. You may need at first weekly, then bimonthly and eventually monthly, vitamin B-12 injections with folic acid to feel your best. Occasionally, the sublingual or nasal gel form of B-12 may do the job.

Many individuals who have taken supplemental hydrochloric acid for years seem to have become dependent on it. When possible, it is preferable to use other approaches to get the stomach working on its own again (like taking bitters or finding a treatable cause of hypochlorhydria, such as helicobacter pylori or adrenal exhaustion). When such a goal cannot be reached, however, supplement dependency may be preferable to an outright deficiency. In fact, the appropriate dose of supplemental hydrochloric acid can safeguard against nutrient deficiencies, intestinal toxicity, and the attendant complications of both conditions.

If you require hydrochloric acid supplements or have ulcers, gastritis, or other persistent upper abdominal digestive symptoms, you should be checked for a helicobacter pylori infection. Your doctor should obtain the appropriate diagnostic tests and, if the results are positive, give you a trial of colloidal bismuth subcitrate and appropriate antibiotics (often metronidazole and tetracycline or ampicillin). It is common that two different antibiotics, taken concurrently, are required along with the bismuth ("triple therapy") to prevent recurrences. (If your doctor cannot suggest a bismuth preparation other than the common over-the-counter type containing sugar, food coloring, and aluminum, an excellent source of bismuth is "Bismagel" [bismuth in aloe vera gel], available by prescription through Clark's Prescriptions in Bellevue, Washington (206) 881-0222. This pharmacy processes mail orders.) Successful treatment of this bacteria may enable your stomach to begin producing normal amounts of acid once again.

Pancreatic and Intestinal Enzymes

After spending time in the stomach, chyme, the liquid slurry of food in the process of being digested, exits through the pylorus and enters the duodenum, the first part of the small intestine. At this point, it is greeted by both enzymes and bicarbonate from the pancreas and bile from the liver and gallbladder. In contrast with the stomach, where an acidic environment is necessary for pepsin's action, pancreatic and intestinal enzymes require an alkaline environment. It is the generous supply of bicarbonate secreted from the pancreas that allows these enzymes to do their work (see Figure 7–1).

The pancreas secretes

1. protein-digesting enzymes: trypsin, chymotrypsin, and carboxypeptidase, which break down protein to

polypeptides (small chains of amino acids). Ribonuclease and deoxyribonuclease digest RNA and DNA.

2. starch-digesting enzymes: amylase, which breaks down carbohydrate polysaccharides to disaccharides.

3. fat-digesting enzymes: lipase, which helps break down fat into glycerol and fatty acids.

These enzymes do their work in the remainder of the duodenum and subsequent sections of the small intestine. To complete the process that pancreatic enzymes initiate, other crucial enzymes located in the villi, the epithelial cells of the mucosa of the small bowel, finish the digestive phenomena. At this point, these digested molecules have already begun their absorption into the brush border microvilli membrane, where they will soon enter the bloodstream and be whisked off to the liver for further processing. Intestinal secretory IgA (components of which come from both immunocytes and intestinal mucosa cells) is an antibody also involved in the final steps of digestion and assimilation. Its primary role is to defend the mucosa from infections and allergies.

Acute digestive symptoms from pancreatic and intestinal enzyme deficiencies can mimic symptoms of hypochlorhydria. Greasy, fatty, floating stools, diarrhea, and stools with a lot of undigested food may be additional symptoms. Acne, food allergies, hypoglycemic symptoms, and abnormal weight gain—or, more commonly, weight loss—may also herald pancreatic insufficiency. The easiest and least expensive definitive test for determining pancreatic enzyme sufficiency is measuring the level of chymotrypsin in a stool sample (fecal chymotrypsin).[10] A chymex urine test is also available to identify pancreatic enzyme output.[11] The Obermeyer test for urinary indican can also show indirect evidence of pancreatic insufficiency.

Several theories have been proposed to explain the causes of pancreatic enzyme insufficiency. Overeating can exhaust the pancreas, and, according to live-food enthusiasts, so can a diet too high in cooked foods that rely on pancreatic enzymes.[12] According to these theories, cooking inactivates and depletes the food enzymes that in raw food aid in their own digestion. Cooked food, lacking its own food enzymes, relies on and eventually depletes the body of its digestive enzymes. Again, a diet too high in devitalized foods, which are deficient in zinc, manganese, vitamin B-6, and magnesium, or insufficient in protein will not provide the pancreas its nutritional building blocks.

Such foods are also usually lacking in fiber, and insufficient fiber is known to diminish pancreatic exocrine output.[13] Too much sugar may do the same. Again, in terms of acid-base balance, if the body has become too acidotic—quite common in the standard American diet—the body will want to conserve the bicarbonate-producing ability of the pancreas to help reverse the acidosis. With the pancreas being stingy about bicarbonate secretion, its enzymes may not function well. In states of diminished vitality, such as adrenal exhaustion or hypothyroidism, the limited amount of energy the body has is reserved for the most important functions; digestive organs are considered less vital.

I am not sure just which theories to believe, but I have seen countless numbers of individuals improve with treatment for pancreatic deficiency, which leads me to believe their conditions are real. It is also important to note that the spasm that helicobacter pylori and giardia infections cause in the duodenum can shut off or drastically compromise the flow of pancreatic enzymes into the small intestine and cause, in effect, a functional enzyme deficiency and a subclinical pancreatitis.

Supplemental digestive enzymes are generally used to treat cases of pancreatic enzyme insufficiency. Many plant/aspergillus-derived enzymes contain protease, amylase, and lipase, and are acid stable, which means they can work in the acidic environment of the stomach as well as in the alkaline small intestine. Some formulas contain another enzyme to digest cellulose (cellulase). Papaya and pineapple provide natural sources of enzymes (papain and bromelain), which are available in capsules or tablets. However, these two enzymes digest protein only—not fat or carbohydrates—and may not be adequate supplementation alone. I have some concern about the safety of glandular supplements (see discussion in Chapter Eleven) and until this is addressed, I am no longer recommending animal-derived pancreatic enzymes or pancreatin.

I have seen many individuals benefit from using digestive enzyme supplements. Some are able to be weaned off them successfully after four to twelve months, probably due to the combined effects of switching to a whole-foods (nutrient- and fiber-rich) diet, following the measures outlined on pages 152–153, and finding and treating underlying disorders.

Gastrointestinal symptoms may be caused by intestinal infections or inflammation diminishing intestinal cell enzyme and intestinal secretory IgA levels. Excessive stress can diminish secretory IgA production as well (see Chapter Eleven). A stool sample can determine and assess intestinal secretory IgA levels,[14] whereas a urine test for intestinal permeability and absorption can assess the health and absorptive capacity of the small intestinal cells.[15] Finding and treating giardiasis and other parasitic infections (see Chapter Seventeen), intestinal yeast overgrowth (Chapter Twelve), the "leaky gut" syndrome (Chapter Thirteen, page 242), and food allergies (Chapter Thirteen)—all common causes of intestinal inflammations—are paramount in returning normal digestive function to intestinal mucosal cells. Using the nutrients that specifically feed intestinal cells also gives these cells the best chance to recover (see Chapter Thirteen, page 243).

Bile and the Liver

The function of bile is discussed in Chapter Nine. Briefly, bile acts to emulsify dietary fat into tiny chylomicrons that can pass through the brush border membrane of the small intestine into the lymph vessels, where it is carried off to its destinations. Poor-quality bile cannot readily be measured, yet some indirect signs may be intolerance to fatty foods, biliousness, constipation, and bad breath. Insufficient quantity of bile may produce very light-colored stools as well. Herbal choleretic and cholegogues can stimulate production and secretion of bile, and, if necessary, ox bile–containing digestive aids are also available (particularly important if you have had your gallbladder removed). The liver-cleansing and rejuvenating programs outlined in Chapter Nine may provide more useful options.

HERBAL DIGESTIVE REMEDIES

In addition to the above practices and supplements, other remedies may also prove helpful. Try an herbal combination capsule—wild yam, sarsaparilla, ginger, and goldenseal; or fennel, wild yam, peppermint, ginger, papaya, spearmint, catnip, and lobelia. Combination herbal digestive formulas are available commercially from health food and herb stores and herbal product distributors.

Drink peppermint, spearmint, papaya-mint, or bancha (kukicha or twig) tea. As mentioned earlier, try bitters or an aperitif. The bitters can be used symptomatically as well to relieve indigestion.

Cooking with ginger can also aid digestion, as can using aloe vera, ½ ounce of juice or ½ tablespoon of the gel. Slippery elm tea and aloe vera juice can work effectively to soothe irritation, inflammation, heartburn, indigestion, even ulcers. "Glyconda" by Eclectic Institute (Sandy, Oregon) and "Gastro Relief" by Enzymatic Therapy (Green Bay, Wisconsin) are effective combination herbal remedies for indigestion. Deglycerhizinated licorice root is an effective healer of stomach and duodenal inflammations and ulcers; take two tablets twenty minutes before meals and at bedtime. Chapter Nineteen discusses these and other digestive herbs.

Uncooked fermented foods and uncooked sprouts are also beneficial. By their nature, they have already begun the digestion of their macromolecules, thereby freeing up some of your digestive energy to work on other foods. Items such as unpasteurized miso and unpasteurized or raw sauerkraut are examples of fermented foods. They contain live enzymes (if you do not boil it) that can aid in their digestion and that of other foods (see recipes in Chapter Five). Include small amounts of fermented, cultured foods (yogurt, for example), or high-enzyme foods (sprouts, for example) with your meals. Fresh papaya and pineapple, as previously mentioned, contain active protein-digesting enzymes. Incidentally, soaking raw seeds and nuts overnight initiates the sprouting process and enhances their digestibility (see Chapter Three for more information).

Examples of fermented foods include:

- Unpasteurized miso—used as a soup base and seasoning.
- Tempeh—a vegetarian protein staple made from soy and grains.
- Unpasteurized sauerkraut.
- Yogurt, buttermilk, or keir.
- Rejuvelac and seed or nut yogurt.
- Sprouts: alfalfa, clover, mung bean, sunflower seeds, other seeds and nuts, some legumes.

Raw foods contain abundant enzymes that aid in their own digestion; they also offer a higher nutrient content than their cooked counterparts. Many health enthusiasts feel that a good part of your diet should consist of raw foods. Too much, however, can bring on gas, bloating, cramps, diarrhea, and other symptoms in many individuals. Cooked food is somewhat predigested (higher temperatures break down cellulose) and is easier to digest, though it no longer contains any live enzymes or as many vitamins and minerals as in its raw state. There are benefits and disadvantages to both raw and cooked foods, and each person must find the ratio that best suits his or her own tastes and dietary needs.

High-acid-containing substances, such as vinegar and fresh lemon juice, can help in the digestion of protein meals; try one to three teaspoons. Take some precautions, however; the regular use of these undiluted acids can contribute to the erosion of tooth enamel. Mix them in your food—salads, for example—or in a little liquid. If highly acidic substances have direct contact with your teeth, swish thoroughly with water and a little baking soda right after the meal. Better yet, brush your teeth with baking soda.

REJUVENATING YOUR DIGESTIVE SYSTEM

There are many interrelated components to successful digestion and assimilation:

- Being hungry and relaxed for meals.
- Chewing well.
- Choosing healthful, whole foods.

- Finding the relative percentages of raw and cooked foods that are appropriate for you.
- Eating sensible amounts and at the right times.
- Drinking only modest amounts of fluids with meals (and not iced or very hot).
- Experimenting with food combinations.
- Being aware of the importance of daily bowel elimination.
- Adequate hydrochloric acid and pepsin secretion from the stomach.
- Adequate enzyme and bicarbonate secretion from the pancreas.
- Adequate bile from the gallbladder and liver.
- Adequate enzymes from the epithelial cells of the small intestine (as well as adequate secretory IgA).

Identify and avoid food allergens, and treat candidiasis, helicobacter pylori, parasites, adrenal dysfunction, and other related conditions. Attending to such digestive supporting measures over which you have direct control will put less of a strain on your primary digestive organs and secretions and enhance your digestive and absorptive capacities. There are accurate and inexpensive tests to measure your stomach and pancreatic enzyme output and safe, effective treatments to enhance and/or supplement your digestive secretions. Proper digestion and absorption of nutrients is paramount to maintaining your health and well-being. In Chapter Eighteen, you will learn in more detail how common eating styles contribute to digestive fatigue and how cleansing diets and periodic fasts can help undo some of the damage and rejuvenate digestive capacities.

SUGGESTED READING

Hoffman, Ronald L. *Seven Weeks to a Settled Stomach*. New York: Simon & Schuster, 1990.

Kaslo, Arthur, M.D., and Miles, Richard. *Freedom from Chronic Disease*. Los Angeles: Tarcher, 1979.

Matsen, John, N.D. *Eating Alive: Prevention through Good Digestion*. Vancouver, Canada: Crompton Books, 1987.

Wigmore, Ann, N.D. *The Hippocrates Diet and Health Program*. Wayne, NJ: Avery, 1984.

Wiley, Rudolf A., Ph.D. *Biobalance: The Acid/Alkaline Solution to the Food-Mood Puzzle*. Tacoma, WA: Life Sciences Press, 1989.

Wright, Jonathan, M.D. *Dr. Wright's Guide to Healing with Nutrition*. Emmaus, PA: Rodale Press, 1984.

CHAPTER 8

THE TOXIC BOWEL

In the preceding chapter, we discussed the processes of digestion and assimilation. In this chapter, we focus on the colon and its role in elimination.

Below the first twenty-five feet of the gastrointestinal tract, where the bulk of digestion and assimilation takes place, lies the colon, the body's disposal system. Although only five feet long, the large bowel is one of the more central of the body's four excretory organs, along with the lungs, kidneys, and skin. The colon suffers greatly from poor care and can subsequently cause many problems, from gas and constipation, to colon and rectal cancer. This chapter presents the subject of bowel toxicity, its recognition, treatment, and prevention. We will begin with a case history followed by a review of the basic workings of the colon, and finally, a plan for colon health.

CLAIRE

Claire, a forty-six-year-old mother of three, came to see me because of her "bowel problems." For the last ten years she had become increasingly constipated. She was "lucky," as she put it, if she had two bowel movements a week, and she relied upon laxatives for that. In addition, she used enemas because her evacuations usually felt incomplete. From all her straining (her stools were a very hard consistency and difficult to expel), Claire had developed hemorrhoids and recurring bleeding from an anal fissure.

Always a very energetic woman and free of health problems for the most part, Claire admitted that this "bowel thing" had eroded her sense of well-being and positive disposition. Furthermore, Claire had read that colon and rectal cancer were more likely to occur in in-dividuals with chronic constipation, and ten years of chronic constipation was enough now to have her more than a little worried. She also began to wonder if her current fatigue in the last few years was related at all to her bowels.

I asked Claire if she could remember any event or circumstances that related to the onset of her initial siege of constipation ten years previously. She recalled that her normal bowel pattern began to change shortly after the birth of her daughter (her third child). That pregnancy went well, other than the eighth and ninth months when she took several courses of antibiotics for a persistent sinus infection. She developed loose stools during this time and for another several months.

However, right at the time her bowels were beginning to normalize, she went on an overnight camping outing, inadvertently drank untreated river water and developed a far more severe case of diarrhea, this time with cramps. She saw her doctor subsequently and was diagnosed with an intestinal parasite and treated with an antibiotic that seemed to resolve her condition. After this episode, her bowels gradually became more and more sluggish, and over the years assumed their current pattern.

I suggested to Claire a number of commonsense measures such as including more fiber-rich foods in her diet (whole grains, legumes, fresh vegetables, and fruits) and limiting such potentially constipating foods as white flour and cheese. I also told her to drink at least four large glasses of water every day and to work in some exercise at least three days a week. I also suggested using flaxseed powder, a fiber powder supplement (she had experimented previously with psyllium powder, only to find it caused her to bloat and become more consti-pated). I also recommended a few stool tests to rule out

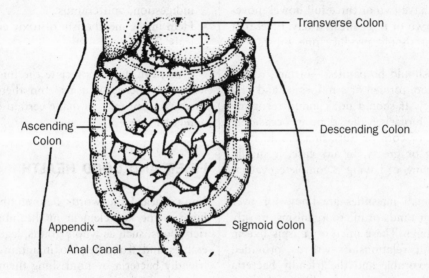

Figure 8–1. The Large Bowel

Transverse Colon

Ascending Colon

Descending Colon

Appendix

Sigmoid Colon

Anal Canal

the possibility of an intestinal yeast overgrowth and a persistent giardia infection (possibly left over from her infection ten years previously). Both these conditions are common causes of constipation (and fatigue), and I obtained a blood screen to rule out hypothyroidism (low thyroid function), another common cause of Claire's symptoms.

On her follow-up visit, Claire reported that the diet and lifestyle changes had been definitely helpful. Her bowels were moving three times a week now, and she was not requiring the use of laxatives and enemas as often. I reported to her that her tests showed the presence of the giardia parasite as well as an intestinal yeast overgrowth and that treatment of these conditions (see in Chapter Seventeen, "Parasites," and Chapter Twelve) would most likely return her bowel condition and her energy level to normal. (Her thyroid test proved to be fine.) Within one month of the treatment program,

Claire was having daily, effortless bowel movements without laxatives or enemas and was feeling her energetic, positive self again.

Claire's story brings to light many aspects of colon care. Let's now review some basic fundamentals of colon health.

A SHORT LESSON IN PHYSIOLOGY

The colon, or large intestine, is a muscular tube that serves as a temporary holding tank for what the upper gastrointestinal tract does not digest and assimilate (see Figure 8-1).

A thick liquid, or chyme, is transformed in the colon to solid or semi-solid feces, which are propelled along by waves of muscular contractions (peristaltic action) until they are expelled. The majority of the peristaltic action necessary for a bowel movement is caused by stomach and duodenal reflexes, when these parts of the upper gastrointestinal tract are distended from food.

Transit time, or the time it takes for food to travel the length of the entire gastrointestinal tract (twenty-five feet of small intestine and five feet of colon), is approximately eighteen to thirty-six hours. Several health authorities feel that if you eat two or three full meals every day, you should also have two or three full bowel movements. If you do eat two or three meals a day, I feel that at the very least you should produce one substantial evacuation daily.

The elimination should be painless—in fact, rather effortless—and the stool formed or semiformed and of a bulky, soft consistency. It should not contain recognizable undigested food morsels (other than an occasional poorly chewed piece of corn or nut), nor should it be terribly foul smelling or greasy. In any case, it should leave you with a feeling of having a complete evacuation.

The large and small intestines are home for over four hundred different kinds of microorganisms, mostly bacteria and some fungi. These microorganisms live in harmonious, symbiotic relationship with us, provided the conditions are favorable and the friendly bacteria (*Lactobacillus acidophilus* and *Lactobacillus bifidus*) are sufficient in quantity. The acidophilus bacteria live primarily in the small intestine, the bifidus primarily in the colon. These bacteria feed on the fermentable carbohydrates in our diet (found in grains, beans, vegetables, fruits, and lactose from milk products). They also feed on constituents of our intestinal mucus. In turn, they perform many crucial tasks for us.

LACTOBACILLI OR FRIENDLY BACTERIA

Lactobacilli produce natural antibiotics (acidophilin, lactocidin, and acidolin) to fend off such bacterial pathogens as salmonella, shigella, staphylococcus, *E. coli,* clostridia, and *Helicobacter pylori*.[1] The lactic acid that they form from the fermentation of carbohydrates discourages the growth of unfavorable organisms. Yeast *(Candida albicans)* is also inhibited by lactobacilli. In performing this service, the friendly bacteria prevent the intestinal overgrowth of harmful organisms and the secretion and absorption in the bloodstream of microbial toxins. In essence, they prevent intestinal, bladder, and vaginal infections and bowel toxicity.

Lactobacilli also:

- Synthesize B vitamins and vitamin K.
- Synthesize butyric acid (butyrate), which is a primary fuel and healer for cells lining the colon and an im-

portant anticancer agent that serves in the prevention of colon and other cancers.
- Synthesize acetic acid, which inhibits cholesterol synthesis in the liver and helps lower serum cholesterol levels.
- Improve lactose metabolism.
- Promote regular bowel functioning, countering both diarrhea and constipation, as well as gas, bloating, indigestion, and cramps.
- Help in the metabolism of toxic environmental chemicals.

You can now appreciate the importance of friendly intestinal microorganisms, and there are specific measures you can take to make certain their population remains strong.

FIBER AND GOOD HEALTH

You've heard the words before: fiber, bulk, roughage. Fiber is the key element in the intestinal arena. Fiber-rich foods, such as whole grains, legumes, and fresh vegetables and fruit, help to maintain the populations of friendly bacteria by nourishing them and by promoting normal transit time.

Milk products with lactose and lactobacilli-containing foods, such as yogurt and fermented foods (unpasteurized miso, raw sauerkraut, and tamari-shoyu), help to increase intestinal lactobacilli populations as well. Vegetarians and lactovegetarians, with a preponderance of high-fiber foods in their diets, have been found to possess a much higher percentage of lactobacilli and a much lower percentage of clostridia, or harmful bacteria, in their stools when compared with those who eat a considerable quantity of flesh foods and refined carbohydrates. The incidence of colorectal cancer is also correspondingly lower in vegetarians than in the latter group.[2]

Dennis Burkitt, M.D., compared the transit time, stool volume, consistency, and ease of defecation of rural Africans on a very high complex-carbohydrate diet (fiber rich: 100 to 170 grams a day), with that of the wives of British naval officers, whose diets contained a lot of meat, fat, sugar, and refined flour products and processed foods (fiber poor: 20 grams a day). He found that the first group showed transit times of eighteen to thirty-six hours, with large, bulky, effortless stools; the second group, seventy-two to more than 100 hours, with small, compact, dry, and often very difficult stools.[3]

When Burkitt compared the health problems of the two groups, he discovered that the latter, representative of developed nations, exhibited constipation, hemorrhoids, anal fissures, varicose veins, thrombophlebitis, diverticulosis and diverticulitis, gallbladder disease, appendicitis, hiatal hernia, irritable colon, obesity, high blood cholesterol, coronary artery and heart disease, hypertension, diabetes, hypoglycemia, colon polyps, and colon and rectal cancer. The rural Africans only experienced these conditions and diseases when they converted to the dietary standards and lifestyles of westernized cultures.

The benefits of a fiber-rich diet are many:

- Optimal transit time and daily full evacuations and bulky, hydrated, soft, easy-to-pass stools—all of which help prevent constipation, straining, hemorrhoids, fissures, appendicitis, and an overgrowth of undesirable intestinal bacteria.
- Normal pressure within the intestines and the abdominal cavity, which prevents diverticulosis, diverticulitis, hiatal hernia, and hemorrhoids.
- High percentage of favorable intestinal bacteria (lactobacilli) and fewer unfavorable toxin-producing bacteria and yeast, more short-chain fatty acids to help prevent colon cancer and help lower serum cholesterol, which prevents the overgrowth of unfavorable bacteria and Candida, regular elimination and so on.
- Stimulation of the secretion of pancreatic enzymes and bicarbonate, which prevents incompletely digested proteins from reaching the colon, thereby preventing the formation and release of toxins.
- Indirect assistance of digestion and assimilation, which prevents gas, bloating, acute digestive disturbances, and nutrient malabsorption with its attendant short- and long-term consequences.
- Increase in bile solubility, which prevents gallstones.
- Binding and diluting of carcinogenic secondary bile acids, which helps prevent colorectal cancer.
- Binding and excretion of primary bile acids and cholesterol, which produces lower total and LDL serum cholesterol and the increase in HDL cholesterol—all of which can help prevent heart attacks and strokes and peripheral vascular disease.
- Binding of such heavy metals as lead, cadmium, and mercury, which helps prevent high blood pressure and other known consequences of these toxins (see Chapter Fourteen).
- Slowing of gastric emptying, enhancement of a full feeling and a longer maintenance of satiety, which helps prevent overeating and overweight.
- Necessity for thorough chewing, and therefore a slowing down of caloric consumption and a quicker feeling of satiety in relationship to the number of calories consumed, which also helps prevent overeating and overweight.
- Control of sugar release from the intestines into the bloodstream, which helps prevent both diabetes and hypoglycemia.

There are two types of dietary fiber: soluble and insoluble. The soluble fibers dissolve in water and include, for example, plant gums, mucilages, hemicelluloses, pectin, and guar. Examples of soluble fiber are apples, citrus fruit, carrots, oat bran, lima beans, and psyllium husks. Soluble fibers are the ones that nourish the favorable bacteria, lower serum cholesterol levels, slow the rate of sugar entering the circulatory system, and bind heavy metals.

Examples of insoluble fiber are wheat bran, brown rice, rye, lentils, asparagus, brussels sprouts, and flaxseed. Insoluble fibers are the ones known to lessen the incidence of colon and rectal cancer by binding bile acids as well as by increasing stool bulk and speeding transit time. By preventing constipation, they also lessen the chances of hemorrhoids, fissures, diverticulosis, appendicitis, and other conditions. Soluble fibers absorb water as well and help counter constipation by softening stools and giving them a mucilaginous quality to ease their passage. Most foods have both soluble and insoluble fiber in varying percentages (see page 162).

A diet rich in whole grains, legumes, vegetables, and fruits should provide an adequate amount and balance of fiber, but a fiber supplement may be helpful (see page 161).

BOWEL TOXICITY

An inadequate amount of fiber in your diet can cause a decrease in the number of favorable intestinal bacteria and a subsequent increase in unfavorable organisms. This is the beginning of the toxic bowel, recently named dysbiosis. Symptoms of a toxic bowel can be detected within the gastrointestinal tract and throughout the body.

PROCESSES CONTRIBUTING TO TOXIC BOWEL

A colon that is sluggish and is inhabited predominantly by unfavorable bacteria can cause several problems. The longer a stool sits in the colon, for example, the greater the chance that organisms like clostridia will convert primary bile acids to a carcinogen, which, in repeated contact with the intestinal mucosa, can contribute to the development of colon and rectal cancer. Without adequate fiber and water in the stool, the carcinogenic toxin and the primary bile acids have little chance of being diluted and moved along and out of the body. Other bacterial toxins have been implicated in irritable bowel/spastic colon and in food intolerance.[4]

How does a toxic bowel adversely affect the rest of the body? According to Erich Rauch, M.D., author of

SYMPTOMS OF BOWEL TOXICITY

SYMPTOMS WITHIN THE GASTROINTESTINAL SYSTEM PRIMARILY FROM INSUFFICIENT FIBER

Constipation
Hard, dry, or difficult stools
Sluggish or incomplete stool evacuation
Excessive gas
Very foul-smelling stools or gas
Bloating or overfullness of the abdomen
Abdominal pain or cramps
Diarrhea
Irritable bowel or spastic colon
Indigestion, heartburn
Bad breath
Coated tongue

Nausea
Hemorrhoids
Varicose veins
Anal fissures
Diverticulosis, diverticulitis
Hiatal hernia
Appendicitis
Gallbladder disease, including gallstones
Colon polyps
Colon cancer
Rectal cancer

SYMPTOMS OUTSIDE THE GASTROINTESTINAL TRACT DUE PRIMARILY TO INSUFFICIENT FIBER

Elevated blood sugar, diabetes mellitus
Hypoglycemia
Elevated blood cholesterol
Coronary artery disease, arteriosclerosis
Heart attack
Stroke
Hypertension

Heavy metal accumulation, such as lead, cadmium, and mercury
Overeating tendency
Overweight
Allergic tendencies, especially food allergies
Susceptibility to bladder or vaginal infections

SYMPTOMS RELATED TO CIRCULATING BOWEL TOXINS

Offensive breath
Coated tongue
Body odor
Nausea
Headache
Personality and brain changes (depression, moodiness, irritability, nervousness, forgetfulness, insomnia, dizziness)
Fatigue
Acne, boils, folliculitis
Eczema, psoriasis, dermatitis, itchy skin

Sallow complexion
Puffy, flaccid, or thinning skin; loss of skin elasticity
Arthritis
Autoimmune diseases
Muscle aches
Rheumatism
Gum disease
Ulcers and gastritis
Liver problems, diminished detoxification systems

Health through Inner Body Cleansing,[5] and Bernard Jensen, D.C., author of *Tissue Cleansing through Bowel Management*,[6] an unhealthy bowel will produce toxins such as: fusel (an alcoholic product of carbohydrate fermentation), indican, putrescine, neurine, and cadaverine (ptomaine), which enter the bloodstream and contribute to many of the symptoms listed above.

Otherwise classified as bacterial endotoxins, and characterized biochemically as lipopolysaccharides, these toxins bind to cell membranes, disturb cellular metabolic functions, and can cause tissue damage.

According to iridology, which is the study of the iris of the eye for indications of disease and other risks, many health problems are directly related to the colon.

Iridologists map the entire body on the iris, with the colon closest to the pupil (see Figure 8-2). An inflammatory or degenerative lesion on the iris in the location of a particular organ or structure can usually be traced to a corresponding lesion in the colon.[7]

Some authors also attest to the theory that organs and structures adjacent to the colon, such as the uterus, ovaries, prostate, bladder, diaphragm, and spine, can be directly affected, primarily because the pressure of a distended and distorted colon and neural reflexes compromise the healthy functioning of these organs and structures. Such conditions as menstrual cramps, ovarian cysts, cystitis, prostate problems, back and neck pain, chiropractic adjustments that will not "hold," poor posture, shortness of breath, and shallow breathing may result.

To make matters worse, you can become allergic to bowel microorganisms. In bombarding these bacteria with antibodies, your immune system can mistakenly attack your own healthy tissues and produce chronic illness in many systems of the body. Intestinal bacteria— *Proteus mirabilis*, for example, an organism recently implicated in rheumatoid arthritis—share some antigenic determinants with the body. This means that certain aspects of the proteus cell wall resemble aspects of the synovial membrane of our joints. If conditions in the intestine cause proteus to overgrow, overwhelm secretory IgA defenses, and invade the intestinal wall, the antibodies attempting to attack it will inadvertently attack the joints as well. The same kind of link has been made between another bacteria (*Klebsiella pneumoniae*) and alkylosing spondylitis, a severe form of arthritis affecting the spine. There have also been reports of intestinal bacteria actually translocating to joints and causing arthritis.[8]

It is no wonder that an increasing number of health practitioners are focusing on the bowel, as clinical experience and evidence in the scientific literature point to the gastrointestinal system as a contributing, if not primary, source of many of today's common ailments and systemic illnesses. Although some of these theories are not well substantiated, in my experience, intestinal cleansing measures usually prove to be very beneficial.

A toxic bowel, oddly enough, is an appealing concept to some individuals who are led to extreme forms of bowel cleansing and detoxification. Although such protocols have merit when done appropriately, I have seen some individuals who are looking for better health do themselves harm from too intensive or prolonged detoxification programs. Such individuals could often

Figure 8–2. Iridology Chart

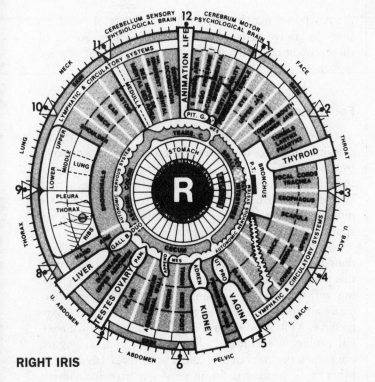

RIGHT IRIS

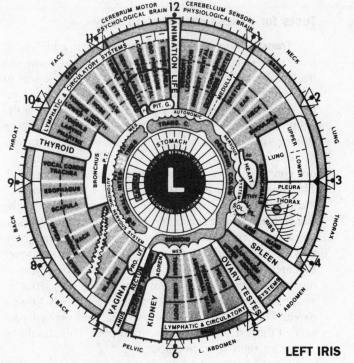

LEFT IRIS

shorten these protocols (or not need to repeat them so frequently) if they looked beyond toxicity and sought evaluation and treatment for other causes of intestinal and systemic symptoms (parasites, *Helicobacter pylori*, pancreatic enzyme insufficiency, hydrochloric acid insufficiency, a "leaky gut" syndrome, food allergies, and yeast overgrowth, to name a few).

DIAGNOSING TOXIC BOWEL

Many doctors still do not search adequately enough for these conditions. For the most part, modern medical thinking has ignored the whole area of fiber, transit time, and intestinal microorganisms, and how they relate to health and disease. For decades doctors ignored published research and failed to relate a fiber-poor diet and slow transit time to diverticulosis, appendicitis, irritable bowel syndrome, colorectal cancer, and heart disease.

It's only in the last several years that modern medicine has promoted the use of a high-fiber diet for the prevention of these conditions. However, many doctors today still consider "normal" a patient who has only one or two bowel movements a week. But what is "normal" is certainly not always healthy. Depending on the beliefs and practices of your doctor, you may have to take it upon yourself to initiate a program to improve and maintain the health of your bowel.

Tests for Assessing Bowel Toxicity

Transit Time and Retention Time In addition to using the symptoms list (see page 158) to assess the health of your bowel, you can perform a simple test to determine transit time. At any one meal, include an ample portion of a test food, one that will be visible in the stool, such as corn on the cob, sesame seeds, beets, or five or six charcoal tablets. For test purposes, *do not* chew as thoroughly as usual. After this initial meal, do not consume test food again until the test is completed. The time between this test meal and the first passage of the test food (its first appearance in your stool) is the transit time. If it is substantially more than thirty hours, you are constipated. If it is less than eighteen hours, you may be exhibiting diarrhea (see "Diarrhea" in Chapter Seventeen). Be aware that you may be having one or more bowel movements a day and feeling no particular abdominal discomfort and yet still be severely constipated. The time between the test meal and the last passage of the test food is the retention time. This should be no longer than sixty-five hours.

Urinary Indican (Obermeyer Test) Your doctor can arrange for you to take a urine test to measure the quantity of indican, a metabolite from the bacterial breakdown of the dietary amino acids tyrosine, phenylalanine, and tryptophan. This is often referred to as the Obermeyer test. If you have a slow transit time and therefore an intestinal overgrowth of putrefactive bacteria, much indican will be made and escape into the bloodstream and be present in the urine. Elevated urinary indican levels may also reflect the possibility of inadequate protein digestion, commonly from insufficient hydrochloric acid and/or pancreatic enzyme production (see Chapter Seven). In any event, elevated urinary indican means protein putrefaction and bowel toxicity, and therapeutic action is indicated.

Stool Culture A specialized microbiological assessment of a stool sample can detect the quantitative presence of lactobacilli, *E. coli*, klebsiella, and other aerobic (oxygen requiring) intestinal bacteria.[9] With this information, treatment to correct bacterial imbalances may be better directed. Testing for anaerobic organisms, which do not require oxygen—the more predominant species in the bowel—could be more helpful. But technical difficulties make this test too specialized for widespread use.

CONDITIONS ASSOCIATED WITH A TOXIC BOWEL

A toxic bowel may be the result of a variety of problems that the above tests do not address. The presence of these conditions may help in the diagnosis of a toxic bowel.

Food Allergies

Any food can be an allergen and cause constipation, cramps, bloating, diarrhea, and other bowel symptoms (see Chapter Thirteen). You can have a reaction to a food item anytime from immediately after ingestion to seventy-two hours later. Delayed food reactions are more difficult to identify but are usually the ones responsible for chronic symptoms.

Although whole wheat and wheat bran are abundant in fiber, many people are allergic or intolerant to this grain. It is a common cause of constipation alternating with diarrhea and cramps. Chapter Thirteen offers many alternatives to wheat. See also the recipes in Chapter Five. Milk products are a common source of intestinal problems. Cultured milk products, such as yogurt, are sometimes tolerated by those who react adversely to other milk products. Some very sensitive individuals need to eliminate dairy altogether because of lactose intolerance or milk protein allergy/intolerance.

FACTORS THAT PROMOTE A TOXIC BOWEL

Excess dietary sugar
Excess dietary animal protein
Constipation
Food allergies
Antibiotic overuse
Intestinal yeast overgrowth

Overgrowth of unfavorable intestinal bacteria
Low thyroid function
Inadequate digestion
Liver/gallbladder sluggishness
Intestinal parasites

Intestinal Yeast Infection

An overgrowth of *Candida albicans*, a fungus in the intestines, is a common cause of constipation, diarrhea, gas bloating, and abdominal pain. This condition is virtually unrecognized by most conventionally practicing physicians.

Hypothyroidism

Low thyroid status commonly causes constipation. This condition can exist despite normal thyroid blood tests (see "Hypothyroidism," in Chapter Seventeen).

Inadequate Digestion

As explained in Chapter Seven, without sufficient hydrochloric acid secretion and pancreatic enzymes, constipation and other ailments can result.

Inadequate Liver and Gallbladder Function

Constipation and many varieties of gastrointestinal distress can occur as a result of this dysfunction (see Chapter Nine).

Intestinal Parasites

Undiagnosed parasites are common causes of constipation, diarrhea, bloating, weight loss, weakness, and allergies (see Chapter Seventeen).

Overgrowth of Unfavorable Intestinal Bacteria

Due to the overuse of antibiotics, toxin-producing bacteria can flourish in the intestines, causing intestinal and systemic symptoms (see page 160). Inadequate fiber intake, too much sugar and animal protein, and poor digestion can also encourage growth of these organisms.

DIET AND LIFESTYLE HINTS FOR HEALING A TOXIC BOWEL

Eat Sufficient Fiber

Your diet may include too much concentrated protein (beef, pork, luncheon meats, poultry, fish, eggs, and cheese), sugar, and white flour products (bread, rolls, muffins, crackers, croissants, tortillas, noodles, pasta, pancakes, cookies, etc.) and not enough of the fiber-rich foods your intestines require. You will need to cut back on some of these constipating foods and make changes in your diet.

For instance, substitute whole grain or whole wheat for your white flour items. Add oat bran cereal and brown rice on a regular basis. Have several pieces of fresh fruit and several raw or lightly steamed vegetables every day. Learn how to make a legume dish that you enjoy, like black bean or lentil soup, chili, or hummus.

With these fiber-rich changes, you will be doing a great service to your colon and your health in general. As you grow more familiar with whole grains, legumes, fresh vegetables, and fresh fruit, you will learn what proportions work best for your own individual bowel function. You may also discover that there are particular foods your bowel will not tolerate at all. Caution: Be sure to make a *gradual* transition to a high-fiber diet; too abrupt a change may bring gastrointestinal distress.

Fiber Supplements Of great help to many individuals is the addition of a fiber supplement to the diet. Fiber supplements are available in powders, capsules, tablets, and wafers, from a variety of sources (psyllium seed, flaxseed, oat bran, rice bran, pectins, guar gum, gum karaya, cellulose gum, glucomannan, carrageenan, agar, triphala, etc.). Any health food store should be well stocked with a variety of these products. Some supplements contain single agents, others are combined; still others contain such synergists as herbs, bentonite clay, acidophilus, and barley malt.

You may need to experiment to find the product that gives you the best results.

Depending on your health problems or susceptibilities, you may require more soluble or insoluble fiber or both, and should choose accordingly (see the following table).

You may have allergies or intolerances to some fiber sources. If you are allergy prone, it may be better to find a number of single-fiber agents that work well so that you do not develop an intolerance from the repetitive use of any one. In all cases, you will need to consume a lot of fluid, because the fiber needs to soak up much water in order for it to function properly (up to two quarts a day). If you stint on raw vegetables and fruit or water-cooked foods such as brown rice, legumes, and soups, you will have to take in maximum fluids. A fiber supplement, even one that is appropriate for you, may cause bloating, discomfort, and constipation if you take too much or do not use enough fluid with it and throughout the day.

It's probably best to take your fiber supplement several hours before or after a meal because of the large amount of fluids required with it. Despite this recommendation, if convenience demands, you may take the supplement with a meal. However, take a little less water with it and make up the difference between meals.

Some studies suggest that grain fiber products (taken with or separate from meals) bind up minerals (especially calcium, iron, and zinc) from your diet and therefore contribute to mineral deficiencies. There is a concern that phytate in grain, especially wheat bran, may be the culprit. Using flaxseed powder or psyllium husks as regular fiber supplements would present less of this risk.

If you are trying to lose weight and need a strategy that will help you eat less, take a low-phytate fiber supplement before meals—it will fill you up and lessen your appetite. If a particular meal is especially fiber poor as well as fat and sugar rich, taking your fiber supplement with it may reduce some of the inherent bowel and blood sugar consequences.

Fiber supplements should not be used on a regular basis in place of the adoption of an appropriate diet. The overuse of refined flours, processed foods, sugar, and concentrated proteins—even when accompanied by a fiber supplement—carries grave consequences. A fiber supplement cannot compensate for a fundamental lack of optimal micronutrients and an excess of fat, protein, and sugar. And avoid the regular use of fiber supplements containing habit-forming laxatives such as cascara or senna.

Drink Fluids

You need an adequate amount of fluids to keep your stools hydrated. Water, juices, herbal teas, broth, and soups, as well as raw vegetables and fruits, will do the job. Drink the majority of your beverages separate from meals. Use cooked whole grains in kernel form, like brown rice, to add to your fluid intake and bowel health. Avoid excessive dehydrating flour products, such as bread.

Eat Sufficient Raw Food

Include more raw food in your daily diet, in particular fresh vegetables, fruits, and sprouts, which contribute not only fluid but fiber.

SOLUBLE AND INSOLUBLE FIBER SOURCES

Higher in Insoluble Fiber	Roughly Equal Amounts of Insoluble and Soluble Fiber	Higher in Soluble Fiber
Whole wheat	Kidney beans	Apples
Wheat bran	Navy beans	Bananas
Brown rice	Green beans	Citrus fruits
Rice bran	Green peas	Blackberries
Rye	Winter squash	Prunes
Cooked lentils	Corn	Carrots
Asparagus		Barley
Brussels sprouts		Oats and oat bran
Flaxseed		Lima beans
		Psyllium husks
		Guar gum

Based in part on information from the Institute of Food Technology, Chicago, Illinois.

Avoid Overeating

Very large meals and snacking between meals place a continual energy demand on the colon, which can eventually force it to function suboptimally. Overdistension of the stomach also shuts down hydrochloric acid production. Eat sensible and moderate quantities. See Chapter Eighteen for cleansing diets and fasts, which give the bowel a chance to rejuvenate.

Respect the Body's Signal to Defecate

Ignoring too often your body's signal to defecate may weaken the strength of the signal or distort your perception of it. Either of these can have a negative impact on bowel function. You may think it fine to ignore subtle signals from your body, but if you do not respond to its light knocks, it may have to crash in the door and force you to pay attention.

Allow for Adequate Exercise

Part of what helps the bowel move its contents along is regular exercise: walking, biking, swimming, running, aerobics, dance, yoga, tai chi, calisthenics. Find any way you can to work in some form of exercise regularly.

Maintain a Balance in Life

A sluggish bowel, or diarrhea, may be a signal that you are overextending yourself, testing your limits to excess, poorly managing the stress in your life, inadequately nurturing your personal needs. Sometimes your body will let you know that you have gone too far long before your mind does. Try making things safer or more nurturing for yourself.

On the other hand, a sluggish bowel may signal a stagnant life, where things have gotten too safe, too comfortable, boring, unchallenging, or uninteresting. Challenge yourself. Risk new things a little more! Be more of who you're holding back. Benefits will abound!

SUPPLEMENTS TO ASSIST BOWEL FUNCTION

Flaxseeds

One tablespoon or more of flaxseeds soaked overnight in a glass of water can provide both fiber function and lubrication to the colon. (You can also add other ingredients and make a blender drink.) You may prefer to grind flaxseeds into a fine powder and add it to yogurt, cereals, fruit salads, and blender drinks. They have a pleasant, nutty taste. Store ground flaxseeds in an airtight, opaque container and refrigerate, but make only a small quantity at a time as they go rancid quite easily. Flax powder is commercially available as well. I prefer the more stable defatted variety produced by the Omegaflo process. It's available from Omega Nutrition (Ferndale, Washington).

Lactobacillus acidophilus and *Lactobacillus bifidus*

These intestinal organisms help normalize digestion, constipation, and diarrhea. You can find acidophilus in several forms. It is one of the cultures in yogurt and kefir. Using some of the fermented foods discussed in Chapter Seven will also provide a dietary source of these organisms. Acidophilus milk is another source, but it usually doesn't contain enough organisms to provide much benefit.

Acidophilus supplements are also available in powder, capsule, tablet, and liquid form and are usually more potent and effective. For powder forms, use up to ½ teaspoon (best taken thirty to forty-five minutes before meals) one to three times a day. Capsule doses are usually one or more taken two to three times a day. The "acid stable" forms can be taken with meals. It is also a sign of quality if there is an expiration date on the bottle. Health food stores carry several brands, and I recommend the ones containing not just *Lactobacillus acidophilus* but *Lactobacillus bifidus* as well (or buy a bottle of each). Some brands are milk free (if you happen to be milk allergic). An independent laboratory study published in 1990 in *Obstetrics and Gynecology*, however, showed that nine out of ten popular *Lactobacillus acidophilus* brands tested actually had no acidophilus at all (they had other types of lactobacilli and all nine of these brands had contaminants).[10] You may want to contact some of these companies to inquire if they have implemented better quality control measures. Some have, and their products will usually give you results.

For my patients who need acidophilus/bifidus therapeutically, particularly those with altered intestinal microorganisms due to antibiotics, steroids (cortisone), chemotherapy, radiation, intestinal infections, diarrhea, constipation, and/or chronically poor diet, I recommend HMF (Human Microflora) by Interplexus of Kent, Washington. It is one of the few brands of acidophilus/bifidus that I know of that is independently certified and that is human specific (rather than derived from animals). It therefore has a very high implantation rate on the intestinal wall. You may need to obtain it through your physician or pharmacist. The dose is one capsule twice a day with meals. One other strain (acidophilus only) with a very high implantation rate is NCFM (North Carolina Food Microbiology) strain acidophilus available as Ultra Dophilus by Metagenics, Inc. of San Clemente, California.

Saccharomyces boulardii

A friendly, nonpathogenic yeast, *Saccharomyces boulardii* is gaining recognition for its use in helping to normalize intestinal bacteria.[11] It is a unique yeast in that, like lactobacilli, it ferments carbohydrates and produces lactic acid, which helps acidify the intestines and reduce the population of unfriendly bacteria and Candida. Saccharomyces is quite compatible with acidophilus and bifidus bacteria and is often the answer for common antibiotic-related intestinal disturbances, such as candidiasis and diarrhea, when acidophilus and bifidus supplementation is not effective. It has particular application for the prevention and treatment of the most severe intestinal complication of antibiotics, *Clostridium difficile*-related pseudomembranous colitis. It is becoming some physicians' first choice over lactobacilli. The yeast has been used successfully in AIDS-related and other severe forms of diarrhea, and may increase immunity by enhancing levels of secretory IgA, a protective antibody of our mucous membranes. Use one or two 300-milligram capsules two to three times a day.

Fructooligosaccharides

Fructooligosaccharides are also gaining a reputation for favorably influencing intestinal bacteria.[12] FOS, as they are called, are naturally occurring compounds present in a variety of fruits, vegetables, and grains, and especially in Jerusalem artichokes.

FOS are food for *Lactobacillus bifidus* and *acidophilus* and therefore are indicated in the treatment of constipation, diarrhea, foul-smelling stools and gas, bowel toxicity, and the myriad conditions that lactobacilli influence. They can be synthesized and taken in powder or liquid form as a food supplement, which is how they are primarily used therapeutically. FOS are resistant to digestive enzymes and therefore are not absorbed and do not raise blood sugar levels. As they are about half as sweet as table sugar, they can also serve as a sweetener. Use up to eight grams daily (approximately one teaspoon twice a day) for treatment, and if necessary take one to four grams daily as maintenance. Too much will cause diarrhea.

Whey

Whey can nourish your favorable bacteria and therefore help normalize digestive and bowel symptoms. Avoid whey, however, if you are allergic to milk.

Green Juice

The juice from green leafy vegetables, spirulina, and other algae products can act as a bowel cleanser and help in some cases of constipation (see Chapter Five). Liquid chlorophyll can also be beneficial (see page 168 and Chapter Nineteen).

Lemon Juice or Lemon Water

Lemon juice is very cleansing to the intestinal tract. Add the juice of half a lemon to a cup of hot water and drink. Or very thinly slice an organic lemon and let it sit in two to three cups of water overnight. Warm and drink. Do this first thing in the morning. (Caution: Lemon juice can erode teeth enamel if contact with the teeth is prolonged. Thoroughly rinse mouth immediately afterward, or better yet, brush teeth with baking soda.)

Aloe Vera Juice

One to two ounces of aloe vera juice (or the gel—one to two tablespoons) taken once or twice a day can also act as a bowel cleanser and help in cases of constipation (see pages 446–447).

Flaxseed and Slippery Elm Teas

Both teas can act as bowel lubricants. Steep with other flavorful herbal teas, as these are quite bland. Or use one or two teaspoons of the slippery elm powder in a glass of water. Slippery elm has the added advantage of soothing irritated gastrointestinal membranes, helpful in cases of ulcer, gastritis, and colitis.

Figs

Fresh figs (if dried, soaked overnight in water) can help improve constipation without the excessive laxative effect that prunes have.

Vitamin C, Magnesium, and Pantothenic Acid (Vitamin B-5)

While necessary for health, too much vitamin C and magnesium may produce diarrhea. Using just enough to loosen the stool slightly without producing diarrhea can serve as one treatment for constipation. Realize, however, that this approach does not treat the cause and should be used only temporarily until more cause-oriented measures become effective. Because constipation can be one sign of adrenal exhaustion, vitamin C and vitamin B-5, which both help adrenal function, may help treat this particular cause of constipation.

OTHER WAYS TO HELP YOUR BOWEL

Abdominal Massage

A massage can ease constipation and sooth a variety

SUPPLEMENTS AND MEASURES TO ASSIST BOWEL FUNCTION

Treatment of underlying conditions affecting
   the colon
Adequate dietary fiber and/or fiber
   supplements
Sufficient fluid intake
Sufficient raw food
Appropriate amounts of food
Respecting the body's signal to defecate
Adequate exercise
Flaxseeds and flaxseed tea
Lactobacillus acidophilus and *bifidus*
Saccharomyces boulardii
Fructooligosaccharides
Whey
Green juice
Lemon juice or lemon water

Slippery elm tea
Figs
Vitamin C
Magnesium
Pantothenic acid (Vitamin B-5)
Abdominal massage
Foot reflexology
Slantboard exercises
Footstool
Raising arms
The belly roll
Temporary measures:
   Laxatives
   Prunes/prune juice
   Enemas
   Colonic irrigations

of intestinal complaints. Try this technique for five to ten minutes once or twice a day: While lying down, press rhythmically with either the palm of your hand or a rubber ball on the lower right part of the abdomen near the hipbone. Work slowly up the right side of your abdomen to just below your rib cage. Then massage straight across your abdomen toward the left side. Go down the left side of your abdomen to the area by your left hip. Next, come across right above your pubic bone to the starting point. Do not press so hard as to cause pain, but press firmly enough in the areas that permit. Relax your abdominal muscles first so that you can work more deeply. A bath or hot water bottle or heating pad on your abdomen will enhance relaxation. Using any kind of massage or vegetable oil on your hands may enhance the massage (try castor or olive oil). Massage can increase awareness of your intestines and abdomen as well as improve your bowel function. A castor oil pack placed over the abdomen can help heal and normalize bowel function (see page 168).

Stimulating Foot Reflexes

Thoroughly massage the arch and heel areas of the foot with a rolling pin or a foot massage roller for ten to twenty minutes to stimulate reflexes to the colon. (Health food stores usually stock foot rollers.) Be careful not to bruise your feet. Many massage therapists practice reflexology and can give you pressure treatments to

stimulate all of your organs. Practitioners of shiatsu, acupressure, and acupuncture can also stimulate points on your body related to bowel and other organ functions (see Chapters Twenty and Twenty-one).

Slantboard Exercises

The exercises given in Chapter Twenty can help reverse a prolapsed or sagging transverse colon, a condition that iridologists and other natural health practitioners feel is one cause of constipation and a result of years of poor diet and enervation.

Footstool

Position a footstool (or a stack of two or three thick phone books) in front of the toilet, so that while seated on the toilet with your feet on the stool, your knees are well above the level of your hips. This positioning helps to open the pelvis and take further advantage of gravity, allowing for a fuller, easier bowel evacuation. Some individuals actually prefer squatting on the toilet seat. Although this may seem rather odd or extremist, nature actually intended us to use the squatting position for defecation. Many health practitioners, among them Bernard Jensen, D.C., have related a number of bowel ailments to the use of the standard toilet. Using a footstool does not require the agility or potential knee strain of squatting, and it works almost as well. Try this even if you have no bowel problems at all. You will likely see a significant difference and become a footstool convert.

Raising Your Arms

Raising your arms above the head while on the toilet causes the abdomen to lift and may allow for a fuller bowel movement.

The Belly Roll

Although straining a little to have a bowel movement may help, too much may also create tension and contribute to hemorrhoids and other pressure-related conditions. Try making rhythmic downward rolls of your abdominal muscles, as in a belly dance. In this way, your external abdominal muscles will advance stool downward without straining and creating any dangerously increased internal pressure.

Prunes, Prune Juice, and Herbal Laxatives

These may be useful in cases of acute constipation. However, they do not rejuvenate bowel function. In fact, herbal laxatives may weaken the colon if used regularly.

CLEANSING TECHNIQUES FOR THE BOWEL

Enemas

Useful in easing acute constipation, enemas should be regarded as an emergency measure. In cases of extreme bowel toxicity, regular enemas are sometimes recommended as part of a long-term bowel restoration program. I might add here, in keeping with the comments of Andrew Weil, M.D., in *Natural Health, Natural Medicine* that many individuals become addicted to the idea of needing an enema to feel clean. Because of the frank possibility of psychological addiction and a common tendency to overuse, do not use enemas more than occasionally unless you're under the care and supervision of a health professional or unless your bowels do not move. Otherwise, enemas can be used as part of a short-term cleansing or detoxification program (see Chapter Eighteen). When possible, they should be done after a natural bowel movement to prevent dependence.

Colonic Irrigations

Colonic irrigations are also prescribed for those with severe constipation, bowel/liver toxicity, or other intestinal dysfunctions and as part of a colon-cleansing program. Many patients, colon therapists, and other health professionals attest to the extraordinary benefits of this four- to five-gallon, hour-long flushing of the colon. As with enemas and laxatives, there is a high potential for misuse and addiction, and guidance from a health professional competent in this area is recommended. Any measure that replaces your own bowel evacuation mechanisms for too long can create a dependence. Moreover, colonics can deplete your friendly bacteria and electrolytes, both of which need to be replaced. Naturally, it's advisable to improve dietary and lifestyle factors that would render such future interventions unnecessary.

INTESTINAL CLEANSING

The concept of intestinal toxicity is somewhat foreign to modern medicine. However, it is a basic tenet of natural medicine and many books have been written on the subject.[13] I've often witnessed the benefits of intestinal cleansing and its safety, and I continue to recommend it. What I'm presenting here is a combination of elements from programs developed by several practitioners of natural medicine in the United States. These are the programs I know the best, and they don't generally require medical supervision. I must at least mention the Mayr method from Europe, which has a far longer history of successful use; but due to space limitations, and the need for professional supervision for part of that program, I refer you to Dr. Rauch's book.[14]

An intestinal cleansing program can further the benefits already accrued from implementation of measures discussed previously. For individuals who are eating a standard fiber-poor American diet or who have sluggish bowel function, intestinal cleansing is a prerequisite for more complete and intensive cleansing and detoxification of the body. In addition, it's a necessary step before proceeding on to liver detoxification. Together, intestinal and liver cleansing provide the foundation for cleansing the remainder of your body, explanations and protocols for which you will find in Chapter Eighteen.

To prepare for an intestinal cleansing program, begin to adjust your diet, fluid intake, and other habits that we have just discussed to improve transit time and enhance your bowel function. Specifically, diminish your consumption of refined flour products, cheese, and animal flesh products. For four to seven days before your actual cleansing program begins, drink up to two quarts of lemon water a day, most of it separate from meals. If you are allergic to lemons, plain water will do.

Do not jump into a bowel-cleansing program without first taking these measures, or you may inadvertently take a few precious steps backward. On the other hand, an intestinal cleansing program can also be used as a type of periodic crisis intervention to undo the effects of too many dietary infractions and excesses. While in force, it can also motivate an individual to make the dietary and lifestyle changes that will minimize future bowel disturbances.

Intestinal cleansing programs recommended by practitioners of natural medicine usually have three fundamentals in common: a fiber supplement, a combination herbal supplement or a clay supplement (both designed to further cleanse and detoxify), and a lot of water. Other supplements complementary to cleansing include olive oil cream or castor oil (to be applied topically to the abdomen), acidophilus, chlorophyll or the juice from green leafy vegetables, aloe vera juice, and a skin brush (all available in most health food stores).

An intestinal cleansing may seem a rather intimidating endeavor, particularly if you read some of the available health food store literature, which describes the successful removal of old, encrusted fecal matter from twisted, distorted colon walls. Whether or not these particular claims stand up to scientific scrutiny, I cannot say. However, there is much clinical evidence to support these programs, as individuals improve so dramatically in so many ways.

Intestinal cleansing can actually be very easy, requiring only a bit more effort than you might already be putting forth. Sometimes it's as simple as taking a fiber supplement two or three times a day and drinking up to two quarts of fluid a day. And some programs call for the addition of a tablespoon of bentonite liquid clay or a few herbal tablets. This program can last from four to twelve weeks. You would follow a wholesome diet, such as the one outlined earlier in this chapter (see page 161). Such a regimen could conveniently be carried out during the course of your usual daily routine. To enhance an intestinal cleansing program, you could do an abdominal massage, apply a castor oil pack or olive oil cream on your abdomen before bedtime, skin brush once or twice a day, use an acidophilus supplement, include chlorophyll or aloe vera juice in your diet, and take an occasional enema.

The more toxic your bowel is, the more you may require these extra measures or, in fact, one of the more intense programs involving fasting and enemas, colemas, or colonics, which would require a great deal of planning and special time set aside.[15] Depending on your condition and your experience with cleansing, the more intense detoxification regimens are best done under the supervision of a health professional. Regardless of the type of cleansing you choose, if you have any known internal medical disorders, consult a health professional.

A Simple Intestinal Cleansing Program

You will need:

- A fiber/bulk agent, such as psyllium husk powder or combination fiber product containing, for example, psyllium husk, barley fiber, guar gum, oat bran, and fruit pectin. Triphala or flaxseed powder are other options.
- Bentonite liquid or Kalenite internal cleansing tablets (acacia gum, plantain leaf, blessed thistle, cloves, red clove tops, cornsilk extract 4:1, yellow dock root extract 4:1, butternut bark) or colon-cleansing formula tablets (chickweed, Irish moss, cloves, plantain, rosemary, bayberry bark, and cornsilk extract). These herbal agents do not contain any laxative herbs, such as cascara and senna. They are available in most health food stores.

1. First thing in the morning, drink eight to twelve ounces of any of the following *warm* liquids: lemon water, herbal tea, or plain water.

2. Initially once a day for three days, then two or three times a day (best done at least forty-five minutes before or two hours after meals), do the following: In a 12-ounce jar with a tight-fitting lid, mix 1 teaspoon (level initially, then heaping) of a fiber/bulk product with 6 to 8 ounces of water (you may add a small amount of juice for taste). Add 1 tablespoon bentonite liquid. Screw on the lid securely and shake vigorously. You'll want to drink this immediately, as the fiber/bulk agent quickly thickens. Beginning the second week and for subsequent weeks, increase to 2 tablespoons of bentonite with each dosage. If you are using Kalenite or a colon-cleansing herbal formula instead of liquid bentonite, take one tablet initially each time you drink the fiber mixture. During the second week, increase to two tablets. For subsequent weeks, take three tablets with each dosage.

If all this mixing of substances and taking tablets seems a little more than you can handle, I suggest a more simplified plan. Find a fiber/clay/herb combination powder such as Perfect Seven (from Agape Health Products in Seal Beach, California) and take it with water according to the instructions in step 1 above. There are no additional substances or tablets. Perfect Seven contains psyllium seed and husk, milk-free *Lactobacillus bifidus*, montemorillonite clay, alfalfa leaf, cascara sagrada bark, rose hips, buckthorn bark, capsicum, garlic, and goldenseal.

3. Follow with approximately 6 to 8 ounces of water. You need to drink at least two quarts of fluids (mostly separate from meals) throughout the remainder of the day.

A Few Words of Caution

If you have not used a fiber/bulk agent before, start out with a level teaspoon or less. Drink copious amounts of fluids and see if it suits your system. It is common in the first few days of this program to experience abdominal fullness or bloating. However, over time you should begin to feel quite comfortable. The use of herbal laxatives during the first few days of the program should minimize this discomfort, but they should be unnecessary by the second week.

Unfortunately, some fiber products may be constipating, excessively bloating, or irritating to your intestines. You will need to experiment with different products to find the ones that are suitable for you. Once you have succeeded, increase the dose to a heaping teaspoon. After the first week, increase the frequency to twice a day, and perhaps three times a day during the third and subsequent weeks. Twice a day may be sufficient. If the fiber product has a significant number of herbal ingredients and therefore less fiber per teaspoon, you may need more than a heaping teaspoon per dose (check the label for instructions).

Your bowel movements should become very full, bulky, soft, effortless, and lacking any foul odor. They should be cleaner, too, leaving minimal residue. Initially, you may discover unusually dark colors or odd shapes to your feces, even ropes of mucus. Eventually they will become normal appearing.

If the recommended amount of fluid seems virtually impossible to you to drink, do the best you can. The fiber/bulk agent requires that you significantly increase your fluid intake, so try to push your limit slightly. If necessary decrease the dose of fiber slightly. You may find that what you can drink, though less than optimal, will be sufficient for vastly improved elimination. Try not to drink too much after dinner or before bedtime, as you do not want to be awakened too often to urinate.

Continue the program at least three to four weeks, although you have the option of continuing eight to twelve weeks. If you do decide to proceed past four weeks, use the herbal colon detoxifiers after this time period rather than the bentonite, as bentonite may chelate nutrients as well as toxins. If, however, you have chosen the simplest cleansing and are using a fiber powder containing bentonite or montemorillonite clay, you may use this for eight to twelve weeks as the clay content is not excessive.

An Enhanced Cleansing Program

To enhance the above basic cleansing program, I recommend the following:

Chlorophyll With each meal, take three or four alfalfa tablets (do not use if you have any kind of lupus disease) or wheat or barley grass, or algae (spirulina, chlorella, or blue-green algae) tablets. You can also find these forms of chlorophyll in powder form and can mix them in juice or in a blender drink as part of your total fluid intake requirement for each day.

If you prefer, you can derive chlorophyll by juicing leafy green vegetables (parsley, kale, chard, spinach, etc.) and celery stalks, zucchini, and other green vegetables (perhaps sweetening with a little carrot juice). One to two ounces of wheat grass juice can also substitute. Liquid chlorophyll (available in health food stores) or undiluted green juice is very potent. Begin with small amounts, since too much too soon in your cleansing program may cause nausea, headache, intestinal upset, and a general toxic feeling.

Aloe Vera Juice See suggestions on page 164.

Acidophilus See suggestions on page 163.

Dry Brush Skin Massage Before bathing or exercising, do a dry brush skin massage with a natural-bristle skin brush, as described in Chapter Eighteen. Stimulating the excretory function of your skin enhances total detoxification.

Castor Oil Pack or Olive Oil Cream At bedtime place a castor oil pack (see Chapter Twenty), or rub olive oil cream on your abdomen. One product particularly designed for this use is Vivalo Creme. These oils, which are absorbed by the skin quite effectively, are said to stimulate the excretion of bile into the intestine. Olive oil also stimulates the pancreatic enzyme and bicarbonate secretions. Both have a soothing and beneficial effect when applied topically.

Enemas A daily enema, preferably taken after your own natural bowel movement, can be useful in intestinal cleansing. It can also be beneficial even if done just once or twice a week during this cleansing program (see page 166 and Chapter Eighteen for a more detailed discussion of cleansing).

Slantboard Exercises Slantboard exercises can help reverse the deleterious effect of gravity, particularly in cases of a sagging or prolapsed transverse colon. You can do these exercises for five to ten minutes once or twice a day.

SPRING CLEANING

From this chapter you can see how important it is to maintain healthy bowel functioning. By following the suggested cleansing programs, adding recommended supplements, and making the necessary diet and lifestyle changes, you can lessen bowel toxicity and improve your general health.

As a routine health maintenance practice, I suggest for many of my patients a yearly three- to four-week basic or enhanced intestinal cleansing program. This is akin to a spring cleaning, something useful to avoid unneeded and potentially harmful accumulations, particularly when living in a society of so many dietary excesses. Such a cleansing may serve as a preventive measure as well as a reminder of what good bowel functioning should be. More important still, it can motivate you to follow the healthful eating and living habits that will not only keep your intestines but your whole body functioning well.

SUGGESTED READING

Berry, Linda, D.C. *Internal Cleansing: A Practical Guide to Colon Health.* Botanical Press, 1985. (P.O. Box 742, Capitola, CA 95010).

Bland, Jeffrey, Ph.D. *Intestinal Toxicity and Inner Cleansing.* New Caanan, CT: Keats Publishing, 1987.

Burkitt, Dennis, M.D. *Western Diseases: Their Emergence and Prevention.* Cambridge, MA: Harvard University Press, 1981.

Gray, Robert. *The Colon Health Handbook: New Health Through Colon Rejuvenation.* Oakland, CA: Rockridge Publishing, 1983.

Jensen, Bernard, D.C. and Bell, S. *Tissue Cleansing through Bowel Management: From the Simple to the Ultimate.* Escondido, CA: Bernard Jensen International, 1980.

Rauch, E. *Health through Inner Body Cleansing: The Famous Mayr Intestinal Therapy from Europe.* Heidelberg, Germany: Carl F. Haug, 1988 (available from Medicina Biologica, Portland, OR).

Trenev, Natasha, and Chaitow, Leon. *Probiotics: The Revolutionary "Friendly Bacteria" Way to Vital Health and Well-Being.* New York: Thorson's Publishers Ltd., 1990.

CHAPTER 9

THE SLUGGISH LIVER

Intimately related to the bowel is the liver, one of the most important and multifaceted components of the gastrointestinal system (see Figure 9–1). The liver is a vast metabolic factory responsible for the processing of proteins, carbohydrates, and fat and the synthesis of many essential substances such as bile, glycogen, and serum proteins. It also serves as the body's primary site of detoxification, protecting us from both environmental and metabolic poisons.

William's story, below, demonstrates the multitude of symptoms that can be produced by a dysfunctioning liver—symptoms that are often difficult to trace. In the process of working through this case history, we will review some basic facts about the liver, how to assess its functioning, and how to restore and maintain it.

WILLIAM

At twenty-eight, William had recently gone back to college in an undergraduate program in computer sciences. He had left school nine years before because he hadn't been able to keep up with his studies. He'd been working in his father's auto mechanic shop since. During this time, he had also married and now had a four-year-old stepson. He sought my assistance for what he referred to initially as difficulties in applying himself to his school work. But this turned out to be only the tip of the iceberg.

William's chief complaint was fatigue. Even with twelve hours of sleep, it was a major feat for him to simply get out of bed every morning. And he needed a two-hour nap most days of the week. It had only been because he'd been working for his father—an understanding and lenient father, at that—that he'd been able to take a two-hour lunch break and sleep during most of it.

But now that he was back in school again full time, while still working fifteen hours a week, he told me that he was unable to "stop his life anymore." He couldn't get in those much-needed naps. He realized that he was spending most of his energy fighting his fatigue. However, what disturbed him just as much as his fatigue was an inability to concentrate, a failing memory, and an increasing sense of disorientation. He'd recently found himself getting lost on streets he'd traveled for over twenty years. And he'd begun to forget names of people he'd known his whole life. He also told me that he felt more tired and disoriented after meals unless all he'd eaten was fruit. And with fewer than twelve hours of sleep, William's irritability had become explosive.

William felt it important to report several more symptoms: He had to urinate six to eight times during the first three hours after awakening; and his socks smelled like ammonia by the end of the day, and his whole body itched. He was too thin and needed to eat incredible amounts to keep from losing weight. He also experienced excessive intestinal gas, burping, and there was undigested food in his stool. And he had developed extreme allergic reactions to various chemical fumes (perfumes, exhausts, paints, etc.). He had once wondered whether his exposure to lead and other toxic metals in his father's shop had any bearing on his symptoms, but he realized that all these symptoms predated by many years his time as an auto mechanic.

He had been treated by many doctors over the years. But none of them could find any explanation for his multitude of symptoms and diminished level of functioning. The only "finding" on his many physical exams was his abnormally orange-hued skin color, which he'd had nearly his whole life. All laboratory tests, including standard liver function tests, were always normal. By conventional medical standards, William had no disease, which was why he couldn't seem to get much help from his doctors. Nevertheless, he was not well by any means. If it hadn't been for his willpower, youth, and strong constitution, he would never have been able to go back to school or keep a job. He had symptoms involving nearly every system in his body—nervous, gastrointestinal, endocrine, genitourinary, and immune systems—plus his skin, his muscles, and his metabolic energy production.

Taking an optimal wellness approach to William's case, I began to think about the possible underlying conditions that could have so many diverse simultaneous effects. What conditions could produce this form of systemic toxicity? Laboratory testing demonstrated several food allergies (see Chapter Thirteen), intestinal yeast overgrowth (see Chapter Twelve), and serious digestive deficiencies—pancreatic enzyme and stomach hydrochloric acid deficiencies (see Chapter Seven). Treating these conditions helped his gastrointestinal symptoms significantly—he gained fifteen pounds and began feeling a little better overall.

But William's other major symptoms were not much improved, at all. Testing his liver's ability to clear toxins gave us a major clue. The metabolic toxicity scale and the liver detoxification capacity set (both presented later in this chapter) showed a serious functional impairment of his liver.

William protested that his liver could not have anything to do with his problems. He had never used recreational drugs, hardly ever drank alcohol, and had never had hepatitis. And he reminded me that his previous liver function tests had always been normal. I explained to William that "normal liver function" tests actually meant no evidence of liver injury or inflammation. But even with no evidence of injury, his liver's functional capacity to metabolize toxins was reduced. These accumulating toxins circulating throughout his body were poisoning him to a certain degree and triggering a multitude of symptoms.

I placed William on a nutritional program to enhance liver detoxification, and to simultaneously reduce his load of metabolic toxins. He followed the program diligently and made such a dramatic turnabout in just three weeks that his excitement was difficult to contain. He could think clearly once again, focus his mind and remember! He could awaken without a struggle and have a surplus of energy well into the evening! His coping tolerance for both everyday stresses and unusual

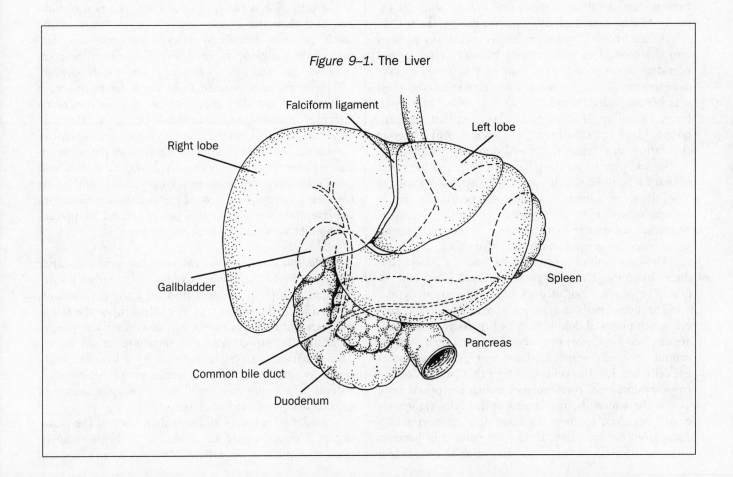

Figure 9–1. The Liver

Falciform ligament

Right lobe

Left lobe

Gallbladder

Spleen

Pancreas

Common bile duct

Duodenum

ones was higher than it had ever been. He told me that he was really enjoying life for the first time. And also, for the first time, he was able to make realistic plans for the future. He ended his visit by informing me that his unusual urinary frequency was much less, the ammonia odor was diminishing, and his orange skin was returning to a normal flesh color and was no longer itching. Primarily by restoring the detoxification functions of his liver, William was feeling a sense of well-being for perhaps the first time.

A SHORT LESSON IN PHYSIOLOGY

The largest solid organ in the body, the liver is located in the upper right section of the abdomen, hidden and protected under the lower part of the rib cage and extending slightly across the midline (see Figure 7–1, page 144). The liver weighs approximately five pounds and uses over 12 percent of your total energy supply. The body can function without the stomach or colon, but not without the liver. Given that it operates on a dual blood supply, the liver is designed quite perfectly as the body's primary filter/detoxification site for impurities in the blood, whether chemical, bacterial, or allergic. The liver awaits such toxins, which are absorbed into the bloodstream from the intestinal tract, the lungs, and the skin. Its capacity to deal with such assaults, however, is limited.

A toxic bowel, you now understand, leaks poisons into the bloodstream that travel by way of the portal vein directly to your liver. If your liver is forced to take over too much of your bowel's work, particularly when it is burdened by the other tasks it is called on to perform, its ability to detoxify the body will be compromised. Harmful substances will escape into systemic circulation, and injure tissue and diminish health.

In addition to its detoxification role, the liver is a primary metabolic site. It serves as a vast factory for the biosynthesis of numerous substances essential for life. It also processes most of our food, converting nutrients and other substances to their active forms, and providing storage for several nutritional elements.

The basic unit of the liver is the lobule, a small cylindrical structure. There are nearly 100,000 lobules in the liver. The primary cell of the lobule is the hepatocyte.

The liver lobule consists of a central vein and two cell-width plates of double rows of hepatocytes that radiate out like the spokes of a wheel. Between each plate lie venous sinusoids, which are lined with porous endothelial cells and Kupffer cells. It is here that blood, coming from the intestinal tract, enters through the portal vein.

In the sinusoids, the large Kupffer cells vigorously engulf bacteria, toxins, and other foreign matter that come from the intestines. In fact, 99 percent of bacteria escapees are trapped here. It is interesting to note that if the quantity of particulate matter or other colon debris increases, there will be a corresponding increase in the number of Kupffer cells. But this response, of course, has its limitations, and a toxic bowel will eventually overwhelm these capacities and cause harmful substances to escape past the liver into the general circulation.

One unique feature of the liver is its dual blood supply—from both the portal vein and the hepatic artery. Approximately 1½ quarts of blood flows through the liver each minute. So, virtually millions of cells are at work continually processing blood.

The Metabolic Factory of the Hepatocytes

The liver's hepatocytes are endowed, like most cells, with tiny organelles that perform a vast array of tasks, one of which is the formation of bile. Anywhere from 600 to 800 milliliters of bile can be produced daily, which is secreted into the hepatic duct, which transports bile to the gallbladder, a muscular, golf ball–sized sac nestled under the liver. Although initially very watery, bile ends up as a much smaller volume after being concentrated in the gallbladder.

Bile is composed primarily of bile salts—cholesterol, lecithin, and bilirubin, a breakdown product from red blood cells. When food, especially fat, enters the stomach and then the duodenum—the upper part of the small intestine—hormonal reflexes trigger the contraction of the gallbladder, which expels bile into the common bile duct and quickly thereafter into the duodenum.

Here, the concentrated fluid has a detergent action on the fat in our diet and, with the help of pancreatic enzymes (lipase) and intestinal churning, the bile emulsifies large globules of fat into microscopic particles (chylomicrons). The bile salts bind these particles, including the fat-soluble vitamins A, D, E, and K and prostaglandin-forming essential fatty acids, and allow for their absorption by way of the intestinal mucosa into the lymphatic vessels. At this point, around 94 percent of the bile salts recycle back to the liver.

Bile Imbalances Several potential problems arise here. The first is gallstones. Cholesterol is rather insoluble, and is kept in solution through adequate amounts of lecithin. If the percentage of cholesterol in the bile is too high and the lecithin too low, cholesterol can precipitate initially into crystals and then into actual stones. This imbalance can be brought on by a high-fat, high-sugar, low-fiber diet. Food allergies in susceptible individuals is another presumed cause of gallstones and gallbladder pain, even after surgery.

Similar imbalances and/or a deficiency in the quantity of bile can trigger an additional problem—namely, poor absorption of the fat-soluble vitamins and essential

FUNCTIONS OF THE LIVER

DETOXIFICATION

Toxic chemicals	Hormones	Microbes
Drugs	Allergens	Microbial metabolites
Alcohol	Antigen-antibody complexes	Microbial antigens

METABOLISM

Production:	Blood-clotting factors	Fat to energy
Bile	Glucose tolerance factor	Glucose to fat
Cholesterol for sex	Glutathione	Fat to phospholipids
hormones and adrenal	Conversion:	Beta-carotene to vitamin A
hormones	Glucose to glycogen	Synthesis of nonessential
Globulin	Glycogen to glucose	amino acids
Albumin	Amino acids to glucose	

STORAGE

Glycogen	Vitamins B-12, A, D	Iron
Blood		

fatty acids. Thus your varied symptoms of nutrient or essential fatty acid deficiencies may not stem from dietary inadequacy, but from poor absorption due to problems in the liver and gallbladder.

Cholesterol Synthesis Hepatocytes also synthesize cholesterol, which serves several important functions in the body. Cholesterol is the basic molecule from which adrenal hormones and our sex hormones—estrogen and testosterone—are produced. Besides being an actual constituent of bile, it is the precursor of bile salts. Cholesterol also serves as an antioxidant in cell membranes, helping to prevent free radical pathology.

The Lymphatic System Hepatocytes play a role as well in the synthesis of lymph. In fact, they are responsible for producing half of our total lymphatic fluid. This circulatory system is separate from our arteries and veins, but anatomically adjacent and intimately related. Thus, the lymphatic system serves as a transport system for fat-soluble nutrients absorbed from the gastrointestinal tract.

It also works as a drainage system for foreign organisms and matter that have escaped the bloodstream or are too large to enter it. Once trapped in lymph nodes, they are attacked and eliminated by immune cells. Lymphatic channels are found throughout the body and have their headwaters, in part, in the liver, adjacent to hepatocytes.

Plasma Proteins The liver synthesizes 95 percent of our plasma proteins—albumin and globulin. Albumin functions as a carrier, transporting numerous hormones, nutrients, and other substances. Globulin serves as a backbone for most of the immune system's antibodies. The liver forms factors responsible for coagulation (clotting of blood), and it can synthesize any of the nonessential amino acids.

Processing of Food

You may be surprised to learn how important the liver is in regulating blood sugar levels. The liver converts glucose to glycogen, the storage form of sugar, and therefore removes excess sugar from the blood. Conversely, by converting glycogen back to glucose, the liver can bolster low blood sugar levels. It accomplishes this same effect as well by converting protein to glucose (gluconeogenesis).

The liver is responsible for producing 60 percent of the usable energy derived from the metabolism of dietary fat. Because it cannot utilize all of this energy, it donates a good part to metabolic processes in need elsewhere. The liver converts dietary fats to other fatty substances for cellular membranes.

Nutrient Storage and Conversion

The liver stores vitamins B-12, A, and D and the mineral iron (as ferritin). It converts B vitamins, for example, vitamin B-6 (pyridoxine), to its active form, pyridoxal-5 phosphate, and beta-carotene to vitamin A. Individuals who do not respond to the therapeutic administration of B-6, other B vitamins, and/or beta-carotene may have hepatocyte activation failure.

In addition, the liver combines niacin and glutamic acid to make glucose tolerance factor (GTF), which potentiates the function of insulin at the cellular level. It also combines glutamic acid, cysteine, and glycine to form glutathione, a critical antioxidant.

Detoxification

We have briefly mentioned the roles that Kupffer cells and hepatocytes play in detoxification. Kupffer cells scavenge not only intestinal bacteria but also endotoxins from bacteria and fungi and large antigenic/allergic molecules and antigen-antibody complexes. Hepatocytes contribute significantly to the liver's overall detoxifying ability through their elaborate microsomal enzyme systems known as cytochrome P-450.

These systems initiate biochemical reactions that lead to the detoxification and eventual urinary or intestinal excretion of potentially toxic chemicals and compounds. (Under stress, these systems can paradoxically create carcinogens and free radicals that can lead to disease.) Some of the potentially poisonous compounds that hepatocyte metabolism protect us against are pesticides, herbicides, industrial chemicals, food additives, hydrocarbons, metals, pharmaceutical medications, plant toxins, and alcohol.

One can only marvel at the fact that hepatocytes will, on demand, fabricate the specific enzyme needed to

SYMPTOMS OF A SLUGGISH LIVER

Premenstrual syndrome (depression, irritability, mood swings, fatigue, tender breasts, fluid retention, etc.)	Very dark urine
Fibrocystic breasts	Yellowish skin and sclera
Food allergies	Tender or swollen liver
Chemical hypersensitivities (see Chapter Fourteen)	Gallbladder problems
Overweight	Achy joints and muscles
Acne	Sore feet
Elevated blood cholesterol	Slow wound healing
Fatigue	Itching
Depression	Peeling skin
Headache	Dry skin
Dizziness	Burning feet
Nausea	Rashes
Bad breath	Psoriasis
Constipation	Bitter taste in the mouth
Bloating	Unexplainable worry or nightmares
Greasy, fatty stools	Hypoglycemia (see Chapter Ten)
Intolerance of fatty foods	Bowel toxicity (see Chapter Eight)
Light or clay-colored stools	Fat-soluble vitamin deficiency (A, D, E and K—see Chapter Six)
	Essential fatty acid deficiency (see Chapter Three)

metabolize a specific toxin. It's important to understand that the effective functioning of all our enzymes depends on adequate dietary nutrients. Zinc, for example, fuels ninety known enzymes. A deficiency of zinc will, among many things, cause a shutdown of vital hepatocyte detoxification systems.

The liver enzyme systems metabolize not just harmful external substances but our own hormones as well, such as estrogen, testosterone, insulin, cortisol, and adrenaline. Some cases of premenstrual syndrome are a result of the liver's inefficient breakdown of estrogen. In the formation of urea, hepatocytes detoxify and remove ammonia, a by-product of intestinal bacteria that in severe liver malfunction causes coma and death.

With hundreds of essential functions occurring simultaneously, you can appreciate how an impaired or sluggish liver could trigger a host of symptoms. See how many of the symptoms on page 174 you can identify in yourself. The following scored questionnaire is designed to assess symptoms of impaired liver detoxification mechanisms.

LIVER DETOXIFICATION CAPACITY TESTING SCALE

Rate each of the following symptoms based upon your health profile for the past thirty days.

POINT SCALE:
0 = Never or almost never have the symptom
1 = Occasionally have it, effect is not severe
2 = Occasionally have it, effect is severe
3 = Frequently have it, effect is not severe
4 = Frequently have it, effect is severe

DIGESTIVE TRACT
____ Nausea or vomiting
____ Diarrhea
____ Constipation
____ Bloated feeling
____ Belching, or passing gas
____ Heartburn   Total: ____

EARS
____ Itchy ears
____ Earaches, ear infections
____ Drainage from ear
____ Ringing in ears, hearing loss   Total: ____

EMOTIONS
____ Mood swings
____ Anxiety, fear, or nervousness
____ Anger, irritability, or aggressiveness
____ Depression   Total: ____

ENERGY/ ACTIVITY
____ Fatigue, sluggishness
____ Apathy, lethargy
____ Hyperactivity
____ Restlessness   Total: ____

EYES
____ Watery or itchy eyes
____ Swollen, reddened, or sticky eyelids
____ Bags or dark circles under eyes
____ Blurred or tunnel vision
(does not include near- or farsightedness)   Total: ____

HEAD
____ Headaches
____ Faintness
____ Dizziness
____ Insomnia   Total: ____

HEART
____ Irregular or skipped heartbeat
____ Rapid or pounding heartbeat
____ Chest pain   Total: ____

LIVER DETOXIFICATION CAPACITY TESTING SCALE

JOINTS/
MUSCLES
___ Pain or aches in joints
___ Arthritis
___ Stiffness or limitation of movement
___ Pain or aches in muscles
___ Feeling of weakness or tiredness   Total: ___

LUNGS
___ Chest congestion
___ Asthma, bronchitis
___ Shortness of breath
___ Difficulty breathing   Total: ___

MIND
___ Poor memory
___ Confusion, poor comprehension
___ Poor concentration
___ Poor physical coordination
___ Difficulty in making decisions
___ Stuttering or stammering
___ Slurred speech
___ Learning disabilities   Total: ___

MOUTH/
THROAT
___ Chronic coughing
___ Gagging, frequent need to clear throat
___ Sore throat, hoarseness, loss of voice
___ Swollen or discolored tongue, gums, lips
___ Canker sores   Total: ___

NOSE
___ Stuffy nose
___ Sinus problems
___ Hay fever
___ Sneezing attacks
___ Excessive mucus formation   Total: ___

SKIN
___ Acne
___ Hives, rashes, or dry skin
___ Hair loss
___ Flushing or hot flashes
___ Excessive sweating   Total: ___

WEIGHT
___ Binge eating/drinking
___ Craving certain foods
___ Excessive weight
___ Compulsive eating
___ Water retention
___ Underweight   Total: ___

OTHER
___ Frequent illness
___ Frequent or urgent urination
___ Genital itch or discharge   Total: ___
                                               GRAND TOTAL: ___

Scores in the range 51–75 may indicate early signs of metabolic toxicity.
Scores in the range 76–100 may indicate a moderate level of metabolic toxicity.
Scores greater than 100 may indicate severe signs of metabolic toxicity.

Used with permission from Health Comm, Inc., 5800 Soundview Dr., Gig Harbor, WA 98335 (206) 851–3943

FACTORS INFLUENCING LIVER FUNCTION

Just what causes the liver to become sluggish? As with most organs in the body, when adverse influences overcome supportive ones, a deterioration of function ensues.

Supportive Influences

- Adequate and balanced macronutrient intake (protein, fats, and carbohydrates; see Chapter Three)
- Adequate general micronutrient intake (vitamins and minerals)
- Adequate digestion and assimilation so that macro- and micronutrients reach the liver (see Chapter Seven)
- Adequate thyroid function
- Genetic presence of necessary enzymes

Adverse Influences

- History of viral hepatitis (or mononucleosis that has affected the liver), especially chronic hepatitis
- History of alcoholism or significant regular use of alcohol
- History of drug abuse
- History of chemical hepatitis or significant or regular exposure to chemicals: pesticides, herbicides, halogenated compounds (PCB, PCP), industrial chemicals, formaldehyde, paints, fuels, solvents (see Chapter Fourteen)
- Use of pharmaceutical medications with potential liver toxicity: anabolic steroids, oral contraceptives, cancer chemotherapy, radiation to the liver, high-dose acetaminophen and/or aspirin, griseofulvin, ketoconazole, phenothiazine, and chlorpromazine
- Fiber-poor, refined diet
- Excessive fat and protein-rich diet
- Excessive calories in the diet
- Bowel toxicity (see Chapter Eight) and/or "leaky gut" syndrome (see Chapter Thirteen)
- Candida overgrowth (see Chapter Twelve)
- Dietary sources of free radicals: rancid oils and fats (fried foods, heated polyunsaturated oils, broiled cheese, charred meats; see Chapter Three)
- Trans-fatty acids (margarine, refined oils) and partially hydrogenated vegetable oils (see Chapter Three)

ASSESSING YOUR LIVER FUNCTION

Common liver function tests include serum measurements of SGOT, SGPT, gamma GTP, alkaline phosphatase, LDH, and bilirubin. Serum protein electrophoresis, BSP retention, and prothrombin time also provide important information.

The liver has an immense capacity to tough out dietary and chemical abuse. Until things have gone way too far, or any one particular assault becomes extremely toxic or invasive, these laboratory tests may be completely normal, even when significant liver symptoms exist. However, the salivary caffeine[1] and urinary hippurate[2] clearance tests can detect any altered detoxification capacity of the liver when more standard tests demonstrate no abnormalities. I use these two tests frequently to provide objective documentation for a multitude of symptoms that otherwise would be difficult to explain. (I give take-home test kits to my patients, and they mail saliva and urine samples directly to the laboratory.)

There are two primary steps in liver detoxification to prepare toxins for excretion from the body: phase 1–oxidation (measured by caffeine clearance) and phase 2–conjugation (measured by hippurate clearance). If clearance for either phase is diminished, an individual would be unable to effectively excrete toxins, would then accumulate them, and would suffer from symptoms of metabolic poisoning. Appropriate nutrient/herbal supplementation would then be indicated to regulate detoxification enzyme function.

If either phase shows excessive clearance, nutrient support would still be indicated to fuel those overworking systems, in addition to liver-specific and general antioxidant measures to address the extra free radicals normally generated from phase 1 reactions.

Excessive clearance would also, of course, indicate overexposure and call for you and your physician to search for the sources of toxins (environmental pollutants, bowel toxins, alcohol and other drugs, hormones, and immune complexes from food allergens).

By reducing the toxin load to your hepatocytes, you would hopefully reduce free radical production and lessen not only your current symptoms but your future risk of malignancy, atherosclerosis, and other free radical–induced degenerative disease. I often recommend the Ultra Clear metabolic detoxification program, which addresses the nutrient needs of both diminished and overworked liver detoxification systems (see page 180).

An estrogen fractionation test[3] to determine the percentages of estradiol, estriol, and estrone can demonstrate specifically if the liver is detoxifying estrogen adequately or not. An abnormal ratio derived from these numbers can imply that liver function is not normal and requires supportive measures. (Some physicians use this ratio as a preventive diagnostic test for breast cancer.)

Early liver abnormalities can be suspected as well, by means of pulse, face, or tongue diagnosis by a practitioner of Oriental medicine (see Chapter Twenty-one), by electronic screening or biokinesiology (see Chapter Thirteen), or by reflexology (see Chapter Twenty).

Assessment by Symptoms and History

As with many conditions we have discussed, a review of your symptoms and history can be as important as any test a doctor can perform. Such a review may be far more important if the available laboratory tests are normal. Knowing what factors are detrimental to your liver and what symptoms can be produced may provide the medical detective with the necessary clues to solve many a dilemma. In the face of "normal" standard laboratory data, so common with sluggish livers, such clues provide a vital rationale for the implementation of valuable therapeutic trials.

RESTORING YOUR LIVER FUNCTION

A unique feature of the liver is its ability to regenerate. It has the capacity to heal itself, particularly when supported with effective therapeutic agents and practices. Even cases of chronic hepatitis or chemical injury to the liver have responded to safe and usually effective liver restoration measures. If you have symptoms of a sluggish liver or simply want to enhance its reserve for preventive purposes, consider incorporating several of the following items.

Seven Steps to Restoring Your Liver

1. Diminish the use of or exposure to agents which adversely affect liver function.
2. Follow the measures supportive of liver function.
3. A toxic bowel presents a major stress to the liver and requires treatment. Optimize colon function (see Chapter Eight), with particular attention to transit time, beneficial microorganisms, intestinal permeability (see Chapter Thirteen), intestinal candidiasis (see Chapter Twelve), and parasites.
4. Use liver-protecting agents and nutrients that stimulate the liver's enzyme detoxification systems.

The liver-protecting agents are:

- Milk thistle (*Silybum marianum*)
- Lipoic acid
- Catechin
- Vitamin C and other antioxidants (vitamin E, beta-carotene, glutathione, selenium)
- N-acetylcysteine or cysteine
- Liv. 52

Use two or three of the above agents simultaneously: milk thistle, vitamin C (and the other general antioxidants), and perhaps cysteine. (For more details, see "Enhancing Your Liver Function," page 179 of this chapter.)

Note: The herbal agents in this category (milk thistle, catechin, Liv. 52) may cause nausea, headaches, intestinal upset, or a general toxic feeling if you start at too high a dose. Begin modestly, then work up according to the recommendations of the doctor supervising your treatment.

Nutrients specific for activating or enhancing the liver's detoxification capacity include B-complex vitamins (B, B-2, B-3, B-5, and folic acid), minerals (molybdenum and zinc), and amino acids (glycine, cysteine, N-acetylcysteine, and glutathione). A potent multiple vitamin/mineral supplement and a whole-foods diet would include most of these, as would the Ultra Clear program (see page 180).

Milk thistle and Liv. 52 (see pages 179 and 180) also stimulate liver detoxification. One or two liver tablets (glandular extracts of the liver),[4] with meals three times a day (also available as intramuscular injections) are often recommended by nutritional physicians for liver support (see precautions, page 181). In addition, they often recommend vitamin B-12 (intramuscular injections, nasal gel, or sublingual tablets) if they suspect poor intestinal absorption. Fresh carrot juice and nutritional or brewer's yeast (if there is no yeast allergy) are also helpful.

5. Cleanse and stimulate overall liver functioning with choleretic agents, which stimulate bile production and increase solubility; cholegogues, which stimulate the gallbladder to contract and release bile; and lipotropic factors, which assist general hepatocyte metabolism and prevent fatty accumulation in the liver.

A common choleretic agent is milk thistle, which can be taken alone in one or two capsules three times a day, or in a combination formula with curcumin (turmeric, see Chapter Nineteen) and artichokes.

The botanicals known as cholegogues include celandine, fringe tree, dandelion root, Russian black radish, Oregon grape root, and beet leaf. They are available combined in tablets, capsules, and tinctures. Take one or two capsules three times a day with meals, or five to twenty drops three times a day. Again, start out with a smaller dose and work up.

You should also be sure to include other dark leafy greens in your diet, as well as artichokes, beets, radishes, and young dandelion greens. These vegetables are liver cleansers.

The most important lipotropic factor is methionine. Others include choline, vitamin B-6, betaine, and folic acid. These are available combined in tablets or capsules with the choleretics and cholegogues (OptiLipotropic[5] or SLF[6]). The dose is generally one or two capsules three times a day, with meals (using the dose precautions in item 4 above). These agents can also be found separately.

Carnitine, a lipotropic factor not usually included in lipotropic formulas, is used in cases of alcohol abuse.[7] Recommended dosage is 500 to 1,000 milligrams three times a day.

6. Cleanse the liver in a somewhat different manner using the Liver Flush and Purifying Diet (see page 180).

Periodic short fasts (see Chapter Eighteen) allow an even more effective rest period and therefore potential rejuvenation for the liver. Other recommended cleansers include chlorophyll and aloe vera (see Chapter Nineteen). You may also want to try placing a castor oil pack on your abdomen over the area of the liver (see Chapter Twenty).

7. Enhance liver function for general preventive purposes. As with the intestinal cleansing program described in Chapter Eight, a preventive program for the liver can combat dietary abuses and assaults by environmental toxins and maintain proper functioning. Use a combination lipotropic/cholegogue/choleretic agent for one to two months every year, and do the liver flush and purifying diet periodically. Or do the Ultra Clear metabolic clearing program once a year. A periodic short fast is also helpful. If your liver is particularly at risk, due to environmental toxin exposure, medications you are currently taking, or other factors, supplement with liver-protecting agents, especially milk thistle and general antioxidants.

ENHANCING YOUR LIVER FUNCTION

Liver-Protecting Agents: A Closer Look

Liver-protecting agents offer an extremely effective way to treat liver disease, prevent liver injury, assist liver detoxification, and maintain the health of this vital organ.

Milk Thistle (Silybum marianum) This agent stands at the top of the list, with an impressive track record in Europe, where it has been prescribed for years for many liver conditions.[8] The active ingredient silymarin is known to be a superior agent in preventing liver destruction and enhancing liver function.

As a potent antioxidant, and inhibitor of lipoxygenase (an enzyme that leads to inflammation), silymarin inhibits free radicals and leukotrienes, the actual biochemical agents that injure the liver in most toxic substance exposures. It also inhibits both the pathological decomposition of membrane lipids and the synthesis of inflammatory prostaglandins that occur during free radical pathology. Moreover, silymarin stimulates both the protein synthesis of new liver cells and the production of increased quantities of bile.

In cases of amanita and carbon tetrachloride poisoning, pharmaceutical-grade silymarin has prevented liver necrosis and death when administered intravenously. This botanical can be used orally for cirrhosis, acute and chronic hepatitis, chemical- and alcohol-induced fatty infiltration, cholangitis, pericholangitis, psoriasis, chemical hypersensitivity, sluggish liver symptoms, and any symptom created by overloaded detoxification systems.

Try to find tablets or capsules with standardized extracts 70 percent silymarin calculated. (See Chapter Nineteen for more of this herb's properties and uses.)

Lipoic Acid Considered by some authorities to be a member of the B vitamin family, this biocatalyst is necessary for multiple enzymatic functions, some of the more important of which are oxidative decarboxylation and the production of key substrates in the Krebs cycle, our main energy production pathway.[9] Lipoic acid has been used successfully in cases of exposure to mercuric chloride, arsenobenzoles, lead and other heavy metals, carbon tetrachloride, and aniline dyes.

Like silymarin, lipoic acid is used to treat alcohol-induced liver disease, hepatic coma, and amanita poisoning. It has been effective in cases of altered hepatic carbohydrate metabolism, as well as viral hepatitis, drug- and chemical-induced liver damage, and chronic hepatitis. It is also a potent antioxidant, and is used in peripheral and diabetic neuropathies.

Catechin A naturally occurring flavonoid, catechin has some of the properties of silymarin and lipoic acid. As an antioxidant, it inhibits free radical oxidative damage. It also combats intestinal toxins, stabilizes cell membranes, and has been used for viral hepatitis and alcohol- and chemical-induced liver damage. (Catechin has other uses related to its flavonoid function; see Chapter Nineteen.)

Vitamin C (Ascorbic Acid) Vitamin C has been used effectively to reduce recovery time in the treatment of mononucleosis and acute or chronic viral hepatitis. In these cases, it is administered intravenously in very large doses, up to 50 grams a day, and orally up to bowel tolerance (the dose that causes diarrhea).

Vitamin C has also been used as part of an antioxidant defense in cases of chemical hypersensitivity and food and inhalant allergies, as well as for general health maintenance. Overdosing may cause diarrhea, and the buffered form (ascorbate) may be easier on your stomach (see Chapter Six).

N-acetylcysteine Used successfully in treating acetaminophen-induced liver toxicity, this amino acid derivative has not only antioxidant properties but also immune-enhancing, cholesterol-lowering, and infection-reducing effects (see Chapter Six).

Liv. 52   Liv. 52 is an Ayurvedic combination herbal remedy introduced in India in 1956 and used successfully to treat a variety of liver diseases: alcoholic liver injury, cirrhosis, viral hepatitis (both acute and chronic), drug-induced liver injury, heavy metal and chemical toxicity, radiation-induced liver damage, and general toxicity.[10] In repeated studies, Liv. 52 reverses abnormal liver function tests in such diseases. It quickens the return of well-being and shortens the recovery time for most individuals who have such disorders.

Liv. 52 functions as an antioxidant, and it protects and restores the detoxification and metabolic functions of hepatocytes. It may also stimulate and regenerate normal liver architecture. Its ingredients are: *Capparis spinosa* (capers), *Cichorium intybus* (chicory), *Solanum nigrum* (wonderberry), *Cassia occidentalis* (myrobalan), *Terminalia arjuna* (senna), *Archillea millefolium* (yarrow), *Tamarix gallica* (manna), and *Mandur bhasma* (organically complexed iron). These ingredients are further processed in a solution containing *Phyllanthus amarus*.

For more information, contact Jivan Botanical Laboratories of Seattle, Washington, or Probiologic of Bellevue, Washington.

The Ultra Clear Detoxifying Program

The Ultra Clear metabolic clearing/detoxification program is a seven- to twenty-one-day protocol designed to nourish and enhance the liver's detoxification functions. The program involves fasting using the Ultra Clear beverage, a rice-based hypoallergenic powder formulated not only to regulate liver detoxification, but to minimize allergic and digestive stress. Ultra Clear is an ideal program for those suffering from symptoms of liver toxicity, chemical hypersensitivity, chemical exposure, food allergy/intolerance, and digestive disturbances. It is also one of the least painful and safest ways to accomplish some of the benefits of fasting (see Chapter Eighteen).

The program involves fasting for three to seven days using the Ultra Clear or Ultra Clear Plus beverage five times a day, followed by one to two weeks on a hypoallergenic diet supplemented with Ultra Clear three times daily. Ultra Clear products are available through health professionals and pharmacists. For more information, contact: Metagenics, 1010 Tyinn Street, #26, Eugene, OR 97402 (800) 338-3948.

Liver Flush and Purifying Diet*

This one- to seven-day cleansing regimen consists of a tasty morning juice and oil drink and a diet of fresh fruits and vegetables. It gives the liver a break from processing heavier foods, allowing it a relative rest so that its metabolic functions can be rejuvenated and enhanced. While on the purifying diet, you may feel much lighter and more energetic. You may also develop a new way of looking at eating and learn to modify your abusive or unwise eating patterns.

Liver Flush Tea
1 teaspoon fenugreek seeds
1 teaspoon fennel seeds
1 teaspoon peppermint leaves
1 teaspoon flaxseed
4 slices fresh gingerroot cut about ⅛ inch thick
Licorice root (optional)

Boil the gingerroot three minutes in 1½ to 2 pints of water. Then add the other ingredients and let steep 10 to 15 minutes while you prepare the liver flush.

Liver Flush
Mix together in a blender:

Juice of 1 or 2 grapefruits or several oranges (or blend the whole peeled and sectioned fruit, removing most of the seeds first); or use apple juice
4 to 6 tablespoons fresh lemon or lime juice
2 to 3 tablespoons cold-pressed virgin or extra virgin olive oil or unrefined almond or sesame oil
1 to 3 cloves of garlic or ½ to 1 teaspoon liquid deodorized garlic
A sprinkle to ½ teaspoon cayenne pepper (optional)

Drink the liver flush (it is surprisingly tasty). Then drink a glassful of the liver flush tea, without honey, while it is hot. This is your breakfast. During the day, drink four or more cups of the tea, with honey as desired.

An hour or two after your liver flush "breakfast" have some fresh citrus (oranges or grapefruit, or their juice) or other fresh fruit (apples, pears, apricots, grapes, etc.) or some freshly made vegetable juice (mixture of carrot, celery, beet, etc.). You may repeat this between lunch and dinner.

Lunch can be a fruit or vegetable salad; the same for

---

*Adapted from R. Stone, Dr. Randolph Stone's Polarity Therapy: The Complete Collected Works, CRCS Publications, P.O. Box 1460, Sebastopol, CA 95473.

dinner. Avoid mixing fruits and vegetables at the same meal. Eat leafy greens and other vegetables, such as lettuce, carrots, turnips, summer squash, zucchini, spinach, onion, celery, cabbage, avocado (a small amount), broccoli, cauliflower, string beans, radishes, cucumbers, beets and their tops. Add sprouts to your mix of vegetables—alfalfa, fenugreek, clover, mung bean, lentil. Eat your vegetables raw as much as possible. But you may also steam the vegetables or make them into soups if your digestion cannot tolerate much raw food, or if the weather is cold.

Another choice is to make gourmet fruit salads with apples, pears, grapes, peaches, prunes, figs, bananas, raisins, mangoes, papayas, pineapples, berries, melons, etc. Some sources suggest eating melon separately from other fruits. You may add lemon juice and herbs, and just a touch of good oil, if needed, to your salads. You may also add a small amount of ground flaxseed or sesame seeds.

Do not eat meat, fish, chicken, eggs, legumes (unless sprouted), starches (potatoes, rice, bread, cereal, winter squashes), sugar (small amounts of honey or maple syrup are permissible), milk or milk products, coffee, regular caffeinated tea, or alcohol. Avoid any unnecessary medications, either prescription or over-the-counter. A *small* amount of raw nuts or seeds may be eaten if you get too hungry, but too much will cancel the cleansing effect of this diet.

OPTIONAL: 1 or 2 ounces of aloe vera juice twice a day; one or two capsules/tablets of OptiLipotropic or SLF three times a day. A nightly castor oil pack placed on the abdomen over the liver is also supportive.

It is common to suffer nausea or headaches on this diet if your liver or bowel is toxic. Correcting a constipation problem first, as much as possible, will make this purifying diet easier. Using minimal amounts of garlic and oil in the liver flush drink will also ease the process; increase these as tolerated. The discomfort you may feel in the beginning should be temporary.

You get a better cleansing the more days in a row you do this diet (seven to ten days maximum). But if you do not feel well on this diet or cannot afford to lose much weight, do it only for a short time. A one-day purifying diet is still very good. And if you cannot tolerate the liver flush, simply do the diet; it will still be effective. Find the right length of time and frequency for doing this diet according to your response—that is, the way you feel on it. This is usually determined by your level of toxicity, your metabolism, and the demands of your daily schedule.

SUGGESTED SCHEDULE. Try this regimen for one to two days every week or two, or for two to three days every three to four weeks. Or do it for four to seven days in a row, perhaps once or twice a year. You cannot live on this diet; it would weaken you eventually. Do it periodically, as advised here, or use it as a rescue measure after dietary debaucheries.

Individuals with severe hypoglycemia should stabilize blood sugar before attempting this diet. Diabetics or any persons with an internal disorder should not attempt this diet without professional guidance.

THE MARVELOUS LIVER

The liver is a vast metabolic factory with many important functions. It also detoxifies hormones, environmental pollutants, and other substances. Some of these toxins are transported in the blood to the kidneys and are excreted in the urine. Many are sent through the bile to be excreted through the intestines.

The liver relies on a dependable bowel to remove these toxins. When bowel function diminishes, these toxins are reabsorbed and sent back to the liver. Eventually the liver becomes overwhelmed and its other functions are compromised. Sooner or later the toxins enter the general circulation, creating a condition of impure blood, and multiple symptoms of systemic toxicity can arise. But the liver is very forgiving, and significant liver function can be compromised before symptoms become apparent.

Liver function can often be restored, however. Ingesting the right nutrients and avoiding dietary excesses and harmful substances, both dietary and environmental, are key to maintaining and restoring liver function. Reversing a toxic bowel is also imperative, and with carefully chosen therapeutic agents and reparative measures, the liver can once again perform its essential marvels, safeguarding and maintaining the body's well-being.

SUGGESTED READING

Note: Contact The American Liver Foundation (998 Pompton Ave., Cedar Grove, NJ 07009) for a packet of information regarding many aspects of the liver. I am unaware of other material on the liver suited for the lay public. The following titles are more technical reading:

Bland, Jeffrey S., Ph.D., and Bralley, Alexander. "Nutritional Upregulation of Hepatic Detoxification Enzymes," *The Journal of Applied Nutrition*, vol. 44, Nos. 3 & 4, 1992, pp. 1–15. Reprints available from and published by International Academy of Nutrition and Preventive Medicine, P.O. Box 18433, Asheville, NC 28814.

Guyton, Arthur C., M.D. *Textbook of Medical Physiology.* Philadelphia: W.B. Saunders, 1971, pp. 861–869.

Murray, Michael T., N.D. *Phyto-Pharmica Review*, Volume 1 (Fall, 1987). Available from Phyto-Pharmica, P.O. Box 1348, Green Bay, WI 54305, (414) 435–4200.

Pizzorno, Joseph E., N.D., and Murray, Michael T., N.D. "Hepatoprotection: Clinical Indications for the Use of Lipotropic Factors," in *A Textbook of Natural Medicine.* Seattle, WA: John Bastyr Publications, 1987, Section IV, pp. 1–8.

Ruckpaul, Klaus and Rein, Horst (eds.). *Basis and Mechanisms of Regulation of Cytochrome P-450.* Academy of Sciences GDR. London, New York, and Philadelphia: Taylor and Francis, 1989.

CHAPTER 10

HYPOGLYCEMIA

In this chapter, we will discuss the subject of hypoglycemia, or low blood sugar, a condition fraught with much misunderstanding. Hypoglycemia has been commonly recognized in diabetics who overmedicate with insulin or other blood-sugar-lowering agents. However, for the broader population, many physicians still regard it as a fad.

Nevertheless, millions of Americans are indeed affected by this condition, and its recognition and proper treatment will bring them much-needed relief. For those of you who are already familiar with hypoglycemia, you may be happily surprised to learn that the condition need not be a lifelong problem. Frequently, it is a symptom of an underlying condition, and when this is corrected the hypoglycemia can often be eradicated. We will begin with the case history of Larry, one of my patients.

LARRY

A construction worker, Larry had been one of the top men on his crew, up until the last year, when his job performance began to decline steadily. He had become more irritable and moody, less able to concentrate, and less able to stick to a task, especially under pressure. His physical stamina seemed normal until about eleven o'clock in the morning. But after that, he just didn't seem able to keep up with the demands of the job. If Larry hadn't had such a good track record and such a good rapport with his foreman, he would have been fired long before. However, his foreman was getting to the point where he wasn't going to tolerate Larry's moods, inappropriate outbursts, and his ineffectiveness on the job much longer.

Larry told me that his foreman had noticed that, initially, Larry only showed signs of poor physical performance and emotional instability in the late afternoon. More recently, however, his foreman thought that Larry now seemed stable and capable for only a few hours in the morning.

Larry also seemed to suffer from frequent headaches in the late mornings or late afternoons, and had gotten in the habit of using aspirin every day. He also mentioned being temporarily light-headed when rising quickly from a sitting or lying position. He frequently felt depressed and didn't know why. Normal stresses would often seem too much for him. Many of these symptoms, he noticed, would subside if he remembered to snack every few hours, but his work made this nearly impossible.

A bachelor, Larry rarely cooked for himself. Breakfast usually consisted of a packaged breakfast drink and cereal with milk. He'd frequently have coffee and doughnuts while driving to work, sometimes an apple. One or two mornings a week he'd have eggs, bacon, and toast. On those days he'd generally feel a little stronger. Lunches and dinners were fast foods—burgers, fries, soft drinks, milk shakes, tacos, fried chicken.

He ate some kind of sweet every day after lunch and about half the time after dinner, usually cookies. He drank two or three beers after work and usually one or two with dinner. After work or on weekends, he no longer seemed interested in doing anything that required much physical or mental effort.

Larry took his foreman's suggestion to have a physical exam and blood tests. His doctor told him everything was "normal," but his symptoms still persisted. This is when he came to see me.

A Classic Case of Low Blood Sugar

An analysis of Larry's diet revealed that he consumed approximately 30 to 35 teaspoons of sugar a day. About 75 percent of his sugar intake could be attributed to the obvious sweets: milk shakes, cookies, doughnuts, cola drinks, and desserts. The rest came from hidden sugar, found in fast foods and added to such items as ketchup, breads, alcoholic beverages, breakfast drinks, canned foods, and salad dressings.

The analysis also disclosed that he consumed far below even the minimum daily requirement for many vitamins and minerals, nutrients essential for healthy carbohydrate metabolism and stable blood sugar levels. By virtue of Larry's highly refined and processed diet, his sugar intake was excessive and his vitamin, mineral, and fiber intake deficient. These factors predisposed him to a hypoglycemic condition.

How many of the symptoms and predisposing factors on the following pages apply to you?

Before we can fully understand these symptoms with respect to sugar metabolism, a few definitions are in order. Carbohydrates are classified "simple" or "complex" depending on their molecular structure.

1. REFINED means processing foods in a way that removes vitamins, minerals, and fiber. White flour, enriched flour, and white rice are refined products. (Unbleached white flour is still refined.)

2. UNREFINED means minimally processed. Such foods contain the vitamins, minerals, and fiber with which nature endowed them. Whole wheat flour, brown rice, and any whole grain or whole-grain flour are unrefined carbohydrates.

3. SIMPLE CARBOHYDRATES, or sugars, such as table sugar (sucrose), honey, maple syrup, fruit sugar (fructose), and corn syrup are characteristically sweet. They are found in both refined and unrefined products.

4. COMPLEX CARBOHYDRATES, or starches, such as wheat, rice, corn, winter squash, potatoes, and lentils, are characteristically not sweet tasting. The grains in this category may be refined or unrefined. Both white and wheat flour are complex carbohydrates.

5. In the body, both simple and complex carbohydrates are converted to **GLUCOSE**, or blood sugar, which provides fuel for the brain, muscles, and other tissues. Glucose is stored in the liver and muscles as **GLYCOGEN**, which can be easily reconverted to glucose for energy.

By now you can see that one needs to determine whether a carbohydrate is simple or complex, refined or unrefined. The health and disease implications of these differences are immense. You will recall from Chapter Three that the carbohydrate portion of our diet should be mostly complex and unrefined. In this chapter, we will concentrate on the differences between complex and simple carbohydrates as they relate to blood sugar levels.

A complex carbohydrate, such as rice, consists of very long strands of simple sugars (polysaccharides), strands too long to be absorbed across the small intestine lining into the bloodstream. Digestion must occur in order for these long strands to be broken into separate single sugar molecules (monosaccharides) small enough to enter the bloodstream. Various amylase disaccharidases and other enzymes perform this task. This process takes time and produces a slow, gradual rise in the level of blood sugar as more and more simple sugar molecules are broken off from the long strands and absorbed into the bloodstream.

As the blood sugar level gradually rises, this signals the pancreas to release a corresponding amount of insulin into the bloodstream. Insulin contributes to the nourishment of the body's cells by facilitating the penetration of cell walls by the sugar molecules. In so doing, it accomplishes its other role of preventing the accumulation of too much sugar in the blood (diabetes mellitus; see Chapter Seventeen).

Stated another way, a gradual rise of blood sugar from the ingestion of complex carbohydrates causes a gradual release of insulin from the pancreas, which in turn brings about a gradual return of the blood sugar level to approximately what it was before you ate. With the blood sugar level fluctuating gently in this normal manner, the body's cells—most especially in the brain— are supplied with a generally consistent level of fuel. By virtue of this slow-release system, complex carbohydrates seem to be an ideal food for this metabolic design (see Figure 10–1).

WHAT IS HYPOGLYCEMIA?

A simple sugar such as sucrose (table sugar) is so small that it can be absorbed intact into the lining of the small intestine, where it quickly enters the bloodstream. When you eat food containing this simple sugar many sugar molecules rush into the bloodstream, causing an abrupt rise in the blood sugar level.

This is often aggravated by the fact that many sugared foods are also refined. They lack the fiber provided by unrefined grains that could slow the entry of sugar into the bloodstream. Without this protective effect of fiber, brain cells that have become saturated with a sudden increase in levels of sugar can produce various manifestations of abnormal brain cell metabolism. These symptoms include aggressiveness, sudden mood changes, and hyperactivity. They also include some changes that may not necessarily seem adverse—a sudden lift, quicker thinking, increased energy, giddiness.

In susceptible individuals, these suddenly elevated

SYMPTOMS OF HYPOGLYCEMIA

SYMPTOMS THAT ARISE IF MEALS ARE DELAYED OR MISSED

Fatigue or sleepiness
Headaches
Depression
Anxiety
Nervousness
Hyperactivity
Irritability
Crying for no apparent reason
Mood swings
Unexplained feelings of insecurity or fear
Poor concentration
Poor memory
Difficulty making decisions

Insomnia
Nightmares
Weakness
Difficulty working under pressure
Heavy breathing
Intense hunger; always needing to nibble
Nervous stomach
Dizziness, light-headedness
Blurred vision
Hallucinations
Convulsions/seizures
Heart palpitations
Excessive or unexplained sweating

SYMPTOMS THAT MAY OR MAY NOT BE RELATED TO MEALS

Chronic fatigue
Chronic nervous exhaustion
Hyperactivity
Unusual episodes of needing to sleep
Nervous stomach
Caffeine dependence

Craving for sweets
Difficulty coping with normal stresses
Depression
Allergies
Poor libido
Insomnia

PREDISPOSING FACTORS

Significant consumption of sugar, honey, maple syrup, molasses, dried fruit, or other concentrated
     sweets
Regular consumption of junk food, fast food, or processed foods
Inadequate consumption of complex carbohydrates
Inadequate protein consumption (especially if vegetarian)
Inadequate protein digestion
Alcoholism (active or recovering)
Regular alcohol consumption
Cigarette smoking
Significant caffeine consumption (coffee, soft drinks, black tea, various medications)
High-stress work or lifestyle
Frequently missed or delayed meals
Frequent depleting or overexerting exercise or other physical activity
Adrenal weakness

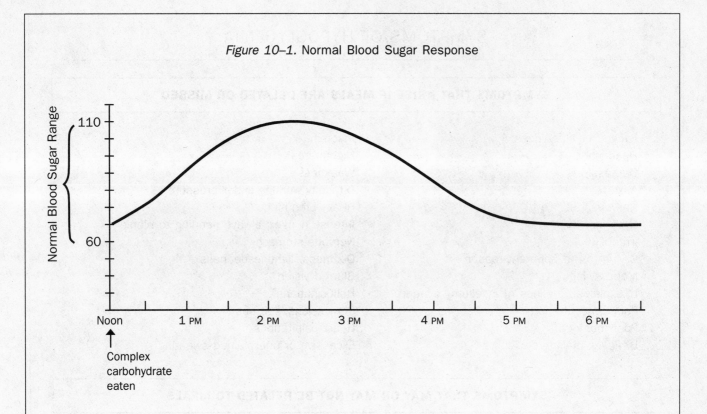

Figure 10–1. Normal Blood Sugar Response

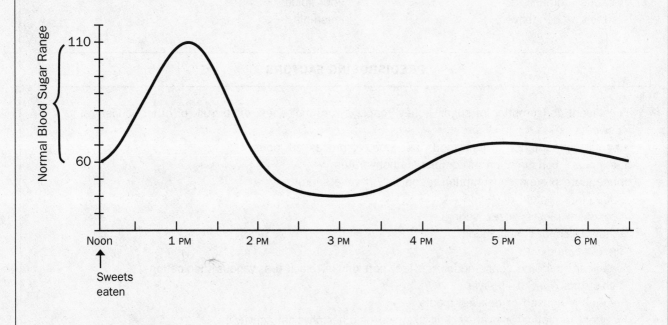

Figure 10–2. Hypoglycemic (Low Blood Sugar) Response

levels of blood sugar create an abnormal, emergency situation for the pancreas, which then secretes an abnormally high level of insulin. When blood sugar levels meet this surge of insulin, they drop abruptly. Consequently, soon after a sweet snack or a dessert loaded with simple sugars is ingested, the brain can become relatively deprived of glucose, its main fuel, and begin to dysfunction. Depression, fatigue, irritability, anxiety, headaches, lack of mental acuity, cravings for sweets or caffeine or alcohol, heart palpitations, tremors, blurred vision, unexplained sweating, insomnia, and an inability to cope with normal stresses are just some of the effects. This constellation of symptoms is known as hypoglycemia, or reactive hypoglycemia. Figure 10–2 shows an example of a hypoglycemic response.

Another Critical Factor in Hypoglycemia

The conventional explanation of hypoglycemia refers to a deprivation of sugar in the brain, or "starved" brain cells. But there is another explanation as well. After the ingestion of sugar, an excessive influx of insulin may be secreted by an overreactive pancreas. The blood sugar level then usually falls dramatically, and electrolytes such as potassium and chloride are driven into the cells. However, the increased concentration of electrolyte particles now within cells obligates extracellular fluid to osmose into cells to restore the intracellular concentration to normal. In other words, the cells swell with increased fluid. When this swelling occurs in brain cells, the brain dysfunctions, causing symptoms of hypoglycemia.[1] This additional mechanism of hypoglycemia may be at work in individuals who produce normal, or only slightly abnormal, results on glucose tolerance tests.

The Adrenal Glands, the Liver, and Hypoglycemia

The adrenals are endocrine glands, just like the insulin-producing beta cells of the pancreas. They are situated just above each kidney. A biochemical factory, the adrenals produce many hormones, two of which are epinephrine (adrenaline), which affects heart rate and blood circulation; and cortisol, which enhances metabolism and blood volume, and counters allergy and inflammation. When the blood sugar level begins to drop too low or too quickly, the adrenal glands are stimulated to action. Both adrenaline and cortisol antagonize the effect of insulin in an effort to keep the blood sugar level from dropping so low that the brain cannot function well. These hormones—as well as glucagon from the pancreas and growth hormone from the pituitary—also help mobilize stored sugar from the liver's reservoir of glycogen when blood sugar levels are too low.

The liver also has the capacity to convert protein to sugar (gluconeogenesis) and will be signaled to perform this function to prevent blood sugar levels from falling too low. Realize, however, that gluconeogenesis can be impaired by excess alcohol and other liver toxins.[2] It also depends upon effective protein digestion and assimilation. The conversion process cannot go on efficiently if hydrochloric acid or a pancreatic enzyme insufficiency exists (see Chapter Seven). Such insufficiencies would prevent the delivery of needed amino acids to the liver. Thus, poor protein digestion is a third although lesser known cause of hypoglycemia.

Our bodies are designed with these emergency systems to accommodate transient levels of low blood sugar, from occasional delayed or missed meals, from occasional excess of sweets or of exercise, and from transient vitamin and mineral deficiencies. These backup systems provide the support to maintain adequate fuel for the brain, muscles, and other tissues. However, months or years of poor eating habits and overwork eventually impair these emergency backup systems. Whether an individual consumes sweets or not at this point, he or she will likely be suffering many hypoglycemic symptoms.

Take Larry, for example. By the time he came to see me, Larry suffered from an overactive pancreas. It was secreting too much insulin and driving his blood sugar down too fast or to levels so low that his overworked adrenals could no longer rescue his falling blood sugar levels. On top of this, Larry's sluggish liver was inefficient at converting protein and/or glycogen to glucose.

Larry did not suspect that these interrelated conditions were producing his fatigue, moodiness, headaches, and other symptoms. Even his doctor had no idea—after all, Larry's standard adrenal and liver function tests, and even his glucose tolerance test, were all normal. As with many laboratory screening tests, the adrenals and liver must be severely impaired before standard tests show any abnormality. Unfortunately, there is a large gray zone where the organ is not functioning well and causing symptoms and yet the standard tests still read normal. Modern medicine doesn't generally recognize this gray zone. "If the tests are normal, the patient must be fine!"

The Effects of Caffeine and Stress

1. CAFFEINE can have a depleting effect on the adrenal glands. In addition to its direct effect on the central nervous system, it whips the adrenals to release hormones that indirectly raise blood sugar levels, placing further stress on the already overburdened adrenals. Caffeine contributes powerfully to nervous and adrenal exhaustion. This means you need to minimize or eliminate caffeine in your diet if you're trying to overcome hypoglycemia.[3]

2. LIFE STRESSES that produce excessive worry, anxiety, and tension all take their toll on the adrenals and draw on their reserve.[4] Adrenals overworked by such responses will be in danger of failing when called upon to rescue low blood sugar levels (or meet other demands). In an effort to stabilize blood sugar and strengthen carbohydrate metabolism, managing your levels of stress may be nearly as important as your nutrition (see Chapter Fifteen). Weakened adrenals will cause many of the same symptoms produced by hypoglycemia (see Chapter Eleven).

Nutritional Deficiencies in Hypoglycemia

The adrenal glands house a biochemical factory capable of producing hormones and other end products of metabolism only if all the "production line" parts are in sufficient and consistent supply. Dietary nutrients serve as cofactors or coenzymes—essential substances that activate the enzyme systems upon which biochemical reactions depend. Without enough vitamin C and vitamin B-5 (pantothenic acid), and other B-complex vitamins in the diet, the adrenal production line would shut down. One consequence would be the failing of a key emergency backup system much needed to combat the effects of stress and to help maintain normal blood sugar levels.

Knowing that several of the B-complex vitamins, especially B-6, are crucial to the utilization of carbohydrates and the release of energy, you can see how a deficiency of these nutrients could contribute to hypoglycemia. The vitamin biotin, for example, is a critical cofactor for glucokinase, an enzyme involved in the initial step of glucose utilization by cells.

The mineral chromium is another nutrient essential for carbohydrate metabolism and necessary for insulin function at the cellular level. Chromium is also a key nutrient in the control of sugar craving (see Chapter Six). Vitamin B-6 (pyridoxine), choline, and methionine are necessary for a healthy liver. Without these lipotropic factors, the liver would not be very effective in releasing sugar into the bloodstream in time of need.

Protein is another vital nutrient for maintaining stable blood sugar levels. An inadequate supply of amino acids can negatively affect the functioning of almost every system of the body, particularly the relationships of the liver, the pancreas, and the adrenal glands to blood sugar levels.[5]

I cannot emphasize enough the importance of eating whole foods to provide these and other nutrients for the body's metabolic needs. A refined, processed, and fast-food diet such as Larry's lacks sufficient quantities of essential nutrients for optimum carbohydrate metabolism and other body processes.

You can now understand how stable and sufficient blood sugar levels are necessary for your brain to function well and for you to feel good. A diet with adequate complex carbohydrates helps accomplish this result. Eating an excess of sugary foods or other simple carbohydrates can, paradoxically, rob your brain of blood sugar—one of its most important fuels—and send your metabolism on a roller-coaster nightmare. These events tax your adrenal, liver, pancreatic, and pituitary backup systems and can eventually deplete your reserves and make you susceptible to more serious illness. A whole-foods diet is essential to provide adequate amounts of complex carbohydrates, protein, essential fatty acids, vitamins, and minerals upon which carbohydrate metabolism equally depends.

TESTS FOR HYPOGLYCEMIA

If your symptoms seem to suggest that you may have a hypoglycemic condition, trust your body sense and follow the treatment recommendations for stabilizing your blood sugar (see box on page 194). Stick with it for at least three or four weeks. If you find you're making good progress, congratulations! If not, you likely have one or more of the masquerading or aggravating conditions (see page 193). You should talk to your doctor about obtaining appropriate laboratory testing.

In my own practice, if I suspect a hypoglycemic condition, I will recommend a three- to four-week trial of dietary and vitamin therapy, along with lifestyle changes to reduce stress. I will also obtain laboratory tests to confirm any suspicions I may have of any masquerading or aggravating conditions. I rarely ask patients to go through the five-hour glucose tolerance test unless they need black-and-white data to consider the necessity of changing their diet.

A glucose tolerance test is taken after an overnight fast. A bottle of sugar water is ingested on an empty stomach, and blood is then drawn every hour for five hours. Blood sugar levels are measured on each sample, and the results are usually plotted on a graph. A fall in the blood sugar level in any one hour's time of more than 20 milligrams per deciliter, or a level at any time less than 60 milligrams per deciliter, may be diagnostic. Be aware, however, that many individuals with symptoms of hypoglycemia produce normal test results.[6]

A glucose-insulin tolerance test may be more diagnostic, in that insulin levels are measured along with blood sugar levels every hour for up to five hours.[7] Elevated insulin levels, suggesting an overreactive pancreas and altered brain function, may be present when blood sugar levels are not terribly low and may, therefore, confirm the need for changes in the diet. This test is extremely useful for predicting or diagnosing borderline or latent diabetes. I recommend it when there is a family history of diabetes and when diabetes is a concern or suspicion.

Another method of testing for hypoglycemia, less arduous though less reliable, is to test blood sugar and insulin levels (one blood draw only, as opposed to the six required for the glucose tolerance test) when you're experiencing your hypoglycemic symptoms. See if you can recognize a consistent time of symptom onset before or after eating in your customary way, and try to arrange with your doctor to have a test done at this time.

TREATMENT OF HYPOGLYCEMIA

Treatment involves primarily a combination of dietary and lifestyle measures that minimize shock to the pancreas and adrenal glands and stabilize carbohydrate metabolism.[8] The program calls for

- A decrease in the consumption of simple sugars (refined or natural), caffeine, alcohol, and white flour.
- At least three meals a day, with usually two or three additional snacks.
- A whole-foods diet that provides a balance of complex carbohydrates and protein (as well as adequate fat) and abundant vitamins and minerals.
- Supplemental vitamins and minerals that can facilitate and accelerate recovery.
- Adequate exercise.
- Lifestyle changes that allow for a reduction of stress in your daily life, and more appropriate ways of handling unavoidable stress.

Dietary Suggestions for Treating Hypoglycemia

The degree to which one needs to restrict certain items or include others will vary, as will the length of treatment, since no one individual's metabolic needs exactly match another's. Review the following to assess your specific needs and circumstances.

1. Do not miss meals. Have at least three a day, punctually, so that your blood sugar levels do not have an opportunity to fall. It would be preferable, in fact, to have five or six small meals a day. If you are most symptomatic in the mornings or late afternoons, your midmorning or midafternoon snack/meal may be a lifesaver (see Chapter Five). If you opt for eating six times a day, be sure to scale down your portions so that you do not consume excessive calories. When your condition stabilizes, three meals a day should be sufficient, and regular snacking is generally no longer advisable.

Some hypoglycemic individuals have no appetite on arising in the morning because dinners are generally late in the evening and large. If this applies to you, try to have at least several dinners during the week before 6:30 P.M. and/or try to eat more at lunch and less at dinner. If you need to snack before bedtime, make it a small one.

If this approach does not improve your morning appetite, perhaps liver and bowel toxicity and/or poor digestion and assimilation are to blame. It can be unwise to eat when not hungry, but in terms of hypoglycemia, it may be even less wise to wait until lunch before eating. Have a wholesome snack midmorning when you feel hungry enough, or at least start the day with a protein powder mixed with water or diluted juice. (Choose a protein powder that is not excessively sweetened.)

2. Begin to replace your refined carbohydrates with unrefined, complex carbohydrate foods (whole grains, legumes, and starchy vegetables). Have some several times a day. One advantage to complex carbohydrate foods is that their slow release avoids shocking the pancreas.

Be aware, however, that these foods have varying speeds of sugar release (and therefore stimulate varying degrees of insulin secretion), known as glycemic index.[9] From the list that follows, you will see that white bread will stimulate insulin secretion more than whole meal bread, which will stimulate secretion more than quick-cooking whole-grain cereal. The least stimulating, and thus the most stabilizing to blood sugar levels, are legumes such as lentils and kidney beans.

You may find that eating foods closer to the form in which they are found in nature—in other words, less processed—will be more filling, more stabilizing to your blood sugar, and more strengthening. For instance, have an apple instead of applesauce, or a whole-grain cereal that takes five to thirty minutes to cook rather than a ready-to-eat whole-grain dry cereal.

You may also discover that different combinations have different effects. For example, you may feel that oatmeal and fresh fruit stick to your ribs much longer than toast and fruit, or that bread and beans keep you going longer than bread and cheese. Experiment to determine what foods and combinations of foods help you and your metabolism feel more stable.

If this higher percentage of complex carbohydrates in your diet seems to cause stomach or intestinal upset, you may need to slow down your transition. You should also check to see if you have an intestinal yeast overgrowth or food allergies (see Chapters Twelve and Thirteen).

If weight gain is a concern and you hesitate to use as much complex carbohydrates as is recommended here, go with what you consider reasonable. Once your carbohydrate metabolism is strengthened and your blood sugar is stabilized, and you're feeling better, then tackle the weight issue. ("Weight Control" in Chapter Seventeen discusses the importance of checking for low thyroid status, food allergy, candidiasis, and other conditions that can contribute to a weight-gaining metabolism.) A fair percentage of my patients concerned about their weight have been surprised to discover that this high–complex carbohydrate diet actually helps them lose weight.

3. You may need to experiment with your diet to determine your protein needs. If the percentage of carbohydrates recommended doesn't help you feel better or makes you feel worse, try using more protein and less carbohydrate, particularly less grain if that has been a predominant carbohydrate in the diet.

Many hypoglycemic individuals initially include some form of animal protein with at least two of their meals. Also, experiment with having protein meals at different times of the day. See if a breakfast of turkey

GLYCEMIC INDEX OF COMMON FOODS

FOOD	GLYCEMIC INDEX*
Glucose	100
White bread	95
Puffed wheat	80
Whole meal bread	77
Potato flakes	74
Spaghetti	64
Shortbread	64
White rice	56
Quick-cooking whole wheat	54
Custard	43
Cooked lentils	30
Cooked kidney beans	23

*Higher glycemic index scores (less desirable) indicate quicker entry of sugar into the bloodstream and increased pancreatic stimulation to release insulin. Lower glycemic index scores (more desirable) indicate slower entry of sugar into the bloodstream and less pancreatic stimulation to release insulin.
Source: Adapted from D.J.A. Jenkins, et al. "The Glycemic Response to Carbohydrate Foods." Lancet 2 (1984), 388. © by The Lancet Ltd., 1984.

and steamed carrots helps you feel and function better than, for example, oatmeal and toast. As a mainstay of the initial treatment, many physicians will recommend drinking a protein powder mixed with liquid several times a day to ensure adequate protein ingestion. This can be especially useful and convenient as a between-meals boost or a light meal. Having enough protein is especially important for vegetarians.

In addition to a protein deficiency, strict vegetarians often suffer from a vitamin B-12 deficiency, which may be improved dramatically within one to two days after the administration of a B-12 injection. The resultant increase in energy, as well as the accompanying emotional transformation, can be a diagnostic sign that your diet is deficient and/or your absorptive capacity impaired.

4. Although excessive fat is a well-known hazard, you must consume at least enough fat calories to keep your metabolism functioning properly. If your diet has been excessively low in fat, include a modest amount of fat-containing foods, such as fish, chicken, perhaps a small amount of extra-lean beef, or some nut butters. Or, if milk products have not previously been a major component of your diet, and if you have no milk allergies, add some cheese.

You can also add a small amount of unrefined oil, such as flax, sesame, olive, or high-oleic sunflower, or a small amount of butter to grains, legumes, and vegetables. The fats help slow the release of sugar into the bloodstream, making meals "last" longer. The essential fatty acids can also help strengthen the adrenal glands (see Chapter Three for a discussion of fats and oils).

5. Minimize the use of sugar (white, brown, or raw) and the many foods containing hidden sugar. If you simply must have a sweet upon occasion, be sure not to eat it on an empty stomach. Having some food in your stomach can slow down a potentially abrupt rise in blood sugar levels and, therefore, minimize a subsequent hypoglycemic reaction. Of course, the less you eat of the sweet, the milder the potential adverse reaction.

Although a whole-grain sweet, such as a cookie or cake made with whole wheat flour rather than white flour, can potentially trigger just as significant a hypoglycemic reaction as a sweet made with white flour, the whole-grain snack is the wiser choice. If you're addicted to sugar or feel you need a lot of support to break the habit, consider the suggestions given in Chapter Three. You may find, however, that with the vitamin and mineral supplement program subsequently outlined, you'll begin to get the upper hand on sugar.

6. Minimize the use of refined carbohydrates, such as white bread, white rolls, white noodles, white crackers, white rice, and any other refined grains or flours. Enriched or unbleached flour does not substitute for the whole-grain products, which are closest to what nature provides. Whole grains, by virtue of their inherent fiber, can slow down the entry of sugar into your bloodstream, promote regular bowel function, and give you a feeling of satiety with fewer calories. Whole grains are also very rich in vitamins and minerals. If you are not allergic to wheat, use whole wheat bread, noodles, crackers, and rolls. Also, use whole wheat flour in your pancake and cookie batters. As alternatives to wheat, try brown rice, rye, oats, millet, buckwheat, barley, cornmeal, quinoa, amaranth, spelt, kamut, and teff.

7. Minimize the use of dried fruits. These are not good snacks for hypoglycemics (unless needed in an emergency), as they represent extremely concentrated forms of fruit sugar. Although fruit sugar (fructose) does not directly cause as rapid a rise in blood sugar as table sugar (sucrose), it gets converted to glucose, which does

cause such a response. Reconstituting dried fruits is an acceptable alternative. Try cooking a small quantity with whole-grain cereals or soaking them and using them with the soaking water as sweeteners for any baked dishes or, in moderation, in blender drinks. In these forms they serve as more gentle sweeteners.

8. Minimize the use of fruit juices. Fruit juice is actually a refined food originating from the whole fruit, with the fiber processed out. This means that the fruit sugar enters the bloodstream rapidly. It's a mistake for hypoglycemics to make a habit of drinking fruit juice regularly. Once a day with breakfast, for example, may be acceptable if the hypoglycemic condition is not severe. If you must drink fruit juice, particularly if you are making a transition from a sugared soft drink addiction, dilute it with water—perhaps 50 percent juice and 50 percent water—to lessen the concentration of sugar. Learn to use cooled herbal teas as beverages. Try a combination of lemon grass, licorice root, and peppermint, for example, or Celestial Seasonings Lemon Zinger. If necessary, add a very small amount of apple juice to the tea. Vegetable juices are even better for hypoglycemic individuals, as they generally contain much less sugar. One exception, however, is carrot juice. It is quite high in sugar (see Chapter Five) and should be diluted with green juice.

9. Be careful not to overeat fresh fruit, for the reasons we've just discussed. Although fresh fruit is not as sweet as dried fruit or fruit juice, too much can trigger hypoglycemic reactions in sensitive individuals. Initially, one piece of fruit a day may be all you can tolerate, although in more severe cases even less may be advisable. As your hypoglycemic condition improves, you can add back more fruit. If you're trying to kick a candy bar or sugar habit, fresh fruit is a splendid alternative initially whenever you feel like something sweet. Eventually, and if necessary, you'll be able to get by with less fruit until your condition stabilizes.

10. Minimize the use of caffeine in any form— coffee, soft drinks, chocolate, nonherbal teas, and even over-the-counter medications such as pain and diet pills. Caffeine can cause abrupt elevations in blood sugar levels and a subsequent abrupt fall, and in this way can overtax the adrenals. Drink herbal teas and coffee substitutes made from roasted grain, rather than decaffeinated tea or coffee products.

11. Minimize the use of alcohol. Alcohol can biochemically stress the pancreas and adrenal glands in much the same way sugar does. Although a little alcohol consumption may not be so terrible for one's overall health (provided alcohol addiction and liver disease are not concerns), an initial abstention or at least restriction may contribute to a quicker recovery from hypoglycemia. As your blood sugar condition stabilizes, you may be able to introduce a little more alcohol, if desired.

However, watch carefully to see how this affects you. You may be surprised to find that your nightly "harmless" glass of wine with dinner upsets your metabolism to an unacceptable degree.

12. Vitamins and other supplements can greatly enhance recovery from hypoglycemia and other related disorders.

The right supplements in optimal amounts will usually improve one's state of health much more quickly than dietary and lifestyle measures alone. Within ten to fourteen days on the appropriate supplements and dietary and lifestyle regimen, most people will experience enough improvement to know they're on the right track.

A Supplement Program for Treating Hypoglycemia

The following supplement program should accelerate your recovery and return to well-being:

- Chromium, an essential mineral, can be taken in tablet, capsule, or liquid form initially in a dose of 200 to 300 micrograms three times a day (best fifteen or more minutes before meals, although with or after meals is acceptable). Chromium, glucose tolerance factor (GTF), helps the body stabilize blood sugar levels whether they are too high or too low. Because of this, it is instrumental in correcting a biochemical imbalance that causes sugar craving, and is invaluable in helping to beat the sugar habit. The trivalent form of chromium, as well as the polynicotinate and Chromate™ forms, have proven very effective. It's best to find a yeast-free form, unless you know you have no allergies to yeast. Eventually, 200 micrograms a day, the amount found in a high-potency multiple vitamin-mineral, may suffice.

- Biotin, approximately 1,000 micrograms three times daily with meals, will enhance glucose utilization, generally improve hypoglycemia symptoms, as well as tend to reduce sugar craving. Biotin is largely synthesized by friendly intestinal bacteria, and if you have used antibiotics (which kill these bacteria), this vitamin is particularly important to use. Once your condition has stabilized, 300 micrograms daily should suffice.

- A supplement of B-complex vitamins, approximately 25 to 50 milligrams three times a day, is usually best with meals. As discussed earlier, B-complex vitamins improve carbohydrate metabolism, adrenal function, and stressed-out nerves. They also ease withdrawal symptoms in cases of sugar and caffeine addiction. In addition, part of the B-complex family aids liver metabolism, another important component in stabilizing blood sugar levels. I would advise you to begin with a yeast-free B-complex supplement to avoid unnecessary reactions and treatment complications should you happen to be allergic. A high-potency yeast-free multiple vitamin/mineral containing the doses recommended above would be equally suitable. After several months or more of such high doses, lower the amount to 25 milligrams one or two times a day for a good maintenance level.

- Extra vitamin B-5 (pantothenic acid or the most preferable form, calcium pantothenate) can work as another adrenal enhancer. Additional amounts may be helpful for some people, particularly if chronic fatigue and characteristic hypoglycemic symptoms have not responded appropriately to the B-complex dose within a period of one month. Take up to 500 milligrams one to three times a day with meals for an extra boost for one to three months or more, then reduce gradually. Eventually you should be able to do without this extra B-5 and get along with what is in your B-complex or high potency multiple.

- Extra vitamin B-3 (niacinamide) can be particularly helpful for depression and anxiety associated with hypoglycemia and stress. It acts like Valium or Librium in the brain without producing the dulling side effects or addictive potential of these two drugs. A dose of 500 to 1,000 milligrams three times a day, usually with meals, may be required, although most individuals get the desired effect at 500 to 1,000 milligrams morning and evening.

  High doses (2,000 to 3,000 milligrams) daily for more than two months may cause a temporary, minor, and reversible inflammation of the liver in a very small percentage of people, and physician monitoring of such high doses is advised.

  As with vitamin B-5, you should be able to do without this extra B-3 eventually and maintain with what is in your B-complex or high-potency multiple. Niacin is another form of vitamin B-3 and will have a similar antianxiety effect. However, it will usually cause a very pronounced flush within minutes after ingestion and, depending on what form you choose, may pose more of a liver risk than niacinamide (see Chapter Six).

- Vitamin C, in doses up to 1,000 milligrams three times a day (with or without meals), can work as an adrenal enhancer and a stimulant to liver metabolism, among other functions. Too much vitamin C, however, causes diarrhea; if this occurs, reduce the dose.

- Brewer's yeast, even if it does not contain chromium, is usually beneficial for its other components—B-complex vitamins, minerals, and amino acids (see Chapter Five). If you are not taking extra chromium, be sure to find a yeast supplement that has chromium-GTF. Take one or two tablespoons once or twice a day in vegetable juice or in blender drinks, or sprinkled on popcorn or other foods. Brewer's yeast is particularly useful as an in-between meal snack to boost blood sugar. Start with ½ teaspoon a day to prevent gas and digestive upset, and gradually build up the dose. **Note:** Individuals who are allergic to yeast may feel worse on this supplement and should avoid it. (See Chapter Twelve.)

- Calcium and magnesium can also help the nervous system, although deficiencies of these minerals do not have a direct effect on hypoglycemia, as do chromium and the B vitamins. Take up to 1,000 milligrams of calcium and 500 milligrams of magnesium a day (usually found together in the same tablet, liquid, or powder). The citrate, malate, and ascorbate forms are well absorbed (see Chapter Six). In cases of insomnia, be sure to use at least half or even all of this dose at bedtime. Up to 500 milligrams of calcium can be found in some high-potency multiple vitamin/mineral formulations. **Note:** Too much calcium can cause constipation, while too much magnesium can cause diarrhea.

- Amino acids can, in certain specific applications, be beneficial in the treatment of hypoglycemia.

  —Glutamine, for example, can be taken to reduce sugar craving if chromium, biotin, and B-complex do not seem effective enough. Take 500 to 1,000 milligrams two or three times a day. Glutamine can also decrease alcohol craving, another characteristic useful in stabilizing blood sugar. This amino acid is best taken at least 1½ hours before or after any protein foods, or on an empty stomach. Entry into the brain is enhanced if amino acids are taken with some carbohydrates (crackers or very diluted fruit juice).

  —If depression and insomnia, with their resultant biochemical and emotional effects, are two of your hypoglycemic symptoms, or if these have developed as a result of a change in your diet, try 5-hydroxy tryptophan, a derivative of tryptophan. Take 100 to 400 milligrams at bedtime (see page 139).

  —Tyrosine may also be useful for depression. Take 500 to 1,000 milligrams first thing in the morning (see page 139).

These three amino acids can have a dramatic effect. I do not recommend prolonged use without the care and supervision of a qualified health professional.

A general protein powder, containing a broad spectrum of amino acids, can be used as a snack or light meal to provide a lift. Mix with water or diluted juice, or in blender drinks. Choose one that has minimal sweetener.

- Chapter Nine offers several supplements and procedures designed to help the liver more directly in its role of stabilizing blood sugar levels. If you have symptoms suggestive of a sluggish or toxic liver, consider the pertinent information presented there.

From a health food store or nutritionally oriented health care practitioner, you may be able to obtain a vitamin/mineral supplement formulated for the particular needs of individuals with hypoglycemia. Such a supplement would simplify this treatment program by providing many or most of the above-recommended nutrients, and may be the only one you will need. I often suggest Glucobalance (Probiologic, Bellevue, Washington), which contains 1,000 micrograms of chromium and 3,000 micrograms of biotin.

If you are not able to find such a specialized supplement, you could still manage very easily with a B-complex of the above-recommended dosage or a high-potency multiple vitamin/mineral containing the previously recommended doses of B-complex, along with separate biotin, chromium, and vitamin C supplements. I suggest starting out simply. Then, if necessary, add extra items appropriate to your needs and symptoms one at a time. Remember, however, that in the beginning you should place equal emphasis on diet and supplements.

13. Regular exercise helps immensely to raise one's stress tolerance level. Its physiological effects benefit nearly every organ and biological system in the body. Exercise can help lower a diabetic's insulin requirements and help stabilize the metabolism of a hypoglycemic individual so that the low blood sugar reactions become less severe and less frequent. It can also help diminish cravings and addictions. Exercise, with its effects on the adrenal glands, central nervous system, and carbohydrate and fat metabolism, will serve you well in your program to recover from hypoglycemia. But, as in any endeavor, overdoing it will work against you. Find the appropriate level of intensity, duration, and frequency for you.

14. Stress management may be another vital addition to recovery from hypoglycemia (see Chapter Fifteen).

As time goes by and symptoms diminish, your supplement program should assume less importance. Dietary and lifestyle measures will, of course, remain the primary thrust of blood sugar maintenance. If implemented with appropriate stress management and regular exercise, hypoglycemia should no longer be a pressing concern.

MASQUERADING OR AGGRAVATING CONDITIONS

If you find that you continually need to take high doses of many supplements and have to watch your diet intensively, if you have to eat every few hours in order to minimize hypoglycemic symptoms, or if your good efforts seem to have little or no effect, it may be that other conditions are masquerading (producing identical symptoms as) or aggravating hypoglycemia. These include food allergy/intolerance, chemical hypersensitivity, inappropriate vegetarianism/protein inadequacy, hypothyroidism, an overgrowth of yeast (Candida albicans), and depleted adrenal reserve. It is quite common for an individual to have both hypoglycemia and one or more of these other conditions.

Food Allergy/Intolerance, Chemical Hypersensitivity, and Hypoglycemia

Brain swelling can occur from mechanisms unrelated to blood sugar or insulin levels or solute (particle) concentrations. For example, just as an allergy can cause a rash—an inflammation and swelling of the skin—it can also cause an inflammation and swelling in the brain. This produces symptoms identical to those of hypoglycemia: headaches, fatigue, depression, irritability, foggy thinking, and so on. Commonly eaten foods used repetitively every day or nearly every day such as wheat, milk, eggs, corn, beef, peanuts, and orange juice are often the culprits (see Chapter Thirteen).

Chemicals in our environment, both indoor and outdoor, can also produce hypersensitivity reactions, brain swelling, and hypoglycemic symptoms. Some of these chemicals include auto exhaust, vapors, and combustion products from gas stoves and gas and oil heat, cigarette smoke, cleaning fluids, some perfumes, copy machine fumes, and formaldehyde from particleboard and other sources (see Chapter Fourteen).

According to the bioecologic theory of allergy and maladaptation outlined by William Philpott, M.D., and Dwight Kalita, Ph.D., in *Victory Over Diabetes*, "hypoglycemia" may represent the pancreatic overstimulation of a process that can result eventually in the phase of exhaustion or inhibition of the pancreas known as diabetes mellitus. Sugar is not the only substance that can trigger an overstimulation of the pancreas; any food or chemical to which you are allergic can tax the body's system in this manner.

Vegetarianism, Protein Adequacy/Digestion, and Hypoglycemia

In my practice, I have observed many individuals who have changed to a vegetarian diet, and felt remarkably better, only to develop a lack of physical and mental stamina along with many hypoglycemic symptoms over time. Some vegetarians may experience hypoglycemic symptoms as a result of a subclinical protein deficiency. With marginal protein intake, it would require less than excessive amounts of sugar, honey, or even fruit to trigger hypoglycemia. Many protein-deficient in-

DIETARY RECOMMENDATIONS TO HELP STABILIZE BLOOD SUGAR

1. Eat breakfast, lunch, and dinner, as well as small snacks between meals. Do not miss meals. Frequent small meals and snacks initially may be most helpful. Regular snacking between meals is recommended only until your condition stabilizes.

2. Have cooked grain daily (if tolerated), such as millet, buckwheat, brown rice, oats, whole-grain bread or whole-grain pasta, etc. Have as cereals, side dishes, casseroles, in soups, etc.

3. Have legumes regularly as soups, casseroles, dips, side dishes: lentils, split peas, navy, pinto, kidney, soy, aduki, black, or garbanzo beans, etc.

4. Have adequate protein daily. At least once and sometimes twice a day at first have fish, poultry, other flesh foods, and eggs. If you are vegetarian, you must ensure adequate protein intake. (To increase protein content of salads, add tofu, almonds, toasted sesame seeds, cooked beans, hard-boiled egg, or cheese.)

5. Because each individual has unique requirements, experiment with varying amounts of protein and at different times of the day to see how you best feel and function. Some people may feel better with a whole-grain cereal for breakfast, for example, while others may feel better having a breakfast of a higher protein and lower carbohydrate content, such as turkey and steamed carrots.

6. Have an abundance of vegetables in salads, with dips, in soups, casseroles, etc. Have vegetables both raw and steamed.

7. Occasionally add a little cold-pressed unrefined oil or butter to grain dishes, legumes, and vegetables. This will enable the meal to stay with you longer and slow the rate of sugar entering the bloodstream.

8. Snacks:

   - unsalted almonds, filberts, sunflower or pumpkin seeds, walnuts, etc.

   - almond or sesame milk or other blender drink (see Chapter Five).

   - rice ball (recipe in Chapter Five).

   - occasional glass of milk or piece of cheese (if not milk allergic).

   - 1 or 2 tablespoons of protein powder in vegetable juice, water, or very diluted fruit juice; especially useful if you want to minimize calories.

   - raw vegetables alone or with a dip (see recipes in Chapter Five).

   - primary or true brewer's yeast (if not allergic): 1 or 2 tablespoons mixed in vegetable juice, water, or diluted fruit juice. Start with ¼ to ½ teaspoon and gradually over one week work up to one or two tablespoons.

   - vegetable juices; if you use carrot juice, dilute it with other vegetable or green juice because it is very sweet.

   - Jerusalem artichoke and avocados are of specific benefit.

9. Vitamin B complex (approximately 25 milligrams), chromium (250 to 300 micrograms), biotin (1,000 micrograms), and vitamin C (500 to 1,000 milligrams) three times a day with meals can

DIETARY RECOMMENDATIONS TO HELP STABILIZE BLOOD SUGAR

be very helpful in speeding recovery. These can sometimes be found combined together in a specialized multiple vitamin/mineral formula. Nutrients may need to be tailored according to individual needs and medical history. Glutamine (500 milligrams) three times a day away from any protein meals is additionally useful if sugar craving persists.

10. Regular exercise helps stabilize carbohydrate metabolism.

11. Learn to manage stress more successfully and consistently, which may require reducing stress and examining lifestyle and priorities.

12. Minimize sugar and anything containing sugar—white, brown or raw. Sugar as dextrose, sucrose, glucose, maltose, corn sweetener, and corn syrup is listed on bottled salad dressings, ketchup, boxed cereals, canned fruit, etc. Find sugar-free alternatives. Avoid obvious sources like chocolate, ice cream, cookies, candy, soda, and cake.

13. Minimize honey and all other natural sweets. If you need to use a little honey, make sure it's raw. In baking, sweeten with soaked dried fruit (raisins and dates) and the soaking water for some of the sweetener; a little molasses or honey, too, if necessary. As the hypoglycemic condition improves, more natural sweets can gradually be allowed, but still in moderation.

14. Minimize coffee, black teas, soft drinks (including diet) and other caffeine-containing substances.

15. Minimize white flour, white rice (enriched or unbleached), enriched flour or white pasta, and any refined grains. Have mostly whole wheat or whole-grain flour products. Whole-grain dishes (with brown rice, millet, buckwheat, etc.) as opposed to wheat flour products, such as bread and noodles, produce a more stable effect on blood sugar levels. Legumes are even more stabilizing.

16. Minimize fruit juices. If you must have fruit juice, dilute it with water. Try lemon grass iced tea, vegetable juice, diluted carrot juice, lemon water, herbal tea, or spring water.

17. Do not overeat fruit—have only occasionally at first, and especially minimize raisins, dates, and other dried fruit eaten as snacks. You can add a small amount of dried fruit to whole-grain cereals (while cooking) to sweeten them.

18. Minimize the use of alcohol.

19. Food allergy is sometimes the cause of hypoglycemia, and the allergic food may not necessarily be sugar or refined carbohydrates. Also, rule out hypothyroidism, deficiencies of pancreatic enzymes and/or hydrochloric acid, adrenal insufficiency, yeast overgrowth, and nutrient deficiencies.

dividuals feel remarkably better in a short time when they begin eating animal protein again.

This seeming failure of some vegetarians may result from an insufficient knowledge of the vegetarian principles of protein adequacy. However, inadequate protein digestion from hydrochloric acid and pancreatic insuffi-

ciencies might also be the culprit (see Chapter Seven). Alternatively, an individual may have a metabolism that is not suited to strict vegetarianism over a prolonged period of time, particularly if he or she has type O blood (see Chapter Three). Heredity may play a role in one's suitability for a strict vegetarian diet and one's metabolic need for vegetable or animal protein. Then again, many hypoglycemic vegetarians who eat a limited number of foods in an extremely repetitive fashion—foods such as soybeans, tofu, brown rice, cheese, yogurt, and eggs— turn out instead to have one or more food allergies.

Hypothyroidism, Yeast Overgrowth, and Hypoglycemia

Both yeast overgrowth *(Candida albicans)* and hypothyroidism can produce symptoms very similar to hypoglycemia. In fact, hypothyroidism can predispose you to hypoglycemia. These conditions, of course, have their own unique symptoms as well. See Chapters Twelve and Seventeen, "Yeast Overgrowth," and "Hypothyroidism," respectively, for complete discussions.

Depleted Adrenal Reserve

You will recall that the adrenal glands can help rescue low blood sugar. In Larry's case, they can be weakened by sugar abuse and other demanding stresses. Many individuals can adequately reverse a mildly weakened adrenal state by the treatment recommendations for hypoglycemia outlined in this chapter. However, extreme fatigue, weakness, unremitting hypoglycemic symptoms, and depression not improved by conventional nutritional or medical measures may reflect a depleted adrenal reserve (see Chapter Eleven).

REVERSING HYPOGLYCEMIA

Hypoglycemia is a reversible condition. It is usually a symptom of excess refined carbohydrates in the diet, and/or insufficient complex carbohydrates, protein, and/or specific vitamins and minerals. Caffeine, alcohol, and too much or poorly managed stress are also significant contributing factors. A careful review of your symptoms can help you pinpoint this condition, but laboratory testing may be needed. A commonsense diet and improvements in your lifestyle will usually reverse your symptoms. If these measures are unsuccessful, other conditions may be causing your hypoglycemic symptoms. Check for food allergy, pancreatic insufficiency, hydrochloric acid insufficiency, a malabsorption syndrome, hypothyroidism, and/or adrenal insufficiency (see Chapter Eleven). Hypoglycemia is not something you should have to live with; the condition is usually treatable, and your efforts to restore balance and regain health and vitality should prove worthwhile.

SUGGESTED READING

Airola, Paavo, N.D. *Hypoglycemia: A Better Approach.* Phoenix: Health Plus, 1977.

Barnes, B., and Barnes, C.W. *Hope for Hypoglycemia: It's Not in Your Mind, It's Your Liver.* Fort Collins, CO: Robinson Press, 1989.

Cheraskin, E., and Ringsdorf, W.M., with Brecher, A. *Psychodietetics: Food as the Key to Emotional Health.* New York: Stein and Day, 1974.

Fredericks, C., and Goodman, H. *Low Blood Sugar and You.* New York: Constellation International, 1969.

Philpott, William, M.D., and Kalita, Dwight, Ph.D. *Victory Over Diabetes.* Keats, 1983.

Tintera, J.W., M.D. "Endocrinologic Approach to the Etiology and Treatment of Hypoglycemia," in *Hypoadrenocorticism.* Mount Vernon, NY: Adrenal Metabolic Research Society of the Hypoglycemia Foundation, 1974, pp. 115–134.

Wright, Jonathan, V., M.D. *Dr. Wright's Book of Nutritional Therapy.* Emmaus, PA: Rodale Press, 1979, pp. 197–208.

ADRENAL EXHAUSTION

As our body's primary shock absorber, the adrenal glands determine our response to stress. In this chapter, we will discuss adrenal function and review the critical roles the adrenals perform to maintain and safeguard our health. We will list the causes, signs, and symptoms of adrenal exhaustion, cover medical testing, and finally present a program for adrenal restoration. Let's begin with the case history of Barbara, one of my patients.

BARBARA

The first thing Barbara said as she sat down in my office was, "I am totally exhausted." A thirty-eight-year-old grade school teacher, she was barely able to meet the demands of her work. Barbara was nearly desperate in her plea for help. She told me that by the end of each school day, her muscles and joints ached, her throat hurt, and she would develop a low-grade fever. She couldn't even imagine having the strength to prepare dinner for her family, or keep house. Fortunately, her husband did all the domestic activities. The elder of their two children pitched in as well.

When Barbara was able to get nine hours of sleep, she would arise in the morning with the feeling that if she pushed herself hard enough, she could manage through the day. But she felt hardly any joy, spontaneity, or creativity—qualities she considered essential to teach and to parent. For this reason especially, she was depressed, for she was falling far short of her expectations. But she was depressed all the time anyway, she said, even if she'd had a rare good day at school and everything was going well in her family.

If anything out of the ordinary happened—like having a cookie, having a pleasant dinner with friends, staying up past 10:00 P.M., shopping for groceries, or making love with her husband—then her usual end-of-the-day symptoms would be even worse. She usually needed several days or more to recover. If she drank milk or orange juice, she would suffer from migraine headaches—sometimes she'd get them regardless. Wheat would drastically increase her fatigue, and she would get ill from certain perfumes as well as from automobile exhausts.

As a result of these symptoms, Barbara attempted to control each day. She had absolutely no reserves to deal with unforeseen events. She said she couldn't continue on this way. If she didn't get some relief soon, she was going to have to take a medical leave of absence from her work.

I asked Barbara when she last felt well. She replied that she'd been functioning fairly normally until eighteen months before, when she'd been diagnosed with mononucleosis. She never seemed to recover fully from the mono, she continued, and it was in the following months that her current symptom picture began to develop. After a year of not getting any better, she was treated with an antidepressant. This medication had given her a little relief, but the overall effect was not substantial.

Barbara had been on the antidepressant for several months when I saw her the first time. After hearing her out, I questioned her about her earlier history. Her second child had been born nine years before her arrival in my office, a colicky and finicky baby who kept Barbara up many nighttime hours with her crying over an eighteen-month period. To make matters worse, when her son was just over a year old she'd been in a motor vehicle accident and suffered a whiplash injury to her neck that required months of physical therapy. Three

THE ADRENALS: STRESS AND SYMPTOMS

ADRENAL STRESSORS*

Trigger emotions
  Anger
  Fear
  Worry/anxiety
  Guilt
Depression
Overwork (physical or mental strain)
Late hours/insufficient sleep
Chronic, severe, or prolonged infections
Surgery
Trauma/injury

Excessive exercise
Temperature extremes
Toxic exposure
Chronic inflammation
Chronic pain
Chronic illness
Chronic/Severe allergies
Light cycle disruption (awake at night, asleep during the day. This is a problem for those who work at night, especially the midnight to 8:00 A.M. shift)

SYMPTOMS ASSOCIATED WITH AND CONSEQUENCES OF ADRENAL DYSFUNCTION**

Excessive fatigue
Weakness
Nervousness/irritability
Mental depression
Apprehensions
Inability to concentrate
Moments of confusion
Poor memory
Feelings of frustration
Light-headedness
Dizziness that occurs upon standing
Low blood pressure
Insomnia
Premenstrual tension
Craving for sweets
Headaches
Alcohol intolerance
Sternomastoid/Trapezius pain and spasms
  (muscles in area of upper back/neck/
  shoulders)

Hypoglycemia
Excessive hunger
Epigastric discomfort
Dyspepsia (indigestion)
Alternate diarrhea and constipation
Palpitation (heart fluttering)
Poor resistance to infections
Food and/or inhalant allergies
Dry and thin skin
Scanty perspiration
Tenderness in adrenal area
Low body temperature
Unexplained hair loss
Difficulty building muscle
Difficulty gaining weight
Tendency to inflammation
Increased susceptibility to cancer
Increased susceptibility to osteoporosis
Increased susceptibility to autoimmune hepatitis and to other autoimmune diseases

*Adapted from: E. Ilyia, The New Definition of Stress Evaluation: Adrenal Stress Index (Monograph). (Kent, WA: Diagnos-Techs, Inc., 1991), 2–4.
**Adapted from: J.W. Tintera, "The Hypoadrenocortical State and Its Management." New York Journal of Medicine July 1, 1955 vol. 55, No. 13, reprinted in J.W. Tintera. Hypoadrenalcorticism (Mount Vernon, N.Y.: Adrenal Metabolic Research Society of the Hypoglycemia Foundation), 3.

years later, when it seemed that life was finally beginning to settle down to normal, a lengthy and nasty legal battle was sprung upon them involving her husband's ex-wife. These difficulties were not yet over when Barbara suffered a herniated disk in her lower back, which once again necessitated months of physical therapy.

When the Battery Runs Down

Everyone encounters stress in their lives. However, when the intensity and chronicity of stress surpasses the level beyond which an individual can cope, something's going to break down. If you race a horse too frequently, if you keep running and whipping her when she's tired, very soon she won't be able to perform at all. If you keep your headlights on all night and run down your battery, the only way to get your car going is by a jump start. But if your battery is too depleted, even a jump start won't do the job.

It wasn't surprising, with years of continual stress—pregnancy and lactation, sleep deprivation, injuries, illness, overwork, emotional anguish, and anxiety—that Barbara lost her strength and her health. The events of her life had forced her to keep performing beyond her limits. She never seemed to get enough of a break to rest and build up her strength.

THE ADRENALS: OUR BODY'S BUFFER ZONE

It is our adrenal glands that buffer stress and enable us to stand up to life's onslaughts. These glands give us the capacity to perform and to adapt flexibly to the demands of every day. It is also the adrenals that enable us to go beyond our usual limits of endurance when needed and help us to recover in a reasonable amount of time. But plainly, Barbara had little capacity left to perform, adapt, or recover. It was my strong suspicion that she was suffering from adrenal exhaustion. I wasn't the first physician who suspected a problem with her adrenal glands. Barbara had numerous symptoms that fit the adrenal depletion picture in addition to nearly nine years of continuous stresses of varying magnitude.

Check the list of Adrenal Stressors on page 198 to see how your symptoms and stress history stack up. (Also use the Holmes/Rahe Social Readjustment Rating Scale, page 290, to quantify your stress points.)

THE FUNCTION OF THE ADRENALS

The adrenal glands, each approximately the size of your thumb, sit on top of the kidneys (their position is on each side of the spine approximately at the level of the lower ribs). The adrenal cortex is central to this discussion. It is the part of the gland that synthesizes a number of hormones from cholesterol, the two very important ones being cortisol and DHEA (dehydroepiandrosterone). The adrenal medulla is the part of the gland that secretes adrenaline. Cortisol is akin to the drug cortisone (prednisone, prednisolone, etc.), and although cortisone has developed an unfavorable reputation for its well-known adverse side effects, our well-being depends on the adrenals' ability to produce adequate amounts of cortisol. DHEA is also essential. See the boxes on pages 200 and 201.

Testing Barbara's Adrenals

One of Barbara's previous physicians had tested her adrenal function with a blood cortisol level. The sample was drawn at 8:00 A.M., which is when the level should be at its highest of the day. It was a "low normal."

Her physician subsequently performed an ACTH (adrenocorticotropin) stimulation test. ACTH is the pituitary gland hormone that stimulates and controls functioning of the adrenal cortex. The pituitary gland is located in the brain and synthesizes several hormones, each controlling one of the body's many endocrine glands. Injecting ACTH should nearly double the blood cortisol level within an hour in an individual with normal adrenal function. Barbara's adrenal function was therefore declared "normal," because her cortisol level doubled.

The problem with the ACTH stimulation test is that it doesn't really measure the usual day-to-day functional capacity of the adrenals. By this, I mean the effect the adrenals have on an individual's everyday energy, stamina, mood, clarity of thought, immune function/resistance, and circulation. An injection of ACTH provides an abnormally high and very powerful adrenal stimulation, much like the pituitary might produce under the most extreme levels of fear or anxiety, such as running for your life.

This means the ACTH stimulation test will therefore almost always be able to squeeze the double-normal levels out of even very tired adrenals. The adrenal cortex would need to be nearly nonfunctioning, as in Addison's disease, to fail this test and gain adequate attention from most physicians. This test recognizes only normal function or no function, nothing in between. It is clearly not sensitive enough to recognize the spectrum of diminishing adrenal function, which is where Barbara's and many other individuals' adrenal function lies. Thus it is unable to explain why they are not well.

Another problem with standard blood cortisol testing is its lack of specificity for "free" cortisol as opposed to protein-bound cortisol. It is only the free, unbound fraction that is biologically active and is therefore the only fraction that accurately reflects adrenal status. The standard blood cortisol test measures both bound and

FUNCTIONS OF CORTISOL[1]

- Mobilizes and increases amino acids, the building blocks of protein, in the blood and liver.

- Stimulates the liver to convert amino acids to glucose, a primary fuel for energy production.

- Stimulates increased glycogen in the liver. Glycogen is a storage form of glucose.

- Mobilizes and increases fatty acids in the blood (from fat cells) to be used as fuel for energy production.

- Counters inflammation and allergies.

- Prevents the loss of sodium in urine and thus helps maintain blood volume and blood pressure.

- Maintains resistance to stress (infections, physical trauma, temperature extremes, emotional trauma, etc.).

- Maintains personality and emotional stability.

However, in excess, cortisol

- Diminishes glucose utilization by the cell and increases blood sugar levels.

- Decreases protein synthesis.

- Increases protein breakdown, which can lead to muscle wasting and osteoporosis.

- Causes shrinking of lymphatic tissue, diminishes lymphocyte numbers and functions, and lessens secretory antibody production. This immune system suppression may lead to increased susceptibility to allergies, infections, and cancer.

---

unbound cortisol. If the result is "low," you can believe it; if it is "normal," it can mislead you into thinking the adrenals are fine when in fact they may be functioning far below normal.

In my experience, measuring free cortisol and DHEA levels in saliva has proven to be the most dependable method of assessing adrenal function.[2] This test has enabled me to explain why so many of my patients have been unwell for so long—the "walking dead," as many of them refer to themselves. And it has given me a base line from which to help these individuals return to the "living" and rediscover their well-being.

I utilize the Adrenal Stress Index Test,[3] which measures free cortisol at four specific times during a day (8:00 A.M., noon, 4:00 P.M., and midnight) and DHEA/DHEA sulphate at the noon and 4:00 P.M. collections. Saliva samples are collected at these times during an individual's normal day—during real-life conditions—without the added stress of being in a doctor's office or

laboratory. On the other hand, having blood drawn has been shown to cause cortisol elevations all by itself, and thus interferes with accurate adrenal assessment.

Comparing these four samples to the norm and looking at the cortisol/DHEA ratio can reveal both overstimulated and depleted adrenal states.[4] Such information can pinpoint the most effective treatment recommendations, whether diet/nutritional therapy, herbal medicines, stress management, and/or pharmaceutical hormones.

Under stress, healthy adrenals will respond by increasing the output of both cortisol and DHEA to higher than normal levels. Such temporary adaptive elevations enable an individual to maintain homeostasis and preserve health in the face of stress. However, if stress becomes chronic, eventually the adrenals can no longer maintain the production of extra DHEA. With continued elevated levels of cortisol and falling DHEA levels, an elevated cortisol-to-DHEA ratio ensues. This signifies an initial stage of adrenal exhaustion and has potentially devastating effects on health (see Figure 11–1). These include:

- Diminished immune function[5] through:
  —Decreased levels of secretory IgA (mucosal antibodies)
  —Increased absorption of antigens (foreign substances)
  —Decreased natural killer cell activity
  —Decreased levels of interleukin 2
  —Decreased T lymphocyte counts leading to increased susceptibility to infections, allergies, autoimmune disease, and cancer
- Reduced REM (rapid eye movement) sleep and therefore sleep that is not restful or restorative[6]
- A catabolic state where tissue breakdown exceeds tissue repair/building, which leads to muscle wasting, weight loss, and bone loss/osteoporosis[7]
- Greater percentage of body fat and smaller percentage of muscle mass;[8] fat accumulation around the waist
- Diminished insulin sensitivity and therefore reduced glucose utilization at the cell level leading to elevated blood sugar levels and possibly diabetes[9]
- Salt and water retention, leading to edema
- Elevated blood fat levels, leading to atherosclerosis[10]

People whose test results show a significant cortisol elevation at midnight commonly experience an endogenous, or biochemically induced depression in contrast to one produced by circumstances.[11] It also sometimes correlates with insomnia. Figure 11–2 shows the results of Barbara's Adrenal Stress Index test.

Barbara's 8:00 A.M. cortisol level should be the highest of the day (between 13 and 23 nanomolars), giving her a strong start and enabling her to meet the day's demands. What is most striking here is the significantly low cortisol level of 4 at 8:00 A.M. She also experienced a low level of 2 at 4:00 P.M. and a borderline low of 4 at noon. Considering Barbara's history—especially her daily struggle to get out of bed, even with more than eight hours of sleep—and the need she experienced to push herself all day long, her uniformly low cortisol levels come as no surprise. Over time, continued stress and lack of effective intervention usually first results in the abnormally elevated cortisol/deficient DHEA state, and later in Barbara's more deteriorated state of both cortisol and DHEA depletion.

To help restore Barbara's depleted adrenal glands, I recommended most of the measures on pages 203–205. These make up the the bulk of my adrenal restoration program.

FUNCTIONS OF DHEA

- Functions as an androgen, a male hormone, with anabolic activity (*anabolic* refers to building or synthesis of tissues).

- A precursor that is converted to testosterone, a male anabolic hormone.

- A precursor to estrogen, a female anabolic hormone.[12]

- Reverses immune suppression caused by excess cortisol levels,[13] and therefore improves resistance against viruses, bacteria, *Candida albicans*, parasites, allergies, and cancer.

- Stimulates bone deposition and remodeling, which prevents osteoporosis.[14]

- Improves cardiovascular status by lowering total and LDL ("bad") cholesterol levels[15] and lessens the incidence of heart attack.[16]

- Increases muscle mass, decreases percentage of body fat.[17]

- Reverses many of the unfavorable effects of excess cortisol and therefore creates an improvement in energy/vitality, sleep, premenstrual symptoms, and mental clarity, as well as quicker recovery from any kind of acute stress (insufficient sleep, excessive exercise, mental strain, etc.).

Figure 11–1. The Adrenal Stress Index Test

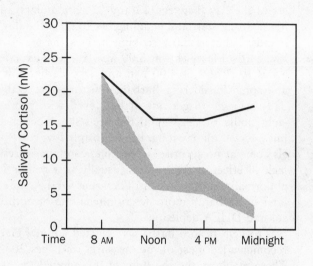

Salivary Cortisol Values: (nM-Nano Molar)		Normal Range
7:00–8:00 A.M.	22–Normal	13–23 nM
NOON	15–Elevated	4–8 nM
4:00–5:00 P.M.	14–Elevated	3–8 nM
11:00–12:00 P.M.	16–Elevated	1–3 nM

DHEA Sulfate & DHEA Value (ng/ml)	Normal Range
2–Depressed	3–10 ng/ml

Adapted by permission of Diagnos-Techs, Inc., Clinical and Research Laboratory, Kent, Washington.

Figure 11–2. Barbara's Adrenal Stress Index Test

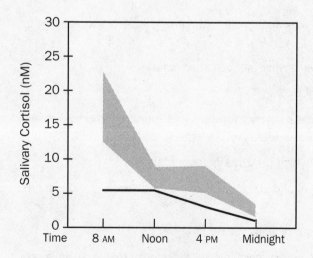

Salivary Cortisol Values: (nM-Nano Molar)		Normal Range
7:00–8:00 A.M.	4–Depressed	13–23 nM
NOON	*4–Depressed	4–8 nM
4:00–5:00 P.M.	*2–Depressed	3–8 nM
11:00–12:00 P.M.	1–Normal	1–3 nM

DHEA Sulfate & DHEA Value (ng/ml)	Normal Range
1–Depressed	–10 ng/ml

Adapted by permission of Diagnos-Techs, Inc., Clinical and Research Laboratory, Kent, Washington.

ADRENAL RESTORATION MEASURES

DIET

Eat a whole-foods diet with minimal sugar, minimal caffeine (adrenal stimulants), minimal alcohol, and adequate protein—the diet recommended for the treatment of hypoglycemia (see Chapter Ten). Because food allergy is a weakening condition and one source of adrenal stress, determining what foods you are allergic to and avoiding them can be important. Fasting and detoxification/cleansing diets should be avoided, at least initially.

HERBS

- **Ginseng** (Siberian/Eleutherococcus) is one of the more important herbs for the adrenals because one of its constituents can be made into pregnenolone, a precursor to cortisol and DHEA. In addition, it has steroid-like activity of its own and increases resistance to a wide range of stressors. It can prevent shrinking of the thymus gland, which maintains the body's immune function, and prevents adrenal hyperplasia. It can also help prevent adrenal atrophy in cortisone treatment. I recommend it in both high and low cortisol states. Take a 100-milligram capsule twice a day. If its effects are too stimulating, especially at bedtime, take the second dose before 3 P.M. or take only a morning dose. See Chapter Nineteen for further information and precautions.

- **Licorice root** is an equally important adrenal herb because it increases cortisol half-life and is extremely useful in correcting low cortisol states, giving the adrenal glands a relative rest and a chance to restore. It can prevent shrinking of the thymus and immunosuppression from the administration of cortisone. It may also lessen the dosage of cortisone needed to achieve a therapeutic effect. Take up to ¼ tsp. of a 5:1 solid extract three times a day. The solid extract is available from Scientific Botanicals of Seattle, Washington. (See Chapter Nineteen for further information.)

- **Wild yam** is known for its progesterone activity, and thus it is often useful for hyperestrogen states and premenstrual syndrome. Progesterone also lessens the undesirable effects of too much cortisol. In addition, a fermented constituent of yam (diogenim) may provide actual DHEA activity. For the tincture of wild yam, use up to 25 drops daily.

VITAMINS/MINERALS

- **Vitamin C** is essential for the structural support of the small arteries and veins in the adrenals, especially if the gland is overstimulated and hypertrophied or hyperplastic. Take 500 to 1,000 mg two or three times a day (too much can cause gas and diarrhea). Bioflavonoids (hesperidin methylchalcone or naringin—250 to 300 mg three times a day) are also helpful in this regard, along with vitamin C. These bioflavonoids are far more absorbable than those from citrus sources.

- **Vitamin B-5** (pantothenic acid/calcium pantothenate) is involved in the production of metabolic energy (ATP) for the adrenals and elsewhere in the body through a series of biochemical reactions called the Krebs cycle. Use 500 to 1,000 mg a day in divided doses. I also suggest a vitamin B complex of approximately 25 to 50 mg twice a day.

- **Magnesium** is an important cofactor in many biochemical reactions, particularly those that produce metabolic energy. Urinary excretion of magnesium is increased in hypercortisol states, making a magnesium deficiency quite likely. Use 300 to 400 mg daily in divided doses. I suggest the fumarate, citrate, glycinate, or malate forms (see Chapter Six).

ADRENAL RESTORATION MEASURES

- **Additional Supplements: Vitamin A**, at least 10,000 I.U. daily; **zinc**, 15 to 30 mg daily; **vitamin E**, 400 I.U. daily; and unrefined **flax oil**, 2 to 4 capsules or 1 or 2 teaspoons daily, are all additional helpful nutrients. (See Chapter Six for discussions of these nutrients, and Chapter Three for a discussion of flax oil.)

- **A multiple vitamin/mineral preparation** may contain most of the above nutrients, which would simplify any adrenal supplementation program. You may, however, require extra vitamin C and bioflavonoids (as well as the adrenal-specific herbs).

AMINO ACIDS

- **Tyrosine**, an amino acid, can be overutilized and eventually depleted in hypercortisol states. This can lead to deficiencies of dopamine, norepinephrine, and epinephrine (adrenaline). Such deficiencies, usually caused by continual stress, impair the adrenal medulla's "fight or flight" response. Use 100 to 500 mg of tyrosine twice a day (see Chapter Six).

- **Phosphoserine.** High midnight cortisol levels (which suggest endogenous depression, as well as possible insomnia) indicate that the hypothalamus and pituitary glands have not turned down their output of ACTH stimulation to the adrenal glands for the night. These master glands in the brain normally have a very finely tuned sensitivity to circulating cortisol levels. Taking phosphoserine (a combination primarily of the amino acid serine and the mineral phosphorus) can help the hypothalamic and pituitary membranes regain their ability to suppress adrenal output at night.[18] Look for some improvement in depression and insomnia within several weeks. However, several months is sometimes necessary for a significant response. I suggest using Seriphos by Neesby of Fresno, California. Take three capsules anytime before 3:00 P.M.

STRESS MANAGEMENT

- Get adequate sleep. Try to go to bed as early as you can in the night. Eight hours of sleep beginning at 10:00 P.M. is usually much more restoring to the adrenals than eight hours of sleep beginning at 1:00 A.M. Nap if you feel the need, as many days a week as you can, but not if this interferes with your sleep at night (see "Insomnia" in Chapter Seventeen).

- Relax several times during the day and early evening, even if it is just a few minutes doing a breathing or skilled relaxation exercise, listening to a relaxation tape, or meditating. Such exercises can help offset some of the adrenal-damaging effects of stress (see Chapter Fifteen). Listen to music you love. Get help with your children so you have some time to yourself.

- Rank a list of your most important activities and commitments each day. Then, let go of the rest. Do not take on any new plans or projects that may be taxing for at least the next several months.

- Ask for and allow yourself to accept nurturing and affection. Do things that you consider fun. Above all, do anything that makes you laugh. Laughter not only heals the soul, it also helps heal the body. These are necessary nutrients for well-being, and healers of depleted and overstimulated adrenal glands.

- Work on resolving emotional conflicts. You may want to get professional help in dealing with your feelings of worry, anger, fear, sadness, guilt, or grief. Emotions powerfully affect the adrenal glands and immune system—for good or ill. Thus the process of improving emotional health is

ADRENAL RESTORATION MEASURES

a major factor in your optimal wellness program. Increasing self-esteem and self-knowledge are also inherent in this process (see Chapter Fifteen).

EXERCISE

Do light to moderate exercise if possible. If you get exhausted or if you feel depleted or ill afterward, you're doing too much. Pushing yourself only weakens your adrenal glands even more. You may once have been a marathon runner or triathlete, but if you find you can't even walk a mile now without getting overtired, simply begin at a level you can handle—even if it's walking one block. As your health improves, you'll gradually be able to increase your exercise program.

NATURAL LIGHT

Get outdoors for at least an hour a day if possible. Direct sunlight is not necessary—and too much, of course, is undesirable. But there is a growing body of research suggesting the benefits of full spectrum natural light for the adrenal glands as well as the immune system. If you do not spend much time outdoors, consider purchasing full-spectrum lighting for your office or home (see page 317). There have been some reports attesting to the adrenal benefits of green light. Obtain a Par 38 dichromatic 150-watt spot or flood green light (Sylvania or General Electric) to have as an ambient light in your home.

PROBLEMS WITH ADRENAL GLANDULAR SUPPLEMENTS

Adrenal glandular tablets or capsules are derived from the adrenals of cattle and often contain adrenaline-like compounds that drive cortisol production mechanisms. In the case of low cortisol output due to very depleted adrenals, adrenal glandular tablets would produce only a "whipping the tired horse" effect and further deplete the glands. Also, in the case of a hypercortisol state, they would increase further the already elevated cortisol levels; again, just what you want to avoid.

So, although people taking these types of adrenal supplements often feel better in the short run, they may actually be worsening their adrenal dysfunction. In addition, antihistamines containing ephedrine, pseudoephedrine, and ephedra/ma huang would have the same effect.

There is perhaps an even more compelling reason not to use adrenal glandular (or any glandular) substances: viral contamination. Eighty percent of the domestic animal herds in England have been found to contain a "slow" virus (one that takes years for its symptoms to show), which causes a form of dementia in humans, bovine spongiform encephalitis, that is similar to Alzheimer's disease.[19] It is not likely that this virus has contaminated herds in the United States or in Argentina or New Zealand—frequent sources of glandular products. But until adequate detection techniques are widespread, and government protective agencies decide to investigate this concern, I suggest you avoid using raw glandulars, which are essentially uncooked animal tissues.

Additional Cortisol and DHEA

Besides the above primarily self-care measures, individuals like Barbara with severe adrenal exhaustion often require a prescription of small doses of cortisol in the form of hydrocortisone.[20] I recommend up to 20 milligrams a day in divided doses. Such a dose is approximately half of what normal adrenal glands produce every day. It has never, in my experience, produced any of the common side effects caused by pharmacologic doses, usually over 40 mg daily of hydrocortisone, the equivalent of over 10 mg of prednisone.

If, like Barbara's, an individual's DHEA is too low, or the cortisol/DHEA ratio is too high, supplemental DHEA is often needed. I recommend individualized doses, gradually working up to the desired level. For women this might be up to 10 mg twice a day; for men, up to 20 mg twice a day. Some of my patients have required somewhat higher doses. If using the more absorbable alcohol-based DHEA tincture, reduce the maximum doses by one-half.

In addition to its own functions, DHEA can be converted in the body to estrogen. Too high a DHEA dose in women causes breast tenderness or spotting between periods. DHEA can also be converted into testosterone (the male hormone) and, in women, too much DHEA can trigger acne and male pattern hair growth. A woman's appropriate dose is one that brings the desired results without any of the adverse side effects. Too much DHEA can suppress cortisol production to abnormally low levels. Monitoring these hormone levels with periodic follow-up testing is essential, to assure adequate levels and to safeguard against overdosing.

DHEA should not be taken routinely by women who have conditions that can be worsened by supplemental estrogen, such as endometriosis, fibroids of the uterus, or estrogen-sensitive breast cancer. Nor should it be taken routinely by men for conditions worsened by testosterone, such as prostate cancer. Although the immune systems of these individuals with low DHEA levels could benefit from increasing these levels, supplementing with any doses of DHEA beyond physiologic levels carries potentially serious risks. Close periodic monitoring of levels and supervision by a qualified health professional are essential.

By supplying safe doses of cortisol and DHEA to a body deficient in these essential hormones, an individual begins to feel normal again, with strength and mental powers returning. This "borrowed" health enables them to manage their stress, and any other ailments they may be battling, more effectively. This, in turn, eases the demand on the adrenals, which allows these glands a partial rest and gives them a chance to restore their strength.

These hormones also directly allow the adrenals to rest by lowering the pituitary's ACTH stimulation to some extent. Just like a tired horse, exhausted adrenal glands will only grow weaker if they are continually overstimulated, overstressed, and whipped into action. By providing safe, temporary small doses of hydrocortisone and/or DHEA, this potentially damaging ACTH stimulation is lessened.

Once the adrenals are thus rested, they can begin to restore their strength. Over time—four to twelve months commonly—supplemental hormones can be slowly tapered and discontinued as the adrenal glands start to function better on their own again. However, this rejuvenation program is equally dependent on a diligent maintenance of the adrenal restoration measures discussed above, most especially stress management. Lifestyle changes are an inherent part of bringing your body to a state of optimal wellness. Avoiding excessive and prolonged hormone supplementation will also help make successful weaning possible.

AGGRAVATING CONDITIONS

There are many conditions that, if present, can be additional sources of adrenal stress and need to be identified and treated in order to achieve the best outcome. Food allergy, hypoglycemia, inhalant allergies, yeast overgrowth, intestinal parasites, chronic sinusitis and other infections, and chronic inflammation and pain are common drains on adrenal strength. On the other hand, adrenal exhaustion will also render an individual susceptible to some of these very same conditions.

An optimal wellness approach must fully consider this cause/effect continuum and pinpoint all associated conditions. Barbara, my adrenal exhaustion patient, was indeed suffering from more than just one of the ten common denominators of illness (see Chapter Sixteen). My diagnostic evaluation of her condition also disclosed hypoglycemia, food allergy, and yeast overgrowth.

However, I had evaluated enough patients to recognize that for Barbara, the resolution of her adrenal status was critical. The treatments for her other conditions could then have a better chance of succeeding. Nevertheless, this isn't always the case. I've had patients whose chronic sinusitis was the most deep-seated condition, and it was only after resolving it that adrenal depletion and other conditions could be successfully addressed.

RESTORING THE ADRENALS: A GOLDEN OPPORTUNITY FOR STRESS REDUCTION

Stress abounds in our world today, and our adrenals serve as shock absorbers to help protect our bodies from the physical and mental wear and tear of our lives. But like any gland or organ in our bodies, there's a limit to how much the adrenals can withstand. Past a certain point, they will begin to weaken and affect our health in very serious ways.

Without adequately functioning adrenal glands, it would be difficult to feel or function anywhere near your best. You'd be subject to a multitude of physical and mental symptoms that your doctors might have a hard time pinpointing. They might even tell you that it's all in your head.

If you have adrenal dysfunction you can make a substantial improvement in how you feel with the self-care measures outlined in this chapter. I cannot stress enough the critical role stress management will play in your recovery. However, also consider seeking the assistance of a medical professional to help in adrenal assessment and restoration. The body's delicate balance of hormones and chemical messengers needs skilled professional monitoring.

SUGGESTED READING

Gaby, Alan, M.D. "DHEA: The Hormone That Does It All," in *Preventing and Reversing Osteoporosis: Every Woman's Guide.* Rocklin, CA: Prima, 1994.

Jeffries, W.M. "Cortisol and Immunity," *Medical Hypotheses*, March 1991, 34(3):198–208.

Jeffries, William McKendree, M.D. *Safe Uses of Cortisone.* Springfield, IL: Charles C. Thomas, 1981.

Seyles, Hans, M.D. *Stress Without Distress.* New York: NAL Dutton, 1975.

Tintera, John W., M.D. *Hypoadrenalcorticism.* Mount Vernon, NY: Adrenal Metabolic Research Society of the Hypoglycemia Foundation, 1974.

CHAPTER 12

YEAST OVERGROWTH

Candida albicans (yeast) is nothing new to the medical profession. At one extreme, it can cause skin rashes or vaginal infections (mucocutaneous candidiasis). At the other extreme, in individuals whose immune systems are severely compromised, yeast can invade the bloodstream (candidemia) and cause death. In this chapter, I will present an aspect of yeast overgrowth largely unrecognized by the medical profession, one that certainly is not fatal, but which can nonetheless be devastating. As in the case of Lindsey, one of my patients, it is often the underlying cause of multiple symptoms in individuals who are chronically unwell. It is known as Candida-related complex, or polysystemic candidiasis, and we will discuss its symptoms, causes, medical testing, and treatment.

LINDSEY

As Lindsey sat down in my office, she began to cry. She was afraid that I would be another in a series of doctors to tell her nothing was wrong. Twenty-six years old, the mother of two and a homemaker, she was barely able to cope with daily life. She complained of exhaustion, depression, inability to concentrate, fuzzy thinking, headaches, muscle weakness, joint pains, terrible abdominal bloating and excessive gas, episodic diarrhea, irregular and strange menstrual periods, recurrent vaginal yeast infections, no sex drive, continual runny nose and congested sinuses, an irritated throat, itchy ears, and a heightened sensitivity to cigarette smoke and chemical odors. She also had an overwhelming craving for sweets.

Lindsey had been treated by ten physicians in the past fourteen months, from general internists to several specialists, but none had been able to offer any substantial treatment. Their diagnoses were simply descriptions of her symptoms: vasomotor rhinitis (runny nose) or spastic colon (diarrhea) or urticaria (hives) or pruritis ani (itchy anus) or pharyngitis (irritated or sore throat) or arthralgia (joint pain). These findings never took into account any underlying condition. The treatments were no better. She continued using various pills, salves, sprays, and suppositories to temporarily suppress specific symptoms but none of these made any significant improvement in her health.

All the exams and test results were normal. The majority of these doctors suggested that she see a psychiatrist. Lindsey had a hard time believing that her symptoms were all in her head. She had never been even vaguely hypochondriacal in the past. She was depressed, certainly, but this was not her primary illness. It had come as a normal reaction to her body's "falling apart" and her inability to function adequately in her life. Although antidepressants might help, she thought, they were essentially another temporary Band-Aid approach, not addressing the core issue.

I asked Lindsey when she'd last felt well. She replied it was during her first pregnancy, when she was twenty-one. After the birth of her first child, things began to go downhill. It was after her second child, when she was twenty-four, that her health truly began to deteriorate. At that point, she decided to get serious about her diet. The fact that she could lose only a fraction of the weight she had gained from her pregnancy was an additional motivator. She gave up sugar, white flour, red meat, coffee, and fast foods. She began to feel a little better.

However, when her husband did not care to make similar dietary changes, Lindsey felt she lacked support. Not long after, she gave in to her sugar compulsion, which she described as "dangerous." It was during this time, when she could hardly live a normal life, no longer muster the strength to perform some of the bare necessities in her home, that she began seeing one physician after another.

I questioned Lindsey further about her past history. When she was fourteen, her mother had brought her to a dermatologist to see if he could do anything for her acne. The doctor gave her an antibiotic (tetracycline) to take daily. As the medication seemed to do its job reasonably well, Lindsey was told to continue it for several more months. Her skin stayed reasonably clear as long as she took the tetracycline. Everyone was happy—Lindsey, her mother, and the doctor. Lindsey took the antibiotic for eighteen consecutive months.

During this period of time, she was also put on oral contraceptives to alleviate her excruciating menstrual cramps. She stayed on the pill until she was twenty and ready to have a family. Lindsey mentioned that her diet from age thirteen to the present consisted largely of cakes, cookies, milk shakes, soft drinks, chips, hamburgers, and pizzas.

I suspected from Lindsey's symptoms and history that an overgrowth of *Candida albicans* was responsible for the deterioration of her health. She likely had an overcolonization of yeast organisms in her intestines, vagina, and sinuses, which was causing not only local symptoms in these specific areas, but polysystemic symptoms in her dermatologic, nervous, musculoskeletal, endocrine, and immune systems. The laboratory results I obtained, and above all her response to treatment, confirmed my suspicions.

DO YOU HAVE YEAST-RELATED ILLNESS?

Intestinal infections can be responsible for numerous symptoms involving more than just the gastrointestinal system, and yeast overgrowth is one that is extremely common. It can trigger minor irritations and cause debilitating states. The following list of symptoms and conditions can be caused by or associated with yeast overgrowth—of course, many items listed have other causes as well. If you can identify with enough of these symptoms/conditions, you should pursue further diagnostic confirmation of a yeast-related illness and/or a therapeutic treatment trial.

SYMPTOMS OF YEAST-RELATED ILLNESS

GASTROINTESTINAL

Constipation	Cramping	Excessive gas
Bloating and distension	Diarrhea	Mucus-filled or bloody stools
Colitis	Intestinal growling	Enteritis
Irritable bowel syndrome	Crohn's disease	Esophagitis
Indigestion	Spastic colon	Itchy anus
Decreased appetite	Heartburn	Canker sores
Coated tongue	Oral thrush	Chronic gum inflammation
Cracked/fissured tongue		

RESPIRATORY

Chronic stuffy or runny nose	Shortness of breath/difficulty taking a deep breath	Chronic sneezing or coughing
Asthma		Recurrent or chronic sore throat
Itchy throat	Recurrent infections (sinusitis, tonsillitis, bronchitis, pneumonia, ear infections)	Recurrent colds and flus
Congested or allergic sinuses		
Snoring		

MENSTRUAL

Premenstrual symptoms:
depression, emotional
fragility, irritability, anxiety,
fluid retention (including
puffy face and fingers),
breast tenderness,
abdominal bloating,
nausea, headaches, etc.

Delayed periods
Irregular periods
Bleeding between periods
Scanty or profuse bleeding
Infertility
Fibrocystic breast disease
Passing clots

Painful periods
Decreased libido (sex desire)
Endometriosis
Miscarriages
Under normal breast development

BRAIN AND NEUROLOGICAL

Fatigue and lethargy
Crying
Nervousness
Grumpiness
Suicidal thoughts
Behavior and learning
problems
Memory impairment
Impaired ability to reason
"Spacey" or unreal feeling
Dizziness, light-
headedness
Insomnia
Autism
Multiple sclerosis

Lack of mental or physical
stamina
Mood swings
Agitation
Explosive irritability
Loss of ability to concen-
trate
Hyperactivity/poor attention
span
Drunk feeling (without alcohol
consumption)
Clumsiness/lack of
coordination
Schizophrenia
Manic-depressive syndrome

Depression
Anxiety
Restlessness
Hostility
Decreased intellectual
functioning
Tantrums
Increasing lack of self-
confidence
Headaches (all varieties,
including migraines)
Shaking
Catatonia
Psychoses
Myasthenia gravis

UROGENITAL

Women:
Vaginal itching
Burning
and/or discharge
Vulvar itching and
inflammation
Vaginal or pelvic pain
Painful intercourse
Infertility

Men:
Impotence
Recurrent prostatitis or
inflammation of the
prostate

Both men and women:
Recurrent urethritis/cystitis
Bladder irritations
Painful urination
Frequent urination
Bladder cramping
Loss of sex drive

SKIN

Rough, dry, or scaly skin
Rashes of all kinds
Chronic or recurrent fungal
  infections of the skin/nails
Recurrent staph infections of
  the skin

Acne
Generalized itching
Psoriasis
Folliculitis
Rosacea
Tingling

Hives
Eczema
Easy bruising
Acne
Burning
Numbness

EAR

Ringing in the ear
Recurrent ear infections

Stuffed or clogged ears
Ear pain

Itching ears
Diminished hearing

MUSCULOSKELETAL

Arthritis
Joint stiffness
Muscle weakness
Fatigue

Arthralgia
Joint swelling
Muscle swelling

Joint pain
Muscle pain/aching/
  discomfort

INTOLERANCE OR ALLERGY TO BEVERAGES AND FOODS CONTAINING DIETARY YEASTS AND MOLDS

Alcoholic beverages
Soy sauce
Mushrooms

Aged cheeses
Brewer's yeast
Peanuts

Vinegar
B vitamins with yeast
Bread and other yeast-raised
  items

CHEMICAL INTOLERANCES

Cigarette smoke
Gasoline odor
Paints

Exhaust fumes
New carpets
Solvents

Perfumes
Marking pens
Cleaning agents, etc.

INHALANT ALLERGIES

Mold
Hay fever

Mildew (overall worsening
  of condition in damp,
  cold season)

Dust, etc.

HEART/CIRCULATORY SYSTEM

Rapid heartbeat   Mitral valve prolapse   Cold hands and feet

SENSES

Disturbances of smell, taste, vision, and hearing (i.e., increased sensitivity to noise or light, deafness, salty or metallic taste, blurred vision, watery eyes)

AUTOIMMUNE DISEASES

Rheumatoid arthritis	Multiple sclerosis	Systemic lupus
Myasthenia gravis	Autoimmune hemolytic	erythematosus
Thyroiditis	anemia	Scleroderma

OTHER

Multiple allergies to foods	Cravings for sweets, alcohol,	Hot and cold sweats
Underweight	bread, and cheese	Fluid retention/edema
Overweight	Tendency to bleed easily/slow	Elevation of blood alcohol
Anorexia nervosa	clotting	levels (without alcohol
Cancer	AIDS	consumption)
General feeling of ill health		

Adapted from The Missing Diagnosis, *2nd ed., by C.O. Truss, M.D. and* The Yeast Connection and the Woman *by W.G. Crook, M.D. (Professional Books, Inc., 1995).*

A BRIEF LESSON ON YEAST

Candida albicans is normally present in the gastrointestinal tract of healthy individuals. It shares its living space with millions of bacteria, a large percentage of which in healthy individuals include lactobacillus bacteria, friendly organisms that synthesize vitamins for our benefit and help fight undesirable intestinal bacteria, high cholesterol levels, and even some cancers. They keep the bowel functioning normally and discourage the overgrowth of yeast. We need sufficient lactobacilli to maintain good health (see Chapter Eight).

Unlike these friendly bacteria, the Candida yeast are normally present in very small numbers and do not apparently serve us in any way. They live off us, but are normally harmless. However, any condition or circumstance that enhances the growth of Candida populations or weakens the lactobacilli population or the immune system can upset the balance and trigger a yeast-related disorder.

Complications of Antibiotics

Over a period of years Lindsey's balance was altered

by several mechanisms. The initial assault came with the extended course of antibiotics she was prescribed for her acne. As you probably know, antibiotics kill bacteria and are prescribed for the infections they cause. Following is a list of common antibiotics.

COMMON ANTIBIOTICS

BROAD SPECTRUM

Achromycin™	Doxycycline	Panmycin™
Amoxicillin	Duricef™	Pediazole™
Ampicillin	EES	Principen™
Anspor™	E-Mycin™	Retet™
Asulfidine™	Eryc™	SAS 500™
Augmentin™	Erythromycin	Septra™
Azo Gantanol™	Flagyl™	Sulfisoxazole
Bactrim™	Floxin™	Sumycin™
Biaxin™	Ganatanol™	Suprax™
Ceclor™	Gantrisin™	Tegopen™
Ceftin™	Geocillin™	Terramycin™
Cefzil™	Ilosone™	Tetraclor™
Cepotex™	Keflex™	Tetracycline
Cipro™	Keftab™	Tetracyn™
Cleocin™	Lorabid™	Velosef™
Cloxacillin	Minocin™	Vibramycin™
Dicloxacillin	Noroxin™	Zithromax™

NARROWER SPECTRUM

Bicillin™	Penicillin	V-Cillin™
Macrodantin™	Pen-Vee K™	Wycillin™

These antibiotics are used to treat such common infections as

Strep throat
Tonsillitis
Middle ear infections (otitis media)
Sinusitis
Cellulitis
Abscesses of the skin, teeth, or organs
Kidney infections
Bladder infections (cystitis)
Bacterial pneumonia
Pelvic inflammatory disease (PID)
Uterine infections (endometritis)
Dysentery
Intestinal parasites
Prostatitis
Surgical wound infections
Osteomyelitis
Gonorrhea
Syphillis
Chlamydia

Although antibiotics have been extremely useful in the practice of contemporary medicine, they are often overprescribed and abused. Physicians commonly prescribe them for colds and flu ailments that are usually viral in origin and for which antibiotics are not effective. Some individuals are accustomed to receiving antibiotics for any cold or flu, and if not given antibiotics, they feel that they have been mistreated. Many physicians are aware of this attitude and feel pressured to prescribe antibiotics even when they're not entirely appropriate.

Another reason for the overuse and inappropriate prescription of antibiotic drugs is that most physicians, in their training, rarely learn how to enhance the immune response without using a pharmaceutical agent. It is almost a reflex for a doctor to reach for an antibiotic to treat an infection. In addition, even if antibiotics may not be entirely necessary, many physicians feel that they generally do no harm.

However, it has become apparent that extended use of antibiotics—for recurrent or prolonged infections, for instance, or for conditions like acne—triggers in users like Lindsey the potential for a new chronic illness. This is a yeast-related polysystemic condition that has potentially devastating mental, physical, and even social consequences.

The antibiotics listed above kill bacteria, not yeast. Broad-spectrum antibiotics kill a wide range of bacteria, including friendly lactobacilli in the intestines and the vagina. Too many antibiotics will kill enough lactobacilli to enable yeast to flourish and proliferate.[1] It is common knowledge that women often develop vaginal yeast infections after using antibiotics. Yeast overgrow, invade the vaginal mucosa, and cause an inflammation, with accompanying discharge, burning, or itching. Lindsey grew intimately acquainted with this condition before the age of eighteen.

During antibiotic use, it follows that a process similar to that described as occurring in the mucosa of the vagina would also take place in the colon and digestive tract, one of the larger surface areas of mucous membranes and home for yeast in the body. Many physicians, however, are entirely unaware of this disruption of intestinal ecology, or if they do recognize it, they are usually unaware of its implications.

Complications of Sugar and Other Dietary Hazards

In addition to antibiotics, dietary factors can also contribute to an imbalance and subsequent yeast overgrowth. An analysis of Lindsey's diet revealed that she ate foods extremely high in sugar and fat and low in vitamins, minerals, and protein. Lindsey's sweet tooth provided yeast with a superior food for their growth and proliferation. Simply stated, sugar is one of yeast's favorite foods. Sugar or sucrose also happens to weaken the immune system.[2] It decreases the ability of white cells, specifically, phagocytes, to engulf invaders. A high-fat diet also weakens immune function by diminishing lymphocyte function.

In addition, the immune system (see Chapter Sixteen) requires numerous nutrients that Lindsey's deficient diet did not adequately provide (vitamins A, B-6, and E; beta-carotene; biotin; folic acid; the minerals selenium, iodine, and zinc; and essential fatty acids).[3] You can begin to understand how Lindsey's diet and antibiotic dependency were setting up the conditions that would later allow yeast to cause a downward spiral of her health.

Complications of Hormones, Oral Contraceptives, and Pregnancy

About ten to fourteen days before a woman's menstrual period, progesterone levels rise until the monthly flow starts, at which point progesterone levels drop abruptly. This hormone stimulates Candida, and whatever symptoms the yeast produce the remainder of the month are much aggravated during this high-progesterone premenstrual time. (Yeast overgrowth happens to be one very common and unrecognized cause of premenstrual syndrome; see Chapter Seventeen.)

Menstruating women have a built-in monthly mechanism that stimulates yeast and are therefore somewhat more susceptible to this condition than men, children, and nonmenstruating women. If other factors are in balance, however, this monthly stimulation will not amount to anything significant. If they are not in balance, this time of the month can be a nightmare for some women.

Unfortunately, women have several additional opportunities to enhance their yeast populations.

1. The stimulation of synthetic hormones in oral contraceptives, predominantly the progesterone fraction, can contribute more to the disruption of the body's ecologic balance than a woman's natural premenstrual progesterone surge. If used for two or more years, oral contraceptives, as in Lindsey's case, can help trigger the Candida illness.[4]

2. Pregnancy presents two extremely favorable conditions for Candida yeast to grow and proliferate, namely, continuous, high levels of progesterone and higher than normal blood sugar levels—the sweeter state of a normal pregnancy. What could make yeast happier? You will recall Lindsey mentioning that her health began to deteriorate only after her first pregnancy. The more pregnancies a woman experiences—in addition to past antibiotics and oral contraceptive use, sugar abuse, and a nutrient-poor diet—the greater the chance that during or soon after the pregnancy the yeast will overcome her metabolic defenses. If a woman has not already developed a yeast overgrowth from her Candida-promoting diet and medications, the pregnancies will almost certainly tip the balance in favor of yeast.

Other Factors Favoring Yeast Overgrowth

Many other agents and conditions have the potential to weaken immune functioning and therefore contribute to yeast overgrowth.

We have already discussed the effect of sugar (a simple carbohydrate) on Candida growth. Even complex carbohydrates can feed the yeast in certain circumstances, such as when the bowel is irritated from food allergy, chronic anxiety, or other causes and moves food too fast to be digested properly. It is a rapid transit time, in effect, diarrhea, that delivers undigested carbohydrates to the yeast in the colon, nourishing and perpetuating their overgrowth.

Cortisone is another well-known immune system suppressant. Various oral preparations of cortisone, such as prednisone and prednisolone, are administered on a continuing or episodic basis for such chronic diseases as asthma, arthritis, lupus, and colitis. Sometimes intramuscular injections of cortisone (Kenalog, for example) are given for allergic conditions. Cortisone can cause devastating secondary problems when administered in high doses for too long. One side effect is the stimulation of yeast populations. The polysystemic effects of yeast can, in turn, actually exacerbate the very conditions for which you may be taking cortisone.

Medications such as Imuran are given to recipients of organ or bone marrow transplants, or to individuals with certain autoimmune diseases, to prevent the immune system from attacking and destroying the transplanted tissue or the autoimmune-involved tissues. These medications work by suppressing immune function and, like cortisone, help pave the way for yeast to flourish.

The chemotherapy and radiation treatments given to cancer patients destroy white blood cells. With low numbers of white cells, an individual becomes extremely susceptible to infections, including those from yeast overgrowth. These treatments can also cause gastrointestinal ulcerations and weaken mucosal defenses, allowing yeast to gain a stronger foothold. Any medication that can cause gastrointestinal ulcerations or gastrointestinal inflammations—aspirin, cortisone, and nonsteroidal anti-inflammatory drugs like Advil, Anaprox, Feldene, Motrin, Naprosyn, and Plaquenil—can also fortify yeast. And medicines given to ulcer patients—acid antagonists such as Tagamet, Zantac, and Prilosec—decrease acidity to levels low enough for yeast to grow.[5]

Environmental chemicals also burden the immune system (see Chapter Fourteen). The more chemical expo-

FACTORS INFLUENCING YEAST OVERGROWTH

Antibiotics

Oral contraceptives

Pregnancies

Cortisone and other immunosuppressant drugs

Sugar

Typical American diet (high-fat, high-sugar, nutrient-poor diet)

Environmental chemicals

Chemotherapy and radiation treatments

Free radicals

Food and other allergies

Malabsorption of nutrients

Deficiencies of hydrochloric acid, pancreatic enzymes, and bile

Excessively fast bowel transit time—chronic diarrhea

Hypothyroidism

Adrenal dysfunction

Chronic viral infections

Parasitic infections

Deficiency of intestinal secretory IgA

Diabetes

Anti-inflammatory drugs and other medications that can produce gastrointestinal ulcerations

Ulcer medications or acid blockers/antacids used for prolonged periods

Major surgery

Physical trauma

Emotional trauma

Poor coping mechanisms to life's stresses

sure accumulates, the greater the likelihood of immune breakdown and, therefore, yeast overgrowth. Individuals who have an occupational exposure to chemical toxins are at highest risk, but anyone can accumulate significant exposure. I refer to such toxins as pesticides, herbicides, solvents, paints, formaldehyde, pentachloro- phenol, combustion products of natural gas and coal (sulfur and nitrous oxides), petrochemicals (exhaust fumes), and heavy metals such as lead, cadmium, arsenic, mercury, aluminum, and nickel.

The preponderance of chemicals in our environment, even at "safe" levels, puts us all at risk. They are in the air we breathe, the water we drink, the soil our food is grown in, and even in the silver/mercury fillings in our teeth.

Allergies, whether inhalant, food, or chemical; viral infections, such as Epstein-Barr, HIV, and chronic or recurring flus; intestinal parasitic illnesses; and free radicals all consume some of the immune system's reserves and therefore potentially compromise its ability to control yeast populations. The more severe these conditions, the more they sap the immune system and trigger the potential for yeast overgrowth. In addition, if allergic inflammation happens to involve the intestines (common symptoms would be gas, bloating, diarrhea, alternating diarrhea and constipation, and cramps), it becomes easier for yeast to penetrate deeper into the intestinal mucosa. This can also happen as a result of parasitic invasions, from a deficiency of intestinal secretory IgA, or from free radical damage in the intestines.

Hypothyroidism/hypometabolism (see Chapter Seventeen) and adrenal exhaustion (see Chapter Eleven) are common causes of a weakened immune system. Nutrient deficiencies due to a poor diet or to digestive deficiencies will also weaken immune function and predispose an individual to a yeast overgrowth. Digestive deficiencies (hydrochloric acid, pancreatic enzymes, and bile) can in themselves directly increase susceptibility to yeast overgrowth.

For some individuals, major surgery seems to be a primary trigger of yeast overgrowth, even if antibiotics are not administered. It is likely that the trauma of this event alters immune function, perhaps by a mechanism similar to that of emotional trauma. Mental and emotional strain and anguish have documented weakening effects on the immune system (see Chapter Fifteen).

Two final factors predispose people toward a yeast overgrowth:

1. Diabetes—because of the high blood sugar state that yeast enjoy.
2. Beef, poultry, lamb, and pork products that come from animals fed antibiotics. Unless specified organic or chemical free, or unless your state has forbidden such practices, you can assume your meat and poultry products are tainted and contribute to the stimulation of yeast growth. This is, however, minimal in comparison to antibiotic medication that you take directly. By itself meat eating alone would not cause yeast overgrowth or sabotage treatment results.

THE CUMULATIVE EFFECT

It should be clear by now that a yeast overgrowth need not be caused by any one factor, but in all likelihood is the result of a combination of factors. These factors can be current or have been active in the past. For example, you may have taken an extended course of antibiotics or birth control pills a decade ago, without any apparent complications. Your immune system and lymphoid tissue were more than competent at the time to handle the increased yeast load, and your liver was able to sequester and eliminate any yeast antigens that managed to escape into the general circulation.

In recent years, however, you may have suffered an emotional or physical trauma or had major surgery. Perhaps you have had young children, or a chronically ill parent, or a difficult marriage or divorce, or conditions that make it difficult for you to get the sleep you need. Perhaps there are severe financial strains or continual deadlines that haven't allowed you to exercise or relax and just plain have fun for far too long. Perhaps you've been exposed to too many chemicals over the years, and your liver and immune system have reached their tolerance level.

Perhaps too much sugar or too much fast food has crept into your diet. Perhaps antibiotics have come into the picture again for a minor infection, or have been given prophylactically to prevent infection for dental or other surgery. Maybe your blood sugar is running a little high thanks to an overweight condition or a chromium deficiency. Many factors can influence your immune system and yeast populations in a cumulative fashion, so that a recent stress may have been the "last straw" that throws you into a polysystemic Candida condition.

YEAST TOXIN DAMAGE

Yeast attach themselves to the walls of the gastrointestinal tract or any other mucous membrane in the body. When conditions are right, they transform their "bud" form into the mycelial state, where filament-like roots invade deep into the mucosa in search of nourishment. The mycelia release phospholipase, an enzyme that attacks cell membranes of the mucosa, splitting fatty acids, generating free radicals, and causing inflammation in the intestine. Wherever the yeast colonize, they cause symptoms, whether an itchy anus or vagina, diarrhea, heartburn, or sore throat. They can also colonize the sinuses and trigger sinus, ear, and eye symptoms.

The yeast release toxic by-products that enter and circulate throughout the bloodstream and cause disturbances in organs and tissues distant from the growing yeast colonies.[6] Such diverse conditions as bronchial asthma, mucous colitis, schizophrenia, lupus erythematosus, sinusitis, emotional lability, premenstrual tension, bleeding between periods, kidney stones, and recurrent infections can all be caused by tissue injury from yeast. The good news is that they can all be treated successfully with the yeast protocol.

The specific tissue or organ damaged by the yeast toxins will determine which symptoms will occur.[7] If the damage is in the brain, then depression, schizophrenia, irritability, mood swings, fatigue, poor memory, fuzzy thinking, and headaches are all possible symptoms. If the damage is in the lungs, then asthma, chronic coughing, and other symptoms may result. If the damage is to the skin, then itching, hives, and rashes are likely reactions.

Yeast toxins can cause damage either by direct injury or by impaired tissue response to hormones.[8] The mechanism may be hormone masking, or tricking the body's hormone receptors into thinking the toxins are hormones or bacterial protection, enhancing staph and other bacteria.[9] In the case of hormone masking, receptor sites for thyroid hormone may be taken up by yeast toxins and therefore bring on a state identical to hypothyroidism. Many menstrual abnormalities and symp-

toms of hypoestrogenism can occur from toxins taking up receptor sites for estrogen. It is also felt that yeast can bind cortisone, progesterone, and other hormones for its own use and by this mechanism bring on endocrine deficiency states. It can do this by decreasing adrenal steroid and testosterone synthesis. (You will learn shortly how autoimmune damage of thyroid, ovarian, and other tissues brought on by a yeast-impaired immune system can also explain these symptom pictures.)

One of the yeast toxins, acetylaldehyde, is known to adversely affect red blood cell flexibility, making the cells abnormally rigid and thus impairing circulation and diminishing oxygen transport.[10] Such a mechanism may explain many of the mental symptoms as well as the cold hands and feet often experienced by those with the yeast syndrome. Mental symptoms are also precipitated by acetylaldehydes binding to the amine groups of neurotransmitters. Acetylaldehyde also interferes with acetyl

YEAST TOXIN DAMAGE

Hormone masking/impairment of tissue response to hormones

Hypothyroid symptoms

Ovarian/hypoestrogen symptoms

Hypoadrenal symptoms

Symptoms of testosterone deficiency

Loss of bacterial protection

Recurrent staph infections

Acetylaldehyde production

Decreased absorption of vitamin B-6

Decreased metabolism of beta-carotene

Decreased red blood cell flexibility, which leads to impaired circulation

Neurotransmitter impairment

Interference with magnesium and protein metabolism

Interference with delta-6 desaturase enzyme, which causes a functional essential fatty acid deficiency and increased production of unfavorable and inflammatory prostaglandin hormones (see Chapter Three)

Decreased suppressor cell function, which triggers multiple allergies, polyendocrinopathies and other conditions

Impaired T-cell response and low T-cell counts

Co A function and metabolism of glucose, both inherent components of energy production. Moreover, it is known to interfere with both the absorption of vitamin B-6 and the metabolism of beta-carotene, magnesium, and protein.

Yeast toxins interfere with delta 6 desaturase enzyme pathways during the synthesis of prostaglandin hormones, thereby potentially giving rise to inflammatory conditions. With widespread inflammation in the small bowel, caused by yeast disruption of the mucous membrane, incomplete digestion and poor assimilation of nutrients ensues, contributing often to weight loss and pronounced weakness.

The inflammation also creates a "leaky gut," where large undigested food molecules and other foreign substances are able to get into the circulation and trigger multiple allergies and intolerances (see Chapter Thirteen). Yeast are also known to produce alcohol in the body from the fermentation of carbohydrates.[11] Several cases of drunkenness due to such a Candida brewery have been documented.

Figure 12–1 shows yeast toxin injury to the immune system. The immune system consists partly of lymphocytes: B cells, which produce antibodies to foreign organisms or substances, and T cells, which can directly attack foreign invaders. Of the T cells, there are helper cells (H), which among other functions stimulate B cells to make antibodies, and suppressor cells (S), which are capable of arresting B-cell antibody production. There are also killer (K) cells, which directly attack foreign invaders or cancer cells. A delicately balanced feedback control relationship exists between T and B cells.

Through the circulation, yeast toxins proceed to inhibit the function of suppressor cells by mechanisms not entirely understood. The abnormally elevated helper/suppressor ratio in many Candida-afflicted individuals reflects this disturbance. The helper cells are then unimpeded or unopposed in their function of stimulating B-cell antibody production. B cells go wild, so to speak, and begin making antibodies to substances that ordinarily would not be considered foreign—to foods, for instance.

In addition to becoming hypersensitive or allergic to foods, a yeast-impaired immune system has less than the normal tolerance for ordinarily "safe" levels of common chemicals, such as gas and oil fumes, cleaning fluids, chlorine, perfume, and pesticide residues on produce. In such cases the chemical hypersensitivity syndrome can often develop.

The yeast-impaired immune system can become so confused that it can produce antibodies that attack the body's own tissues. The ovaries and thyroid are prime targets—resulting in the premenstrual syndrome and hypothyroid symptoms, respectively. Multiple endocrine glands can be targeted, giving rise to a polyendocrinopathy and multiple complex symptoms.[12] The yeast syndrome has been related to autoimmune diseases like rheumatoid arthritis, multiple sclerosis, myasthenia gravis, systemic lupus erythematosus, scleroderma, uveitis, thyroiditis, and autoimmune hemolytic anemia.

Although yeast may not be the precipitating cause for every autoimmune disorder or for such conditions as colitis, Crohn's disease, asthma, allergies, malabsorption, hypothyroidism, and chemical hypersensitivity, yeast treatment can often bring about remarkable improvement in these conditions and play a significant role in their successful management.

RECOGNIZING A YEAST PROBLEM

In order to determine the presence of a yeast-related illness, an assessment of symptoms and history and laboratory testing are needed.

Symptoms and History

First and foremost, you must ask: "Do my symptoms suggest a yeast problem? Do I have enough symptoms to 'fit' the yeast picture or the particular events in my history that are known to favor yeast overgrowth?"

The symptom list on pages 209–212 for yeast and the description of this syndrome throughout the chapter should provide adequate information for you to make this assessment. Remember that toddlers, children, teens, adults, and seniors can all be affected and manifest mental, emotional, behavioral, and physical symptoms due to yeast overgrowth.

You may also want to consult the "Candida Questionnaire Scoresheet" in *The Yeast Connection*, by William G. Crook, M.D. (Future Health, 1989). And in *The Missing Diagnosis*, by C. Orian Truss, M.D., one of the original researchers and authors on the subject, you will find very useful descriptions of individuals in whom a yeast-related illness should be suspected.[13]

Laboratory Testing

Cultures. Several laboratory tests can aid in the diagnosis of yeast-related illness. A quantitative Candida stool culture will tell if more than normal amounts of yeast are growing in the stool.[14] An abnormally high stool yeast count will usually correlate with Candida-related illness. About 20 percent of the time, in my clinical experience, an individual who turns out to have this condition does not show it on the stool culture. For this reason, I usually obtain the stool culture in combination with a test for intestinal antibody levels specific to Candida, as well as a blood test for Candida toxins. These

Figure 12–1. How Yeast Toxins Injure the Immune System

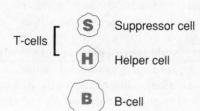

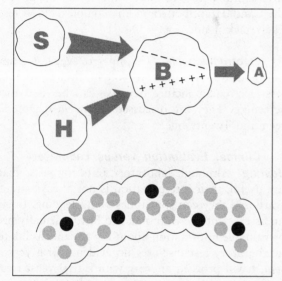
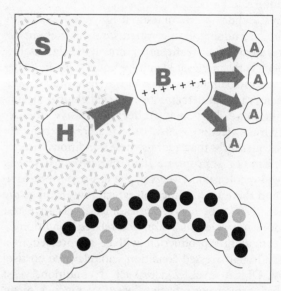

Diagram 1: Yeast and intestinal lactobacilli bacteria in balance; normal immune function.

Diagram 2: Overgrowth of intestinal yeast, release of toxins into the bloodstream, and altered immune function.

In diagram 1, a balance between intestinal lactobacilli bacteria and yeast allow for normal immune lymphocyte function: helper cells stimulate the B cells to make antibodies, whereas suppressor cells appropriately oppose B-cell antibody production. Antibody production is in balance.

In diagram 2, intestinal yeast overgrowth and yeast toxins released into the bloodstream inhibit suppressor cell function. Stimulation of antibody production by helper cells is now unopposed, and inappropriate antibody production occurs. Here we have a heightened state of allergy, as well as an increased susceptibility to autoimmune conditions.

additional tests can also help your doctor determine when a high count on the stool culture does not necessarily indicate Candida-related illness (see below).

A careful review of symptoms will help determine the locale of yeast outside the intestines, but vaginal, nasal, throat, and skin cultures or smears may also be indicated. If the cultures are positive, they will certainly guide treatment and are therefore worthwhile. Some-

times, however, they will show no yeast when in fact yeast are present but "burrowed." Treatment will then need to be guided by symptoms and other tests.

Candida-Specific Intestinal Secretory IgA. The immune system secretes antibodies (secretory IgA) that stand guard in the mucous layer to defend mucosal cells from invasion. A stool sample can disclose levels of

Candida-specific intestinal secretory IgA, antibodies responsible for defending against yeast attaching to intestinal wall cells.[15] The latter test obtained along with a stool culture can determine, for example, if yeast are attached to intestinal mucous membranes, which would challenge the immune system, and cause an IgA elevation. Whether the stool yeast culture shows overgrowth or not, yeast treatment is indicated here. If the IgA is elevated and the culture count is not, this would indicate a false negative on the culture. So it would seem, for the time being, that the IgA test is more reliable than the stool culture.

The Candida-specific intestinal IgA test is also very useful in determining if an elevated stool yeast count necessitates aggressive treatment or not. If the IgA is low in tandem with an elevated culture count, this indicates the presence of abundant yeast not attached to the mucous membrane, and therefore not challenging the immune system. This may reflect excessive dietary carbohydrates feeding yeast, or rapid transit time. In this case, measures that address these conditions directly might be more appropriate than prescribing a strong antifungal medication. However, the IgA test is not foolproof, and there are instances in which low readings are false negatives and, hence, misleading. A negative test result does not rule out a Candida-related condition.

Intestinal IgA production will be suppressed in a chronic adrenal stressed condition with elevated cortisol and low DHEA levels. Under such a condition, yeast could be aggressively infecting intestinal mucous membranes, and yet, due to immune system depression, the IgA levels would be very low. If necessary, obtaining cortisol and DHEA levels will clear the confusion (see Chapter Eleven).

Candida Antigen Titer Test. The Candida antigen titer test demonstrates if yeast antigens (toxins) are present in the bloodstream and in what concentration.[16] Any amount of yeast antigen found in the blood is abnormal and means that the body's protective mechanisms are overwhelmed. The higher the blood concentration of antigen, the worse your symptoms and state of health are likely to be. The accuracy of the antigen titer test makes it superior to the Candida stool culture. It is not foolproof, however, so I generally use it in combination with the stool and the IgA test. One weakness of the test is that when no yeast antigen is found, toxins may still be present but bound to antibodies in an antigen/antibody complex. This complex can still cause problems similar to the toxin alone. A negative result may indicate the need for other methods of assessment.

Candida Antibodies and Immune Complexes The Candida antibody blood test measures the amount of antibodies—IgA, IgE, IgG, IgM—immune system cells have generated to fight yeast.[17] The higher your antibody count, the more likely it is that you're in a battle with yeast. High counts of Candida immune complexes usually indicate the same thing. Interpretation can sometimes be difficult, because a high Candida IgG does not necessarily mean a current overgrowth, a low level of IgG could mean either no infection or immune suppression, and an elevated IgE count may be the result of yeast allergy, not overgrowth. It is best to test all the antibodies and immune complex levels. If you need laboratory documentation of an existing yeast problem and the stool culture, stool IgA and antigen tests are all negative, the Candida antibody/immune complex blood tests will likely pick it up.

Electrodiagnosis The Interro, Vega, Computron, Eclosian, and Dermatron Voll machines—all more or less electroacupuncture devices—can be used for yeast screening. They are discussed briefly in Chapters Thirteen and Twenty-one.

Clinical Evaluation versus Laboratory Testing Although laboratory tests for yeast diagnosis are useful, their interpretation is not always straightforward and they can sometimes be misleading. In general, an assessment of symptoms and history usually provides as valuable information about my patients as lab tests. If a laboratory test discloses no evidence of a yeast problem, I will proceed anyway with a trial yeast treatment program if the person's history and symptoms lead me to suspect strongly that yeast is the underlying factor. Since this is not dangerous, the results are actually the final and best diagnostic test. I will not deny my patients treatment simply because of a lack of laboratory confirmation.

On the other hand, knowing that the treatment program is involved and sometimes prolonged or may even initially leave you feeling worse, lab tests that uncover the problem can make you feel more confident about your course of treatment and more willing to stick with it.

If yeast overgrowth is indeed related to your symptoms, you will usually have some indication that the treatment is significantly helping by the third or fourth week of the program. This improvement will provide the strongest motivation to continue the treatment. In effect, positive results of treatments are a confirmation of an accurate diagnosis.

TREATING YEAST OVERGROWTH

The treatment indicated for yeast-related symptoms varies according to the degree to which the yeast has overgrown and the degree to which immune function has deteriorated. Simply using yogurt for several weeks may be adequate to reverse symptoms. However, a six- to twelve-month program involving dietary, medical/therapeutic, and lifestyle/personal adjustments and treatment of concurrent conditions may be necessary to reverse symptoms and reestablish the body's balance. If your yeast symptoms are confined to the gastrointestinal tract or vagina, a shorter and less involved program will usually be successful. If yeast toxins are circulating throughout your bloodstream and causing polysystemic symptoms, you will most likely require more involved treatment.

Dietary Changes

Eating whole foods that nourish you and not the yeast provides a basis for treatment, whether your chronic or recurring symptoms are localized or systemic. Before we present the specifics of the Candida-control diet in the tables that follow, there are a few things you may find helpful.

Avoiding sweets and eating an adequate amount of protein foods, an abundance of fresh vegetables, appropriate portions of unrefined complex carbohydrates and fat-containing foods, and perhaps a small amount of fresh fruit, provides the basic dietary guidelines for the program. Of course, individual needs vary. Some people will initially need to consume less complex carbohydrates and fruit. Others will need to minimize yeast- and mold-containing foods because of a yeast/mold allergy.

Minimizing sugar and other concentrated sweets is universal for all people with yeast infections. In addition, Candida-afflicted individuals should minimize their intake of the common dietary health hazards discussed in Chapter Three and listed in Group F (page 225) of the following tables.

Contrary to what you may have heard or read elsewhere, the diet may not have to be extremely restrictive—I allow occasional departures. So it shouldn't be difficult to remain on the diet for the initial three-to-four-week trial. If it proves to be helpful, then staying on it another three or more months may seem very reasonable to you.

CANDIDA-CONTROL DIET GROUP A:
PROTEINS AND LOW/MODERATELY LOW-STARCH VEGETABLES (EAT FREELY)

Protein Foods	Low-Starch Vegetables	Moderately Low-Starch Vegetables
Eggs	Celery	Carrots
Fish	Cabbage	Beets
Shellfish	Broccoli	Rutabaga
Turkey	Cauliflower	Turnips

Protein Foods	Low-Starch Vegetables	Moderately Low-Starch Vegetables
Chicken	Leafy greens (e.g., lettuce, spinach, parsley, chard, kale, collards, beet greens, watercress, Bok choy)	Parsnips
Duck		Eggplant
Beef		Artichoke (Jerusalem globe)
Lamb		
Pork		
Rabbit		Avocado
Wild game		Bamboo
Water chestnuts	Brussels sprouts	Mushrooms
Other flesh foods	Squash (e.g. zucchini, summer, crook neck)	
Milk/milk products (if there is no milk allergy; e.g., unsweetened yogurt, cottage cheese)	Asparagus Radishes Bell peppers (green, red, yellow)	
Seeds and nuts (e.g., almonds, sunflower seeds, filberts, walnuts, sesame seeds, cashews, pine nuts, macadamia nuts, Brazil nuts, pecans, pistachios, peanuts)	Onion Leek Garlic Sprouts Tomatoes Green beans	
Seed and nut butters		

For most Candida-afflicted individuals, I recommend adequate, but not excessive, protein intake and as many of the low-starch and moderately low-starch vegetables as desired. None of these foods will feed the yeast to any significant degree. In fact, eating primarily from this group will starve the yeast.

Some physicians actually recommend that for the first few weeks of treatment their Candida patients eat solely animal proteins and low-starch vegetables. Some advise the addition of yogurt in those who are not milk allergic. For some individuals, eating in this manner for a relatively short period of time can be extremely therapeutic. Others may find it weakening. For anyone, however, such a diet for too long can be too high in protein and fat and insufficient in complex carbohydrates and the nutrients they provide.

It is my experience that a diet drastically low in carbohydrates is unnecessary for most people fighting yeast overgrowth. I reserve it for those who have a more serious yeast illness, for those who have multiple allergies to the grains in Group B, and for those who can afford to lose some weight.

Many people on the Candida-control diet tend to oversnack on seeds and nuts. Be careful here. If you seem to return to this group again and again to satisfy a craving, or if your digestion of these foods does not seem up to par, try soaking a small quantity of raw seeds and nuts overnight in water, strain, let dry, and store in the refrigerator. The soaking initiates the sprouting process, which renders nuts and seeds significantly easier to digest. Soaking will not work for all varieties, however. Try it with almonds, sunflower seeds, and filberts to start. Generally, eat most seeds and nuts raw and occasionally, dry-roasted.

GROUP B: COMPLEX CARBOHYDRATES (EAT ENOUGH TO MAINTAIN ENERGY—RESTRICTIONS VARY)

STARCHY VEGETABLES	LEGUMES	WHOLE GRAINS
Potatoes	Lentils	Brown rice
Sweet potatoes	Split peas	Wild rice
Yams	Black-eyed peas	Millet
Winter squash	Beans (e.g., navy,	Buckwheat
(e.g., acorn,	garbanzo, pinto,	Oats
butternut,	mung, kidney,	Barley
buttercup, blue	lima, adzuki,	Corn
hubbard)	black)	Rye
		Wheat
		Triticale
		Amaranth
		Quinoa
		Kamut
		Teff
		Spelt
		Whole grain
		rice cakes
		crackers
		cereals
		pastas
		pancakes
		waffles
		muffins
		bread
		popcorn
		bulgur
		couscous
		tortillas
		essene bread

The amount of complex carbohydrate allowed on the Candida-control diet depends primarily upon the variables just mentioned: weight, food allergies, and degree of illness.

You will recall that complex carbohydrates, when digested, break down in the intestines into simple sugars that can feed the yeast, particularly if diarrhea is a problem. But even with normal transit time, I advise many of my patients to reduce this group of foods somewhat—(smaller portions and no second helpings)—but to still

consume enough to retain their energy and strength. For some, this means one helping a day. For instance, try one moderate-sized bowl of oatmeal, or one moderate-to-large baked potato, or one moderate helping of brown rice. The remainder of their foods would come primarily from Group A, and some, perhaps, from C and D. However, many individuals need more than one helping a day and make adequate progress without much carbohydrate restriction at all.

If you reduce the carbohydrates too much, you can become very tired, even exhausted, weak, or "spacey," and will be unable to function normally. Some people become so zealous in their attempts to starve the yeast by reducing carbohydrates that they seriously endanger their health by losing far more weight than they can afford to. This occurs most commonly, but not exclusively, in lean individuals who have difficulty gaining weight or maintaining their less-than-normal weight. Although initial carbohydrate reduction can be useful, it must be done appropriately. Take caution not to compromise your health, and above all, work closely with a health professional familiar with the treatment of yeast.

Allergies to grains are extremely common and can often sabotage Candida treatment results. If you are not making expected progress while on the yeast treatment, try to restrict some of the more common and repetitive grain items in your diet such as wheat, corn, rice, etc. Your repetitively used grains are the ones to suspect for allergy. Try a one-to-two-week elimination of suspected allergic grains, using instead those less common to you. It may prove worthwhile to do a trial elimination of all grains, substituting mostly starchy vegetables and some legumes for a week or two. You may need to use a trial-and-error approach to find the carbohydrates you can best tolerate.

If you are motivated enough, you can begin your yeast-control diet by restricting grains. Then, after you have experienced some improvement, reintroduce them one at a time for a three- to four-day test period to see if your symptoms recur. You can therefore decide which ones to include or avoid in your diet. You may need to do this trial elimination outside of the grain family with some of your other common repetitive foods. (See the self-testing instructions for food allergy on page 245.) And, of course, laboratory tests can reveal your allergic foods as well (see Chapter Thirteen).

GROUP C: YEAST AND MOLD-CONTAINING FOODS (ALLOWABLE IF NOT ALLERGIC— RESTRICTIONS VARY)

Bread and other yeast-raised baked items
Brewer's yeast
Enriched flour
Alcoholic beverages

Vinegar (including mayonnaise, mustard, ketchup, and prepared salad dressings)
Aged cheeses (e.g., blue cheese, cheddar, Swiss, brie, Camembert, Limburger)
Fermented dairy products (yogurt, kefir, buttermilk, sour cream)
Fermented foods (pickles, sauerkraut, tempeh, miso, soy sauce, pickled vegetables)
Mushrooms
Peanuts and peanut butter
Coffee
Canned soups and juices
Yeast-containing vitamins and minerals

Some individuals with yeast-related illness develop an allergy or sensitivity to their Candida and experience varied allergic reactions when ingesting food or beverages that contain dietary yeasts or molds, which are also in the fungus family and thus can cross-react. If you are allergic to your Candida, then you will also likely be allergic to some dietary yeasts and molds. Such allergic reactions can include sinus congestion, headaches, excessive fatigue, fuzzy thinking, gas, bloating, and itchiness, which can occur within an hour or two after ingestion and up to twenty-four hours or more afterward. An almost immediate reaction of this type to alcoholic beverages can be especially—but not exclusively—characteristic of yeast allergy. Be aware, however, that some yeast-afflicted individuals who are not allergic to Candida can tolerate these foods without any aggravation of their symptoms.

If you are not sure whether you have a yeast/mold allergy, try the following: After approximately two weeks of avoiding all the Group C yeast/mold-containing foods while on the Candida-control diet, reintroduce to your diet, on a trial basis, Group C items of your choosing—only one at a time, however. If an item triggers a reaction, whether immediate (symptoms occur within an hour after eating it) or delayed (symptoms occur in one or two days), you can conclude that you are allergic to it. Avoid its use for several months at least, until you've become less sensitive and can tolerate it. If you react to any item, wait until the reaction clears before reintroducing the next item. If there is no reaction by the end of day three, you can conclude you are not allergic to it and allow it in your diet. Then reintroduce the next item on your list. Follow the self-testing instructions for food allergy on page 245.

Realize that the category of "Yeast-Raised Baked Items—Bread, Etc." in Group C includes muffins, buns, rolls, croissants, some crackers, coffee cakes, and other items. If you react to these foods, try rice cakes, corn tortillas, essene bread in very small amounts, sourdough, whole wheat, or rye bread made without any yeast, whole grain pasta, chapatis or tortillas—beware, some brands contain a little yeast—yeast-free muffins or cornbread made with whole-grain flours, yeast-free whole grain crackers (wheat, rice, or rye), and such whole-grain cereals and dishes as brown rice, bulgur, buckwheat, millet, quinoa, spelt, and the like.

If you react to vinegar or products containing vinegar, avoid these items; for salad dressing use fresh-squeezed lemon juice, plain or with unrefined oil (with or without herbal seasoning). Also realize that many B-complex vitamins and some mineral supplements contain yeast; you can easily find yeast-free supplements. If you are not milk allergic, instead of using the aged cheeses listed under Group C, use younger cheeses that have minimal mold content (cream cheese, cottage cheese, jack, feta, ricotta, mozzarella).

Fermented dairy products such as yogurt, buttermilk, and kefir contain beneficial bacteria, and are generally helpful if unsweetened. But these foods can also trigger reactions as well due to yeast allergy and of course, due to milk allergy. Other fermented foods with helpful bacteria, such as miso or "raw" sauerkraut, may also trigger symptoms, but if they do not, they may certainly be included in the diet. Most Candida-afflicted individuals should be able to use herbal teas, canned soups, and juices (if low in sugar and sodium, and preservative- and additive-free), and seeds and nuts, especially if soaked. However, severely allergic individuals may react to the small amount of mold on these items.

If you find that you do not experience a reaction upon reintroduction of a particular food, feel free to add it to your diet. Contrary to what you might have learned elsewhere, you may therefore be able to include on your Candida-control diet some of the following items: vinegar and vinegar-containing products, soy sauce (tamari/shoyu, the sugar-free kind), peanut products, coffee, and whole grain breads. Nevertheless, too much bread is inadvisable, and coffee is not generally recommended. If you must have a small amount daily, and it doesn't seem to cause symptoms, you can use it on your yeast-control program.

Even if you seem to be able to handle some alcoholic beverages without an adverse reaction, it may be inadvisable to use them regularly. The reasons are twofold. First, many alcoholic beverages contain a significant quantity of sugar. And second, the generation of acetylaldehyde from the metabolism of alcohol may add to the yeast assault with Candida-derived acetylaldehyde. This would place undue strain on your liver's detoxification mechanisms and thus aggravate Candida symptoms.

If you have so many symptoms that it's not at all clear what eliminating or reintroducing these yeast/mold foods is doing to you, the health professional monitoring your treatment may advise you to minimize them all until the picture clears somewhat. Some sources recommend that all yeast- and mold-containing foods be avoided for months. In my experience, this across-the-board restriction is unnecessary. It also has the unfortunate effect of deterring many individuals from staying with the treatment for the required time span. Let your symptoms—or lack of symptoms—be your guide. The health professional monitoring your treatment should be able to help you sort out any confusion.

GROUP D: FRUITS (SMALL AMOUNTS OF 1, SMALLER AMOUNTS OF 2, RESTRICT 3)

(1) LESS SWEET	(2) MORE SWEET	(3) MOST SWEET
Berries (e.g., blueberries, huckleberries, raspberries)	Melons	Dried fruits (e.g., dates, raisins, bananas, apricots, pineapples, mangoes, papayas, figs, prunes)
Grapefruit	Apples	
Fresh figs	Pears	
	Plums	
	Peaches	
	Oranges	Fruit juices
	Nectarines	
	Grapes	
	Bananas	
	Apricots	
	Cherries	
	Pineapple	
	Berries (e.g., strawberries, blackberries)	
	Grapefruit juice	
	Very diluted fruit juices	

Fresh fruit contains simple sugars that yeast feed on, although not as readily as the concentrated sweets. If your condition is not too serious, allow perhaps just one piece of fresh fruit daily (the less the better in the initial phase of treatment). Generally speaking, the less sweet fruit tastes, the less sugar is available for the yeast. So choose blueberries, for example, over strawberries, or grapefruit over oranges. Avoid snacking on dried fruit—raisins, dates, prunes, apricots, and the like—as these contain very concentrated sugars. However, dried fruits may be used to sweeten hot cereals if they are cooked with the cereal, and therefore reconstituted, and if not too many are used. They can also be used to sweeten baked items.

Avoid fruit altogether initially for the first three to four weeks if you know that fruit affects you adversely, if your condition is serious, or if you won't miss it at all. But if it does not seem to impede your progress, allowing some fruit on your individual treatment program may not be a terrible violation. It's potentially much less damaging then indulging in concentrated sweets.

GROUP E: CONCENTRATED SWEETS (RESTRICT)

Refined sugar: Cake, cookies, candy, candy bars, donuts, pastries, ice cream, pudding, sodas, pie, etc.
  (e.g., table sugar, corn sweetener, high fructose corn sweetener, corn syrup, dextrose, glucose)
Maple syrup
Molasses
Malt syrup (barley or rice malt)
Honey
Dried fruit

This is the most important group to avoid. The concentrated sweets, whether refined or "natural," provide immediate nutrients for the yeast and feed them better than anything else. If you can avoid the obvious sweets (cookies, candy, soft drinks, etc.) then the small amount of sugar in such foods as ketchup or salad dressing should not be a problem. However, it is best to find versions of such items that are sugar-free or minimally sweetened. Read the ingredient lists on food labels, and remember that the closer sugars appear to the beginning of the list, the higher the sugar content.

It may be easier than you think to reduce your sugar intake. Once you begin the medication part of the yeast treatment, sugar cravings diminish greatly (they sometimes vanish). In addition, the use of a multiple vitamin/mineral preparation formulated to help lessen sweets cravings may prove invaluable. Try Glucobalance (by Probiologic of Bellevue, Washington) or include its key ingredients: B complex, chromium, and biotin, discussed on page 193. Glutamine, if necessary, may also be helpful in reducing sweets cravings (see page 192).

If you can get along fairly well without sweets, yet occasionally experience overwhelming pangs of deprivation, allow yourself an occasional treat (not on an empty stomach, however)—ideally not more than once or twice weekly. If this episodic indulgence does not upset your progress, and helps you maintain the diet and treatment program most of the time, perhaps it's not such a terrible thing. Preparing your own sweet treats (with the smallest amount of sweetener possible) could also minimize the harm (see Chapter Five). If such an occasional treat does cause a significant setback, then you will understand the necessity of avoiding sweets altogether (for several months at least).

You may wonder if aspartame-sweetened beverages are allowable. Aspartame does not, to my knowledge, feed yeast, and small amounts may be permissible. Be aware, however, that aspartame may promote a craving for sweets. Those genuinely interested in optimal nutrition should minimize aspartame-sweetened nonfoods such as artificial chemical beverages (soft drinks), which do nothing to build health and can in fact damage it.

Stevia may be used regularly if you just cannot get by without a sweetener (see page 66).

GROUP F: COMMON DIETARY HEALTH HAZARDS (RESTRICT)

Sugar
White or refined flour products
Fried foods
Fast foods
Junk foods
Soft drinks
Caffeine
Margarine
Refined oils
Chemical additives (preservatives, dyes, etc.)

Avoid the items listed above whether you're on or off a Candida-control diet. They are generally hazardous to your health (see Chapter Three).

Helpful Hints While on the Candida-Control Diet

1. CONSTIPATION: If you restrict too many Group B carbohydrate foods, whether for Candida control or for food allergy, it is possible that you will become constipated as a result of reduced fiber intake. Psyllium husk or flaxseed powder or other bulk/fiber combination powders should remedy the problem: use one or two teaspoons shaken up vigorously in six to eight ounces of water, taken usually just once or twice daily—generally away from meals, although this is not a requirement. Drink another six to eight ounces of fluid immediately after and several more glasses throughout the day. If psyllium or flax does not agree with you, see Chapter Eight for other options.

2. MILK PRODUCTS: Cow's milk products quite often cause allergies for many individuals—especially those with type O blood. You may need to go through a trial elimination and reintroduction period to discover this. Some milk-allergic individuals will react adversely to ice cream or milk and yet be able to tolerate some cheese and yogurt. Some can tolerate only yogurt, while even more severely allergic individuals cannot. Most people who are milk-allergic, or are "lactose intolerant," seem to be able to tolerate butter. Some individuals will react adversely to aged cheese but will be able to handle fresh or younger cheeses, which can indicate a mold allergy.

Several sources suggest that, regardless of allergy, cow's milk products (lactose) feed the yeast. Others, admittedly more extreme, feel that most milk products are generally unfit for human consumption. Whether or not these assertions are true, I cannot say. As with so many other facets of this treatment, you must experiment to see how your body responds. However, if you restrict milk products for a long period of time, and are eating animal protein regularly, it would be wise to include non-dairy calcium-rich foods in your diet (see pages 87–88) and perhaps add a calcium-magnesium supplement (see Chapter Six).

3. WEIGHT CONTROL: Many overweight Candida-afflicted individuals are pleased to observe significant weight loss on their yeast-control program without their necessarily having to cut calories. Restricting sweets, partially restricting complex carbohydrates and portion size, and identifying and avoiding food allergens are key. All these are helped by the Candida treatment's overall normalizing effect on the metabolism. I often see this treatment program trigger a whole self-care transformation with many of my patients. They not only improve their diet, but they begin to exercise more regularly, and learn to manage stress more effectively. And as they get healthier, they shed many pounds as an unexpected and very welcome result.

4. VEGETARIANISM: Because vegetarians commonly derive a good percentage of their protein from foods that are also high in carbohydrates—grains and legumes, as in Group B—their carbohydrate intake may be somewhat higher than is optimal for a Candida-control diet.

If you are a vegetarian, this increased carbohydrate load may not present a problem if you are able to identify and eliminate food allergies (especially in groups B and C). Be very rigorous about other aspects of the Candida-control diet—particularly concentrated sweets from Group E, and even the fruit listed in Group D; and be aggressive about therapeutic antifungal and immune-enhancing measures (see pages 226–231). Try to lower the percentage of grains and legumes in your diet somewhat. Get more protein from eggs and yogurt—if they are part of your vegetarian diet and you can tolerate them. Also, try hypoallergenic protein powders, free-form amino acids, seeds and nuts, nut butters, and seed and nut yogurts.

If this doesn't help, and you feel frustrated despite having tried everything in this chapter as well as the recommendations of your health care practitioners, try adding some fish or other animal protein, at least as a temporary medical/therapeutic measure. I would consider this recommendation early on in the treatment program if you are chronically ill or in a much weakened state—and especially if you have type O blood (see page 97). You may require supplemental hydrochloric acid and/or digestive enzymes if the sudden increase of protein seems to cause digestive discomfort (see Chapter Seven).

5. DISCIPLINE/BALANCE: Remember that the first three to four weeks can be crucial. Try to be as disciplined with your diet as you can. Your efforts will bring about substantial progress. This, in turn, will help confirm the diagnosis, and encourage you to continue with treatment. In subsequent weeks and months, you should be able to relax your diet somewhat without losing ground.

An overly restrictive diet may be dangerous or too difficult or unacceptable to carry out for as many months as your condition requires. However, too many dietary indiscretions will sabotage the treatment program. You and the health professional counseling you should be able to come up with a reasonable middle ground.

Medical/Therapeutic Agents

In concert with the yeast-control diet discussed above, a broad range of medical and therapeutic agents are used to discourage and kill yeast directly, to stimulate the immune system to control yeast, and to normalize metabolic processes.

With so many treatment options available, you may wonder where to begin. Every Candida-afflicted individual has unique needs, and every health practitioner has particular preferences in the choice and style of treatment. Along with the yeast-control diet, I generally place my patients on an antifungal agent—either a combination herbal formula, caprylic acid, or nystatin—along with a high-potency, quality acidophilus/bifidus supplement, and a yeast-free, high-potency quality multiple vitamin/mineral supplement with approximately 50 milligrams of yeast-free B complex. This threesome generally provides the backbone of therapeutic agents: nystatin, the herbal formula, or caprylic acid to kill yeast, acidophilus/bifidus to build friendly bacterial populations, and vitamins and minerals to support the immune system and help correct metabolic imbalances and deficiencies. The program usually begins with the diet, caprylic acid, the acidophilus/bifidus, and the vitamin/mineral. If indicated, particularly in cases of constipation or slow transit time, measures to increase bowel and liver function are implemented. After several weeks on this regimen, I may introduce nystatin.

This combination of agents may not be appropriate or effective for everyone. Individual tailoring of the yeast-control program is a must, taking into account initial response, concurrent conditions, and the capacity to manage an involved program. For this reason, an experienced health professional's guidance is indispensable.

Nystatin Nystatin is a drug, available by prescription only, that taken orally coats the membranes of the gastrointestinal tract and kills the yeast with which it comes in contact. Hardly any nystatin enters the bloodstream, and most of it exits with the stool, so it is considered very safe and nontoxic, even for infants.

Nystatin tablets are widely available and are useful if your yeast colonies reside primarily in the lower bowel, or if you're traveling and away from a refrigerator for more than a week.

If you have sinus, mouth, throat, esophagus, or even stomach symptoms due to yeast, pure powdered nystatin for oral use is indicated over the tablets, because the pills won't dissolve in time to coat most of these areas. The powder is very versatile. You can also use it vaginally, nasally, rectally, and topically, which also makes it preferable to tablets.

However, nystatin powder requires refrigeration, which may present a problem if you need to travel. You can keep a small supply unrefrigerated for up to one week—provided it is not exposed to excessive heat. Some individuals choose to use the more convenient tablet doses during the day when away from home and the powder for morning and nighttime doses.

Nystatin oral powder is generally available in the strength of approximately 500,000 units per 1/8 teaspoon—the equivalent of one nystatin oral tablet. The powder may be taken straight—swallowed with saliva—or mixed with a few ounces of water according to the following adult dosage schedule.

NYSTATIN DOSAGE SCHEDULE

FIRST WEEK
1/8 teaspoon or 1 tablet three times a day

SECOND WEEK
1/4 teaspoon or 2 tablets three times a day

THIRD WEEK
3/8 teaspoon or 3 tablets three times a day

FOURTH WEEK
1/2 teaspoon or 4 tablets three times a day

Due to the yeast die-off phenomenon (see below) or because of the extrasensitivity of your system, you may need to begin with even smaller doses, take a longer time to move up to the next dose level, or restrict your dose to no more than 3/8 teaspoon two or three times a day. Tailor the dosage to your response. Don't be too concerned if you can't follow the schedule exactly.

If your yeast overgrowth symptoms are primarily in the large intestine, it probably doesn't matter when you take the nystatin in relation to meals and beverages. Just divide the three doses throughout the day. However, if you have mouth, throat, esophagus, stomach, or other upper digestive tract symptoms, take the medication separately from meals if you can, at least one hour or more before meals and at bedtime. In this way your food or fluid intake won't wash off the nystatin coating. Swish and gargle the dose before swallowing for mouth and throat symptoms.

THE NYSTATIN "SNIFF" If you have sinus, Eustachian tube, bronchial/lung, or brain symptoms, try sniffing nystatin powder directly into your nostrils. Put a small amount on the tip of your finger or on a Q-Tip and sniff it vigorously high up in the nostrils, one nostril at a time, closing off the opposite nostril. Do this two to four times a day. Some authors recommend shaking the nystatin jar, then immediately removing the lid and sniffing the nystatin cloud that arises.

Others find it easier to use a medicine dropper, taking a squirt of your oral dose of nystatin dissolved in water into each nostril. Let it trickle back while sniffing a little. Experiment, after it has trickled back some, with leaning forward abruptly, bringing your head between your knees. If the nystatin water does not leak out, it should find its way into the deeper recesses of your sinuses. If yeast are growing in the sinus or nasopharyngeal areas, you may find significant if not dramatic relief from this approach. If helpful, continue this nasal administration. Discontinue if not helpful, or if irritating.

NYSTATIN ENEMA Some physicians recommend an occasional enema with one teaspoon of nystatin dissolved in a quart of water. If you're unfamiliar with this procedure, see Chapter Eighteen, and consult your physician or an experienced nurse.

NYSTATIN DOUCHE AND OINTMENT You can use nystatin powder as a vaginal douche in the same dosage as for the enema. You can also put nystatin powder in empty clear gelatin capsules and use them as vaginal suppositories, one every twelve to twenty-four hours. If you suffer skin symptoms due to yeast, you can make your own antifungal ointment, mixing up to 1 teaspoon of nystatin powder in a small cup with a cream or ointment that is nonsensitizing and nonirritating to your skin. Keep it refrigerated.

YEAST "DIE-OFF" AND HOW TO MINIMIZE IT Before beginning nystatin (or other antifungal) therapy, it is essential to understand the die-off phenomenon. As yeast are killed, they can temporarily release more toxins into the circulation and make you feel worse before you feel better. Symptoms may range from mild to severe and include fatigue, nausea, headaches, flu-like aches and pains and malaise, itching, diarrhea, hives, and nearly any symptom the yeast are known to produce.

Not every individual will experience die-off, and those who do generally suffer only mild to moderate symptoms. Taking approximately 500 milligrams of vitamin C with each dose of nystatin may be beneficial. In addition, Advil or other ibuprofen medications will relieve die-off symptoms. (Avoid these medications, however, if you have ulcers, colitis, or Crohn's disease.)

I have found that the greater the constipation or transit time, or the longer the suffering from polysystemic Candida symptoms has continued, the more likely a die-off will occur, and the more severe it will probably be. If you fall into either of these categories—particularly if your bowel evacuations are not full and daily—it is advisable to prepare for nystatin therapy by doing a bowel-cleansing program for one to two weeks and continuing it along with nystatin therapy for three to four weeks. (Bowel cleansing, using simply a fiber/bulk agent like psyllium husk or flaxseed powder twice daily, is discussed in Chapter Eight.) Adding approximately 1 tablespoon of bentonite clay liquid to the bulk/fiber water mixture can enhance intestinal detoxification, but this is not essential. Be sure to drink four to six large glasses of water throughout the day. You can also start the yeast-control diet and acidophilus during this colon preparation period.

Once you begin nystatin therapy, with improved transit bowel time, yeast toxins will likely have less opportunity to find their way into the circulation. Consequently the treatment program will proceed more comfortably. In *The Yeast Syndrome* (Bantam, 1986) authors John Parks Trowbridge and Morton Walker suggest enemas if die-off symptoms are significant, and some sources recommend colonic irrigations to minimize the yeast and toxin load.

If die-off symptoms continue to limit your ability to tolerate antifungal therapy, you might try taking the bentonite or the bentonite and psyllium together with the nystatin as the clay can bind the toxins. Experiment and see what works best for you.

If die-off symptoms are too severe, halt the nystatin and work instead to increase your liver's ability to detoxify yeast antigens. Herbs such as barberry, goldenseal, and Oregon grape root (see Chapter Nineteen) activate the tissue macrophages in the liver that sequester yeast antigens. Berberine complex and Phyto-biotic, by Phytopharmica/Enzymatic Therapy of Green Bay, Wisconsin, contain these three herbs. At least two to three weeks of treatment with berberine products, along with bowel cleansing and the yeast-control diet, should help you better tolerate die-off symptoms.

If necessary, you can always lower the nystatin dose and lengthen the weekly dose intervals until you are more comfortable. Some physicians—not myself, however—suggest the opposite: increasing the dose and thereby accelerating the treatment program. Their theory is that small doses agitate the yeast, whereas larger doses deal an eradicating blow.

Switching temporarily to a ketoconazole (Nizoral) or fluconazole (Diflucan) may reduce yeast to the point where, within two to four weeks, nystatin may be well tolerated. These medications, unlike nystatin, enter the bloodstream effectively and work systemically with very little die-off. However, they have a potential for toxicity, especially to the liver, and need to be monitored closely by your physician. I prescribe these drugs not only for managing die-off but also for particularly difficult cases (see the discussion on page 230).

Be aware that continued adverse symptoms from the use of nystatin may not be related to die-off at all, but a definite sign that you are allergic to the drug itself or that nystatin is simply the wrong agent for your body. A menstrual period may come early or late after a course of nystatin (or other antifungal agents). This is not usually an adverse effect, but an indication that the yeast's influence over your hormonal status is being altered. Consult a physician experienced in the treatment of polysystemic candidiasis.

TREATMENT TIME FRAME FOR NYSTATIN You should begin to experience significant improvement on nystatin by the third or fourth week. Many people feel better sooner, but some need to persevere several weeks longer before substantial improvement begins, particularly if there are coexisting conditions such as severe food or inhalant allergies, endocrinopathies, or chemical sensitivities.

If nystatin does contribute significant relief, continue its use at the normal dose level (½ teaspoon three times a day) for at least three months. Longer treatment is often necessary when lifestyle and dietary factors are not optimal, when concurrent conditions are not treated adequately, and when the immune system is slow to recover. Most of my patients average four to six months of active treatment. A few have taken nystatin for twelve months or more.

You will suspect that it's time to discontinue use when you can tolerate dietary infractions that used to set you back, and when it's been well over a month since you experienced any yeast-related symptoms. Nevertheless, you should not make this decision without the guidance of a health professional experienced in the treatment of yeast.

One additional point: I have seen nystatin work exceptionally well for some individuals and then, after several months of use, cause adverse symptoms such as abdominal pain and diarrhea. As with any medication, it is possible to develop a sensitivity or intolerance to nystatin. You would need to discontinue its use and replace it with a different antifungal agent.

Other Antifungal Agents

1. Caprylic acid. Many physicians, particularly naturopathic doctors, use caprylic acid products as the antifungal agent in a yeast-control program. Caprylic acid is a long-chain fatty acid naturally occurring in co-

conut. It is toxic to yeast and safe for humans when taken in prescribed dosage limits. It has the potential to trigger die-off, but generally less so than nystatin. I often use it to prepare for nystatin therapy. Sometimes I prescribe it along with nystatin, and sometimes it's the only antifungal I prescribe.

Most health food stores stock a variety of caprylic acid products. They come in 300- to 680-milligram capsules, sometimes less when combined with synergistic agents. I often recommend Mycopry 680 by Neesby of Fresno, California. Start with one capsule once a day with a meal; increase the dose in three days to one capsule twice a day, then in three more days to one capsule three times a day. Work up accordingly to a maximum adult dose of 1,300 to 2,000 milligrams three times a day with meals. This means two to three capsules per dose.

If die-off does not seem to be a problem, you can accelerate more quickly to the full dose. But if it is an issue, go more slowly. You may need to stay at this dose up to sixteen weeks. In my experience, I have found that approximately 20 to 30 percent of my Candida patients need no other antifungal agent besides caprylic acid.

2. Herbal antifungal agents. Many herbs act as antifungal agents. I am familiar with several combination formulas and sometimes recommend them instead of caprylic acid or nystatin. In addition to countering yeast, they also enhance immune function; both actions are necessary for an effective yeast-control program. A.C. Formula (by Pure Encapsulations of Sudbury, Massachusetts) contains barberry, grapefruit seed extract, undecylenic acid (from castor beans), lavender, tea tree oil, and red thyme. I suggest one or two capsules twice daily with meals.

Phellostatin (a primarily Chinese herbal formula by Health Concerns of Alameda, California) contains phellodendron, codonopsis, white atractylodes, anemarrhena, plantago, pulsatilla, capillaris, cnidium fruit, houttuynia dioscorea, licorice, and cardamom. I suggest up to three tablets three times daily, best between meals.

Yeastplex (by Herb Technology/Khalsa Health Center of Seattle, Washington) contains Chinese amur corktree bark, celandine, and citrus extract. I suggest up to two to three capsules three times daily. Some health food stores and nutritionally oriented physicians carry some of these products. Or you can contact the companies directly.

Single antifungal herbal agents can also be added to the program, such as pau d'arco/taheebo, which is also immune enhancing (see Chapter Nineteen); mathake tea (terminalia catappa), a tropical almond from the South Pacific Islands available from Ecological Formulas/Cardiovascular Research of Concord, California; grapefruit seed or citrus seed extract, which has antibacterial and antiparasitic actions as well; or garlic.

GARLIC. This medicinal food contains two potent antifungal agents, allin (a precursor to allicin) and haeoni, the stronger of the two. Fresh raw garlic contains these active ingredients, as does garlic oil.

However, cooking or processing garlic into capsules, tablets, or liquid will usually cause a loss of the antifungal properties, unless the garlic is frozen cryogenically (freeze-dried) before being crushed. Aging the garlic before processing also appears to retain antifungal properties.

Use one to two garlic tablets with meals or work into your daily diet approximately three to four small cloves of garlic. Too much garlic, however, may injure red blood cells and produce some stomach discomfort. If garlic seems particularly helpful as part of your yeast-control program, and you are compelled to use more than recommended amounts for an extended period, consult your physician for a blood test to be sure the amount you use is safe. In addition to its antifungal properties, garlic enhances health in many other ways (see Chapter Nineteen).

BERBERINES. As another example of just how multifunctional herbs can be, consider berberine-containing herbs (barberry, goldenseal, or Oregon grape root). Berberine has effective antifungal properties and activates macrophages (immune system white cells). It has antibacterial activity as well, important for eradicating bacterial overgrowth in the small intestine, which some physicians believe commonly coexists with yeast overgrowth and causes consequences similar to those of the yeast mycelia.

Berberine inhibits the bacterial and yeast enzymes (decarboxylases) involved in the toxic amine production that contributes to leaky gut syndrome. In addition, this one single agent enhances all normal digestive secretions. Choosing herbal products with such a broad range of therapeutic activities will shorten active treatment time with pharmaceuticals and in some cases make them unnecessary.

3. Additional antifungal agents. Many practitioners promote the use of various other agents to kill or inhibit yeast overgrowth. These are protein-digesting enzymes, tanabilt, dioxychlor,[18] food-grade hydrogen peroxide,[19] intravenous hydrogen peroxide, and oral and intravenous ozone. I've spoken with individuals who have experienced "miracle" responses to some of these agents.

I've also spoken with people who have had poor responses. Question your health practitioner thoroughly about the efficacy and safety of any antifungal agent recommended. And, remember, the response depends on accurate diagnosis and the recognition of other conditions that can influence the outcome of any therapy.

Agents That Counter Intestinal Imbalances

Lactobacillus Acidophilus and Bifidus. Friendly intestinal bacteria (lactobacilli) help discourage the growth of yeast. They serve as one of the primary components of the Candida-control program because of their ability to normalize the ecology of your intestines. Intestinal yeast overgrowth is one manifestation of intestinal dysbiosis (disordered intestinal microbial balance), and supplementing the diet with these favorable organisms is an important part of reversing this condition. I recommend a refrigerated lactobacillus acidophilus and bifidus supplement which most health food stores and some pharmacies carry in powder, liquid, and capsule form. For the powdered lactobacillus products, take initially ½ to 1 teaspoon two to three times a day, preferably thirty minutes before a meal or well between meals. After two or three months, use half that dose for maintenance. For capsules, initially take one capsule two times a day (once daily for maintenance). Lesser-strength and lower-quality products require higher doses. For milk-allergic individuals I recommend milk-free acidophilus/bifidus products.

In addition to oral use, acidophilus and bifidus can be used vaginally to treat and prevent vaginitis. Prepare as a douche (with 1 tablespoon unsweetened yogurt or 1 teaspoon acidophilus/bifidus powder dissolved in 1 quart of warm water), or inject the yogurt carefully into the vagina using an applicator or infant syringe. Or use acidophilus/bifidus capsules as vaginal suppositories. Some health practitioners recommend using acidophilus or bifidus powder in a retention enema. (See page 163 for a more detailed discussion of lactobacilli.)

SACCHAROMYCES BOULARDII Like lactobacilli, *Saccharomyces boulardii* produce lactic acid and inhibit the growth of yeast and unfavorable bacteria. I recommend it for cases where lactobacilli supplementation and antifungal agents do not seem helpful (particularly for diarrhea), and where antibiotic use has been a cofactor in yeast overgrowth. *Saccharomyces boulardii* is available in capsules. Use up to 500 milligrams three times daily. (See Chapter Eight for more details.)

FRUCTOOLIGOSACCHARIDES These are food-derived sugars that feed lactobacilli, encourage their repopulation, and assist the normalization of bowel function. They are not absorbed and therefore do not raise blood sugar levels. The product is inexpensive, and using up to 3,000 milligrams two or three times daily (1 teaspoon dissolved in a few ounces of water) may eventually lessen the need for more expensive lactobacilli supplementation. (See Chapter Eight for more details.)

A Program to Enhance Your Immune Function

Using antifungal agents without taking measures to improve and preserve your immune function may bring you only temporary relief from recurrent or chronic yeast-related illness. A comprehensive program to enhance and preserve immune function is often necessary to obtain lasting results. Such a program will include the following:

1. A whole-foods yeast-control diet as discussed earlier in this chapter and in Chapter Three.
2. Antifungal agents.
3. Medical/therapeutic agents that enhance immune function.
4. Personal and lifestyle adjustments.
5. Treatment of coexisting conditions to relieve the immune system of its burden.

Some individuals will require work in just one or two of these areas, but others will require work in all areas for the return of health and well-being.

Many substances can be drawn upon to help build and preserve immune function in yeast overgrowth sufferers: vitamins, minerals, trace elements, amino acids, essential fatty acids, herbs, mushrooms, chlorophyll products, homeopathic Candida drops, constitutional homeopathy, acupuncture, Candida vaccines, enzymes, staphage lysate, and some pharmaceutical drugs. You will find a discussion of specific immune-enhancing agents in Chapter Sixteen.

In my own practice, I generally start most patients on a high-potency yeast-free multiple vitamin/mineral supplement that contains many of the nutrients needed for immune function. Then, as needed, I add other agents specific for their needs. Because vitamin A and the mineral zinc are so important in mucous membrane health and resistance and cellular immunity, I may suggest additional amounts of these nutrients for resistant cases—up to 50 milligrams a day of zinc and up to 35,000 I.U. of vitamin A. Taking 300 to 1,000 micrograms of biotin three times a day is recommended by many practitioners to inhibit mycelial formation of yeast (it also helps stabilize blood sugar levels).

Alpha-linolenic acid found in flaxseed oil and gamma-linolenic acid found in primrose, borage, and black currant oils are essential fatty acids that promote the production of immune-stimulating prostaglandin hormones (see Chapter Three). Such hormones also act as anti-inflammatory agents and help reestablish normal metabolic conditions. Free-form amino acid supplements can provide immune system support and a quite valuable form of easily assimilated protein for individuals who have lost weight, are in weakened states, and/or do not digest and absorb food very well. And if I do not start out a patient on one of the immune-enhancing antifungal combination herbal formulas, I will eventually suggest one.

In order to know what any one individual requires and therefore to optimize this most essential aspect of the treatment program, I need to evaluate each individual for signs and symptoms of nutrient and immune deficiencies, coexisting conditions, personal predilection and/or belief in a particular treatment choice, response to each stage of treatment, and so on. With such a wide choice of treatments available, it is indispensable to work with a health professional experienced in these mostly natural, nontoxic, immune-enhancing therapies. Optimally, such a practitioner will suggest a combination of multifunctional agents that on one hand will do the job effectively while, on the other hand, minimize the number of supplements needed, and thus keep costs down.

Personal and Lifestyle Changes

A large percentage of my patients do not require extensive use of immune-enhancing agents because of the emphasis I place on a whole-foods diet and habits of living that strengthen the body's resistance. Getting a handle on stress and learning a skilled relaxation exercise can increase immune factors that will help you overcome yeast overgrowth.

Much of my time with patients involves counseling to help them stop putting such a drain on immune strength. In this age of fast living, financial pressures, and social instability, I must always remind my patients about nature's laws, and those who abide by them seem to require much less specific immune-enhancing agents and, in fact, can bring the yeast treatment to a successful conclusion much sooner than those who do not. You will find further comments on personal balance and nature's laws in Chapter Sixteen.

More Pharmaceutical Intervention

If you are following treatment guidelines relatively well, yet are not making expected improvements, and if your history and symptoms and test results are too suggestive of yeast overgrowth for you to abandon treatment, you and your physician might consider the following:

1. Nizoral (ketoconazole), one tablet a day with a meal. Nizoral is absorbed systemically and attacks yeasts that have burrowed too far into the mucosa for nystatin to reach. Your physician should know that if you have a deficiency of stomach acid, you may need to

take supplemental hydrochloric acid in order to absorb Nizoral. If you do not respond to this drug, it may mean that there is hydrochloric acid insufficiency and not drug resistance.

Your doctor should avoid Nizoral if you have or have had a past history of hepatitis or other significant liver disease. Periodic liver enzyme monitoring is essential if you will be on this medication more than a month. I avoid this medication if another potentially liver-toxic drug is being used. Your doctor and pharmacist should know that Nizoral can interact dangerously with several common medications (erythromycins, Seldane, Hismanol, and probably Claritin); so avoid such combinations.

2. Diflucan (fluconazole) has been heralded recently as another potent systemic-acting antifungal that is effective in reaching burrowed yeast. It has less potential for toxicity than Nizoral. However, like Nizoral, the chances for a toxic liver reaction increase if other potentially toxic drugs are being used. It should not be taken in combination with Seldane, Hismanol, erythromycins, and probably Claritin. Close physician monitoring is essential. Take a 100-milligram tablet once a day if you are an adult under 125 pounds, or a 200-milligram tablet if you are over 125 pounds. Continue this medication for up to four weeks or more to treat recalcitrant Candida infections.

Diflucan therapy is costly, so consult your physician about tapering the dose later on to perhaps every third or fourth day while using other antifungal agents the days in between.

TREATMENT OF CONCURRENT CONDITIONS

In treating yeast overgrowth, you should investigate for coexisting conditions: intestinal parasites (especially *Giardia*), food allergy, leaky gut syndrome, inhalant mold allergy, hypochlorhydria, pancreatic enzyme deficiency, helicobacter pylori, hypothyroidism, adrenal exhaustion (or overactivity), other endocrinopathies, chronic viral infections/chronic fatigue syndrome, chemical injury or hypersensitivity, heavy metal poisoning (especially mercury toxicity from silver mercury amalgam dental fillings), bacterial overgrowth syndrome, and hormone hypersensitivity (particularly to progesterone).

Identifying and treating these conditions will be necessary for you to reach your full health potential. See the respective chapters and index entries for a discussion on these other conditions.

You may also need to determine if your regular sexual partner has a yeast overgrowth condition and is reinfecting you. Although I have found this phenomenon to be extremely rare in my practice, recognition and treatment of this condition may be necessary to prevent unexplainable recurrences. If you are still symptomatic after what seems like sufficient Candida treatment and have ruled out concurrent conditions (particularly if you are still very sensitive to dietary yeasts and molds), you should be tested for Candida allergy. You may not need more antifungal agents, but rather Candida allergy shots, a candida vaccine.

POSTTREATMENT GUIDELINES

When you are able to discontinue nystatin (or whatever antifungal agents you've been using), remember the factors that led to the yeast overgrowth in the first place and take care not to repeat any previous patterns that would invite a recurrence. I've seen too many of my patients who started feeling cocky at the height of their recoveries and reverted to their old habits—too much sugar, alcohol, and fast foods; overwork; insufficient rest and relaxation; excess stress. Within three to four months they usually developed a far more serious Candida condition than before.

After your recovery, please continue to care for yourself and your immune system. There may be occasions beyond your control—when you must use antibiotics, for instance—but even then you will be able to avoid a yeast recurrence by proper diet and by taking one nystatin tablet (or ⅛ teaspoon of the powder) with each antibiotic dose. Tell your doctor how susceptible to yeast overgrowth you are and request a prescription for as many nystatin tablets as antibiotics. You can substitute antifungal herbs or one to two caprylic acid capsules for nystatin. Use an antifungal agent for at least two weeks more than the antibiotic. Acidophilus/bifidus is also strongly encouraged during your weeks of antibiotic use and for at least three weeks after the course is completed.

The use of oral cortisone (or any immunosuppressive drugs), or an extended course of an anti-inflammatory agent, can also cause a yeast recurrence, and these preventive measures are advisable here as well.

If, because of pressures or holiday festivities, you find yourself bingeing on sweets or eating them regularly again, it's best to compensate with antiyeast measures.

If you become pregnant, be sure to eat and live as healthfully as you can, and take acidophilus/bifidus and/or unsweetened yogurt. Miso, yogurt (if tolerated), and other foods with friendly bacteria are encouraged in all these circumstances.

You and your physician should be able to work out a long-term posttreatment guideline program. Follow the laws of nature as best you can, compensate with the antifungal agents and acidophilus when necessary, and consider some immune-enhancing agents. Being immediately attentive to the recurrence of yeast-related symptoms will shorten subsequent re-treatment programs.

CURING YEAST OVERGROWTH— A WHOLE PERSON APPROACH

Any discussion of yeast overgrowth and its treatment provides an exemplary model of whole-person health care. Like many complex conditions, yeast overgrowth juxtaposes the areas of nutrition, immune competence, intestinal ecology, bowel and liver function, pharmaceutical agents, botanical and other complementary agents, environmental and lifestyle factors, stress control, and personal balance. Such a comprehensive approach is often the only way to return you to good health and to help you maintain it.

SUGGESTED READING

Burton, Gail. *Candida Control Cookbook*. New York: NAL, 1989.

Crook, William G., M.D. *Chronic Fatigue Syndrome and the Yeast Connection*. Jackson, TN: Professional Books, 1992, and *The Yeast Connection and the Woman*, Jackson, TN: Professional Books, 1995.

Crook, William G., M.D., and Crook, Cynthia P. (illustrator). *The Yeast Connection: A Medical Breakthrough*. Jackson, TN: Professional Books, 1986.

Crook, William G., M.D., and Jones, Marjorie, R.N. *The Yeast Connection Cookbook*. Jackson, TN: Professional Books, 1989.

DeScheppar, Luc, M.D. *Candida, Its Symptoms, Cause,* *and Cure*. Available from 2901 Wilshire Blvd., Suite 435, Santa Monica, CA 90403, 1987.

Nolan, Donna. *Ending Fatigue and Depression*. Redmond, WA: McCormick and Co., 1987.

Remington, Dennis, M.D., and Higa, Barbara. *Back to Health: A Comprehensive Medical and Nutritional Yeast Control Program*. Provo, UT: Vitality House International, 1986.

Rockwell, Sally. *Coping with Candida*. Available from P.O. Box 15181, Seattle, WA 98115, 1984.

Trowbridge, John Parks, M.D., and Walker, Morton. *The Yeast Syndrome*. New York: Bantam, 1986.

Truss, C. Orian, M.D. *The Missing Diagnosis*. Birmingham, AL: C.O. Truss, 1985 (available from P.O. Box 26508, Birmingham, AL 35226).

RESOURCES

Candida Research and Information Foundation, P.O. Box 2719, Castro Valley, CA 94546, (510) 582-2179 (provides referrals, a newsletter, books, meetings, and much practical information)

Echo, Box 126, Delano, MN 55328 (promotes the use of food-grade hydrogen peroxide)

Institute for Child Behavior Research, 4182 Adams Ave., San Diego, CA 92116, (619) 281-7165 (primary interest in nutritional, environmental, and toxicologic causes and treatment for autism and other mental illnesses; Candida is one link)

International Health Foundation, P.O. Box 3494, Jackson, TN 38303 (provides referrals, educational seminars, a newsletter, and literature documentation on yeast overgrowth)

Price Pottenger Foundation, 5871 El Cajon Blvd., San Diego, CA 92115, (619) 582-4168 (provides referrals, books, and much nutritional and health education)

CHAPTER 13

FOOD ALLERGIES

RECOGNIZING FOOD ALLERGIES

Healing the True Causes of Your Allergies

Food allergy/intolerance is extremely common in the United States. Up to perhaps 50 percent of symptoms seen in the offices of general or family medicine practitioners are related to food sensitivity. Symptoms may be mild to debilitating. Some food allergy reactions occur immediately, but the majority may be delayed up to several days, making food allergen identification more difficult. Your doctor can perform several effective tests to help diagnose your food sensitivities, and many effective self-testing measures are also available.

Eliminating food allergies will usually make a significant difference in how you feel day to day and may even lessen your chances of developing a chronic illness. Some food allergies are "fixed" and lifelong, but most are temporary.

In this chapter, we will learn what food allergies are, how to recognize them, and how to manage them. We will cover self-testing approaches as well as laboratory/technical methods of diagnosis. Just as important, however, is the recognition and treatment of the multiple conditions that predispose us to food allergies. By uncovering and reversing these problems, one stands a good chance of becoming less allergic, and efforts to avoid allergic foods become less and less necessary. The case of Jaynine is woven throughout the first part of this discussion.

JAYNINE

Before coming to my office, Jaynine had been treated by several physicians, each of whom had diagnosed her problems as hypochondriasis. Her list of symptoms was formidable: mental fatigue, muscular fatigue and weakness, difficulty concentrating, mental fogginess, dizziness, nausea, diarrhea, constipation, cold hands and feet, difficulty waking up in the morning, water retention and total-body bloating, prickly sensations in her face, and a feeling of psychological withdrawal. She told me that at times she felt eating brought on these symptoms, and "if only I didn't have to eat, I would be fine."

Jaynine's doctors found nothing wrong with her, since her physical examinations and blood tests showed no evidence of disease. They maintained that most of her problems were the result of a psychological disturbance and referred her to a particular psychiatrist. On finding that Jaynine's symptoms were not improving significantly with medication and psychotherapy, this analyst then sent her to me.

Before seeing me, Jaynine had visited another nutritional doctor, who diagnosed hypoglycemia and hypothyroidism and suggested several kinds of vitamins and supplements to correct these metabolic abnormalities. Jaynine tried to follow this approach but was forced to discontinue it because of the nausea she experienced when taking the vitamins.

She said that she had been relatively well until three or four years ago, when she suffered four or five flu episodes, two of them severe. The illnesses occurred over an eight-month period. During this period of time, she was placed on multiple courses of antibiotics. She felt that she had never fully recovered her health after these episodes. It was also during this period that she suffered a shoulder separation and several other injuries in an automobile accident. For a period of approximately ten months, she had regularly used over-the-counter nonsteroidal anti-inflammatory painkillers, such as ibuprofen.

Over the course of the next three years, Jaynine began to develop the symptoms described above. At the time of her first visit to me, these problems were preventing her from holding a job or having relatively normal social interactions. She felt severely limited in her ability to function in life. At thirty-three years of age she found herself chronically ill.

From a medical point of view, the results of her physical examination and standard blood tests were all normal, yet it was clear to me that she was not at all well. I did not believe she was a hypochondriac. Her history clearly pointed to food allergy or food intolerance. After listening to Jaynine and reviewing her test results, I agreed with the other nutritional doctor that she exhibited hypothyroidism and hypoglycemia. I also suspected, however, that he had failed to consider her food allergies, and that the supplements he had prescribed for her, though quite appropriate for the diagnosed conditions, were made from substances to which Jaynine was allergic. Thus, they only aggravated her condition.

In looking at Jaynine's diet, we found that nearly every day she consumed wheat products (in the form of bread, crackers, noodles, cookies, crusts, some gravies, pancakes, waffles, cereals), cow's milk products (milk, cheese, cottage cheese, yogurt, butter, sour cream, nonfat dried milk, and some baked goods containing milk), and beef.

I told Jaynine that one relatively easy and cost-free method of diagnosing food allergies was the elimination diet.[1] We made a list of all the foods and beverages that Jaynine consumed regularly and repetitively—three or more days a week. Then, for a defined period of time, she eliminated those foods entirely from her diet while substituting nutritionally equivalent items (see "Self-Testing for Food Allergy on the Elimination Diet" on page 245).

The foods an individual craves are also important to list and eliminate.[2] Jaynine craved milk. She thought she could never do without it. But since at this point she was ready to do just about anything to get well, she was willing to omit all wheat, milk, and beef products from her diet for two weeks (see "Alternate Foods for Allergen Avoidance," pages 250–252).

Jaynine's Recovery Begins

The results of this experiment were quite astounding to Jaynine. In four days, she said she lost eight pounds and was able to see her ankle bones for the first time in two years. Her ankles had previously been quite swollen with allergic edema. The weight loss was all water! During the first four days of the experiment, her craving for wheat was intense, and she experienced what she learned subsequently were withdrawal symptoms. However, four to five days into her new diet she found that her cravings and withdrawal symptoms had dissipated. By the end of the second week, she began to awaken early in the morning feeling bright-eyed and well rested. Nothing short of a miracle, she declared.

After three full weeks of this specific food elimination experiment, Jaynine was able to go to bed without socks. Previously, her cold feet and hands had necessitated special measures. Her head "pressure" and dizziness had cleared significantly, the diarrhea and constipation had subsided, and her bowels "felt like themselves" again. Her chest constriction had lightened, and she could once again take full, deep breaths. Her throat did not seem so constricted anymore, and her taste for sweets had diminished.

The most gratifying changes were the significant reductions of mental fatigue, muscular fatigue and weakness, the mental fogginess and difficulty she'd had concentrating, and her tendency to be psychologically withdrawn. She said she felt like a member of the human race again. She had begun to make more social plans and was even preparing to look for work again. Remembering the initial frustration and difficulty she had felt at having to eliminate the mainstays of her old diet, Jaynine was glad she'd been willing to make the effort.

MULTIPLE MANIFESTATIONS OF FOOD ALLERGIES

Food allergy reactions can show up in nearly any organ or part of the body, either by excitation (stimulation) or inhibition.[3] They are capable of giving rise to any set of symptoms these tissues or organs are able to produce. See how many symptoms from the survey on pages 235–237 you can identify in yourself.

Jaynine's Self-Testing Program for Food Allergens

We proceeded with the next part of Jaynine's program. One by one, according to self-testing instructions for food allergy (see page 245), Jaynine reintroduced the foods she had eliminated. To her surprise, within ten to fifteen minutes of eating wheat, she was overcome with abdominal bloating, "foggy" thinking, and fatigue.

After several days, when these symptoms had cleared, she tried introducing milk products. Within forty minutes, she had a bout of diarrhea, and cold hands and feet. The following morning, she had swollen ankles.

When she reintroduced beef, Jaynine could not initially discern any noticeable reactions at all. But she continued to follow the self-testing instructions. Approximately thirty-six hours after her test meal of beef,

SYMPTOMS OF FOOD ALLERGY/INTOLERANCE[4]

NERVOUS SYSTEM

Depression
Drowsiness
Fatigue
Faintness
Weakness
Poor memory
Poor concentration
Dopiness
Unclear thinking
Feelings of unreality or
    depersonalization
Withdrawal
Personality changes
Melancholy

Confusion
Crying
Stammering
Lack of confidence
Silliness
Intoxication
Hyperactivity
Minimal brain
    dysfunction
Dyslexia
Anxiety
Panic
Irritability
Restlessness

Fidgeting
Uncontrolled rage and
    outbursts
Insomnia
Headaches
Hallucinations
Schizophrenia
Delusions
Dizziness, vertigo
Nightmares
Crankiness
Hot flashes
Twitching
Seizure disorder, epilepsy

MOUTH AND THROAT

Sores or ulcers in mouth
Cold or canker sores
Swollen gums
Difficulty swallowing

Increased or decreased
    salivation
Bad taste in mouth
Metallic taste in mouth

Sore throat
Hoarseness
Swelling in throat
Mucus in throat

SINUSES AND NOSE

Stuffiness
Drippiness
Postnasal drip

Itching
Sneezing
Reduced sense of smell

Obstruction
Sinus pain and tenderness
Recurrent sinusitis

EARS AND HEARING

Itching
Earache
Hearing loss
Stuffed feeling

Ringing
Increased sensitivity
    to sound

Recurring infections,
    especially in children
Ménière's disease

GASTROINTESTINAL

Bloating
Indigestion
Acid stomach
Nausea
Abdominal cramps
    or spasms
Diarrhea

Constipation
Alternating bowel function
Spastic colon/irritable
    bowel
Colitis
Increased belching or
    flatulence

Hunger pains
Reduced or increased
    appetite
Itchy anus
Crohn's disease
Peptic ulcer

MUSCLES AND JOINTS

Muscle cramps or spasms
Muscle pain
Polymyalgia
Muscle tremors or jerks

Muscle weakness
Muscle stiffness
Myositis (inflammation
    of muscles)

Fibrositis
Stiff, swollen joints
Arthritis, osteoarthritis,
    rheumatoid arthritis

URINARY

Nephrotic syndrome
Frequency of urination
Bed-wetting

Urgent need to urinate
Painful or burning
    urination

Need to urinate during
    the night

GENITAL

Painful menstrual periods
Irregular menstrual periods
Premenstrual symptoms

Increase or decrease in
    sexual drive

Genital itch
Recurrent vaginitis

SKIN

Local or generalized
    itching
Hives
Pallor

Increased or decreased
    perspiration
Acne
Eczema

Nonspecific rashes
    or lesions
Blotches
Dark circles under eyes

LUNGS

Difficulty breathing
Asthma

Coughing

Hyperventilation

HEART AND BLOOD VESSELS

Chest pain or
  tightness
Angina
Palpitations, especially
  after eating
Rapid or irregular
  heartbeat

Generalized swelling
Faint feeling
Inflammation of veins
  (phlebitis)
Inflammation of arteries
  (arteritis)

High blood pressure
  (hypertension)
Low blood pressure
  (hypotension)

EYES AND VISION

Sensitivity to light
Blurred vision
Double vision
Itching or redness

Burning
Pain
Sandy or gritty feeling
Heavy feeling

Excessive watering
Flashing lights
Spots, floaters
Dark circles under eyes

BLOOD

Decreased immunity
Abnormal clotting
Anemia (low hemoglobin
  or hematocrit)

Leukopenia (low white
  blood cell count)

Thrombocytopenia (low
  platelets)

MISCELLANEOUS

Feeling worse after
  eating
General feeling of ill
  health
Flu-like state that is
  not the flu

Abrupt changes of state
  of health
Feeling totally drained or
  exhausted
Sudden fatigue or chills after
  eating

Underweight or
  overweight
Fluctuations of weight
Alcoholism
Diabetes
Anorexia nervosa

she awoke with head pressure, a cold and achy feeling, and abdominal cramps that culminated in an episode of diarrhea. It was now totally clear to us both that Jaynine needed to avoid wheat, dairy products, and beef.

Jaynine's story is an excellent demonstration of the concepts of food allergy/intolerance. What is normally wholesome and healthful food for one individual can cause allergies in another and trigger a variety of symptoms, ranging from rashes and sinus problems (the most commonly recognized allergic symptoms) to multisystem complaints like Jaynine's.

WHY DO WE GET ALLERGIES?

An allergic reaction is an inflammation or irritation of tissues caused by an interaction between a "foreign," sensitizing substance (an antigen) and one of a variety of the body's defense mechanisms. In Jaynine's case, the antigens (allergens) were milk, wheat, and beef.

There are four known types of allergic/hypersensitivity reactions.[5] Type I immediate onset allergy mechanism is characterized by the binding of IgE antibodies to a specific antigen (a food or inhalant, for example). When white blood cells are sensitized by the specific IgE antibodies and then contact the specific antigen, the cells release powerful substances. These are highly destructive and inflammatory agents such as lysosomal enzymes, histamine, toxic oxygen radicals, arachidonic acid, leukotrienes, kinin and bradykinin-like substances, and dehydroascorbic acid.

Such substances inadvertently damage the organism's own tissues, thereby giving rise to a potentially vast array of symptoms, which usually appear within thirty minutes: sinus congestion, nasal discharge, itchy eyes, hives, edema, asthma attack, intestinal spasms, and anaphylaxis, to name a few.

Underlying Causes of Allergic Reactions

To give you a better understanding of why Jaynine was so ill, I will briefly describe some of the mechanisms of these inflammatory agents derived from allergic or allergic-like reactions. The lysosomal enzymes digest and destroy tissue. Histamine causes leakage from capillaries and produces tissue swelling, constriction of bronchioles, excessive mucus production, and more.

Toxic oxygen radicals destroy cellular membranes, accelerate the aging process, and contribute to arteriosclerosis, arthritis, and other problems discussed in Chapter Three. Arachidonic acid becomes quickly converted into the prostaglandin-2 hormone series (PGE-2), and leukotrienes are released, which act as potent inflammatory mediators (see the discussion of prostaglandin hormones in Chapter Three). Kinin, bradykinin, and other "slow-release" substances are fiercely injurious and produce inflammation. It has been estimated that in over 75 percent of food-allergy reactions, cells are actually destroyed.[6]

Many of the body's destructive agents can be engaged without the presence of elevated antigen-specific IgE antibodies.[7] In terms of the classical meaning of allergy—which by definition is Type I IgE antibody mediated, with immediate onset of symptoms and easily diagnosed by skin tests—these non-IgE reactions may not be truly allergic but rather allergic-like.[8] Types II to IV reactions involve IgG antibodies, IgG immune complexes, IgM and IgA antibodies, and cellular (T-lymphocyte) mediated responses, all of which have delayed onset of symptoms (up to forty-eight and sometimes seventy-two hours or more after eating the allergic food) and are rarely diagnosed by conventional skin tests.

Nevertheless, the destructive effects of these allergic-like reactions are just as significant as those caused by classical IgE mediated allergies, perhaps more so because they're often hidden or masked and may be an underlying mechanism contributing to some serious chronic and even autoimmune diseases.[9] In autoimmune phenomena, the immune system considers a part of one's own body to be "foreign," attacks it, and attempts to destroy it. Rheumatoid arthritis and systemic lupus erythematosus are two examples of autoimmune diseases.

Oxidized Vitamin C   A slight shift in the acid-alkaline balance of the body also occurs during allergic reactions, favoring a somewhat acidotic state. This effect, along with others, causes a toxic accumulation of an oxidized form of vitamin C (dehydroascorbic), which has been implicated in multiple autonomic nervous system dysfunctions (dysautonomia) with symptoms of increased frequency of urination, bed-wetting, headache, insomnia, increased appetite, cold hands and feet, hot flashes, hypertension, cardiac arrythmias, palpitations, excessive pupillary dilation, constipation or diarrhea or both, disturbed thinking, and more.

High levels of dehydroascorbic have also been associated with shrinking of the thymus gland and diminished T-cell lymphocyte cell count, both of which impair immunity, as well as hyperglycemia (diabetes) and increased lipid peroxidation (free radical pathology).[10]

Allergy and Inflammation

Whether you have an autoimmune condition, hay fever, or food allergies, allergic or allergic-like phenomena all create inflammation. If the inflammation occurs on the skin, a rash will develop. If it occurs in the nose or sinuses, hay-fever-like symptoms will develop. If the site of the inflammation happens to be in the brain, swollen and irritated brain cells can produce a host of symptoms: depression, fatigue, head pressure, dizziness, mental fogginess, difficulty concentrating—all symptoms that Jaynine experienced. Other reactions of cerebral allergy include mood swings, learning disorders, hyperactivity, paranoia, hallucinations, delusions, manic behavior, poor memory, and seizures. The list goes on and on.

If the inflammation happens to be in the joints, arthritis, stiffness, or arthralgias can occur. If in the muscles, there can be myalgias or muscle aches. If in the bladder, the symptoms are increased frequency of urination or recurrent bladder infections. If in the kidneys, unexplained red blood cells or protein can appear in the urine. Inflammation in the bowel can cause diarrhea, constipation, spastic colon, mucous colitis, bloating, nausea, gas, and itchy anus. Any part of the body can be involved. Any two people allergic to the same food can be affected in an entirely different area.

It is a paradox that the body's attempt to fight a "foreign" substance can inadvertently cause inflammation and even destruction of its own tissue and produce such an array of symptoms and diseases. Yet from another point of view, this mechanism may be valuable in that it alerts one to the danger of continued exposure to food allergens. If heeded and corrected, it can prevent unnecessary suffering and chronic disease.

According to Theron G. Randolph, M.D., a pioneer of clinical ecology and Ralph W. Moss, Ph.D., in *An Alternative Approach to Allergies*,[11] undiagnosed food allergies plague more than 50 percent of the population. It is sobering to realize how many people are being told by their physicians that they just have to live with their chronic diseases and conditions, both mental and physical, when much symptom improvement and reduced pharmaceutical intervention could be achieved through proper allergy diagnosis and treatment.

Allergy/Addiction, Adaptation, and Maladaptation

Jaynine's case is a demonstration of Randolph and Moss's concepts of addiction, adaptation, and maladaptation as they relate to allergy. As we have emphasized, repetitive use of the same food is commonly associated with the development of allergies to that food. It is also extremely common to find that the foods to which we're allergic are the same foods we crave.

For Jaynine, wheat was an allergy/addiction. When nearly any addictive substance is withheld from an addict for a relatively short period of time, withdrawal symptoms are likely to develop (maladaptation)—symptoms that are sometimes quite severe and painful. When the addictive substance is then given to the individual, withdrawal symptoms quickly subside, and relief and even euphoria may ensue. Maintaining this stimulated, symptom-free relief state (adaptation) requires intermittent use or ingestion of the addictive substance.

What Jaynine experienced when she eliminated wheat closely fits this classic picture of addiction. Avoidance induced uncomfortable symptoms, which were then relieved by eating wheat. Food-allergic individuals are often unaware of their addictions, yet they are certain to include in their diet a daily dose of the addictive/allergic food or beverage. By such stimulation, they can prevent or postpone the maladaptive state of withdrawal, sustain their "adapted" state, and therefore mask the allergy.

Also contributing to the craving and the addictive nature of many allergic foods are the narcotic-like substances produced by one's own body in the course of some allergic reactions. These are endorphins, methionine-enkephalin, leuenkephalin, and opiate alkaloids.

This habitual ingestion of foods to which one is allergic in order to stay continually in this stimulated, symptom-free state is extremely dangerous. Overstimulation almost always leads to exhaustion or an inhibition of healthy function. According to Randolph and Moss, the stimulatory adaptive mechanism eventually tires and is no longer able to postpone or prevent the withdrawal state. The food or beverage that once produced stimulation then loses its punch. This is when we see the eventual outcome of food addiction: chronic maladaptation, or the inability of the body's biochemical and immunologic processes to correct or balance themselves. It is a disordered state that, as in Jaynine's case, often leads to incapacitating systemic symptoms and chronic illness involving multiple organs and tissues. In the box that appears on the next page, Randolph and Moss have categorized various maladaptation responses.

Consider another example of this phenomenon: An infant develops a series of ailments—first colic and then, over the next six years of his life, eczema and asthma—in reaction to cow's milk. As he gets older, he seems to outgrow the allergy. Regular use of milk no longer seems to cause symptoms (he has adapted). It is soon evident that he loves and even craves milk. After several decades, however, he gradually develops unexplained depression, headaches, and crampy diarrhea, which are eventually traced to his regular use of and addiction to milk products. He has entered the maladaptation phase. He still feels addicted to milk, yet the substance is causing persistent and sometimes disabling symptoms leading to chronic illness.

THE UPS AND DOWNS OF ADDICTION

Directions: Start at zero (0). Read up for predominantly stimulatory levels; read down for predominantly withdrawal levels.

Maladapted Cerebral and Behavioral Responses	++++ MANIC, WITH OR WITHOUT CONVULSIONS	Distraught, excited, agitated, enraged, and panicky. Circuitous or one-track thoughts, muscle-twitching and jerking of extremities, convulsive seizures, and altered consciousness may develop.
	+++ HYPOMANIC, TOXIC, ANXIOUS, AND EGOCENTRIC	Aggressive, loquacious, clumsy (ataxic), anxious, fearful, and apprehensive; alternating chills and flushing, ravenous hunger, excessive thirst. Giggling or pathological laughter may occur.
Adapted Responses	++ HYPERACTIVE, IRRITABLE, HUNGRY, AND THIRSTY	Tense, jittery, "hopped-up," talkative, argumentative, sensitive, overly responsive, self-centered, hungry, and thirsty; flushing, sweating, and chilling may occur, as well as insomnia, alcoholism, and obesity.
	+ STIMULATED BUT RELATIVELY SYMPTOM-FREE	Active, alert, lively, responsive, and enthusiastic, with unimpaired ambition, energy, initiative, and wit. Considerate of the views and actions of others. This usually comes to be regarded as "normal" behavior.
	0 BEHAVIOR ON AN EVEN KEEL, AS IN HOMEOSTASIS	Calm, balanced, level-headed reactions. Children expect this from their parents and teachers. Parents expect this from their children. We all expect this from our associates.
Maladapted Localized Responses	– LOCALIZED ALLERGIC MANIFESTATIONS	Runny or stuffy nose, clearing throat, coughing, wheezing. Asthma, itching (eczema and hives), gas, diarrhea, constipation (colitis), urgency and frequency of urination, and various eye and ear syndromes.
Maladapted Systemic Responses	– – SYSTEMIC ALLERGIC MANIFESTATIONS	Tired, dopey, somnolent, mildly depressed, edematous with painful syndromes (headache, neckache, backache, neuralgia, myalgia, myositis, arthralgia, arthritis, arteritis, chest pain), and cardiovascular effects.*
Maladapted Advanced Stimulatory Responses	– – – BRAIN-FAG, MILD DEPRESSION, AND DISTURBED THINKING	Confused, indecisive, moody, sad, sullen, withdrawn, or apathetic. Emotional instability and impaired attention, concentration, comprehension, and thought processes (aphasia, mental lapse, and blackouts).
	– – – – SEVERE DEPRESSION, WITH OR WITHOUT ALTERED CONSCIOUSNESS	Unresponsive, lethargic, stuporous, disoriented, melancholic, incontinent, regressive thinking, paranoid orientation, delusions, hallucinations, sometimes amnesia and coma.

Cardiovascular manifestations, including rapid or irregular pulse, hypertension, phlebitis, anemia, and bleeding and bruising tendencies, may occur at any level. From An Alternative Approach to Allergies, *by Theron G. Randolph and Ralph W. Moss. Reprinted by permission of HarperCollins Publishers, Inc., and Ruth Hagy Brod Agency.*

TIPS ON MANAGING YOUR FOOD ALLERGIES BETTER

Here are several more concepts concerning food allergy that helped Jaynine refine her understanding and enabled her to manage her allergies more successfully:

food rotation, food chemical sensitivity, and the alcohol-allergy connection.

Rotating Foods

Jaynine began to eat rye crackers and corn tortillas

every day as bread substitutes. Within approximately twelve weeks she was dismayed to notice that allergic reactions had begun to develop from these foods as well. One would cause her lips to tingle nearly immediately, and the other would make her feel thick and foggy-headed on the following day.

Thus she discovered one important principle: for people highly prone to food allergy, repetitious use of the same food is likely to produce an allergic reaction.[12] Jaynine carefully began to rotate her most commonly used foods so that she ate the same item no more than once every four or five days.

As she gained experience with this rotation concept, she learned that she could use some foods more often without experiencing allergic reactions. A few foods, in fact, could be used daily without problems. She also found that if she ate only small quantities of some of her "trick" foods, she could escape the reactions triggered by larger portions. However, some of her allergic foods would get her into trouble even in infinitesimal doses. She had to learn to distinguish which foods she could cheat on and which she could not. Thus, although much planning and effort were required for a good number of her foods, rotation kept her out of trouble most of the time. (See "Coping with Food Allergies: The Rotary Diversified Diet," page 255.)

After eight months, Jaynine was relieved to find that wheat and beef, initially two of her severest food allergens, could be included in her diet again without the old reactions. But, as time went on, she got somewhat cavalier and began to eat them every day. In less than four weeks, she noticed a return of her initial allergic symptoms (swollen ankles, fatigue, abdominal cramps). She told me that is when she realized that she had really "blown it."

However, this episode helped Jaynine understand three important principles:

1. A period of avoidance can break a food allergy.
2. The specific food can then be reintroduced without a return of allergic symptoms.
3. However, eating the reintroduced food frequently (more than two times per week) will induce a recurrence of allergic reactions.

Reacting to Chemicals

Jaynine found that several supermarket fruits and vegetables to which she reacted adversely seemed to cause no problems at all when purchased from a health food store or an organic produce market. This was largely because the items had been grown on much healthier soil and without the use of pesticides. She learned that it was not only the foods themselves that could cause reactions, but also the chemicals used in their growing and transporting. Additional problems are caused by common food additive chemicals such as aspartame, sulfites, sodium benzoate, MSG, food coloring, BHA, and BHT.[13]

Over the course of the next few months, as she stayed away from her allergic foods and used mostly organic and additive-free foods, Jaynine tended to stay reaction-free and feel much better. Organic food was sometimes unavailable. Other times, it was too expensive, so she learned how to detoxify the chemical contamination of supermarket produce (see page 246). The cumulative effect of so many chemicals in our food and environment, even so-called safe levels, can injure the immune system and lead to the chemical hypersensitivity syndrome, part of which includes multiple food allergies (see Chapter Fourteen).

Another type of chemical allergy is a sensitivity to salicylate-containing medications and food additives and the naturally occurring salicylates in fruits and other foods. Salicylate sensitivity came to popular attention largely through the efforts of pediatrician and author Benjamin Feingold, M.D.[14] (*Why Your Child is Hyperactive*), who found that drastically reducing the salicylate as well as food additive content in the diet of hyperactive children diminished (or arrested) their hyperactivity. In adults, salicylate sensitivity can bring on hives and other common allergic conditions. A one- to three-week salicylate-free diet may be an extremely revealing test for mental, behavioral, or physical symptoms that have not improved substantially from other measures implemented.

You will find in Dr. Feingold's book a comprehensive list of many salicylate-containing fruits such as apples, oranges, grapes, raisins, currants, cherries, nectarines, plums, prunes, peaches, apricots, and many berries (except for blueberries or huckleberries). Of course, products made from these fruits, such as jelly, wine, and wine vinegar also contain salicylates. Among salicylate-containing nuts are almonds, and salicylate-containing vegetables include tomatoes and all tomato products, cucumbers, pickles, and green peppers. Also, check the ingredient list on packages for additives such as BHA or BHT, artificial food coloring, artificial flavoring, and others.

Alcohol and Allergies

Jaynine discovered how important it was to abstain from alcoholic beverages derived from wheat or the wheat-related family (barley), not because of the behavioral and psychosocial effects of alcohol but because of exposure to wheat. She was not an alcohol abuser (see Chapter Seventeen, "Alcoholism"). In terms of grain-allergy, most beer is identical with bread: both contain wheat. Beer, however, causes a much more rapid absorption of wheat antigens into the bloodstream, thereby exacerbating an existing wheat allergy and most likely rekindling a wheat-allergic cycle.[15] Moreover, alcoholic beverages contribute to food allergies by increasing intestinal permeability to food antigens, thereby causing a "leaky" gut—a condition where abnormally large and antigenic molecules gain access to the circulation and trigger allergies or allergic-like reactions.[16] For many individuals who seem allergic to alcoholic beverages, the offending antigen is brewer's yeast, from which most alcoholic beverages are brewed.

UNDERLYING CONDITIONS PREDISPOSING YOU TO FOOD ALLERGY

Your allergies may be a signal of other underlying conditions. Ideally, you and your doctor should examine your allergic symptoms with a broad perspective and not confine your investigation and management measures to food alone. Consider any of the following conditions that could predispose you to food allergy. Recognizing and treating these underlying conditions can often diminish and sometimes eradicate your allergies.

Underlying Conditions

1. Candidiasis (see Chapter Twelve for a full discussion).

2. Intestinal parasites. Allergies are known repercussions of parasites. Often, however, parasites are missed by conventional parasite testing (see "Parasites" in Chapter Seventeen).

3. Inadequate secretion of hydrochloric acid, pancreatic enzymes, and intestinal secretory IgA (see Chapter Seven).

4. Adrenal weakness or overstimulation (see Chapter Eleven).

5. Mercury, lead, cadmium, and other heavy-metal toxicity (see Chapter Fourteen).

6. Chemical overload and/or chemical hypersensitivity (see Chapter Fourteen).

7. A toxic bowel and sluggish liver (see Chapters Eight and Nine).

8. Chronic use of anti-inflammatory medications such as ibuprofen/Motrin and other nonsteroidal anti-inflammatory agents such as Naprosyn, Feldene, Anaprox, Indocin, Clinoril, Meclamine, Tolectin, and Orudis. These agents, unfortunately, can inflame and ulcerate the intestines and contribute to food allergy/intolerance. Arthritis, which is commonly induced or aggravated by a food allergy, is frequently treated with

these pharmaceutical agents. Paradoxically, these medications then aggravate the underlying intestinal pathology partially responsible for the condition in the first place.

9. Alcoholism or regular ingestion of alcohol (see "Alcoholism" in Chapter Seventeen).

10. Junk food and fast-food diets. These lack the micronutrients necessary for support of all the body's intricate biochemical reactions, some of which defend against allergy (see Chapter Three).

11. Imbalance of acid/alkaline status (see discussions in Chapters Four and Seven).

12. Stress from
   • Emotional and psychological tension overload.[17]
   • Physical trauma.
   • Severe flu or viral episodes or other illnesses.

13. A few foods used repetitively. These may not in themselves be responsible for allergies, but when taken in concert with other factors, allergies may result.

14. "Leaky" gut. The leaky gut is probably the most important and comprehensive underlying cofactor in food allergy/intolerance. It may be the actual allergy-inducing defect caused by the majority of the items listed above. Due to injury, infection, or biochemical deficiencies, an increased permeability—sometimes gaping holes—in the mucous membrane of the intestinal tract allows abnormally large, and therefore "foreign" and antigenic, molecules into the circulation. These molecules, in turn, stimulate allergic/inflammatory phenomena which can take place locally, right in the intestinal wall, causing gastrointestinal symptoms. It can also occur elsewhere in the body, producing symptoms indicative of those sites: joints (arthritis), skin (eczema or hives), lungs (asthma), etc.[18]

The intestinal impermeability test is an effective and noninvasive method of assessing gut leakiness, as well as absorptive capacity.[19] Leaky gut can be caused by and is associated with many conditions: parasites, bacterial dysentery, candidiasis, bacterial overgrowth (all of which are part of intestinal dysbiosis), alcohol, anti-inflammatory medications, nutrient deficiencies, colitis, Crohn's disease,[20] celiac disease,[21] stress, deficient intestinal secretory IgA levels, trauma, chemotherapy, and others. Recognizing and treating these particular conditions and circumstances is the key to restoring your intestinal mucosa (discussion to follow), diminishing your allergic state, and overcoming your symptoms.

15. Hereditary factors. As you can see, allergies exist or develop for a variety of reasons. Genetic predisposition is yet another cause of allergy—whether Type I immediate onset or Types II to IV delayed hypersensitivity. In fact, in his book *Your Family Tree Connection*, Christopher Reading, M.D.,[22] ties inherited food aller-

gies to such inherited conditions as mental illness, Down's syndrome, Alzheimer's disease, and cancer. Even if you have a strong genetic predisposition to allergy and these other conditions, there is much you can do to successfully lessen allergic illnesses.

It might be worthwhile at this point to mention two other "allergic" conditions with a strong genetic relationship:

- Lactose intolerance. Most common among certain populations—for example Asians, Eskimos, Bantus, Arabs, and African Americans—this condition can be acquired by adults of any descent when they "run out" of lactase, an enzyme necessary to digest the lactose present in most milk products. In some individuals, lactose intolerance is caused by intestinal parasites and will subside after parasite eradication (see pages 85–86).

   Those with lactose intolerance require sufficient lactase supplementation with their milk products, although they would do best to avoid milk products altogether. Some people, however, will be able to tolerate cultured milk products like yogurt or kefir, certain cheeses like cheddar, or lactose-reduced milk products without supplemental lactase.

- Gluten intolerance. Also known as "celiac sprue," a fixed hypersensitivity to the gluten-containing grains (wheat, rye, barley, oats, spelt, kamut, and triticale). Those so disposed can usually handle millet and rice. I have seen conflicting data on corn and buckwheat; they may or may not be tolerated. I have seen no data on quinoa, teff, and amaranth. You may need to experiment with these foods. If you have discovered this condition in yourself after years of symptoms, you would do well to rejuvenate your intestinal mucosa as outlined in the next section.

HEALING YOUR GUT AND DIMINISHING YOUR ALLERGIES

A leaky gut can seriously compromise your health—not just from acute and chronic allergic illness, which can be devastating enough, or acute digestive symptoms. Even worse, nutrients may not have found their way into your circulation and cells due to years of malabsorption. A leaky gut is usually characterized by damaged epithelial cells, flattened or inflamed microvillae unable to produce their enzymes and secretory IgA effectively and facilitate the absorption of nutrients.

In effect, you will incur nutrient deficiencies—not blatant enough perhaps to give you beriberi or scurvy, but significant enough to disorder your metabolism and either cause or predispose you to chronic disease and ill health. To make matters worse, a leaky gut will permit bacterial and fungal toxins to enter into your circulatory system, where they do not belong, and disorder your metabolism with predictable consequences.

To restore your intestinal mucosa to health:

1. Minimize, eradicate, or reverse those agents and conditions injuring your gut:
   - Food allergens.
   - *Candida albicans*/yeast overgrowth and other manifestations of intestinal dysbiosis.
   - Parasite infestation.
   - Alcohol consumption.
   - Nonsteroidal anti-inflammatory medication. Look hard for the underlying causes of the conditions requiring this medication so that less or none will be necessary. Have your physician find, if possible, less potentially damaging therapeutic agents for your conditions.
   - Stress overload.
   - Nutrient deficiencies.
   - Pancreatic enzyme or hydrochloric acid deficiency.

2. Use agents to nourish, soothe, and heal the cells of the small intestine and help reestablish healthy functioning.
   - There are many from which to choose. I often recommend that, for at least two to three months, people take folic acid, 400 to 800 micrograms a day; vitamin A, 15,000 to 25,000 I.U. a day; zinc, 15 to 30 mg a day; and vitamin C, up to 3,000 mg a day—all of which can be conveniently found in a hypoallergenic, multiple vitamin/mineral formula. I will also suggest quercetin (an antiallergic, anti-inflammatory herbal bioflavonoid discussed in Chapter Nineteen), 300 to 500 milligrams three times a day.

      Most importantly, I will suggest glutamine, 500 mg three times a day, best taken an hour before or two hours after meals (see Chapter Six). Instead of taking an L-glutamine supplement, I highly recommend a combination formula containing L-glutamine as well as N-acetyl-D-glucosamine, gamma linolenic acid (from borage oil), gamma oryzanol (from rice bran oil), and vitamin E. This product, Permeability Factors (by Tyler Encapsulations of Gresham, Oregon), is designed specifically to nourish and help heal the gastrointestinal mucosa.

      The amino acid L-glutamine is a preferential fuel for intestinal cells, aiding their growth and function. N-acetyl-D-glucosamine is actually made in the intestinal cells from glutamine; however, because many individuals are unable to make this conversion, it is included in the formula. The gamma linolenic acid, as discussed in Chapter Three, counters inflammation, and the gamma oryzanol provides antioxidant protection as well as a normalizing effect on gastrointestinal function. Take up to two capsules three times a day one hour or more before meals.

- I will also suggest the following herbal agents when indicated, most of which are discussed in Chapter Nineteen:
    a. Licorice root (deglycyrrhizinated) tablets or powder; slippery elm tea or capsules; goldenseal capsules (with slippery elm: 2 parts slippery elm, 1 part goldenseal); marshmallow root and plantain capsules (GI Encap by Thorne Research, Sandpoint, Idaho); aloe vera juice or gel. Roberts Formula or Bastyr B (Eclectic Institute, Sandy, OR) contains a combination of several herbs healing to the intestinal tract.
    b. Amino acids (hypoallergenic). Free-form multiple amino acid supplement, particularly helpful if weight loss and weakness are problems and if protein foods are not well tolerated.

You may find one or more of the agents or approaches in the list very helpful to you. I certainly do not recommend that anyone use this entire list all at once. Although some items may be quite useful to an individual, others may cause adverse reactions. It is important to work with a health practitioner experienced in treating food allergies so that the agents most suitable and correct for you are used. The picture, however, may not be black and white to your practitioner—some experimentation may still be necessary.

For the more severely affected and multiple-food-allergic patient, instead of quercetin, I usually recommend a very safe prescription drug called Gastrocrom (cromalyn sodium), to be taken fifteen to thirty minutes before meals. The contents of one or two capsules should be stirred in a small glass of warm water and taken orally.

This medicine can effectively block food reactions and associated inflammation, and enable eating without as severe restrictions.[23] By reducing the damage from allergic inflammation, cromalyn sodium can ultimately help the leaky intestinal mucosa heal.

Also for more serious cases, if DHEA (dehydro-epiandrosterone) levels are low (especially when cortisol levels are high), supplementary DHEA can help lessen the T–helper–to–T suppressor ratio and decrease one's overall hypersensitivity. If cortisol levels are low, adrenal supportive measures—even low doses of supplemental hydrocortisone, if necessary—may help substantially to diminish allergies (see Chapter Eleven).

For those at risk of developing vitamin and mineral deficiencies because of multiple food restrictions, I provide nutritional support initially through intravenous and/or intramuscular nutrient injections until adequate eating has been reestablished.

For those at risk of developing weight loss and weakness due to poor absorption or insufficient calorie intake, I recommend hypoallergenic, easy to assimilate nutrient powders to supplement the diet. One such formula is Ultra Clear Sustain (by Metagenics of San Clemente, California). It provides additional benefits to the food-allergic individual as it is fortified with glutamine, which nourishes intestinal cells; antioxidant amino acids, which enhance liver detoxification mechanisms and protect intestinal cells; and fructooligosaccharides, which nourish the lactobacillus bacteria of the bowel. Another good nutrient formula is ProGain (by Metagenics of San Clemente, California). For the extremely sensitive individual at risk of protein deficiency, I will also recommend a free-form amino acid formula, Aminoplex (by Tysons and Associates of Hawthorne, California).

The following additional agents can be helpful to diminish the symptoms of acute allergic reactions once they have occurred: buffered vitamin C, Alka-Seltzer Gold, vitamin B-6, and bowel evacuation (see page 247).

TESTING AND MANAGEMENT TECHNIQUES FOR FOOD ALLERGIES

There are many self-care approaches to help you detect your allergies. Not every individual has the inclination or capacity for self-testing, and there are a variety of good laboratory tests that can help determine the foods you are allergic to and the ones you can safely eat. The following sections include information on the detection and management of food allergies:

- "Self-Testing for Food Allergy on the Elimination Diet," page 245.
- "Alternate Foods for Allergen Avoidance," page 250.
- "Five-Day Fast for Allergy Relief and Identification," page 252.
- "The Pulse Test for Allergy Identification," page 254.
- "Coping with Food Allergies: The Rotary Diversified Diet," page 255.
- "Professional Testing for Allergies," page 260.

SELF-TESTING FOR FOOD ALLERGY ON THE ELIMINATION DIET

This program outlines a three-step process. First, eliminating the possible allergic foods from your diet. Second, carefully observing any changes in your symptoms—ideally, their reduction. And third, testing each eliminated food one by one and bringing it back into your diet and awaiting a recurrence or worsening of symptoms.

Step 1

To test yourself for possible food sensitivities, make a list of the foods and beverages that

- You eat repeatedly (daily or nearly daily—those you consume on four or more days a week).
- You crave (foods you think you cannot do without—you know the ones).
- You suspect make you feel bad.
- You suspect give you a pickup or stimulate you (these may also be the foods you crave).

Step 2

For ten to fourteen days, eliminate completely from your diet the foods or food groups in the list in step 1. It's best to eliminate all the foods on the list because multiple allergies are quite common. Hanging on to some of your favorites may render this test inaccurate, because even though you've avoided some of your allergic foods, the ones you may still be eating could be causing symptoms that mask any improvement. On the other hand, you need to set up a realistic testing program, one you feel you'll be able to stick to. For example, if there are six foods on the list and you don't feel that you can eliminate all of them, choose two or three to begin with, perhaps the ones that are most repetitive in your diet and the ones you crave most. Although this isn't an ideal test, you may still learn some valuable information.

I encourage you to do your best to eliminate all step 1 foods. In the long run this will give you far more accurate information to help you identify the foods you're allergic to. Study the alternate food choices box on page 250—you may find it much easier than you suspect to eliminate such staples as bread and other wheat products, milk and other dairy products, eggs, citrus fruits, and their juices, chocolate, corn, soy products, peanut products, tomatoes, and yeast—foods with very high allergy potential. And remember, the elimination period will only be for ten to fourteen days!

Important Hints for Your Elimination Diet

- Plan in advance. By knowing your available alternate food choices, by planning your meals and snacks, and by doing the shopping in advance (also your restaurant scouting), you will greatly improve your chances of sticking to the elimination diet and producing successful results. Remember, departing from the diet even once may render your test less accurate. Be as strict as you can for the elimination period. Choose a stretch of days that will not be interrupted by travel or heavy social or work obligations.
- Read ingredient lists carefully. You will discover that many packaged and processed foods contain numerous items from your step 1 list. Using such a product during the elimination trial will sabotage your results. Since milk is used in so many food products, be sure to check the ingredient lists for casein, lactalbumin, or whey (all derived from milk). The alternate food choice box on page 250 may help you identify food products that contain some of the more common food allergens, particularly cow's milk.
- Maintain adequate nutrient intake. The alternate food choice box offers a list of many alternate complex carbohydrates to replace wheat or whatever other carbohydrates you have listed in step 1, and many sources of animal protein to replace beef or chicken or whatever animal proteins you listed. Alternate sources of milk products are also listed. However, for the relatively short period of time you will be on this trial elimination diet, you need not worry about your calcium intake (unless calcium has been prescribed for you for medical reasons, such as hypoparathyroidism).
- Add your regular vitamins, minerals, and supplements to your step 1 list. Test your vitamins as you would the foods and beverages, since vitamin supplements commonly trigger adverse reactions, particularly if they contain wheat, soy, corn, milk, sugar, or food coloring/additives.
- Does your diet consist largely (or regularly) of processed and prepared foods—mixes, sauces, luncheon meats, instant dinners, or any foods that you have not made from scratch and that come in packages with long lists of ingredients? If so, you'd do well to add the following to your step 1 list: sugar, corn, soy, yeast, food coloring and preservatives, and other artificial additives. These ingredients are ubiquitous in the food processing industry and may be potent allergens for you.

    If you are not familiar with an unprocessed, whole-foods diet, see Chapter Three. If you have been following a whole-foods diet, using a minimum of processed foods, and if you're sure that corn, soy, and yeast products have not been repetitive items for you,

you may use them on your elimination diet. However, it would be preferable to avoid them, because they are foods with high allergy potential.

- If coffee and alcohol have been regular items in your diet, they should be added to the step 1 list and eliminated. It is essential to give these beverages just as high a priority in food allergy testing as any other repetitive item in the diet.
- Whenever you feel you just have to cheat and eat one or more of the foods you are supposed to eliminate, please remember that your test results may very likely be affected. For the days of this elimination diet, stick to the rules!
- Include foods on the elimination diet that you have not used often in the past. These items will likely have the least allergic potential and can add to the variety of your diet.
- Whenever possible, use organic produce and chemical- and hormone-free meats and poultry and foods free of additives. If organic produce is not available, scrub your produce thoroughly with soapy water or vinegar or baking soda in water. Clorox is said to be even more effective (see suggestions below).

Additional Food-Testing Suggestions

- Try to avoid drinking tap water, especially during the elimination diet and perhaps as a general rule, unless you have a good water purifier. Use certified pure bottled artesian or spring water if you can. Your local tap water may contain chemicals to which you have been reacting. Although distilled water can be used for testing purposes, it may not be the best choice for long-term use.
- Avoid your most commonly and repetitively used cooking herbs and spices. Reintroduce them eventually, as you will do with your step 1 foods.
- You may feel worse after the first few days on the elimination diet. Most likely you are experiencing withdrawal symptoms triggered by your body's craving for an allergic, addictive food that you haven't used for a few days. Irritability, fatigue, heart palpitations, muscle or joint aches or pains, headaches, excessive perspiration, gastrointestinal symptoms, cravings—these and more can occur as a result of not eating certain allergic foods. Just keep telling yourself that this is temporary, that all symptoms should subside by day four or five. The following supplements may help minimize withdrawal symptoms.

Sample Elimination Diet   The following sample elimination diet excludes twelve extremely common foods, although your list may be much shorter. Thanks to the food alternatives given on pages 250–251 and the food suggestions and recipes in Chapter Five, it really isn't all that difficult to follow such a diet for ten to fourteen days.

If you are eliminating wheat, milk, corn, sugar, coffee, alcoholic beverages, oranges and orange juice, peanuts and peanut butter, white potatoes, chicken, beef, and yeast, try the suggested substitute diet below.

BREAKFAST CHOICES
- Fruit, eggs, rice crackers, rye crackers (no yeast), rice mochi (a dense, chewy bread substitute available in health food stores), or any yeast-free muffin made without wheat or cornmeal flour. You can also use 100 percent rye bread toast or rye crackers or muffins made from one or more of the following: rice flour, barley flour, oat bran, or buckwheat flour.

DETOXIFYING YOUR PRODUCE

1. Fill the kitchen sink with water (approximately four gallons).

2. Add two teaspoons of Clorox, or if the sink holds only two gallons, then one teaspoon of Clorox.

3. Add fresh produce and let soak for fifteen minutes.

4. Then drain the water, fill sink again, and let produce soak another fifteen minutes.

5. Drain again and rinse or spray briefly.

6. If any Clorox smell remains, fill sink again, adding ¼ cup baking soda or vinegar, and let soak again, then rinse.

SUPPLEMENTS THAT MAY RELIEVE WITHDRAWAL SYMPTOMS AND ACUTE ALLERGIC REACTIONS

1. **Buffered vitamin C** (the ascorbate form containing calcium, magnesium, and potassium). Take 1,000 or 2,000 mg all at once—and in some cases more. Too much will cause intestinal gurgling and diarrhea. If this occurs, reduce the dose. For withdrawal symptoms use several times daily, best forty-five minutes to an hour or more before a meal, between meals, and at bedtime. For acute allergic reactions, use immediately upon recognition of the reaction and several times daily as needed.

2. **Alka-Seltzer Gold.** Take two tablets dissolved in sixteen ounces of water not more than twice in twenty-four hours for both allergic and withdrawal symptoms. Alternatively, you can take a mixture of two parts sodium bicarbonate to one part potassium bicarbonate, up to a maximum of one heaping teaspoon twice a day in any twenty-four hours. Use this mixture in at least twelve to sixteen ounces of water, followed by another full glass of water. It is dangerous to overuse these alkalinizing agents.

3. **Vitamin B-6.** Take 50 mg one to three times a day, or try 100 to 200 mg all at once (see Chapter Six for precautions).

4. **Drink a lot of water.**

5. **Take an enema or use an oral laxative such as unflavored milk of magnesia.** For withdrawal symptoms and particularly for acute allergic reactions, these measures may help your system clear the allergen more quickly. (See page 442 for enema instructions.)

- Boxed dry cereal (rice or oats) with no preservatives or additives, or cooked cereal (oatmeal, oat bran, rye, rice, or wheat- and corn-free eight-grain cereal). Use soy, rice, or almond milk on the cereal, which are pleasantly sweet. You can also use goat's milk or fruit juice. If you need a sweetener, use raisins, or currants, or a few dates cooked in with the cereal.
- Try rice cakes with almond, sunflower, or cashew butter, or sesame tahini. Also try goat's milk yogurt, with or without fresh fruit. You might want to add raw or lightly dry-roasted seeds and nuts other than peanuts.
- Fresh fruit other than citrus.
- Pancakes made from buckwheat and rice flours or any flours other than wheat and corn are quite tasty. Some mixes are commercially available. Beware of milk products as a hidden ingredient—always check the label.

LUNCH AND DINNER CHOICES
- Turkey, lamb, rabbit, elk, venison, goose, quail, pheasant, duck, or seafood.
- Steamed vegetables.
- Fresh vegetable salad.
- Baked squash, yams, or sweet potatoes. Wild rice, brown rice, millet, or buckwheat.
- Legumes, as in bean soups or bean dishes.

SNACKS, DESSERTS, AND BEVERAGES
- See Chapter Five.

Your Food Elimination Journal Keep a journal of before and after observations. "Before" refers to the elimination period when you are omitting suspect foods from your diet. "After" refers to the period when you are reintroducing the test foods (step 3). Try to make daily entries noting how you feel physically (presence or absence of body symptoms such as fatigue, pain, swelling, itching, diarrhea, bloating), emotionally (mood swings, depression, anxiety, irritability, anger, fear), and mentally (cloudy or foggy thinking, dull or slow thinking processes).

Before reintroducing a food, determine what your optimal mental ability and speed is for several tasks, such as counting backward from 100 using only odd numbers, or successively subtracting 7 from 100, or repeating a number of five or more digits that someone else is dictating to you. You may also want to test your before and after vision with an eye chart, or test your speech with another person, or compare your before and after balance and coordination.

Record all these findings in your journal before you begin your elimination diet, at the end of the diet, and then after you reintroduce the test foods. Your handwriting itself may be a valuable diagnostic tool, as allergies often affect the neurological and muscular systems of the body. Compare before and after samples of your handwriting; they may show graphic differences. And since allergic symptoms often affect the emotions and behavior, for important additional data ask a family member or good friend to record before and after observations of how you seem to them. In this way, you'll have a very useful record to study and refer to for additional clarification of your experience.

Feeling Better on the Elimination Diet?   After just five days on the elimination diet, you might be experiencing significant relief from your chronic allergic symptoms (although ten to fourteen days may be required). Like many individuals, you may be feeling so happy and so much better that you would be content never to return to your previous foods. Some of these step 1 foods, however, can be used without problems, and those that have been the allergic culprits can likely be reintroduced, after a period of avoidance, without adverse reactions. Proceed now to step 3 if you can say you are better after being on the elimination diet.

Not Feeling Better on the Elimination Diet?   If you've experienced no significant improvement after ten days on the elimination diet, try five to ten more days. If you're still no better, you may unwittingly have been eating allergic foods. You may need to follow the more stringent Caveman diet for five to ten days (see page 249) and, in addition, rotate your foods on a four- or five-day plan as outlined on page 256. If at this time you feel you have made significant progress, proceed to step 3. With multiple food allergies, it may be extremely important for you to remain on a rotation diet for the majority of your foods. You might consider instead other allergy relief and identification measures such as a hypoallergenic meal replacement powder program, for example, the Ultra Clear program (see page 180), or a more extreme approach such as fasting (see page 252 and Chapter Eighteen).

Lack of improvement on either the elimination or Caveman diet, however, may mean that you have another condition with symptoms similar to food allergy or that you have a condition coexisting with food allergy. Many individuals have several conditions at the same time and present quite a confusing picture even to health professionals. You may want to consider any of the following: candidiasis, bowel and liver toxicity, chemical hypersensitivity, poor digestion and assimilation, thyroid or adrenal conditions, or intestinal parasites. The master symptom survey on pages 17 to 29 may lead you to the appropriate condition. If self-help measures do not initially prove to be beneficial, an evaluation from an appropriate health care practitioner may uncover the possibility of underlying disease and help you get over the hump so that your own efforts eventually prove worthwhile.

Step 3

By this time, your allergic symptoms should be gone or greatly reduced. You may now begin to add back to your diet—one by one, in the prescribed manner—the foods you have been eliminating.

1. List all of the foods you eliminated in step 1, designating a number for each food. Put the foods with the highest allergic potential toward the bottom of your list—wheat, corn, milk products, eggs, peanuts, citrus, yeast, soy, tomatoes.

2. Now test your foods one at a time—each one over a four-day test period. Begin with test food #1, the first item on your list. You can also include other foods that you've been eating over the elimination period.

Day 1, Reintroduction Diet   For breakfast, eat a substantial helping of test food #1. Look for any symptoms of allergic reaction that may arise: headache, itching, irritability, foggy thinking, depression, fatigue, excessive cravings, compulsive eating, joint pains, sweats, burning or irritated mouth or throat, and so forth. If the food seems to make you feel unusually good or "high," this could also signal allergy—the stimulatory phase.

If any of these symptoms do arise soon after eating test food #1, you have just identified an allergic food. Record the symptoms and the time of onset in your journal. If allergic reactions are significant enough, use buffered vitamin C or the bicarbonates discussed previously (see page 247). Resume the elimination diet for the following four days or until your symptoms clear. Then proceed to test food #2.

If no apparent reaction occurs after your initial meal with test food #1, have another substantial helping with lunch that day. Again, watch for any symptoms that may arise. If you do detect a reaction, record the symptoms and time in your journal, use buffered C, and so on to counter the reaction. If necessary, wait several days until the symptoms clear and then proceed to test food #2. If no immediate reactions are apparent on day 1, stop eating test food #1 for the remainder of the four-day test period. Continue on with the elimination diet.

Days 2–4, Reintroduction Diet While on the elimination diet the next several days, look for the following:

1. Any symptoms of delayed allergic reactions that may arise.

2. Any symptoms that arise due to withdrawal. You might experience withdrawal particularly if eating test food #1 made you feel unusually good or "high." If withdrawal symptoms arise, they will come possibly on day 2, but more likely on day 3 or 4. These could be symptoms identical to those listed for an acute allergic reaction.

Eating the test food while experiencing withdrawal symptoms should cause the symptoms to vanish fairly abruptly—a telltale sign of an allergy. However, this would interfere with the testing of food #2, because of the new withdrawal symptoms that would likely arise again in two to four days. If needed, use buffered vitamin C or the bicarbonate as discussed previously.

Once all of your allergic or withdrawal reactions have cleared, which may take longer than the four-day test period designated for each food, proceed to test the next food on your list in the same manner as food #1. Subsequently test the remainder of your foods one by one in the same manner.

Once you have finished your food reintroduction testing, you may have three lists in your journal:

1. Foods that triggered relatively immediate reactions—including both adverse and stimulatory symptoms.

2. Foods that triggered delayed reactions, which would include both allergic and withdrawal reactions. You may not be able to distinguish between the two, but that isn't terribly important at this point.

3. Foods that seemed not to cause any noticeable reactions at all.

How to Set Up an Allergy-Free Diet Identifying allergic foods is an extremely important determination that should allow you to nourish yourself with minimal allergic assault. By eliminating the foods in lists one and two above as best you can for a period of three to six months and sometimes up to twelve months or more, you will allow your body to heal more fully and rebuild its immune system reserve. This period of avoidance should be sufficient to "break" the allergy and allow you to eventually reintroduce these foods one by one into your diet without suffering adverse reactions.

Adding a particular food after the avoidance period on a rotation basis—no more often than once every four to seven days and in small to moderate quantities—will allow you to enjoy it and derive its nutritional benefits without becoming allergic to it once again. Your body will let you know if you're eating the food too frequently. In too large quantities, your old symptoms will recur. If you have multiple food allergies and numerous debilitating symptoms, set up a rotating diversified diet where most of your foods are eaten no more than once every four to five days. This will allow you to eat and remain relatively symptom free. After six to twelve months or more, you should be able to relax somewhat on the rotation schedule.

To make this treatment work for you, you need more than commitment and willpower: you need practical, easy-to-understand information and support. See the sections on rotary diversified diet (page 255) and alternate food choices (page 250). Also see the suggested reading section at the end of this chapter, and try to find an allergy support group and/or an allergy-conscious nutritionist/health professional where you live.

If you have been experiencing severe symptoms or debility from food allergy, you would do well to use the items on list three on a rotating basis, not more than twice weekly. The fact that the foods in this group triggered no reactions when reintroduced doesn't mean they can be eaten indiscriminately. Many individuals are able to eat an "allergic" food two days in a row without a reaction, then suffer allergic symptoms (either immediate or delayed) after the third consecutive day. List 3 foods may therefore become allergic once you have surpassed your body's tolerance to them. On the other hand, they may be nonallergic, in which case rotation may be unnecessary.

It takes months to become adept at a rotation diet, familiar with what you need to rotate and what you can use repetitively. Rotation may seem impossible to a beginner. However, if your symptoms are severe enough and you discover just how good you can feel when not suffering from food reactions, you will find a way to make it work. Sally Rockwell's *Rotation Game* and *Mini-Series Guidebooks* can be of enormous help. See the Suggested Reading section in this chapter. Rotation will prevent you from developing new allergies and will keep your old ones at bay.

The "Caveman" or Stone Age Elimination Diet[24]

The Stone Age elimination diet includes all foods that were available to humans before the introduction of most farming and animal domestication practices. It was limited to what could be killed, picked, or dug up.

Because so many individuals have allergies to grains,

a grain-free elimination diet is a valuable option if you have not experienced much improvement on the standard elimination diet. This means no wheat, corn, rice, barley, oats, rye, triticale, millet, buckwheat, or even quinoa, spelt, or amaranth during the test period. It also means no bread, bagels, rolls, croissants, crackers, pretzels, cookies, cereals, noodles, or pasta. Cavemen also did not use milk products, so any and all such items should be eliminated during the five-to-ten-day test period. This includes milk, butter, cheese, cottage cheese, nonfat dry milk, kefir, and even yogurt and goat's milk products. Naturally, you must also exclude table sugar, alcoholic beverages, margarine, artificial food additives such as preservatives, colorings, and flavorings, and other such developments of civilized man.

However, in your new hunter-gatherer mode, you can eat all fruits, seeds and nuts, root vegetables (potatoes, yams, turnips, etc.), fowl, fish, beef, and eggs if these are not on your step 1 list. All the authors I have read on this subject also permit vegetables, which have a generally low potential for allergy. Some of the sources I have studied on the Caveman also permit legumes (beans). You can use natural sweeteners (listed on page 252), herbal teas, sea salt, and any of the items listed for this particular diet, *if* such items have not been regular or repetitive parts of your previous diet.

Use the same restrictions and precautions discussed for the elimination diet. Regardless of your previous diet, it would also be advisable to eliminate the foods most known for their allergic potential: citrus fruit, sugar, soy products (soybeans, tempeh, miso, tofu, soy nuts), eggs, chicken, peanuts, yeast, coffee, and caffeinated teas.

If constipation occurs, use one tablespoon of flaxseed powder mixed in eight ounces of water once or twice daily. Occasional use of herbal laxatives or milk of magnesia would be acceptable (see Chapter Eight for other bulk/fiber options).

ALTERNATE FOODS FOR ALLERGEN AVOIDANCE

While testing for allergies on an elimination diet or when planning meals and snacks to exclude allergic foods, you will find these lists useful. They will enable you to find alternate choices that provide roughly equivalent nutritional value.

For example, if your diet excludes wheat and oats, the whole grains list offers rice, rye, spelt, and other choices. If you cannot have cow's milk, the milk product list offers almond milk, soy milk, rice milk, rice ice cream, etc. If citrus is banned, under the fruit list you will find a large selection of other fruits. These lists may also remind you of foods that have been outside your habitual choices and may help you vary your diet more.

COMPLEX CARBOHYDRATES

WHOLE GRAINS

- Wheat: bread, rolls, muffins, buns, pretzels, bagels, scones, croissants, tortillas, chappati, cereals, pasta, gravies, pancakes, waffles, doughnuts, cookies, cakes, crusts. Bulgur, couscous, semolina, and durham are all in the wheat family.
- Rice: rice cakes, rice bread, rice noodles, rice cereals, mochi, rice pudding.
- Rye: rye crackers, 100 percent rye bread, rye cereals.
- Corn: corn tortillas, corn bread, corn noodles, cornflakes.
- Oats: oatmeal, oat bran cereal, oat bran muffins.
- Millet: as side dish, as cereal, or puffed millet.
- Other: quinoa (also available as pasta), amaranth, flours of rice, cornmeal, buckwheat, barley, oats, spelt, and quinoa, to make bread, muffins, cookies, pancakes, crusts, etc. Also consider

soy, potato, lentil, or garbanzo flour; chestnut or tapioca flour, kudzu root, and arrowroot (kudzu and arrowroot are commonly used as wheat substitutes for thickening gravies and sauces). Try artichoke or buckwheat pasta (both sometimes also contain wheat), or yam noodles. Try spelt (bread, pasta), kamut (cereal), and teff.

When using alternative nongluten flours, experiment with your recipes as they do not produce the same results as wheat flour. Try using different combinations such as rice or potato flours to lighten heavier oat, soy, or buckwheat flours.

STARCHY VEGETABLES

White potato, sweet potato, yam, winter squashes (acorn, hubbard, butternut, buttercup, delicato, pumpkin). Moderately starchy vegetables include such root vegetables as rutabaga, turnip, and parsnip.

LEGUMES (ALSO HIGH IN PROTEIN)

Lentils, split peas, soy, tofu, tempeh, black, adzuki, kidney, lima, and navy beans, garbanzos, peanuts.

PROTEIN (ANIMAL DERIVED) FOODS

Beef, pork, lamb, chicken, Cornish game hens, pheasant, quail, duck, goose, rabbit, elk, deer, and other wild game. Eggs (chicken, duck, goose, and quail eggs). All saltwater and fresh fish, shellfish, and mollusks. Milk products (see below).

SEEDS, NUTS, AND NUT BUTTERS (ALSO HIGH IN PROTEIN)

Almond, filbert, sesame, sunflower, pumpkin, cashew, pine, Brazil, pecan, pistachio, peanut, walnut, chestnut, beechnut, macadamia. There are far more nut butters than peanut. You might want to make or buy almond, filbert, cashew, sunflower, sesame, and pistachio nut butters. Seed and nut milks (see below "Milk Products").

OILS

(Unrefined, expeller pressed) sesame, sunflower, walnut, hazelnut, extra virgin or virgin olive, avocado, flax, almond, pumpkin seed.

MILK PRODUCTS

- Cow's milk: milk, cream cheese, cottage cheese, other cheeses, yogurt, kefir, buttermilk, sour cream, quark, ice cream. (Milk is a common hidden ingredient in baked items like quiches, biscuits, breads, pie crusts, and crackers. It is also frequently included in scrambled eggs, gravies, creamed soups, bisques, clam chowder, pancake and waffle mixes, cream sauces, bologna, hamburgers, meatloaf, sausages, milk chocolate, cocoa drinks, puddings, custards, doughnuts, mashed potatoes, and soufflés.) Dried milk, powdered milk, condensed milk, and evaporated milk all count as well. Any ingredient list with casein, lactalbumin, and whey contains cow's milk.

- Goat's milk, goat's milk yogurt, goat's milk cheese.
- Soy milk, soy cheese, and soy ice cream.
- Rice milk (Rice Dream™ or Amasake™) and rice ice cream (Rice Dream™).
- Almond milk (White Almond Beverage). See Chapter Five for seed and nut milk recipes.
- Ghee (clarified butter) is an acceptable substitute for regular butter.

SWEETENERS

Honey, molasses, maple syrup, malt syrup, rice syrup, fruit concentrate syrup, sucanat, stevia, dates, raisins, currants, figs.

VEGETABLES

Alfalfa sprouts, artichoke (globe and Jerusalem), asparagus, bamboo shoots, mung bean sprouts, beet greens, beets, bell peppers (sweet—red, green, yellow), cabbage, broccoli, cauliflower, bok choy, collard, kale, kohlrabi, carrots, celery, cucumbers, dandelion greens (young), jicama, lamb's quarters, leeks, lettuces, mushroom, onions, okra, parsley, parsnips, radishes, spinach, tapioca, zucchini, crookneck or summer squash, string beans, swiss chard, tomatoes, turnips and turnip greens, water chestnuts, watercress.

FRUITS

Apple, pear, plum, apricot, peach, cherry, nectarine, orange, lemon, lime, grapefruit, tangerine, quince, kumquat, mango, guava, kiwi, pineapple, banana, pomegranate, canteloupe, honeydew, watermelon, casaba and other melons, rhubarb, grapes, strawberries, blueberries, raspberries, gooseberries, loganberries, huckleberries, cranberries, boysenberries, blackberries.

FIVE-DAY FAST FOR ALLERGY RELIEF AND IDENTIFICATION[25]

Fasting has numerous benefits (see Chapter Eighteen). In connection with food allergy, fasting for approximately five days—eating nothing and drinking only fluids—totally (or nearly totally) eliminates food allergens from the body with resultant clearing or vast improvement of allergic symptoms and conditions.

Fasting can also serve as an additional method of food allergy diagnosis. After five days of fasting, your body becomes exquisitely sensitive to any allergic food or reacting chemical in foods. After this, when you ingest an allergic food, your body will respond with characteristic symptoms (headache, stomach cramps, bloating, joint pain, cloudy thinking, depression, and so on). This allergic response will usually occur within minutes or a few hours after the particular item has been eaten.

By testing foods one at a time after the fast, you can identify which ones are "safe" to eat and which are allergic. The heightened sensitivity of your immune system due to the clearing of allergens, and other effects of fasting, tends to accelerate delayed food reactions to within a period of several hours. However, some delayed food reactions will still occur in their normal time frames, rendering this method of diagnosis somewhat more complex.

The first few days of the fast are usually the most difficult. This is partly because you will want to eat, and partly because you may experience some uncomfortable and sometimes difficult withdrawal symptoms. But most of these should pass after the first few days. Follow the recommendations given on page 247 ("Supplements That May Relieve Withdrawal Symptoms and Acute Allergic Reactions"). Symptoms such as anxiety, irritability, depression, cramps, itching, sinus problems, headaches, and nausea are not caused by nutrient depletion or starvation. Rather, they indicate withdrawal from an allergy/addiction. Once this phase has passed, most food-addicted/allergic individuals feel better than they have in a long time. Many wish they did not have to begin eating again!

The Fast

Drink between two and four quarts of fluids daily (artesian or distilled water, freshly made fruit and vegetable juices, herbal teas, vegetable broth). Choose juices and teas that are not common items in your diet and ones that you are fairly certain have never caused and do not presently trigger any noticeable adverse symptoms.

Fasting on pure water alone would produce the most accurate results, but is a bit more difficult. If you have done some detoxification and fasting previously, you may be able to handle a water fast. If you have no previous fasting experience, a water fast may still be manageable; however, professional supervision is recommended.

Fasting is not for everyone. Those who have trouble fasting even on juices may find the Ultra Clear program an easier and effective alternative (see page 180). If you cannot afford to lose any weight or if you are debilitated or have a medical condition such as diabetes, asthma, epilepsy, or mental illness, I would advise you to consult an appropriate health care professional for advice and supervision.

Emptying the Intestines During the fast, it is advisable to empty the intestinal tract daily to aid in clearing allergens and bowel toxins from your system. Take a spring water enema daily (see page 442 for enema instructions if you are unfamiliar with this procedure). Or take two to four tablespoons daily of unflavored milk of magnesia; or do the salt water purge daily (see page 443).

Most food-allergic individuals will clear their symptoms in four to five days. Occasionally, for severe or more chronic cases, more than a week of fasting is required. This should be supervised by a health professional. If symptoms refuse to clear, the cause may not be food, but ambient chemicals or another condition. Here again, professional help is advised.

Specific Food Testing

Make up a list of foods for your testing schedule beforehand. At first you will have two "monomeals" a day, each of which tests one food at a time. Eat enough of any one food at a monomeal to fill you up. The portion may be two or four times the amount that you would customarily eat when the food is taken along with others at regular meals. If you test wheat, test only wheat, such as cooked wheatberries or a cooked wheat cereal with wheat as the only ingredient. And, of course, cook it in water alone and eat it alone with no milk or sugar or anything.

Do not use bread to test wheat because you would also be testing oil, yeast, and molasses or honey. If you had an adverse reaction after eating bread, you would not be sure which of the ingredients had caused it. If you cook a food in oil or butter, you won't know if you reacted to the food or to the oil or butter unless you have already tested them. Similarly, if you season a test item with an herb or condiment or anything else that you have not previously tested, confusion may result. Test things by themselves, and those that do not produce reactions can be used subsequently with seasoning or another item to test the latter.

The foods you rarely eat are those to which you are least likely to be allergic. Conversely, the ones you eat three or more days a week will be more likely to produce reactions. There are two ways to proceed:

1. By taking advantage of the increased sensitivity of your immune system immediately following the fast, you can "go for it"—introduce one by one the foods you most suspect. If previous testing methods have left you with a few uncertainties, introduce these uncertain items immediately after the fast to help clarify your understanding.

When reactions do occur, observe them carefully so you will know just how particular foods affect you. Record this in your journal (see page 247) and use buffered C or alkalinizing salts to help neutralize the reaction.

Using unflavored milk of magnesia can also accelerate the exit of an allergen.

However, one consequence of introducing suspected allergic foods and thus intentionally triggering a reaction immediately after a fast is that you will need to return to the fast because the allergic reaction must clear before testing the next item. This then brings us to the second method of testing for allergens.

2. By initially reintroducing foods of very low allergic potentials—foods that are infrequent items, or the ones that you've found to be quite safe from previous testing methods, or foods other than the most frequent allergens (wheat, corn, eggs, milk, soy, yeast, sugar, oranges, chocolate, peanuts, tomatoes, coffee, beef, chicken, pork)—then you should be able to get through any number of monomeals before encountering the first allergic reaction. When a reaction does occur, you can eat the recently determined safe foods until it clears.

Remember, the further you are from your fasting state, the more days you've been eating, the harder it will be for your immune system to produce the quick, clear-cut allergic reactions, particularly the accelerated delayed reactions, that it displayed immediately after the fast. However, even at this time your testing should yield fairly useful, accurate information if you stick to the monomeals, wait four to five hours between them, and maintain your journal record.

As residual pesticides, preservatives, coloring agents, and other chemicals found in most commercial food may trigger reactions, it's best to use organic and chemical- and additive-free foods for your testing purposes. If you are unable to find organic or chemical-free produce, see the recommendations for detoxifying your produce on page 246. Also, be sure to read "Important Hints for Your Elimination Diet," on page 245, which offers information pertinent to this method of testing.

Just how long can an individual eat two monomeals a day for the purposes of food allergy identification? If you include a balance of proteins, carbohydrates, and fats and use whole foods for your monomeals, you could proceed for many weeks. Of course, if your health begins to deteriorate because of insufficient calories or nutrients, you should temporarily stop the testing. Resume regular meals from your battery of safe foods. When you can, return intermittently to your monomeal tests.

Tobacco allergy is extremely prevalent in our culture. It contributes to dizziness, nausea, weakness, hypoglycemia symptoms, and fatigue. If you are a smoker, test for this sensitivity by quitting for five days or more, then chain-smoke up to six cigarettes. An adverse reaction may indicate that your allergic health problems have been caused not so much by foods as by tobacco allergy.

THE PULSE TEST FOR ALLERGY IDENTIFICATION[26]

For four to seven days, take your pulse before you get out of bed, before each meal, and then thirty minutes, sixty minutes, and ninety minutes after each meal, which should consist of your customary foods. Take your pulse before retiring. Take all pulse counts for a full minute and in the sitting position and not immediately after any vigorous exercise.

Keep a chart of all pulse recordings. If you have a cold or the flu, wait until it subsides. Smoking cigarettes during this testing period may invalidate the test, as it has been estimated that 75 percent of all humans are allergic to tobacco. You can test for tobacco allergy by taking your pulse before you smoke and then again fifteen minutes later.

Take a close look at the very lowest count—usually the one before rising—and the very highest. If the difference is more than twelve to sixteen counts, a significant rise, chances are you're allergic to something in your diet. The meals that produced such a significantly increased pulse at either thirty, sixty, or ninety minutes contain the allergic item or items. If a meal contained only one food, and caused a significant rise, it is fairly straightforward that you are allergic to that food. However, if the meal or meals contained too many food items to determine which ones caused the rise, proceed with the following plan.

Monomeal Pulse Testing

Make a list of all the ingredients of the meals in question. Over two, three, or more days test them one at a time as follows: Eat a small portion of the first item on the list, taking your pulse immediately before, then again at thirty minutes and at sixty minutes after ingestion of the food item. If your pulse has risen significantly at the thirty- or sixty-minute interval, this likely means that you have an allergy to the food.

You must wait at least sixty minutes or however long is required for your pulse to return to normal before testing the next food on your list. If you had no significant pulse rise after this first test item—compared with the pulse rate immediately before its ingestion—you probably have no allergy to this food and only need to wait thirty minutes before proceeding to test the next item on your list.

If your pulse rate on rising is consistently not the lowest in your record, it is likely that dust, some other inhalant allergen, or an environmental chemical in your home or bedroom is affecting you adversely. This also applies if there is a significant rise between your pulse on rising, and your pulse rate before breakfast.

All methods of allergy testing have their limitations.

The weakness of this particular approach lies in the frank possibility that not every allergic reaction will necessarily produce the biochemical responses that will result in a faster heartbeat.

COPING WITH FOOD ALLERGIES: THE ROTARY DIVERSIFIED DIET*

The key to the control of food allergies is the Rotary Diversified Diet. This diet serves three purposes. It is a diagnostic tool, which can unmask hidden food allergies in the course of normal life. It minimizes the development of new allergies, and is thus a preventive measure. And, finally, it helps the patient maintain tolerance to foods he already is able to eat. An individualized program can be worked out for any patient which will help to control the extent and spread of his food allergy. In fact, the Rotary Diversified Diet is more than just a medical maneuver: it is a *life plan* for anyone who wishes to remain well.

This diet was first developed by Dr. Herbert J. Rinkel in 1934. As the name implies, the diet is made up of a highly varied selection of foods. However, these foods are eaten in a definite *rotation*, or order, to prevent the formation of new allergies and to control preexisting ones.

At first, the diet may sound strange to people who have grown used to eating whatever they please, whenever they please. It sets some limits on what you can eat and when you can eat it. On the other hand, it should not be confused with any of the other dietary plans which are currently popular. The Rotary Diversified Diet is not a mass prescription based on sweeping generalizations such as "eat less meat," "eat more carbohydrates," or "do not eat sugar." It is an individualized plan, tailor-made for the patient, and for him alone: what works for him may not work for his neighbor.

When allergies to common foods were first discovered, it was natural for doctors to attempt to control them with diets. The type of diets employed in the early part of this century were either mainly diagnostic plans, designed to ferret out a hidden allergy, or treatment plans which left patients with sweeping prohibitions against "nuts," "fish," or "candies." Patients were not told when or how they could reintroduce such foods back into their diets.

Dr. Rinkel devised the Rotary Diversified Diet to fill the void created by these earlier plans. His original purpose in devising the diet was to avoid cumulative reactions. These are food reactions which occur if a person eats the same food over and over again, meal after meal. The constant, monotonous intake of any food promotes the development of a food allergy in a susceptible person. Dr. Rinkel believed that by rotating and diversifying foods, the probability of such problems building up could be minimized.

As he continued to use and evaluate this diet, however, Rinkel soon began to employ it on patients who readily developed *new* food allergies. In mid-1934 he used the diet on a woman patient who suffered from almost constant migraine headaches. She reported that she had not been free of headache for a single day during the previous ten years. Rinkel confirmed the seriousness of her illness by observing her over a period of several months.*

Rinkel achieved some success in treating her by eliminating first one food to which she was allergic and then another. But then, five to ten days after a suspected food had been eliminated, her symptoms would increase to their previous intensity. Each temporary, partial "cure" was followed by a very disappointing recurrence: What appeared to be happening was that the woman would eliminate one food—wheat, for example—only to develop a new allergy during the next week to her substitute food, oats. The new allergic reaction would bring back the original headache.

To prevent this from happening, Rinkel suggested she try something new. Specifically, he told her to *diversify* her diet, so that she ate many foods. He also instructed her to *rotate* her foods, that is, to repeat them only at specified intervals. If she ate corn at one meal she would have to, in effect, give her body a rest and not eat corn in any form for several more days. (Originally the interval ranged from one to three days: today it is generally longer.)

Within a few years, Rinkel was joined by a small but dedicated circle of allergists also employing the new technique. I myself began using the diet for my patients in the early 1940s. I have put thousands of people on this diet, and have seen the beneficial results it brings in the great majority of cases.

In devising a rotary diet for patients, I follow certain basic rules. Patients are instructed in these rules and given advice on how to follow them when they return home.

Rule 1: Eat whole, unadulterated foods.

Our ancestors generally ate their food in a simple form, without complicated mixtures, sauces, condi-

*From An Alternative Approach to Allergies by Theron G. Randolf, M.D., and Ralph W. Moss. Copyright © 1980 by Theron G. Randolph and Ralph W. Moss. Reprinted by permission of HarperCollins Publishers, Inc., and Ruth Hagy Brod Agency.

*Source: Herbert J. Rinkel, M.D., "Food Allergy, IV: The Function and Clinical Application of the Rotary Diversified Diet," J. Pediat., 32:266, 1948. Rinkel, Randolph, and Zeller, op. cit., p. 238.

ments, and the like. A diet such as this is cheaper, more readily available, easier to prepare, and more digestible than fancier fare.

Today, most of us have the ability to eat both simply *and* with variety. Culinary refinement, while pleasing to the palate, can sometimes be harmful to health, if it is pursued on a regular basis by susceptible individuals. The overrefinement of foods and their packaging for convenience or longer shelf life have led to abuses. Many people do not know what a diet of plain, simple foods tastes like or how good it can be. If a person tolerates beef, he can and should enjoy a steak, a hamburger, or a piece of boiled beef instead of, say, a meatball sandwich. If he eats steak, he has consumed *one food*—beef. He can then have another food, or several other foods, for his next meal. But the meatballs may contain beef, soy, pork, onion, oil, butter, milk, egg, black pepper, and wheat flour used as a "meat-stretcher." The bread will contain more wheat, rye, corn oil, yeast, sugar of some sort, caramel, lactic-acid cultures, and assorted chemicals. If the sandwich is topped with catsup, it will contain tomatoes, vinegar (grain, cider, or wine), corn sweetener, onion powder, spices, and flavorings. Mayonnaise will add more eggs and vinegar, as well as soybean oil and sugar (beet or cane).

Thus, what most people think of as a fairly simple meal—a meatball sandwich such as is available in many restaurants or "take-out" places—actually may contain *more than two dozen different foods*, including some of the most common allergy-causing substances—wheat, corn, beef, beet, milk, cane, yeast, soy, or eggs. Most likely it will also contain an assortment of chemicals as well.

If you are allergic to any one of these common items (and almost all food allergy patients are), you will not be able to discover this fact by sticking to the average American diet. The reason is that you will eat these common foods over and over again, every day, almost without letup. The symptoms caused by one or more of these foods may fluctuate, but they will never really be absent for long, because their cause is not absent for long. If you find that an average meal gives you reaction, it will be virtually impossible to track down the cause of that reaction when you are eating two dozen different foods at a sitting.

Rule 2: Diversify your diet.

In addition to eating whole, simple foods, the patient must learn to diversify his diet. The modern marketplace offers us a wide variety of different foods from various climates and cultures. We should make use of this diversity. Yet most people eat the same few foods over and over again, sometimes quite literally *ad nauseam*. Wheat, milk, beef, corn, beet or cane sugars, and eggs, in their many varieties and disguises, represent the monotonous basis of the American diet. Some people even brag of being "meat and potato men," who must have these two foods in order to feel satisfied (an almost certain sign of food addiction).

Patients can learn to diversify their food choices. The world is filled with an enticing variety of foods which they can exploit for both enjoyment and good health. For example, few people enjoy (or have even tasted) all of the foods in a well-stocked fruit and vegetable market. They become stuck on certain often-repeated favorites, such as carrots, celery, and lettuce, and bypass what is unfamiliar. Turnips and parsnips are rarely eaten as vegetables in their own right, although they make a delicious dish. Some people have never tasted artichokes, avocados, mangos, or papayas. Each of these can form the basis of a satisfying meal.

Some foods are only eaten on special occasions or in special combinations. Cranberries are highly popular at Thanksgiving, but are rarely eaten at any other time of the year; yet they can usually be incorporated into the diet with little trouble, and in many markets they can be purchased fresh throughout the fall season.

The foods of other countries offer interesting possibilities. Many markets now carry bean sprouts (mung or alfalfa) and (soy) bean curd. Bean sprouts can be readily grown in a jar in the kitchen if they are not available in the store. Health food stores usually stock a wide variety of Japanese foods. The larger cities have stores, listed in the Yellow Pages, which sell speciality foods of other nationalities. There is much to be gained by learning to enjoy the cuisine of cultures other than one's own.

In fact, the Rotary Diversified Diet is in some ways less limited, and more enjoyable, than the supposedly unrestricted but monotonous American diet. It calls on you to eat in a controlled, rational way, but within the plan it offers great latitude for innovation and experimentation with food.

Rule 3: Rotate your diet.

Patients are told that they can develop an allergy to any food if they eat it day in and day out and are susceptible to it. This is as true of the more exotic foods as it is of beef, potatoes, or eggs. A colleague of mine once attempted to practice clinical ecology in Taiwan. He soon discovered that the Chinese people of that island had widespread allergies to the foods eaten there, especially soy and rice, but also including others, some of which are rare by American standards.

The whole point of this diet is to let the body recover from the effects of a food before eating it again. In general, it takes up to three days for a meal to pass through the human digestive system. To be safe, we allow four days between ingestions of a particular food.

In general, patients are instructed to have only three meals per day. They can eat as much as they wish, although they are encouraged to eat portions of normal size. (The diet is also an excellent way to lose weight.)

If he follows a four-day rotation, the patient can eat a particular food on Monday and then eat it again on Friday. Thus, if he has wheat on Monday, he will have to count four days following Monday before he can have wheat again. Bear in mind that this means wheat *in any form*: bread, spaghetti, lasagna, cream of wheat, even the breading on a pork chop. It is important to add that, for the purposes of this diet, wheat is identical to rye, barley, malt, and millet. Of course, if the patient continues to eat the average American diet, he could not manage that, since there is wheat (or a related grain) in almost every typical meal. But on the Rotary Diversified Diet, it is not difficult to avoid unknown or unsuspected ingredients in foods.

While four days is what we might call the "legal limit" on food repetition, many patients go on a seven-day cycle. This allows them to eat the same basic diet each week. The diet can be posted on the refrigerator and is easy to follow. All the patient needs to begin a seven-day food cycle are twenty-one foods to which he is not allergic.

Rule 4: Rotate food families.

Foods, whether animal or vegetable, come in families. Some of these are fairly obvious: cabbage, kale, broccoli, and cauliflower, for example, all taste somewhat similar and are clearly related. You probably would not guess, however, that they are in the mustard family, which also includes horseradish and watercress. Similarly, you would not automatically know that cashews, pistachios, and mangoes are in the same group or that beef and lamb are in the same family but that deer and elk are in a separate group.

Food families are important in devising a Rotary Diversified Diet because patients can cross-react to the "relatives" of food to which they are allergic. Thus, if you are allergic to beef you must suspect goat (not to mention veal and milk, both of which are seen as similar to beef by the body—veal being young beef, and milk a product of the female of the species). People who are allergic to potato must suspect other members of its family, including tomato, green pepper, red pepper, chili, eggplant, and tobacco. (Tobacco, however, should be shunned by everybody.)

Another reason why it is important to be aware of food families is to prevent the formation of allergies by a steady consumption of foods which are members of the same family. If you eat tomato on Monday, eggplant on Tuesday, potato on Wednesday, green pepper on Thursday, and tomato again on Friday, you are not re-ally rotating foods—you are eating from the same food family every day, and this could develop into an addiction to one or all of these items.

Thus, the ingestion of foods which are members of the same family must be spaced, but not quite as strictly as foods themselves. The rule is that the patient must *rotate food-family members every two days*. Using the above example, it might be perfectly all right to have tomato on Monday, eggplant on Wednesday, and tomato again on Friday, provided that no other members of this family were eaten in between.

If a patient has a known allergy to a particular food, he must also avoid the other members of that food family, at least for a while. Thus, sensitivity to beef brings with it a ban on beef, beef by-products such as gelatin, margarine, and suet, milk products, veal, buffalo, goat, lamb, or mutton.

Rule 5: Eat only foods to which you are not allergic, at first.

Patients who are emerging from the [testing phase] are given a summary of their food-test reactions. They therefore know which of the most common foods cause reactions and which do not.

Upon going home, one of their goals is to test other foods which were not evaluated in their weeks in the hospital. If a new food causes no reactions, then it can be added to the Rotary Diversified Diet to give greater variety to the meal plan.

On the other hand, the diet serves as a perpetual diagnostic screen, helping patients to avoid unsuspected sources of mental and physical complaints. It can readily detect the first signs of an adverse reaction to any food, since that food is not in one's system at the time it is eaten.

Basically, there are two kinds of food allergies—fixed and nonfixed, or temporary. A fixed allergy is one with which you are probably born, which does not go away with time. These are relatively less common. More frequently, patients can regain tolerance to troublesome foods after a period of some months of avoidance. The greater the reaction to a food, the longer it takes, in general, to reestablish tolerance. The process usually takes from two to eight months, after which the food can usually be eaten again, if used in rotation. Since the incriminated food is often a favorite and is craved in an addictive manner, the hope of regaining tolerance to it offers some consolation to the patient suffering its temporary loss. Until and unless such tolerance is regained, however, the patient cannot safely use an allergenic food. Moreover, it must not be abused by cumulative intake when it is returned. Re-sensitization occurs very readily and very subtly.

One exception to this rule is the so-called universal

reactor. As mentioned earlier, such a person is allergic to *all* or most foods, and will get sick no matter what he eats, although he feels tolerably well on a fast. Naturally, he cannot avoid all foods to which he is allergic or he will starve. In this case, we do the next best thing. He is instructed to eat only those foods to which he has lesser reactions.

In addition, other procedures can be employed to benefit such patients. Some clinical ecologists employ "neutralizing doses" in the treatment of this condition. A "neutralizing dose" is an infinitesimally small amount of the offending substance. If this dose, placed under the tongue, is at just the right dilution, it will have the effect of turning off a reaction. The same substance in a larger dose will, of course, cause a renewal of symptoms. This seems contradictory, but the effectiveness of the neutralizing dose is attested to by many clinical ecologists.

With the exception of universal reactors, all patients are instructed to keep away from the foods which cause their reactions until these can safely be reworked into the diet.

With these five rules in mind, patients are instructed in how to construct a Rotary Diversified Diet to fit their needs. The diet is an essential part of their treatment. Construction of the diet is essential for such patients, and I employ several well-trained registered nurses whose job it is to instruct patients on the construction of the plan.

It has been explained that four days is a sufficient interval between feedings of any particular food, and that a patient can eat any food to which he is not allergic, provided that he sticks by the rules of rotation. Thus, if a patient wishes, he could have quite a few foods at a meal and then repeat that same meal four days later, *provided* he did not have any of those foods in the intervening time.

For the sake of simplicity, however, let us make the time interval in the following sample diet seven days. Also, for the sake of this presentation, let us assume that the patient eats only one food per meal. This is, of course, not necessary. If he has the tolerance, he can eat a number of foods at each meal.

Following the above-mentioned rules, the patient with at least twenty-one tolerated foods can construct a Rotary Diversified Diet for himself. Here is one such sample diet:

	BREAKFAST	LUNCH	DINNER
Sunday	Fresh or frozen melon	Steamed broccoli	Boiled shrimp
Monday	Poached eggs	Cracked wheat porridge	Broiled steak
Tuesday	Natural applesauce (no sugar)	Cooked lima beans	Pork chops
Wednesday	Hot oatmeal	Steamed zucchini (squash) slices	Chicken
Thursday	Orange slices, plus orange juice	Black-eyed peas	Salmon steaks
Friday	Fresh grapes, plus grape juice	Boiled brown rice	Lamb chops
Saturday	Grapefruit, plus grapefruit juice	Baked flounder	Fresh leg of turkey

You will notice that no food is repeated during the week. Also, no two members of a food family are eaten two days in succession. For example, eggs and chickens are in the same family, but eggs are eaten on Monday and chicken on Wednesday. Squash and melon are related, but they too are separated by a day, as are wheat and oatmeal.

Remember, also, that "apples" means apple *in any form*. At this meal, the patient can have whole apples, apple juice, applesauce, and so forth, provided that the dish to be consumed contains *nothing else*. If anything else is added, it must be counted as a separate food. In other words, if the person sprinkles cinnamon on top of the applesauce, this counts as an item in the Rotary Diversified Diet, and it must be eaten in accordance with the rules. This would mean, for example, that the patient could not have cinnamon again for four days, or members of the cinnamon family (avocado, bay leaf, sassafras) for two days. If sugar is added to the applesauce, this eliminates that type of sugar for four days. One of the dangers of eating commercially prepared foods is that labels are not required to state *what kind* of sugar has been added to food. It is therefore best to avoid foods to which sugars have been added.

It must be emphasized that cane, beet, and corn sugar are specific foods,[*] although cane and beet sugar are chemically indistinguishable, both being called sucrose. In contrast to these double sugars, corn sugar is a molecule one-half their size, most commonly called dextrose, glucose, corn sweetener, or fructose (although fructose for intravenous purposes is usually made from sucrose).

Source: Theron G. Randolph, M.D., "The Role of Specific Sugars," in Dickey, ed., op. cit., pp. 310–320.

It is a good idea, for the sake of variety, to eat a food in a number of different forms at any one meal. In addition, if the patient cooks his meat in a tolerated water he can then drink the resulting juice hot as a delicious soup. Salt can be added to taste, since salt is one food to which people rarely develop allergies. However, salt should not be used excessively by anyone.

In the above basic diet, I have chosen fairly "normal" foods for each time of the day. For example, most people already eat such things as eggs, melons, and oranges for breakfast. Americans are also accustomed to eating their heavier, meat dishes in the evening. Remember, however, that this is purely conventional. There is no physiological reason to do this and, in fact, in different cultures people have different ideas about what constitutes an acceptable breakfast food, or when people should eat their biggest meal.

Patients are therefore urged to break with food stereotypes when preparing meals. For example, one can eat a piece of plain poached fish, such as flounder or cod, for breakfast. At other breakfasts, one can have meat or vegetables. Flexibility in this regard helps the patient succeed in following the plan.

The diet given above assumes that the patient is not allergic to any of the listed foods. But what if he is allergic to some of them, as is likely, since this chart contains some of the most common allergy-causing foods? In that case, the patient must substitute other foods of known safety, or foods which he is about to test for compatibility. Let us say, for example, that the patient is allergic to all grains and to pork. In that case, his Rotary Diversified Diet might look like this:

	BREAKFAST	LUNCH	DINNER
Sunday	Fresh or frozen melon	Steamed broccoli	Boiled shrimp
Monday	Poached eggs	Dates (instead of wheat)	Broiled steak
Tuesday	Natural applesauce (no sugar)	Cooked lima beans	Baked yams (instead of pork)
Wednesday	Pineapple (instead of oatmeal)	Steamed zucchini (squash) slices	Chicken
Thursday	Orange slices, plus orange juice	Black-eyed peas	Salmon steaks
Friday	Fresh grapes, plus grape juice	Bananas (instead of rice)	Lamb chops
Saturday	Grapefruit, plus grapefruit juice	Baked flounder	Fresh leg of turkey

Is such a diet balanced? In my opinion, it is. There is an adequate amount of carbohydrate, calories, protein, and other food constituents over the course of a week to maintain health. Does the patient get enough vitamins and minerals on such a diet? In my experience, the consumption of whole (and especially organic) foods, served fresh, will provide better nutrition than the average American diet, even when the latter is supplemented with vitamin pills. In general, I do not recommend vitamin supplements to patients on this diet.

Although some vitamins are made from foods, the majority are manufactured synthetically. The Food and Drug Administration, which regulates this area, does not distinguish between so-called natural and synthetic vitamins, since both have the same structural chemical formulas. If the vitamin is made from sprouted wheat (as are some of the B-vitamin supplements), you may be creating or perpetuating a susceptibility to cereal grain. This is a fact which is overlooked by many vitamin proponents.

I am not against vitamins—far from it. But I believe it is always preferable to obtain vitamins from their natural source, in whole foods, rather than through a supplement, which may contain traces of various chemicals or foods, including additives (cornstarch, milk lactose, and so forth) that can aggravate allergic problems.

The Rotary Diversified Diet represents a profound step forward in man's understanding of how to eat. For millennia, man ate what came to hand, and did well—well enough to survive, at least. In the last few thousand years, however, civilization has altered man's eating patterns and in many ways disrupted our natural balance with the environment. It has taken science to show us how to eat properly under these new conditions. The first big breakthrough was analytical nutrition. This is the nutrition taught in most schools and preached in newspapers, on television, and in numerous books and articles. According to this concept, all food can be reduced to certain neatly defined constituents in pigeon-holed categories—proteins, carbohydrates, vitamins, and the like. An adequate diet, according to this school of thought, is one which provides a given *quantity* of these various nutrients every twenty-four hours. Ross Hume Hall calls this "adding machine" dietetics.

This theory fails to take into account the individual nature of foods and, in particular, the individual nature of each human being. The reaction between the unique individual and his environment is what really matters, especially to a sick person and his physician. This orientation is best referred to as biologic dietetics or nutrition.*

Clinical ecology shows us how to restore the balance between man and his environment under the conditions of advanced civilization. It recognizes the unique aspects of both sides of this interaction, including the still-unexplored way in which the human body can "recognize" a particular food, even in its most disguised forms.

The Rotary Diversified Diet is the outcome of this new perspective. It is a breakthrough in medicine at least as important as the discovery of "adding-machine" nutrition. It is at once our best means of diagnosis, treatment, and prevention of chronic food reactions.

PROFESSIONAL TESTING FOR ALLERGIES

Several kinds of allergy tests exist that may help you identify your food allergies. See "Laboratories for Allergy Testing" at the end of the chapter. The most common procedure ordered by conventional allergists is the "scratch" test. It is quite satisfactory for identifying inhalant allergies, but it's notoriously inadequate for diagnosing food allergies. The scratch test may accurately pick up Type I IgE, mediated food reactions, but it will miss delayed food reactions—the category into which most food allergies fall. Other tests have a much higher degree of accuracy for pinpointing delayed food allergies: the IgG RAST; IgG Food Immune Complex Assay (FICA); cytotoxic test; antigen leukocyte cellular antibody test (ALCAT); ELISA-ACT test; electronic screening; and biokinesiology.

RAST, RASP, and ELISA Methods of Food Antibody Detection

The RAST and RASP (radioallergosorbent test and radioallergosorbent procedure) are blood tests that determine the presence and level of IgG antibodies (actually, the subclass IgG-4) and IgE antibodies in the blood for specific foods and some food fractions. If high levels of these specific antibodies are found, you and your doctor should suspect that the corresponding foods are allergenic for you. Some RASTs measure only IgE levels (available for foods and inhalants). Some laboratories offer a combined IgG and IgE RAST.

Several labs have recently changed over to the ELISA method of antibody detection (enzyme-linked immunoserological assay), which appears to be somewhat more sensitive than the RAST and is less expensive. (The radioactive components of the RAST increase its cost.)

*Source: Theron G. Randolph, M.D., "Biologic Dietetics," in Dickey, ed., op. cit., pp. 107–122.

Cytotoxic Testing

The cytotoxic test, a blood test, determines if blood cell damage or destruction occurs when the cells are exposed to the allergic or toxic substance. This test is said to be sensitive to both the delayed antibody-mediated allergic reactions and the cell-mediated toxic reactions.

Although comprehensive, the cytotoxic test has the highest potential for human error, since it consists of a human technician looking in a microscope who grades the changes in cellular size and shape. Futhermore, any tests that are not run on the spot are subject to gross inaccuracies because of the unavoidable and increasing damage that blood cells incur in the time that lapses between the blood draw and the actual running of the test. Done competently by an experienced technician, the cytotoxic test is considered by many clinicians to be a reliable and very economical test.

ALCAT

The antigen leukocyte cellular antibody test is, in effect, a more technological version of the cytotoxic test. Changes in cellular size and shape are assessed by a sophisticated coulter counter rather than a technician, thus removing the potential for human error. However, ALCAT is more costly than the cytotoxic test.

ELISA-ACT

The ELISA-ACT (enzyme-linked immunoserological assay activated cell test) is a test that, like the cytotoxic and ALCAT, measures the effect of delayed antibody- and cellular-mediated reactions. Whole plasma, not just serum or cells, is used because it contains all immunologic components. Test results, therefore, reflect a dynamic response to the foods tested and less of a static laboratory measurement. The test is considered by some authorities to be one of the most accurate, sensitive, and comprehensive.[27]

An added feature of this type of testing is the assessment of hypersensitivity to a broad range of common food additives, heavy metals, and environmental chemicals. A recently refined method of drawing and transporting blood, which, in effect, produces suspended animation of the cells, makes it possible for the ELISA-ACT to produce accurate results when blood samples are mailed. At this time, I favor this test over others.

Electronic Screening

The allergy tests just discussed provide in vitro (external, out of the body) measurements of blood samples. An emerging in vivo (in the body) technique of allergy identification is electronic screening, placing an electromagnetic instrument at specific acupuncture or meridian points to enable your body to communicate directly—electromagnetically—what it knows about itself. In this case, it will indicate which foods you are allergic to.[28]

Unlike blood tests, electronic screening also has the ability to find phenolic sensitivities. Phenolics are naturally occurring biochemicals found in many foods. If you have multiple food allergies, it may be that several phenolics common to many of your allergic foods are actually the components triggering the reactions.[29]

Electronic screening not only offers information concerning what foods and phenolics you might be reacting to, but provides a homeopathic desensitization treatment (oral drops) of your specific allergic foods and phenolics. Over time, such treatment should curtail your allergies and lessen the need to avoid particular items. Although it is wise to eliminate the foods that are making you sick, because electronic screening operates on an energy level, it may act to circumvent or at least ameliorate the more conventional, allergen-restricting approach.

With the newer computer-assisted electronic screening devices, your body can directly communicate information relating to allergies and toxicities in an extremely cost- and time-effective manner. There is nothing invasive about the testing procedure; not even acupuncture needles are used. It is ideally suited for children.

What makes electronic screening so exciting is its ability to uncover not only what you're allergic to, but why you're allergic. It can help detect conditions that have not yet surfaced, such as subclinical infections, chemical toxicities, and organ or glandular weaknesses. It can also help determine the correct remedies for treatment. Electrodiagnosis is a true tool for preventive medicine.

However, it is important to note that the accuracy of electrodiagnosis depends to a large degree on the skill and experience of the technician or physician administering the test. Although this technology has yet to be accepted by the conventional medical community, some of the devices have met standards required for FDA approval as an investigational device, and thousands of practitioners worldwide and decades of clinical use have established it as one of the more promising and effective modalities emerging today.

Biokinesiology/Applied Kinesiology

Biokinesiology is another useful method for diagnosing food allergies. A form of muscle testing used widely by chiropractors and by other health professionals as well, this technique allows the body to communicate what it knows to the practitioner. In the right hands, it may be able to provide an allergy diagnosis equally accurate, and far less costly than laboratory methods discussed above.

One common example of a muscle test consists of the patient holding a sample of the suspected allergen in one hand, while holding the other arm straight out. The patient attempts to keep it horizontal while resisting the tester, who tries to push the arm down. As crude as this method may seem, a broad range of diagnostic information is available through applied kinesiology. Like electrodiagnosis, many subclinical conditions can be detected with this method and treated.

Because subjective factors can easily render this test invalid and the accuracy of diagnosis depends largely upon the tester, biokinesiology has been subjected to much scientific criticism. Nevertheless, my initial skepticism concerning this method has been largely dissipated by the results I have seen in several patients of mine who were greatly helped by an experienced practitioner of biokinesiology.

Clinical Ecology (Environmental Medicine)/Immunotherapy

Environmental medicine is the specialty of medicine dedicated to the diagnosis and treatment of environmentally induced illness. Environmental medicine has, in recent years, replaced the term "Clinical Ecology"; and "clinical ecologist" has been replaced with "practitioner of environmental medicine" or "environmental medicine specialist"—a recognized specialty certified by the American College of Environmental Medicine.

Practitioners of environmental medicine are doctors who look closely at nutritional status, food allergy/ intolerance, chemical toxicity/hypersensitivity, polysystemic candidiasis, hormone hypersensitivity, autoimmune conditions, and the immune dysregulation these and other factors can produce. They may use the tests previously discussed. But they also have at their disposal the added modalities of intradermal and sublingual testing and immunotherapy.

The application of immunotherapy can boost the immune system beyond levels achieved through self-help techniques. It begins with the precise identification of the substances (allergens) causing allergic reactions. Using intradermal food antigen injections of varying dilution strengths, a specialist will attempt to provoke allergic symptoms and then proceed to find the dilution that neutralizes or reverses the symptoms (provocative neutralization).[30] Both the skin reaction at the site of the injection and systemic symptoms are evaluated for immediate as well as delayed reactions (twenty-four and forty-eight hours later).

Traditionally, only six (or at the most ten) foods a day are tested so as not to cloud the picture or weaken a patient. Conventional allergists will generally use the scratch test (although some will use the intradermal method). They will test up to twenty or even forty or more foods at once, looking only for immediate reactions (not delayed) and will check only for skin reactions (not systemic symptoms). The individualized vaccines from environmental medicine specialists will usually begin to bring relief within a month. However, those from conventional allergists may take up to a year.

For individuals who cannot lessen their exposure to the offending agents, or those whose health has been drastically compromised, or those for whom self-help efforts have been unsuccessful, immunotherapy may contribute to a successful program for recovery. With immunotherapy, many individuals find that they can continue to eat an allergenic food or breathe an allergic inhalant without developing as severe a reaction. To locate a physician practicing environmental medicine in your area, contact the American College of Environmental Medicine or the Human Ecology Action League (see Resource List Organizations).

Taking a shortcut to the above methods is sometimes effective. Standardized antigen drops to common allergens, such as wheat, soy, and milk, have been made into uniform dilutions and are available commercially through naturopathic physicians and other nutritionally oriented practitioners, and sometimes through health food stores. You can begin this standardized type of immunotherapy by obtaining the appropriate antigen drops. Various brands may have varying antigen concentrations and different dosage instructions. As with allergy injections, they have the potential initially to aggravate your symptoms, so it is best to work under the guidance of a health professional. Some individuals find that the standardized strength will be sufficient to improve the condition. Others, however, will require a more individually tailored vaccine administered by an environmental medicine specialist.

Deciding Which Allergy Test Is Right for You

All methods of allergy testing have their strengths and limitations. On the one hand, I have seen many individuals successfully handle their food sensitivities through self-testing measures and their own dietary adjustments. I have also seen many successfully adjust their diets by using the information obtained from laboratory tests. I have also seen people do equally well with electronic screening, biokinesiology, and immunotherapy. All of these methods help people significantly, if not dramatically. However, it is important to remember that, even with these tests, once you learn which foods to suspect, you will need to avoid them and go on an elimination diet.

On the other hand, I have seen individuals frustrated and confused by their self-testing efforts, and others overwhelmed by blood test results that told them to eliminate too many foods and rotate too many others. I have seen others who felt the electronic screening and biokinesiology methods were inconsistent, contradictory, and plainly unhelpful. And I have seen individuals who were dissatisfied with the results of working with an environmental medicine specialist and tailored vaccines.

So, where do you begin? How do you proceed? In general, when I suspect food allergy in my patients, I recommend that they begin with an elimination diet (see page 245), while I start to look for underlying causes of the apparent food sensitivities. Before launching a full-scale and potentially expensive direct investigation of food allergy, it is my practice to check initially for predisposing conditions, since food allergy may be only a symptom of a deeper problem (see page 242). Even if this is the case, depending on the severity of your state, finding and eliminating culprit foods may be essential before you can begin to experience an improvement.

In some instances, there is no treatable underlying cause for your food allergies, and you may just have to eat around them. Using the elimination diet in particular (page 245) and some of the other self-help approaches in this chapter may help you considerably. However, if you feel you're in over your head, be sure to consult a health professional who is familiar and experienced with one or more of the testing approaches discussed. Under "Organizations" in the bibliography, you will find resources to help you locate such physicians.

Allergy test results can be overwhelming and discouraging. This is why they should always be backed up by a thorough explanation and nutritional counseling from an expert so that you have a clear understanding of the workable alternatives and how to proceed. Some allergy-testing laboratories will provide a computerized rotation diet individually tailored to your test results. This greatly facilitates the implementation of allergy-free eating. Such guidelines can be quite comforting, particularly if you score allergic to twelve or more of your most common and favorite foods. Find out in advance what to expect from your health care practitioner regarding assistance in implementing test results.

SUGGESTED READING

Bates, Charles E. *Beyond Dieting: Relief from Persistent Hunger*. Courtenay, B.C./ Olympia, WA: Tsolum River Press, 1994.

Berger, Stuart M., M.D. *Dr. Berger's Immune Power Diet*. New York: New American Library, 1985.

Crook, William Grant, M.D. *Detecting Your Hidden Food Allergies*, 1988. Available from Professional Books, P.O. Box 3464, Jackson, TN 38301.

Donovan, P.M., and Jaffe, R. M. *Health Assurance: Your User Guide.* Reston, VA: HSC Press, 1995.

Faelton, Sharon, and the editors of *Prevention* magazine. *Allergy Self-Help Book.* Emmaus, PA: Rodale Press, 1983.

Golas, Natalie Francis. *Coping with Your Food Allergies.* New York: Simon and Schuster, 1986.

Hills, Hilda C. *Good Food, Gluten Free.* New Canaan, CT: Keats, 1976.

Mandell, Marshall, M.D., and Scanlon, Lynn Walter. *Dr. Mandell's Five Day Allergy Relief System.* New York: Thomas Y. Crowell, 1979.

Randolph, Theron G., M.D., and Moss, Ralph W., Ph.D. *An Alternative Approach to Allergies.* New York: Lippincott/Crowell, 1988; HarperCollins, 1990.

Rapp, Doris J., M.D. *Allergies and the Hyperactive Child.* New York: Cornerstone Library, Simon & Schuster, 1979.

———. *Is This Your Child? Discovering and Treating Allergies.* New York: Morrow, 1991.

———. *Allergies and Your Family.* New York: Sterling Publishers, 1982.

Rapp, Doris J., M.D., and Bamberg, Dorothy, R.N., Ed.D. *The Impossible Child in School, at Home: A Guide for Caring Teachers and Parents.* Available from Practical Allergy Research Foundation, P.O. Box 60, Buffalo, NY 14223-0060. Also available from Life Sciences Press, P.O. Box 1174, Tacoma, WA 98401.

Reading, Chris M., M.D., and Meillon, Ross S. *Your Family Tree Connection.* New Canaan, CT: Keats, 1988.

Rockwell, Sally. *Mini-series Guidebooks: How to Start an Elimination "Caveman" Diet; How to Use a Food and Symptom Diary and Begin to Rotate;* and *Allergy-Free Baking Tips for Special Flours.* Also see *Rotated Allergy Recipes* and the videotape, "Yes, There's Still Food Left to Eat," Available from Sally Rockwell's Diet Design, P.O. Box 31065, Seattle, WA 98103, (206) 547-1814.

Shattack, Ruth R. *The Allergy Cookbook: Tasty, Nutritious Cooking without Wheat, Corn, Milk, Eggs.* New York: New American Library, 1986.

Sheinkin, David, M.D., Schacter, Michael, M.D., and

Hutton, Richard. *Food, Mind and Mood.* New York: Warner Books, 1987 (original title: *The Food Connection*).

RESOURCE LIST ORGANIZATIONS

American Academy of Environmental Medicine, 4510 West 89th St., Prairie Village, KS 66207, (913) 642-6062

Human Ecology Action League, 2250 N. Druid Hills Rd., #236, Atlanta, GA 30329, (404) 248-1898

LABORATORIES FOR ALLERGY TESTING

American Medical Testing Laboratories (ALCAT), One Oakweed Blvd., Suite 130, Hollywood, FL 38020, (305) 923-2990

Antibody Assay Laboratories (RAST), 1715 E. Wilshire, #715, Santa Ana, CA 92705, (714) 538-3225; (800) 522-2611

Diagnos-Techs Clinical and Research Laboratory, Inc. (intestinal permeability test), P.O. Box 58948, Seattle, WA 98138-1948, (206) 251-0596; (800) 878-3787

Immuno Laboratories (ELISA) 1620 West Oakland Park Blvd. Fort Lauderdale, FL 33311, (305) 486-4500; (800) 231-9197

Meridian Valley Clinical Laboratory (ELISA), 24030 132nd Ave., S.E., Kent, WA 98042, (206) 631-8922; (800) 234-6825

MetaMetrics, Inc., Medical Research Laboratory (ELISA), 3000 Northwoods Pkwy., Suite 150, Norcross, GA 30071, (404) 446-5483; (800) 221-4640

National BioTechnology Laboratory (ELISA) 3212 NE 125th St., Suite D, Seattle, WA 98125-9826, (206) 363-6006 (800) 846-6285

Physicians' Clinical Laboratories (FAST and ALCAT), 15613 Bellevue-Redmond Rd., Bellevue, WA 98008, (206) 881-2446

Serammune Physicians Lab (ELISA ACT), 1890 Preston White Drive, Second Floor, Reston, VA 22091, (703) 758-0610 or (800) 553-5472

CHAPTER 14

CHEMICAL HYPERSENSITIVITY AND ENVIRONMENTAL ILLNESS

CHEMICAL INJURY AND HYPERSENSITIVITY

This chapter falls into two parts: Part One, Chemical Injury and Hypersensitivity, in which we will discuss the prevention of environmental illness, and offer practical approaches for minimizing exposure and for strengthening resistance to environmental chemicals. In Part Two, Heavy Metal Toxins, we will explore heavy metals in detail, highlighting the emerging dangers of mercury.

We will first follow the story of Sylvia, a woman suffering from chemical hypersensitivity syndrome, a form of environmental illness. We will define her illness: its recognition, diagnosis, and treatment.

All of us face a constant barrage of environmental chemicals in our daily lives. Four million distinct chemical compounds have been reported in the scientific literature since 1965. Approximately three thousand chemicals are deliberately added to food, and over seven hundred have been identified in drinking water. Add to this the number of pharmaceutical and recreational street drugs, and the chemical exposure we face becomes overwhelming. "Over 400 chemicals have been identified in human tissues, with 48 found in adipose tissue, at least 40 in breast milk, 73 in the liver, and over 250 in blood plasma."[1]

We have heard of many of these compounds before: chlorinated pesticides such as DDT, DDE, chlordane, dieldrin; polychlorinated biphenyls (PCB), polybrominated biphenyls (PBB), halogenated volatile and aromatic compounds, and organic hydrocarbons, fluorocarbons, and synthetic alcohols. Specific agents in these categories include such agents as trichloroethylene, benzene, chloroform, tetrachloroethylene, trichlorethane, kepone, pentachlorophenol, toluene, isocyanate, xylene, heptachlor, epoxide, hexachlorobenzene (HCB), delta BHC, and beta BHC. There is also vinyl chloride, carbon monoxide, natural gas, sulfur dioxide, nitrous oxide, ethylene glycol, and synthetic ethanol. And then there are the inorganic heavy metal toxins such as lead, cadmium, arsenic, mercury, aluminum, and nickel.

It is well known that many of these chemicals cause cancer, birth defects, spontaneous miscarriages, lung disease, liver and kidney destruction, and irreparable neurologic injury. Yet only a fraction of the chemicals in common use today have undergone toxicologic testing.

SYLVIA

Sylvia is a forty-three-year-old housewife, mother of three, and part-time printer who came to me primarily complaining of depression, headache, exhaustion, and weight loss. She had been well until approximately two years earlier, when she began to notice recurrent bladder infections, heightened premenstrual anxiety, unusual reactions to foods she had previously tolerated, and mild fatigue. She had seen a nutritional physician who treated her with vitamins that had not proved very helpful, and she'd seen another physician who diagnosed food allergies and recommended an elimination diet.

When Sylvia stayed away from her problem foods, she did feel significantly better. Eventually, however, she began to develop memory loss, confusion, mild panic attacks, diarrhea, and a craving for alcohol. Her regular doctor could find nothing wrong from her exam and routine blood tests and prescribed an antianxiety medication. Then she saw yet another physician, who treated her for Candida overgrowth, and she seemed more encouraged by this treatment than anything previously. Nevertheless, after a little over one year, she still could not make it through the day without both her antifungal and antianxiety medications.

Her panic attacks became more frequent and severe, and she was eventually hospitalized and put on antidepressant medication. The apparent trigger for this "breakdown" was a combination of worry over her father's sudden hospitalization for heart problems and her anxiety over alleged incest between her husband and daughter. (Her concern about incest ultimately proved to be paranoia on her part.)

Sylvia's previous treatments, though partially helpful, were not getting to the source of her increasing physical and psychological symptoms. According to her husband, these ailments were turning her into someone quite different from the woman he'd known just three years before. A new perspective was obviously required and careful questioning revealed two key pieces of information:

1. Sylvia had had her own part-time printing business. Her work involved the usual chemicals—inks and solvents, which she felt posed no obvious problems to her.

2. Approximately six months before the onset of her symptoms, she and her family had moved to an older home, which she and her husband were still remodeling. They used particleboard subflooring in several rooms, and particleboard cabinets in the kitchen and bathrooms. All the hardwood floors were stained and Swedish-finished.

Elsewhere, stain-resistant synthetic wall-to-wall carpets were installed. They did much painting and wood staining and installed a wood stove as a backup for their new high-efficiency closed-combustion oil furnace. Their basement was unfinished, and part of it had a dirt floor that always felt damp and musty to Sylvia.

Sylvia could correlate her worsening symptoms with prolonged periods she spent at home, especially when the oil furnace was on (in spite of the guarantee that no vapors would leak). She would experience nausea, abdominal cramps, loose stools, fatigue, fogginess, headaches, chest pains, difficulty focusing her eyes, loss of libido, anger, irritability, a feeling of unreality, depression, and paranoia—all of which would diminish eventually if she stayed outdoors. When her symptoms grew unbearable (which was now more and more often), she would sleep in the car. Unfortunately, her husband did not understand her illness, thought she was a veritable mental case, and became increasingly impatient and short-tempered with her.

Sylvia found that her symptoms could be brought on or aggravated by newspapers, perfume, hair spray, auto exhaust, dry cleaners fumes, plastics, the dampness and mold of her basement, going longer than two hours without eating, even laughter and sexual intercourse. She felt and functioned best when on vacation, and after being home less than twelve hours her symptoms would begin to return. The frustration of always feeling ill and dysfunctional, and the fear and uncertainty she felt about her own home and her husband's and friends' reactions to her, were creating additional anxiety and depression. She felt alienated, hopeless, and even desperate.

THE "SPREADING EFFECT" OF ENVIRONMENTAL ILLNESS

Sylvia was suffering from environmental illness, a condition characterized by multisystem complaints, physical, psychological, and emotional, triggered by a multitude of chemical substances, often due to their cumulative effect. People similarly afflicted can go from doctor to doctor looking for answers. Commonly they are labeled as psychiatric cases—partly because of their extraordinary-sounding, apparently unrelated numerous head-to-toe symptoms, but also because of a paucity of evidence upon physical examination or standard blood tests.

What also typifies this illness, to paraphrase Sherry Rogers, M.D. (author of *Environmental Illness Syndrome* and of *Tired or Toxic*),[2] is the "spreading effect." An individual with environmental illness develops increasing hypersensitivity and intolerance to more and more chemicals, even to such seemingly harmless substances as polyester clothing, chlorine and fluoride in tap water, and household cleaning fluids. Eventually common foods and inhalants such as dust and mold become new problems, and increased susceptibility to Candida and viruses results as well.

Even worse, as time goes on, smaller and smaller doses or concentrations of the offending substances seem to produce symptoms. Severe reactions can develop suddenly, overnight even, lending a bizarre color and stigma to this illness. In severe cases affected individuals become "universal reactors" and, until they are treated, become outcasts from the modern world. Consequently, they often develop deep emotional scars and require substantial emotional support as part of their overall treatment.

Toxic chemical and environmental accidents are making the headlines regularly. However, for most of us, like Sylvia, it is not the Bopals or the Love Canals that directly injure our bodies, but the chronic, pervasive pollution of our air, water, soil, and food supply. In other words, it is living, breathing, and eating in our modern world that puts us at risk. Much of our internal chemical intake now comes from indoor air pollution in our homes, schools, work places, department stores, even hospitals. The following table lists common sources of toxic exposure.

COMMON DAILY SOURCES OF CHEMICAL EXPOSURES*

- **Formaldehyde** in urea foam insulation, plywood (particularly interior grade used in paneling), particleboard and pressboard cabinets, subflooring, furniture, fabric finishes, polyurethane foam rubber (used in pillows, cushions, mattresses, and rug padding), mobile homes, fabric finishes, air deodorizers, some toothpastes, mouthwashes, dentifrices, germicidal soaps, some shampoos, hair setting lotions, nail polish and cosmetics, insecticides, chemical fertilizers, smog, flame-resistant fabrics, waxes and polish, adhesives, and natural and synthetic clothes that are crease resistant, wrinkle resistant, water repellant, dye fast, flame resistant, shrink proof, and moth proof (wool).

- **Oil vapors** from oil furnaces and motor-oil-impregnated air-conditioning filters, electric kitchen appliances such as food processors, blenders, can openers.

- **Combustion products** (carbon monoxide and nitrogen dioxide in particular) from gas ranges (particularly in an unvented kitchen) and from gas or oil heating. Kerosene heat is also extremely polluting.

- **Household chemicals** such as dry cleaning chemicals in clothes, mothballs, rug-cleaning and other cleaning fluids, lighter fluids, the contents of most spray cans, solvents, paints, paint thinners, stain removers, varnishes, and other wood finishes; certain detergents, scented soaps, cleansers (especially pine scented), air fresheners, toilet disinfectants, janitorial chemicals, ammonia fluids, bleaches, window-washing compounds, brass- and silver-polishing fluids, furniture polish, even burning petrochemical base wax candles, and tobacco smoke.

- **Ozone** from electric kitchen appliances.

- **Herbicides** from common lawn and garden chemicals, and from municipal spraying.

- **Pesticides** on your fruit trees or garden; pesticide residues on commercial foods, on cottons and woolens as fumigants and moth-proofing; residues in your home from exterminators; bug and fly sprays, flea and roach bombs.

- **Fluorocarbons** from Teflon, spray cans, and freon (which leaks from refrigerators and freezers).

- **Epoxy adhesives** on plastics and electronic equipment (TVs, microwave ovens, home computers, etc.) which release gases when heated up.

- **Automobile vapors** that enter homes and apartments from garages built under or attached to living quarters.

- **Common office paraphernalia** such as carbon paper, carbonless copy paper, ink, mimeographic and duplicating chemicals, solvent-based felt-tipped marking pens, glue.

- **Certain woods** such as fir, cedar, redwood, and pine.

- **Chlorinated and fluoridated water** out of our own taps has even been incriminated in this vast list of agents related to environmental illnesses.

*Source: Adapted from T. G. Randolph and R. W. Moss. An Alternative Approach to Allergies. New York: Lippincott/Crowell, 1980.
    D. L. Dadd. Nontoxic, Natural, and Earthwise. Los Angeles: J.T. Tarcher, 1984.
    D. L. Dadd. The Nontoxic Home. Los Angeles: J.T. Tarcher, 1986.
    P. L. Saifer and M. Saifer. "Testing for Chemical Sensitivity," "Formaldehyde," "Indoor Air Pollution: The Home," "Chemical Sensitivity," and "Phenols." Unpublished reports.

COMMON DAILY SOURCES OF CHEMICAL EXPOSURES

- **Polyethylene** plastic containers; polyvinyls, particularly the very soft and flexible plastics such as those in shower curtains, fake leather, artificial flowers, electric insulation.

- **Polyesters** in clothing, upholstery, drapery, furniture, and stuffing for pillows and quilts.

- **Medications** you commonly take may be derived from by-products of petrochemicals and perpetuate symptoms in those with environmental illness. Such individuals are commonly food allergic as well, and the lactose, cornstarch, and other elements of high-allergic potential used as fillers and excipients in most medications are also capable of perpetuating symptoms.

CHEMICAL ADDITIVES IN FOODS

Between three and four thousand chemicals are added to our foods by the food industry as preservatives, buffers, stabilizers, colorings, and flavorings. Many of these chemicals fall under the category of GRAS ("generally recognized as safe"), a label not necessarily to be trusted.

Benjamin Feingold, M.D. (author of *Why Your Child Is Hyperactive*[3]) and others have shown that a good percentage of hyperactive, attention-deficit, and learning-disabled children are hypersensitive to the preservatives, colorings, and other chemical additives in common foods on supermarket shelves. Removing these chemicals from the children's diets produces enormous improvements in their brain functioning and behavior.

Many chemicals added to foods still have not been adequately tested to determine with certainty whether or not they're safe. How many years were sulfiting agents causing asthma attacks before they were incriminated? Not long ago a chemical used for years to decaffeinate coffee was found to be carcinogenic.

I do not recommend blind trust and acceptance of the FDA and its GRAS stamp of approval. This point is particularly relevant with respect to FDA-approved drugs, several of which have been either banned, restricted, or labeled with new warnings only after reported incidences of injuries and deaths, for example: thalidomide, diethylstilbestrol, Feldene, Selacryn, Encaid, Omniflox, and Zomax. Perhaps equally frightening is the fact that tens of thousands of chemicals in commercial and industrial use haven't even undergone sufficient testing—if any testing at all—by such government agencies as the EPA.

How Exposure to Chemicals Leads to Environmental Illness

Given this vast list of chemical exposures, you can see that you don't need to be a welder, shipbuilder, professional painter, exterminator, farmer, factory worker, electronics fabricator, embalmer, hairstylist, artist, or someone regularly exposed to solvents or to occupational chemical hazards to be at risk for chemical injury and environmental illness.

Many office workers or housewives have been injured from regular or episodic exposures to these everyday "harmless" products. Often a single, potent exposure from painting in an unventilated room or stripping and refinishing a piece of furniture might provoke a reaction. Usually, however, it requires a barrage of previous minor assaults, ever-present and nearly inescapable. These become cumulative and eventually, with perhaps one or more unusual exposures, overwhelm the body's defenses.

When our antioxidant and detoxification systems are in good working order, they protect us from low-level chemical assault. One can only marvel at their design and performance. Most of the sixty thousand chemicals in current use today have been developed only in the last forty years—in other words, we are creating foreign and toxic substances far more rapidly than the speed at which human detoxifying mechanisms can evolve.

Chemical injury will inhibit metabolic energy production at the cellular level.[4] Initially you might experience fatigue, lethargy, and weakness. Decreased efficiency of cellular membrane sodium pumps will occur, causing cells to swell. If this occurs in the brain, effects include poor memory, insomnia, fogginess, and paranoia. With free radical disruption of cell membranes, inflammatory conditions arise. DNA is damaged in cell nuclei, which can give rise to birth defects and cancer.

Chemical injury is often related to an overload of the liver's cytochrome P450 detoxification system. Also, certain toxins have an affinity for specific tissues, such as the liver, kidney, central nervous system, and so on.

According to Theron Randolph, M.D., a pioneer in

the field of environmental medicine and clinical ecology and author of many books and articles, levels of exposure considered to be "safe" have the capability of triggering such disordered biochemical phenomena and producing the symptoms experienced by an ever-increasing percentage of Americans.[5] These symptoms, much like Sylvia's, are often diffuse and nonspecific. Unless tissue damage is apparent, physicians don't usually find anything medically wrong and most do not look for a chemical cause. Many are quick to call such patients psychoneurotic.

In the list of symptoms and conditions associated with environmental illness that appears on the next page, see if there are symptoms you can identify in yourself—symptoms your doctors may have been unable to explain adequately. These may not have been caused by stress or some virus, but rather be the result of chemical injury or chemical hypersensitivity—in other words, environmental illness.

HOW YOU MAY BE FEELING

You may experience generally worse symptoms upon arising, or from fasting, from exercise, and when undergoing emotional stress.

If offending chemical(s) are in your home, you may feel worse when you first get up in the morning or after a weekend at home. You may feel better when you sleep with the windows wide open, even more so if you sleep outside. You feel better when you're away from home—more so the longer you stay away from home.

If offending chemical(s) are present where you work, you may feel worse by the end of the work day, or you may feel worse by the end of the work week. You may recover somewhat over weekends and especially vacations.

You may have symptoms all the time or episodically, without correlation to any specific activity or event.

TESTING FOR ENVIRONMENTAL ILLNESS

If you suspect chemical injury or hypersensitivity, I recommend making an appointment with a physician skilled in environmental medicine. Such a physician may or may not be board certified by the American Academy of Environmental Medicine, but nevertheless should be familiar with the signs, symptoms, and treatment of environmental illness and could offer several types of testing that could help verify the diagnosis (see "Organizations," page 284).

The Candida Connection

I have seen many individuals who have developed hypersensitivities to chemicals primarily because of a Candida overgrowth (see Chapter Twelve). These individuals are often unable to tolerate normal levels of exhaust, paint, glue fumes, and so on. Some of those affected become too ill to work or to enjoy their lives. After Candida treatment, many of them lose their chemical sensitivities and return to full health. Before launching any costly diagnostic testing for environmental illness, if I suspect yeast overgrowth, I will look carefully for this condition.

Liver Testing

In the environmentally ill patient, focusing on liver function is paramount. An initial laboratory screen I often use in my practice (and one any physician could easily obtain) is the liver detoxification capacity test[6] (salivary caffeine and urinary hippurate clearance—discussed on page 177), which measures the liver's ability to metabolize toxins. If the test results indicate an underactive liver detoxification function, the individual would be highly susceptible to toxin accumulation and chemical hypersensitivity, leading to eventual illness. Specific nutrient support could then be implemented to restore the detoxification mechanisms in the liver, which would begin to reverse the illness. A liver with overactive detoxification mechanisms is obviously stressed, and identifying the toxin(s) would be the next step—in addition to nutrient support and antioxidant protection.

Zinc Testing

Since zinc deficiency is a common predisposing factor to chemical hypersensitivity, a blood test to determine red or white blood cell zinc status, or a lymphocyte growth response test, may prove revealing (see page 121). When you realize that this mineral is required in at least ninety biochemical reactions—notably those involving liver detoxification systems, membrane stability, energy production, immune function, gene repair, and neurotransmitter metabolism—you can better appreciate how a deficiency may be involved in so many chemically related symptoms. As it happens, lead, cadmium, aluminum, and tin are heavy metals that commonly displace zinc in numerous enzyme systems. For heavy metal screening, I usually obtain a provocative twenty-four-hour urine test (see page 281). Hair analysis may have some limited usefulness for both zinc and heavy metal screening.

Hypersensitivity Testing

Allergy (delayed hypersensitivity) to a broad range of environmental chemicals and food-additive chemicals (and foods) can be easily picked up by the ELISA-ACT blood test, discussed in Chapter Thirteen.[7] If you see an environmental medicine specialist who has an allergy

SYMPTOMS AND CONDITIONS ASSOCIATED WITH ENVIRONMENTAL ILLNESS*

NEUROLOGICAL/BRAIN

Fatigue, lethargy, exhaustion
Impaired memory
Impaired thinking, cannot concentrate
Confusion, foggy-headedness, dopiness
Headaches
Insomnia
Excessive sleepiness
Irritability

Restlessness, being hyper
Panic attack
Emotional disturbance or instability
Behavioral or personality changes
Unwarranted depression
Claustrophobia
Poor equilibrium
Poor coordination

Dizziness
Numbness, tingling, or burning sensations
Tremors
Seizures, convulsions
Hallucinations
Amyotrophic lateral sclerosis (Lou Gehrig's disease)
Parkinson's disease
Multiple sclerosis

MUSCULOSKELETAL/MOTOR

Fatigue, lethargy, exhaustion
Joint pain, swelling, arthritis
Malaise—just don't feel good, flu-like symptoms

Muscular aches and pains, may be diagnosed as fibromyalgia
Muscular twitching, spasms

Muscular weakness
Slow movements
Lack of coordination

GASTROINTESTINAL

Nausea, queasiness
Vomiting
Diarrhea

Eating may lessen symptoms
Overeating or loss of appetite

Constipation
Abdominal pains or cramps
Weight loss

HEART/LUNGS/CHEST

Chest pain, tightness

Heart rhythm disturbance

Respiratory distress, wheezing

*Adapted from S. A. Rogers. Tired or Toxic. Syracuse, NY: Prestige Publishing, 1990.

———. The EI Syndrome: An Rx for Environmental Illness. Syracuse, NY: Prestige Publishing, 1988.

———. "Diagnosing the Tight Building Syndrome." Environmental Health Perspectives 76: 195–198, 1987.

Z. R. Gard, et al. "The Biotoxic Reduction Program: Eliminating Body Pollution." The Townsend Letter for Doctors. No. 46, April 1967.

D. E. Root, et al. "Diagnosis and Treatment of Patients Presenting Subclinical Signs and Symptoms of Exposure to Chemicals with Bioaccumulate in Human Tissue." From the Proceedings of the National Conference on Hazardous Wastes and Environmental Emergencies, May 1985, Cincinnati, OH (Hazardous Control Research Institute, 9300 Columbia Boulevard, Silver Spring, MD 20910.

VISUAL/HEARING/SMELL/TASTE

Blurred vision
Dimness of vision
Eye oscillation

Eye irritation, kerato-
   conjunctivitis
Pupil reactions

Hearing or smelling
   impairment

SPEECH/THROAT/SINUS

Sore or irritated throat
Loss of voice

Hoarseness, laryngitis
Speech impairment

Nasal or sinus burning

SKIN/NAILS

Flushing
Acne
Rashes, nonspecific
Dryness of skin

Darkening or thickness
   of skin
Sun sensitivity
Increased sweating

Deformity or discoloration of
   nails
Slow or poor healing of cuts

MENSTRUAL/HORMONAL

Aggravated premenstrual or menstrual symptoms

IMMUNE SYSTEM

Unexplained swelling of lymph nodes
Increased susceptibility to Epstein-Barr virus (EBV), cytomegalovirus (CMV), or chronic fatigue syndrome
Increased susceptibility to polysystemic candidiasis
Increased susceptibility to food and inhalant allergies, or extensive allergies (universal reactor: a state where one cannot tolerate normal levels of fumes, exhausts, smoke, marker pens, perfumes, gas or oil heat, synthetic clothes, synthetic auto or plane interiors, building materials with formaldehyde, such as particleboard, etc., new synthetic carpets, new paint, cleaning chemicals, glues)
Increased susceptibility to autoimmune diseases such as systemic lupus erythematosus (SLE)
Increased susceptibility to cancer

laboratory, intradermal (skin) and/or sublingual (under the tongue) testing can be performed on a variety of compounds: formaldehyde, hydrocarbon (auto exhaust), tobacco, perfume, phenols, chlorine, wood smoke, jet fuel, ethanol, natural gas, and several other toxic compounds. Once the hypersensitive substances are identified, you are advised to eliminate or avoid their main sources, if possible, and if needed, receive a neutralizing vaccine when exposure is necessary or inadvertent.

Many individuals with environmental illness have food allergies (see Chapter Thirteen). Testing and treatment for food (and inhalant) allergies reduces the stress on the immune system of environmental illness sufferers and facilitates their recovery.

Also mentioned in Chapter Thirteen is electronic screening, a system capable of recognizing specific chemical toxicities or sensitivities in the body. Some practitioners recommend homeopathic remedies correlated with the electronic screening to treat these conditions.

Formaldehyde Testing

Serum levels of formic acid (a metabolite of formaldehyde) can also be obtained if formaldehyde is suspected. The air in your home or office can be measured for formaldehyde (also for carbon monoxide and other toxic compounds) to help incriminate the offending substances. You can contract directly with a company that performs this service. Your physician can also contact Antibody Assay Laboratories or Immunosciences Laboratory (see page 285), labs that run antibody assays for formaldehyde (as well as for toluene di-isocyanate, trimellitic anhydride, and other compounds).

Toxic Chemical Testing

In addition, several laboratories are equipped to run serum levels for various categories of toxic chemicals (also known as xenobiotics), one of the more direct screens for documenting environmentally induced illness (see page 285). Results—given in parts per billion for PCBs, PBBs, chlorinated pesticides, halogenated volatiles and aromatics, and many such compounds—can be most revealing.

Most of these chemicals leave the bloodstream within weeks. Therefore, unless the exposure has been relatively recent, your serum levels may be very low or even nondetectable and fail to reflect your actual toxic bioaccumulation. As these chemicals are fat soluble and have an affinity for fatty tissues, a measurement of an adipose tissue sample (taken by needle aspiration) performed by solvent extraction and gas chromatography/mass spectrometry may very well show elevated levels. Measurements of your sebum levels for these toxins are also available. (The EPA-sponsored National Human Adipose Tissue Survey collects and analyzes adipose tissue specimens for the presence of toxic substances. It was this survey that originally documented PCB and dioxin in human tissues. When the survey was abruptly discontinued not too long ago, the EPA was flooded with protests from the scientific and medical communities. The decision was subsequently reversed. But according to the October 29, 1988, *Medical Tribune*,

---

LABORATORY METHODS OF DIAGNOSING ENVIRONMENTAL ILLNESS AND RELATED CONDITIONS

Liver Detoxification Capacity (salivary caffeine and urinary hippurate clearance)

Red or white blood cell zinc status or lymphocyte growth response test

Provocative twenty-four-hour urine test for heavy metals

Hair analysis

Hypersensitivity testing for chemicals, foods, and inhalants

ELISA-ACT

Sublingual tests

Intradermal tests

Electronic screening

Antibody levels in blood (antibodies to specific chemicals)

Serum formic acid

Detection in air (formaldehyde)

Measurement of toxic chemical levels

Serum levels of toxic chemicals

Analysis of adipose tissue sample for toxic chemicals

Sebum analysis for toxic chemicals

Immune profile blood screens

Candida testing

funding was made available for only 600 chemical analyses per year instead of the previous 4,009.)

Immune System Testing

Toxic chemicals have allegedly specific effects on the immune system, and therefore specific blood tests profiling the immune system can be used in the diagnosis of environmental illness and the monitoring of its treatment.[8] Such effects are generally but not always demonstrated by a decrease in the total white blood count and a decreased number of suppressor T cells (lymphocytes), leading to increased antibody production. Elevated blood levels of antibodies made specifically to attack one's own tissues are commonly found in environmentally ill individuals. The presence of such tissue-specific antibodies often correlates to specific symptoms.

There is a decreased response by lymphocytes to mitogen stimulation, which is a standard way of measuring immune function, matched by an abnormal response to allergen stimulation. Lymphocyte proliferation studies commonly show that people who are environmentally ill eventually suffer from depressed immune systems. Before this occurs, though, there may be evidence of a chronically activated cellular immune response because of an increase in circulating Tal-positive lymphocytes.

CLEANSING TOXIC CHEMICALS FROM YOUR BODY

The diagnosis of environmental illness refers to either a state of allergy or hypersensitivity and/or a state where there is a body burden—an excess of chemicals stored in the body. Yet, you can be chemically allergic without necessarily having excessive chemicals in your tissues.

However, if you are ill because of excessive chemical toxins in your tissues, you will need to reduce your body's burden of stored chemicals. These poisons lodge in your fatty tissues and, given their half-lives of ten to twenty years or more, can remain with you for years, even decades. As minute amounts are released into your bloodstream, they continually trigger chronic recurring symptoms.[9]

Physiological stresses such as exercise, heat exposure, fasting (even just overnight), emotional stress, and illness will trigger a release of fatty acids from adipose cells and a subsequent release of the chemicals stored there. In the long term, such stored toxins, whether or not they cause significant immediate symptoms, can predispose you to motor neuron diseases[10], such as Parkinson's disease, and immune dysregulations[11] that can lead to cancer and to autoimmune phenomena such as lupus, thyroiditis, and myasthenia gravis.

Several health centers in the United States (see page 285) offer a method of mobilizing and excreting these storage depots of poisons. This program was originally designed by L. Ron Hubbard during his work with drug addicts who could not be cured successfully by therapy and abstention techniques. He traced their problems to stored depots of toxins in fatty tissues that would continually release small amounts of drugs into the bloodstream, giving these individuals repeated "hits," and perpetuating their addictions. This program was designed to drive these fatty accumulations of drugs into the bloodstream where they could be excreted, and thus the addictions could be cured.[12]

The Michigan Detox Program

The efficacy of Hubbard's program was proven for toxic chemicals when a portion of the population of the state of Michigan was inadvertently poisoned by the ingestion of meat and milk products contaminated with PBBs.[13] A fire retardant containing substantial amounts of this chemical had been mistakenly fed to farm animals in place of a nutritional supplement. It wasn't long before the toxin found its way into the state's food supply.

Hubbard's precisely monitored and physician-supervised program included repeated sauna sessions, aerobic exercise, the oral administration of niacin and other food supplements, and water and electrolyte replacement. This combination of activities was designed to mobilize the fat-stored toxins and enhance their excretion. Lasting up to twenty days or more, the regimen produced a dramatic immediate 20 percent decrease not only in PBB fat levels, but also in PCB, DDE (a metabolite of DDT), heptachlor, epoxide, and dieldrin. Even more impressive was a follow-up measurement that verified a continuation of the mobilization and excretion process long after the program had ended. An average of 42 percent reduction in toxins was measured four months after treatment.

Some centers follow Hubbard's protocol exactly, while others have made some changes, adding bowel cleansing, liver restoration, hydrotherapy, and body work.

Factors Contributing to Susceptibility and How to Overcome Them

It's important to realize that not all environmentally ill people have a time bomb of carcinogenic deposits stored in their fatty tissues. Many have become hypersensitive and hyperallergic from the immune dysregulation brought on by the combined effects of candidiasis, food sensitivities, nutrient deficiencies, and repeated minor chemical exposures. These chemical exposures occur from the frequent inhaling or ingesting of the offending substances.

Why does one person in a typical office setting, for example, develop symptoms of environmental illness, while a coworker exposed to the exact same environment does not? This depends on a balance of two factors: the level of your overall health and resistance; and your level of chemical exposure. The stronger you make yourself, the more chemical assaults you will be able to fend off. Conversely, the weaker you have become, the less it will take to bring on an adverse reaction.

Genetic or constitutional factors are contributing factors to whether your resistance is high or not. But the degree of influence you can exert on your health can often outweigh a weak or a strong constitution, depending upon whether it's a positive or negative influence. If you can nourish yourself with a whole-foods diet and nutritional supplements and keep your bowel and particularly your liver detoxification functions in top shape, you optimize your chances of being able to detoxify and excrete the chemicals that come your way—if the assault is not overwhelming.

Antioxidant Protection   On a more biochemical level, it is the antioxidant nutrients and chemical detoxification mechanisms that protect you from chemical injury. Although we discussed both of these in detail in Chapters Three and Nine, briefly, antioxidants are nutrients or enzyme-coenzyme complexes that protect cellular membranes and structures from the free-radical damage that chemicals and other substances can trigger. Detoxification systems are located primarily in the liver, which is able to metabolize many man-made toxic chemicals into forms that can then be excreted through the bile and intestines or the kidneys.

If your exposure is more than ordinary or high risk, regular use of a broad-spectrum antioxidant formula and specific liver-enhancing agents will give you extra protection. An antioxidant formula commonly contains any or all of the following: vitamins C, E, beta-carotene, B-1, B-2, B-3, B-5, B-6; the minerals zinc, copper, manganese, and selenium; and amino acids L-cysteine or N-acetylcystein, methionine, and sometimes glutathione. Also included may be coenzyme Q-10, lipoic acid, and others. Individual antioxidants in higher doses are commonly used, such as vitamin C and beta-carotene. Additional important liver-enhancing agents include silymarin, N-acetylcysteine, Liv. 52, "Ultra Clear," and catechin (see Chapter Nine).

PANTETHINE   One agent not mentioned elsewhere, and particularly useful in cases of formaldehyde sensitivity, is the pantothenic acid (vitamin B-5) metabolite, pantetheine (available from Ecological Formulas of Concord, California). It is a precursor of coenzyme A and a necessary constituent of the formaldehyde detoxification liver enzyme, aldehyde dehydrogenase. This enzyme also detoxifies acetylaldehyde, a toxic by-product of *Candida albicans* and of alcohol metabolism. In cases of genetic weakness of aldehyde dehydrogenase or when there is an enzyme overload because of formaldehyde exposure, Candida, or alcoholism, pantethine may contribute to recovery of this enzyme function. The dose generally recommended is 300 milligrams three times daily.

Looking at the Bigger Picture   I cannot emphasize enough the importance of treating candidiasis and food sensitivities (particularly the former) to help manage and overcome environmental illness or to help prevent its onset. These three conditions (environmental illness, candidiasis, and food allergy/intolerance) are all commonly present in the same individual as interdependent collaborators. Therapy aimed at any one commonly lessens the symptoms of the other two. Simultaneous treatment of all three conditions provides the best results.

You and your doctor should also consider the possibility that other conditions are present, and may need to be treated with other health-supportive measures to achieve the best possible outcome. Additional measures for your treatment program are outlined on page 274. Be aware, however, that trying any of the modalities we've discussed may initially aggravate your condition. Careful and prudent trials and professional supervision are recommended.

Even with all the treatment measures combined after food allergy and Candida treatment, many chemically allergic individuals find that they cannot return to a state of acceptable health until the offending chemical(s) is removed from their environment and their overall chemical exposures are greatly reduced. Some people are forced, at least temporarily, to leave their jobs or move to a chemical-free—or more realistically, a chemically reduced—environment in order to make any progress.

Some individuals can make excellent progress without such radical measures by making commonsense changes in their homes and workplaces (see "Preventing Environmental Illness by Reducing Indoor Chemical Pollution," below). Substantial improvement can also be achieved by treating other contributing conditions and strengthening antioxidant and liver detoxification capacities.

PREVENTING ENVIRONMENTAL ILLNESS BY REDUCING INDOOR CHEMICAL POLLUTION*

The following suggestions contain some commonsense measures to minimize your everyday exposure to chemicals. If you are not environmentally ill, you would probably not require the strictest and most meticulous

---

Adapted from An Alternative Approach to Allergies, *by Theron C. Randolph, M.D., and Ralph W. Moss. Reprinted by permission of HarperCollins Publishers, Inc., and Ruth Hagy Brod Agency.*

ADDITIONAL MEASURES FOR YOUR TREATMENT PROGRAM

- Keep your elimination routes functioning well (see Chapter Eighteen).

- Treat low thyroid status (see Chapter Seventeen, "Hypothyroidism"), if present—particularly if thyroid autoantibodies are present.

- Support adrenal function (see Chapter Eleven).

- Find and treat intestinal parasites (see Chapter Seventeen, "Parasites"). I have seen several individuals make significant progress with chemical hypersensitivity after working on this problem.

- Hydrotherapy (Chapter Twenty) has been reported to help overall health and resistance and enhance the liver's detoxification systems and bowel's eliminative capacity.

- Taking low-temperature saunas (110–120°F) for up to thirty to sixty minutes encourages the excretion of fat-soluble toxins through sweat oils. Immediately following the sauna, shower using a vegetable bath sponge or washcloth and a glycerine soap to scrub the toxins from your skin and prevent their being reabsorbed.

  Such a practice is part of the professionally supervised detoxification program, done five or more days a week for up to three weeks, for those with environmental illness. It can be done on your own once weekly or periodically to prevent toxin accumulation and environmental illness. It is advisable several times weekly if your exposure to toxins is high risk.

  Leave the sauna before you get dizzy or light-headed. Use common sense. Seek professional advice before using a sauna if you have a heart condition or other serious illness. High-temperature saunas—although they have their own benefits and risks—encourage more water sweat and are not suggested for this type of detoxification.

- Psychological and emotional support is an important aspect of treatment. Consider seeking professional help in your wellness program.

- Lay groups and newsletters for the environmentally ill provide extremely useful and practical self-help information and serve as a support mechanism. (See Organizations, page 284.)

---

chemical cleanup measures, but I would advise you to follow as best you can the easier and obvious ones listed below. In this way, you will reduce the cumulative effect and the possibility of becoming environmentally ill. If you are environmentally ill, following the strict and more radical measures that your physician may advise will help you recover more fully.

CHEMICAL COMPOUNDS. Inspect underneath all of your sinks, your closets, pantries, drawers, medicine chests—anywhere you might be storing products that emit potentially sensitizing vapors. These include paints, thinners, solvents, scented laundry and dishwasher detergents, waxes, polishes, insect sprays, weed killers, turpentine, shoe polish, mothballs, air fresheners, some scented soaps, cosmetics and lotions, toilet disinfectants,

window-washing compounds, and so on.

Dispose of what is unnecessary and keep what is essential in glass jars or bottles or other airtight containers with tight-fitting lids. This is especially important for items used most frequently. If possible, store most of these items somewhere other than your most immediate living areas—in a storeroom or, better yet, in a detached garage or shed if you have one.

Replace as many of the above-listed items as possible with nontoxic, nonpolluting alternatives. See Debra Dadd's *Nontoxic, Natural, and Earthwise.*[14] Also contact Washington Toxics Coalition, 4516 University Way N.E., Seattle, WA 98105, which provides information on nontoxic alternatives to everything from cleaning supplies to lawn care products and more. Call (206)

632-1545 to find out which of its sixteen fact sheets you need ($1.00 each).

PLASTICS. Try to reduce the use of plastics—primarily petrochemically derived products. This group is in a lower category of danger than natural gas combustion products, solvents, bug sprays, or weed killers. The most polluting ones are the soft, pliable plastics, especially those that have an odor. Harder plastics are less sensitizing.

Only those who are environmentally sensitive should consider reducing the use of the following items: plastic lamp shades (use glass, metal, or natural fabrics); plastic bowls and dishes (use ceramic, glass, wood); plastic wrap; plastic food-storage containers (use glass or stainless steel containers); plastic pillow and mattress cases, upholstery materials, handbags, brushes and combs, shoes, and anything made of Naugahyde. You may think that it's impossible in our modern culture to avoid plastics. Yet, although plastics are nearly omnipresent, you can, with conscious effort, minimize their use.

FOAM RUBBER. This is another petrochemically derived substance. Such items as foam pillows, cushions, mattresses, and rug padding may be sensitizing. Whenever possible, choose natural materials as alternatives to foam, especially if you are chemically sensitive—100 percent genuine natural latex, and cotton and wool batting are good choices.

CIGARETTE SMOKE. Most of us are already aware that cigarette smoking causes or contributes to cancer, heart attacks and strokes, chronic bronchitis, and emphysema. However, allergic and maladaptive illness is also prevalent among tobacco users. Remember, too, that susceptibility to this type of illness is also prevalent in nonusers exposed to passive ambient cigarette smoke inhalation.

Smoking tobacco contains not only tobacco, but also pesticides and kerosene fuel combustion products, residues, flavoring and taste additives, sugar, and more. Tobacco allergy has been shown to cause headaches, dizziness, fatigue, mental confusion, circulatory changes, high blood pressure, sugar diabetes, and even mental symptoms such as depression, delusions, psychosis, and schizophrenia.

If you are a nonsmoker or an ex-smoker, demand that a part of your home and workplace be kept smoke-free. In addition, continuing to smoke is highly likely to sabotage and render meaningless most of the other measures you might take to reduce indoor chemical pollution.

NATURAL GAS. The combustion products from your kitchen range pose one of the most serious cumulative chemical threats to your health. Your gas oven will produce in one hour at 350° Fahrenheit as much carbon monoxide and nitrogen dioxide as a Los Angeles smog attack. If your kitchen is unvented, the pollution level will be three times the common Los Angeles pollution level. Even if the gas has been disconnected from your stove and is no longer operational, a well-used stove saturated with combustion products from natural gas can induce symptoms if you are chemically susceptible.

The only way to find out if your gas stove is making you ill is to remove it and the pipe from your living quarters and then see if you feel any different over the next few weeks. If you do feel better, and if you feel a worsening of your symptoms when you bring the stove back into your kitchen, it is likely that natural gas is the problem. If so, your best bet is to remove the stove for good and purchase an electric range and oven.

Note that this experiment might be invalidated if your home is heated by a gas furnace (see below). The best time to run your stove test would be in the warm season when the furnace and its pilot light are shut off.

Even if you're not presently gas sensitive, if you have the option of choosing a gas or an electric oven/range, going electric may reduce the chances of future cumulative chemical injury.

HEATING SYSTEMS. Your home furnace and water heater are common sources of chemical pollution. Gas and oil heat, kerosene space heaters, and, for extremely sensitive people, pine or other wood smoke can cause problems. The fumes and combustion products of petrochemicals contribute in a most significant way to cumulative chemical injury.

People who are petrochemically sensitive can react to pine wood fuel or even to pine paneling. There is some speculation, mentioned in Theron Randolph's *Alternative Approach to Allergies*, that crude oil derives from ancient pine forests submerged and crushed within the earth. This may account for the pine sensitivity in some petrochemically sensitive people.

A gas or oil furnace located in a basement, or especially in a closet or utility room on the main floor of a home that has no basement, will inevitably pollute your living quarters. If those with petrochemical sensitivity and illnesses expect to recover, they may have to remove their gas or oil furnaces from their living quarters or basements and relocate them in a detached garage or shed. Using electric or solar heat would also be an option.

Even if you are not chemically sensitive, you would do better to have a nonpetrochemical heating system if you wish to reduce the cumulative chemical pollution in your environment. If it is already petrochemical, try to have it strategically located for maximum protection. Apartment dwellers should try to locate themselves as far from the boiler room as possible. And to switch to an electric water heater, if it is located inside your apartment.

FILTERING SYSTEMS. If you cannot make your environment as clean as you would like, and if exposure to any household or industrial or office chemicals is unavoidable—or if you find yourself unwittingly exposed—be sure to take appropriate measures for your own protection.

Consider investing in an air cleaner/filter, a three-phase unit with a particulate filter, charcoal filter, and "Hepa" filter (see "Nontoxic Household and/or Personal Products," page 285).

Also consider installing a high-quality water filter on your kitchen tap. An activated carbon unit is adequate. However, a combined activated charcoal/reverse osmosis unit would be optimal—this is particularly important for those who are the most chemically sensitive.

For those who become more symptomatic after taking a shower, a carbon filter shower head or a carbon filter installed for the whole bathroom (or centrally) should be adequate to prevent the trihalomethane accumulation from chlorine interaction.

If you need to use strong cleaners or do a painting or furniture-refinishing project, use a painter's ventilator mask, rubber sealed and with vapor filters, rubber gloves, protective clothing and adequate ventilation. Take any commonsense measure that would substantially reduce contact with or concentration of the offending agents.

LIVING PLANT FILTERS. Several plants have been documented by NASA to act as natural detoxifiers and air purifiers that trap ambient formaldehyde, benzene, trichloroethylene, and other gaseous pollutants. You can experiment with this.

Place such utilitarian plants as the green spider and heart-leaf philodendron in your home or office to see if you feel better. To deter mold growth, use sterile soil. Chrysanthemums and Gerber daisies are also effective.

AUTOMOBILE TRAVEL. We expose ourselves to many serious forms of chemical pollution when we're in our cars. Whether you're environmentally ill or not, your car should have an air intake vent that can be closed to shut out or reduce ambient fumes from heavy traffic exhaust, dumps, fresh tar on the road, airport pollution, pesticide and herbicide fogging, and the like. Especially hazardous are diesel exhaust fumes and any exhaust in confined spaces such as tunnels or garages. Sensitive individuals can minimize their symptoms when driving by using an activated carbon air-filter inside the car to help remove the fumes that do gain access to the passenger compartment.

Plastic automobile upholstery may also be a source of pollution. Leather is the least sensitizing; rayon (made from cellulose, a wood by-product) is safe, too. Nylon is less objectionable than the newer, strong-smelling vinyl upholsteries. The very fact that you can smell the vinyl odor indicates that it is releasing substances into the air. You will notice the smell intensifies when the upholstery is heated, as in direct sunlight. These substances can set off symptoms in sensitive individuals just as severely as exhaust fumes. You may also need to remove all "rubber" mats, which are actually plastic, and replace them with carpeting—preferably made from natural fibers and without an imitation rubber backing.

Before buying a car, spend adequate time test-driving and sitting in it to assess the quality of its internal environment. Does it make you feel subtly ill? Are there exhaust leaks? Does the upholstery give off a plastic odor?

WHEN MOVING TO A NEW HOME. If you're planning to move, it's crucial to survey the surrounding area of your intended location for outdoor air pollution. Try to live as far away as possible from major streets, highways, industries, factories, and dump sites. Determine the direction of the prevailing winds so that you do not find yourself downwind from these sources of pollution. Inquire about whether a major road or highway or factory is to be built near your intended home.

Look for a home with a detached garage. Fumes easily find their way into your living quarters from a built-in or attached garage. If your garage is located just below your living area, be sure to let your car cool off outside before parking it in the garage. This way you can protect yourself from emissions that occur after you turn off the ignition while the engine is still hot.

CREATING A BEDROOM OASIS. Create an environmentally sound, pollutant-free atmosphere where you sleep. This may require a supreme effort, such as a complete stripping of the walls and floors. Or it might mean simply removing a few items. The fewer items you keep in the room, the better. Put your desk, books and magazines not in current use, elsewhere. Perfumes, cosmetics, scented powders, and lotions can all be easily stored in another room. Remove synthetic carpets and their pads. The best floor is bare wood, perhaps with scatter rugs made from natural untreated cotton or wool.

Look closely at your furniture. Has it ever been put in storage and possibly fumigated? Has any of it been plastic-coated, or recently stained, varnished, painted, or waxed? Does any of it emit a chemical or synthetic odor? Is any of it made with particleboard? Is your upholstered headboard emitting formaldehyde?

Remove plastic venetian blinds, synthetic curtains, oil paintings, and plastic picture frames. Use metal, glass, or untreated wood frames.

As chemically sensitive individuals are commonly allergic to inhalants such as molds, it is a good idea to remove houseplants as well from the bedroom, although as mentioned above, certain plants can absorb ambient chemicals and purify the air.

Remove from your closets all chemicals, tools, hobby materials, glue, shoe polish, and shelf paper, which is often impregnated with insect repellent. Try to include only natural-fiber garments in your bedroom closet and on your body. Store suitcases and company gear elsewhere.

Remove motor oil–impregnated filters in your air conditioner and replace them with vegetable- or seed-oil-impregnated ones (oils to which you are not allergic). Close off any oil- or natural gas–heated air vents entering the bedroom and use electric space heaters.

Instead of rubber pillows, use down (if tolerated), cotton-batting-stuffed pillows, buckwheat hull pillows (Japanese), or a rolled cotton bedspread placed in a cotton pillow case. Use a futon mattress containing cotton or wool batting, and do not use a plastic mattress cover or, if necessary, put a zippered cotton cover around a conventional mattress with two cotton pads on top. The cotton will serve as somewhat of a barrier between you and "rubber" or fibers of petroleum origin. Or, purchase a Dux (imported from Sweden), a bed designed for ultimate back support that just happens to be made from 100 percent natural materials (Duxiana, Bellevue, Washington, (206) 637-9725). Use 100 percent cotton sheets and cotton or wool blankets. Keep the windows open, if possible.

If after several weeks of sleeping in such an "oasis" you feel that your health has improved, you may want to extend the effect to other rooms in your home or apartment.

Minimizing the Worst Offenders

Please recall that many recommendations in this discussion require meticulous and sometimes extreme measures. These may be appropriate and practical only if your symptoms and disability are equally extreme.

For those with very mild symptoms or those who want to implement changes to prevent becoming environmentally ill, less harmful items such as plastic picture frames, polyester curtains, dishwasher soap, or polyethylene food containers do not carry the same risks as bug sprays or flea bombs (pesticides), weed killers (herbicides), solvents, or an unvented gas range.

By minimizing the worst chemical offenders and using common sense, you can reduce your chemical exposure enormously and still be considered a normal citizen of twentieth-century Earth.

If you're building a new home, you have a wonderful opportunity to make your entire living space nearly chemical free by a prudent choice of nonpolluting building materials. Your architect and builder may be resistant to your ideas and tell you that such materials are unavailable, but do your homework well. (See the appropriate titles in "Suggested Reading" on page 283 and applicable items under "Nontoxic Household and/or Personal Products," page 285) and you'll end up with a relatively chemical-free home and teach them something valuable.

HEAVY METAL POISONING

Another aspect of environmental illness is heavy metal poisoning. This is considered, by some, an even greater threat than the primarily organic chemicals discussed in Part One of this chapter.

Lead, mercury, cadmium, arsenic, aluminum, and nickel are heavy metals that can cause multiple and mystifying disorders, with both physical and mental/behavioral symptoms. In the body, they do their damage in a number of ways. Commonly, they antagonize the functioning of specific essential vitamins and minerals. This results in the malfunctioning of the enzymes dependent on those micronutrients.

Take, for example, just one toxic metal, lead. According to the excellent study by R. M. Jaffe, M.D., Ph.D.:

The amount of lead introduced into our environment since the beginning of the Industrial Revolution is enormous. From 1720 to 1979, close to 55 million tons of lead were added to the industrial supply in the USA. More than 7 million tons of lead have been used as gasoline additives in the U.S. alone. Much of this lead is now widely distributed on the earth's surface. For example, lead has been found at levels of up to 7,500 mg. per kg. of house dust and the earth's crust at levels of only 15 mg. per kg. This means that urban soil and house dust can contain 33 to 500 times the normal concentration of earth lead. The bottom sediment of U.S. lakes now contains about 20 times more lead than they did just 100 years ago.[15]

Heavy metals often displace nutrient cofactors from their proper enzyme systems. As enzymes are poisoned, metabolic processes are uncoupled and shut down—including the sulfur and selenium antioxidant enzyme systems. These metals can therefore trigger rampant free radical pathology and bring about the destruction of cellular membranes and components. They can be directly toxic to human tissues, including the brain, the kidneys, and the cardiovascular system, and are frequently stored there, as well as in the bone marrow.

Common symptoms of heavy metal accumulation in the body include: fatigue, headaches, depression and other emotional problems, behavioral disturbances, lower intelligence, diminished memory and cognitive ability—even dementia. It can also result in peripheral neuritis and neuropathy, abdominal cramps, anemia, high blood pressure, liver and kidney disease, and cancer.

Massive heavy metal exposure from industrial and occupational accidents can cause severe illness, even death. However, persistent low-level environmental exposures do their damage insidiously, producing common, everyday symptoms that may not alert your doctor to the underlying cause.

RECOGNIZING HEAVY METAL POISONING

In evaluating an individual for heavy metal toxicity, we need to assess symptoms as well as exposure to common sources of these metals. If there are symptoms suggestive of heavy metal toxicity, particularly if there are no other conditions apparent, or if an individual has a history of significant exposure to particular toxic metals, I usually find this reason enough to recommend testing. I have been led by symptoms alone to the diagnosis of heavy metal toxicity in a number of individuals who thought they'd had no significant exposure.

The following section discusses the signs and symptoms of heavy metal poisoning, and sources of these toxic metals.*

LEAD POISONING

SOURCES OF LEAD

Paint chips
Dust in and around homes and
  buildings
Lead-based paint
Solder
Leaded glass
Leaded gasoline
Pottery glaze
Newsprint
Dyes
Plumbing (lead-soldered
  pipes)
Landfills

Batteries (production and
  burning)
Inks
Ashes and fumes from burning
  oil-painted wood
Soil and air in and around in-
  dustrialized areas
Drinking water
Sewage sludge
Waste incineration
Lead-soldered cans (food
  from)

SYMPTOMS OF LEAD POISONING

Psychological, emotional, and behavioral problems, such as
  depression, hyperactivity, and others
Decreased memory and learning ability
Fatigue
Poor intelligence and school achievement scores
Colic and abdominal cramping
High blood pressure
Anemia
Immunosuppression—decreased resistance to bacterial and viral
  infections
Paralysis

*Other than the extended discussion and symptom list on mercury, this information comes from a 1993 monograph, "Toxic Minerals and Their Hypersensitivity ELISA-ACT™: Description of Items Tested," by Russell Jaffe, M.D., Ph.D., and Serammune Physicians Lab of Reston, Virginia. © R. M. Jaffe.

Free radical pathology resulting in atherosclerosis and other
  chronic degenerative diseases
Peripheral neuritis (inflammation of peripheral nerves)
Encephalopathy (severe brain involvement leading to seizures,
  mania, delirium, stupor, coma, death)
Permanent brain damage

Problems of Lead Accumulation

The most common form of lead exposure and lead toxicity is through ingestion of lead-containing paint, often used indoors in older houses. Renovation of old homes is often associated with release into the air of small particles containing high lead content. These lead particles can drift in the wind to adjacent homes. This remains a major health problem for children today in the inner cities. Each year in the United States about 200 children die from lead encephalopathy, while 800 have permanent brain damage and another 3,200 have temporary mental impairment. Children are more susceptible to lead poisoning because they absorb 25 to 40 percent more ingested lead than adults per pound of body weight. According to the Agency for Toxic Substances and Disease Registry 1991 report, excess lead in children remains common. Lead in children is correlated with income, as shown in the next table.

FREQUENCY OF EXCESS LEAD IN CHILDREN SIX MONTHS TO FIVE YEARS

FAMILY INCOME	WHITE CHILDREN	BLACK CHILDREN
<$6,000	36%	68%
$6,000–15,000	23%	54%
>$15,000	12%	38%

Lead is a slow, cumulative poison deposited eventually in the bones. Since the Industrial Revolution, its concentration in human bones has increased more than five hundred fold. Lead also strongly reacts with the selenium and sulfur-containing antioxidant enzymes in cells, severely crippling the free radical protective activities of these enzymes and promoting free radical damage.

Studies by Herbert Needleman, M.D., and others confirm that even lower doses than suspected produce long-term learning impairment and neurologic development in children. Barely twenty years ago, lead levels of 80 µg/dl were considered medically acceptable. Today, experts know that only levels less than 8 µg/dl can prevent the adverse effects of lead. No levels or exposures to lead are healthy.

Encouraging studies by Carl Pfeiffer and Arthur Sohler in lead-laden battery workers showed that supplemental zinc and ascorbate (vitamin C) can displace significant amounts of lead and lower the body burden. This also suggests that lead accumulation occurs when ascorbate and zinc intakes are inadequate.

MERCURY POISONING

SOURCES OF MERCURY

Silver amalgams (dental filling)	Floor waxes and polishes
Paints	Wood preservatives
Broken thermometers and barometers	Cinnabar (used in jewelry)
Felt	Some cosmetics
Fresh and saltwater fish and shellfish	Film
Grains/seed treated with mercury fungicide	Photo engraving
Fungicides	Tattooing
Fabric softeners	Plastics
Adhesives	Histology labs
Mercurial diuretics/ointments/antiseptics	Industrial wastes
	Sewage sludge/sewage disposal
	Air and water in and around industrial areas

SYMPTOMS OF MERCURY POISONING

Disorders in the mouth including excess salivation, swollen tongue, ulcerations of the mouth, burning sensations in the mouth or throat, bleeding gums, and erosion of teeth
Psychological and emotional disturbances such as apathy, depression, irritability, anxiety, and insomnia
Cognitive impairment such as poor memory, poor concentration, poor learning
Neurologic symptoms such as tremors of the eyelids, tongue, lips, and extremities; seizures, loss of coordination, headaches, numbness, tingling, and possibly multiple sclerosis
Gastrointestinal complaints such as abdominal cramps
Cardiovascular disturbances such as irregular heartbeat, chest pains, and high blood pressure
Immune suppression predisposing one to yeast overgrowth, viral and bacterial infections, and possibly cancer; possible predilection to autoimmune diseases
General symptoms such as fatigue, poor appetite, frequent urination
Birth defects, stillbirths, and miscarriages
Infertility

Mercury in Dental Fillings

The most common exposure to mercury is through silver-amalgam dental fillings. Mercury accounts for about 50 percent of this compound by weight. Fillings in the mouth have been shown to release mercury vapor,[16] and in a mouth with many fillings, about 560 milligrams of mercury can leach into the body from amalgam fillings over a ten-year period. A debate on the health safety of using silver amalgam in dentistry has been continuing for many years. There are documented cases of mercury toxicity in dental workers due to inhalation of mercury vapor produced during the insertion or replacement of amalgam fillings. The link between mercury exposure and symptoms is more complex. Strong anecdotal information and clinical observations of physicians exist to support a definite link between amalgam fillings and pathological processes.[17]

With such a growing body of evidence and scientific documentation, the governments of at least two countries (Sweden and Germany) are taking active measures to curtail the use of mercury-containing dental materials. This restriction, which has initially been applied to children and pregnant women, will be extended to the whole population.

In spite of the American Dental Association's position that mercury amalgam is a safe and suitable dental material for the majority of Americans,[18] there has been a growing mercury alarm among a growing minority of dentists and the informed public. Not only are they choosing safer, biocompatible dental materials for new fillings, but they are removing and replacing existing mercury-containing fillings as well. In so doing, some individuals are finding relief from chronic health problems, both minor and major.

In their groundbreaking book, *It's All in Your Head: The Link Between Mercury Amalgams and Illness* (Avery, 1993), Hal Huggins, D.D.S., and Sharon Huggins, R.D.H., not only bring this issue to light, but also discuss the potential toxicity of other common dental materials and the abnormal electrical phenomena that occur with mixed metals—gold, silver, mercury, etc.—in the mouth (see other mercury-related titles in "Suggested Reading").

For information on dentists and physicians with specialized training and data concerning the laboratory evaluation and treatment for mercury toxicity, contact the Foundation for Toxic Free Dentistry, the Toxic Element Research Foundation and Compat Labs, Inc., the International Academy of Oral Medicine and Toxicology, and the American Academy of Environmental Medicine. (See "Organizations," page 284, and "Medical Laboratories Performing Environmental Testing," page 285).

Mercury in Housepaint

Mercury used to be a common ingredient in many brands of latex house paint. It was used to prevent mildew. In August 1990, the EPA banned its use in interior latex paint, but companies with mercury-containing latex interior paint were allowed to sell their previous stock. Call the National Pesticide Telecommunication Network (800) 858-7378 to find out the mercury content of any brand you may have once used—and be sure any interior paint you buy from now on was made after the mercury ban.

You will also want to minimize your exposure to dietary sources of mercury, of course. Fish—especially tuna—have comparatively large amounts. Shellfish are scavengers, and those harvested from most industrial coastal areas are likely to contain high levels of heavy metals.

Be wary, too, of pharmaceuticals and cosmetics as additional sources of mercury, such as thimerosal, an antibacterial mercurial compound. Try to avoid thimerosal-containing contact lens–cleaning solutions, and thimerosal-containing multidose injectable vitamins and drugs. Find substitutes for Mercurochrome and Merthiolate. Also, be aware that some eye salves and ointments, calomel, some antiseptic creams and lotions, and some long-acting nasal sprays may contain mercurial compounds. Read labels and ask questions!

CADMIUM POISONING

SOURCES OF CADMIUM	
Paints (artist's and commercial/ industrial)	Coffee
	Meat (liver and kidneys)
Metals (metal plating)	Poultry
Colored plastics	Grains
Fertilizers	Dairy products
Fungicides	Cigarette smoke
Antiseptics	Soil and air in and around
Solder	cities and industrialized
Batteries	areas
Gasoline	Landfills
Refined foods	Sewage sludge
Fish and shellfish	Waste incineration

SYMPTOMS OF CADMIUM POISONING
Fetal growth retardation and developmental abnormalities in the fetus
Learning disabilities
Poor scores on intelligence, achievement, and verbal IQ tests
Predisposition to lung and prostate cancers
Possible predisposition to benign prostate hypertrophy (enlargement of the prostate gland)
Immunosuppression due to white blood cell impairment; increased susceptibility to bacteria and viral infections
High blood pressure

Cadmium and Cigarette Smoke

Cadmium, like lead, is an underground mineral that has become a prevalent problem. Smoking is one of the primary sources of cadmium exposure for the greatest number of individuals in our society. One cigarette a day can measurably increase blood cadmium levels, and smokers usually have about twice the body burden of cadmium as nonsmokers, especially in their livers, kidneys, and lungs. One of the reasons pregnant women need to stop smoking is that cadmium is toxic to the embryo and fetus, as it can cross the placenta and concentrate in amniotic fluid.

Finally, there is a direct correlation between environmental cadmium levels and death rates due to high blood pressure. Cadmium is known to be especially toxic to the kidneys.

ARSENIC POISONING

SOURCES OF ARSENIC	
Insecticides	Wallpaper
Weed killers	Copper-smelting factories and
Ceramics	soil from surrounding areas
Glass	and downwind (sometimes
Paint	for hundreds of miles)

SYMPTOMS OF ARSENIC POISONING	
Peripheral neuropathy (degeneration of the nerves in the hands and feet leading to numbness, tingling, burning)	Headaches
	Fatigue
	Drowsiness
	Seizures
	Liver damage (fatty infiltration and cirrhosis)
Muscular weakness	Kidney damage
Loss of hair	Death
Dermatitis	

Toxic Effects of Arsenic

Despite its reputation, arsenic has a fairly low toxicity level in comparison with other metals. Nevertheless, it is still extremely poisonous and causes toxicity by combining with sulfur-containing enzymes, thus impairing free radical control and detoxification, and interfering with cellular metabolism. Its toxic effects are cumulative.

Copper-smelting factories are the major sources of arsenic in our environment, contaminating our soil, our waterways, and, ultimately, our food supply.

ALUMINUM POISONING

SOURCES OF ALUMINUM	
Cans	Buffered aspirin
Foil	Deodorants
White flour	Tap water
Some cheeses	Food additives

Antacids
Sodium aluminum sulfate in
  baking powder

Some infant formulas
Aluminum cookware and cooking utensils

SYMPTOMS OF ALUMINUM POISONING

Memory loss
Learning impairment
Dementia, including Alzheimer's disease
Encephalopathy (brain degeneration)
Calcium and phosphorus metabolism disturbances leading to os-
teomalacia (softening of the bones) and osteoporosis

Aluminum-related Brain Disorders

Aluminum can be absorbed from the gut and accumulate in the brain, as well as in other tissue. It may
also enter the brain via direct uptake from the absorptive surfaces of the nose and mouth. Once in the body,
aluminum inhibits the production of an essential cofactor (tetrahydrobiopterin) in the formation of brain
neurotransmitters. This inhibitive action may be the major mechanism by which aluminum contributes to Alzheimer's disease, as tetrahydrobiopterin levels are
significantly lower in Alzheimer's patients.

Another aspect of aluminum pathology that has far-
reaching consequences is its ability to increase the permeability of the blood-brain barrier, a protective barrier
restricting the passage of potentially harmful molecules
into the brain. "Aluminum may enhance the permeability of the blood-brain barrier to small behaviorally active peptides (proteins), and this can lead to dementia
(including senile dementia) and other CNS disorders."[19]
The increased permeability may allow the dangerous
deposition of immune complexes in the brain as well.
This may be the relationship between aluminum and
Alzheimer's disease (see page 328 for further discussion).

NICKEL POISONING

SOURCES OF NICKEL	
Tobacco smoke	Air, water, and soil in and
Electronic devices	around industrial areas
Steel and metal alloys (jewelry,	Hydrogenated oils
prosthetics)	

SYMPTOMS OF NICKEL SKIN SENSITIVITY	
Contact dermatitis	Eczematous dermatitis

CONSEQUENCES OF NICKEL CARBONYL INHALATION	
Neuronal (nerve cell)	Heart attack
degeneration in the brain	Cancer of the respiratory
Edema and hemorrhage in	tract
the lung	

Nickel—Pro and Con

Nickel appears to be an essential element for normal
RNA/DNA structure and function. It may also have a
biological role in the metabolism and function of cell
membranes. Humans need only very small amounts of
nickel; however, nickel deficiency in humans is not
known or clearly defined.

Nickel is poorly absorbed from the gastrointestinal
tract, and the retention of newly acquired nickel in the
tissues, other than the lung, is transient and poor, probably due to active excretory mechanisms. Most nickel
found in food is minimally absorbed, but nickel from
drinking water is more readily absorbed.

Metallic nickel is relatively nontoxic, probably due
to its poor absorption and active excretion. However,
nickel compounds can be inhaled (especially those from
cigarette smoke) and retained in lung tissue, where they
tend to remain. Nickel compounds can cause cancer.

TESTING FOR HEAVY METAL TOXICITY

Your doctor may not readily consider that your headaches, fatigue, recurrent depression, and abdominal
cramps may relate to subtle heavy metal poisoning. But
even if he or she is willing to investigate this possibility,
the standard, first-line tests measuring blood and urine
levels of metals will not usually be very useful. Unless a
person has accumulated an enormous quantity of these
metals in the body, blood and urine levels may not be
abnormal. These metals lodge in intracellular spaces (inside cells) rather than in the blood and urine, until very
high amounts have accumulated in the body.

Provocative Chelation

A far more useful method of testing for heavy metals, by many physicians' standards, is provocative chelation, in which a chelating agent such as intravenous
EDTA (ethylenediamine tetraacetic acid) or oral
d-penicillamine is given. These agents and others, such
as DMSA—dimercaptosuccinic acid—pull metals out of
tissues into the blood and urine where they can be excreted. A twenty-four-hour urine sample is then collected, and a measured amount is sent to the laboratory
for analysis.[20] I am currently using a protocol of Russell
Jaffe, M.D., Ph.D., utilizing d-penicillamine.[21]

Hair Analysis

Hair analysis can be used as a screen for heavy
metal accumulation. Hair is an easily accessible site of
heavy metal deposits in the body. Such testing can provide information on intracellular accumulation, as well

as the body's ability or inability to excrete metals. It can help confirm suspicions of heavy metal toxicity long before abnormal levels show up in the blood or urine. Unfortunately, normal levels of toxic metals reflected by this test don't always correlate with the level of deposits in tissues. This means that further investigation needs to be done. If you do hair testing, see that the laboratories conform to the standards set by the College of American Pathologists. Laboratories should participate in federally approved proficiency test programs as defined by the Clinical Laboratory Improvement Act.

TREATING HEAVY METAL TOXICITY

The aim of this treatment is to reduce or eliminate the source of exposure, and then to reduce the body burden of the metals with chelating agents, and to protect the body with antioxidants and other nutrients. As a first step, you need to identify your sources of exposure as discussed above, and then attempt to minimize or avoid them when possible.

A Nutritional Supplement Program

Next, you need to use supplements and foods that have been shown to help you chelate and excrete metals, as well as counter the damage they may be causing. Among the recommended supplements are sulfhydryl amino acids: cysteine or N-acetylcysteine, 500 milligrams three times daily with vitamin C (see below), and methionine, up to 1,000 milligrams a day provide chelating and antioxidant effects. Cysteine/N-acetylcysteine's chelating function is used especially for mercury and arsenic, although its antioxidant effect is appropriate for countering all metals. Garlic's effectiveness may be attributed to its abundant sulfhydryl groups, and may act somewhat like cysteine.

Minerals such as calcium, up to 1,000 milligrams; magnesium, up to 800 milligrams; and zinc, up to 50 milligrams (all daily doses), can also displace toxic metals from the body. Vitamin C (1,000–2,000 milligrams three or more times daily) is also usually taken to help metal excretion, as well as to bolster antioxidant systems.

This basic combination of detoxification nutrients may suffice for minor cases of heavy metal toxicity. However, for heavier burdens of toxic metals, there are additional remedies to consider. Vitamin B-1 (up to 100 milligrams daily) works with vitamin C and cysteine. In addition, selenium (up to 200 micrograms daily); glutathione (up to 150 milligrams daily), vitamin E (up to 400 I.U. daily); and beta-carotene (up to 50,000 I.U. daily) are also used for their antioxidant roles. (See Chapter Six for precautions, food sources, and further discussion of these nutrients.)

When using a strictly nutritional program, I may also recommend that my patients use Porphyra-zyme, a chlorophyll-based tablet (by Biotics of Houston, TX), or chlorella tablets, as chlorophyll is known to promote the exit of metals.

Using a high-potency multiple vitamin/mineral and a combination antioxidant/chelator/detoxification supplement (such as Perque 1 by Seraphim of Reston, Virginia) can simplify the program. You would need to obtain this through your doctor or pharmacy, but other products of this kind can be found in health food stores.

You will still require an extra calcium/magnesium and vitamin C supplement, however. Such a program may require up to six or more months for successful results.

A Dietary Program

A high-fiber diet rich in low-methoxyl pectin, found in core-type fruits such as apples and pears, and in legumes, can bind heavy metals and prevent their intestinal absorption. I also recommend drinking eight ounces daily of vegetable juice (about half of it carrot), primarily for its alkalinizing effect, but also for its other health benefits. This helps normalize the somewhat acidic systems of those with heavy metal toxicity and allows their detoxification enzymes to function more optimally. Including the juice of dark green leafy and other vegetables increases the chlorophyll content of the drink, which also helps encourage the exit of metals.

Drinking up to sixteen ounces a day of vegetable broth is also alkalinizing and may be a substitute, if you do not have a juicer.

A Homeopathic Program

Homeopathic agents, when skillfully prescribed, have also been used successfully for heavy metal detoxification. Infinitesimal dilutions of the involved heavy metal are taken to engage the body's natural counter-excretory mechanisms (see Chapter Twenty-one).

A Chelation Program

Well-known pharmaceutical chelators include EDTA, d-penicillamine, and dimercaprol/DMPS. Known abroad, and also gaining popularity in the U.S., is DMSA (dimercaptosuccinic acid), a remarkably safe and effective chelator used orally.[22] Unlike others, it also takes metals out of the central nervous system (brain). DMSA is used particularly for mercury, lead, and arsenic poisoning, and is possibly effective for cadmium.

I am most familiar with the use of d-penicillamine. In clear cases of heavy metal toxicity, I will prescribe an adult dose of 500 milligrams four times daily every other day for up to six weeks, along with many of the nutritional recommendations mentioned above. I will re-test the urine at that time, through provocative chelation. I have sometimes needed to re-treat a patient for two more four-to-six-week courses.

One of my more exemplary cases involved Jenny. She had worked as a drawbridge operator, and had been breathing car and truck exhaust fumes for years. She complained of chronic headaches and fatigue, and said she required medication to lower her blood pressure.

After three months of treatment, during which we reversed her extremely elevated levels of lead and cadmium, Jenny's symptoms were gone and she no longer required her blood pressure medication.

YOUR SYMPTOMS ARE REAL— AND HELP IS ON THE WAY

In this chapter we have reviewed the vast subject of environmental illness. We have looked at individuals with the chemical hypersensitivity syndrome, those with chemically toxic accumulations in their fat cells, and those with heavy metal accumulations.

Such affected individuals have great difficulty finding the kind of medical care that can uncover and treat the underlying causes of their problems. Like many of those affected with any of the Ten Common Denominators of Illness (see Chapter Sixteen), they are usually treated primarily with symptom-suppressing medication and are often considered nutcases by their doctors. But there is hope. With the self-care measures you can implement, and the tests and treatments recommended by nutritionally and environmentally oriented doctors, you can move toward optimal wellness.

SUGGESTED READING

Ashford, Nicholus, J.D., Ph.D., and Miller, Claudia, M.D. *Chemical Exposures—Low Levels and High Stakes*. New York: Van Nostrand Reinhold, 1991.

Berlin, A., Dean, J., Draper, M.H., Smith, E.M.B., and Spreafico, F. (Eds.) *Immunotoxicology*. Boston: Martinus Nijhoff, 1987.

Bio-Probe Newsletter (for scientific, medical and political information on mercury-related illness), Sam Ziff, editor, 4401 Real Ct., Orlando, FL 32808, (407) 299-4149.

Bower, John. *The Healthy House: How to Buy One, How to Cure a "Sick" One, How to Build One*. New York: Carroll Publishing Group, 1989.

Clarkson, T.W., et al. *The Biological Monitoring of Toxic Metals*. New York: Plenum Press, 1988.

Cohen, Gary, and O'Connor. *Fighting Toxins: A Manual for Protecting Your Family, Community, and Workplace*. Washington, D.C.: Island Press, 1990.

Dadd, Debra. *The Nontoxic Home*. Los Angeles: JT Tarcher, 1986.

———. *Nontoxic, Natural, and Earthwise (How to Protect Yourself and Your Family from Harmful Products and Live in Harmony with the Earth)*. Los Angeles: JT Tarcher, 1990.

Daum, Susan M., Stellman, Jeanne, Ph.D., and Daum, S.M. *Work Is Dangerous to Your Health: A Handbook of Health Hazards in the Workplace and What You Can Do About It*. New York: Random House, 1973.

Earthworks Group. *50 Simple Things You Can Do to Save the Earth* and *50 Simple Things Kids Can Do to Save the Earth*. Schenevus, New York: Greenleaf Publications, 1990.

Government Accountability Project, 25 E St., NW, Suite 700, Washington, DC 20001.

Hall, Ross Hume. *Health and the Global Environment*. Cambridge, UK: Polity Press, 1990.

Household Chemicals—The Hidden Hazards: What They Are, What You Should Know About Them, How to Safely Dispose of Them. State of Washington Department of Ecology, Hazardous Substance Information Office, Mail Stop PV-11, Olympia, WA 98504, (800) 633-5585.

Hubbard, L. Ron. *Clear Body, Clear Mind, The Effective Purification Program*. Los Angeles: Bridge Publications, Inc., 1990.

Huggins, H., D.D.S., and Huggins, S., R.D.H. *It's All in Your Head: Diseases Caused by Silver/Mercury Fillings*. P.O. Box 2589, Colorado Springs, CO 80901, 1985.

Huggins, H., D.D.S. *The Applications Textbook* (1988), and *Balancing Body Chemistry* (1983). HAH Publications, P.O. Box 49308, Colorado Springs, CO 80949-9308. Contact Toxic Element Research Foundation for professional courses. (See "Organizations.")

Levine, S.A., and Reinhardt, J.H. "Biochemical-Pathology Initiated by Free Radicals, Oxidant Chemicals, and Therapeutic Drugs in the Etiology of Chemical Hypersensitivity Disease," *Journal of Orthomolecular Psychiatry*, 12 (3): 166–183, 1983.

Mandell, A., M.D. *Dr. Mandell's Five-Day Allergy Relief System*. New York: Thomas Crowell, 1979.

McGee, C., M.D. *How to Survive Modern Technology: A Crash Course in Protecting Your Health from the Hidden Hazards of Daily Living*. New Canaan, CT: Pivot Keats, 1979.

Mercury Free News. P.O. Box 49308, Colorado Springs, CO 80949-9308, (800) 243-2782.

National Academy of Sciences. *An Assessment of Mercury in the Environment.* Washington, D.C., 1978.

National Research Council, Subcommittee on Immunotoxicology, Committee on Biologic Markers, Board on Environmental Studies and Toxicology, Commission on Life Sciences. *Biological Markers in Immunotoxicology and Environmental Neurotoxicology and Multiple Chemical Sensitivities.* Washington, D.C.: National Academy Press, 1992.

Pearson, D. *The Natural House Book: Creating a Healthy, Harmonious, and Ecologically Sound Home Environment.* New York: Simon & Schuster, 1989.

Penzer, V., D.D.S. "Amalgam Toxicity: Grand Deception," *The Townsend Letter for Doctors* #35: 58–63, Feb./Mar., 1986, 911 Tyler St., Port Townsend, WA 98368.

Queen, S. *Chronic Mercury Toxicity: New Hope Against an Endemic Disease.* Deerfield Beach, FL: Queen and Co. Health Communications, Inc., 1991.

Randolph, Theron C., M.D. and Moss, Ralph W., Ph.D. *An Alternative Approach to Allergies.* NY: HarperCollins, 1990.

Rapp, D.J., M.D. *Is This Your Child? Discovering and Treating Unrecognized Allergies.* New York: William Morrow, 1991.

Rogers, Sherry, A.M.D. *Tired or Toxic.* Syracuse, NY: Prestige Publishing, 1990.

———. *The E.I. Syndrome: An Rx for Environmental Illness.* Syracuse: NY: Prestige Publishing, 1990.

Root, D.D., M.D., M.P.H., and Wisner, R. *Chemical Exposure in the Workplace.* California Medical-Legal Alert, Summer 1987.

Rousseau, D. *Your Home, Your Health and Well-Being.* Berkeley, CA: Ten Speed Press, 1988.

Schnare, D.W., Ph.D. *The Unpolluting of Man.* Foundation for Advancements in Science and Education, P.O. Box 29813, Los Angeles, CA 90029.

Schecter, S. *Fighting Radiation and Chemical Pollutants with Foods, Herbs and Vitamins: Documented Natural Remedies that Boost Your Immunity and Detoxify.* Encinitas, CA: Vitality Ink, 1988, revised 1990.

Stanley, J.S. *Broadscan Analysis of Human Adipose Tissue,* Volume I: Executive Summary. United States Environmental Protection Agency, Office of Toxic Substances, Washington, DC 20460. EPA–560/5–86–035, December 1986.

Stortebecker, P. *Mercury Poisoning from Dental Amalgam—A Hazard to the Human Brain.* Orlando, FL: Bio-Probe, 1985–86.

———. *Dental Caries as a Cause of Nervous Disorders.* Orlando, FL: Bio-Probe, 1982.

Taylor, J., D.D.S. *The Complete Guide to Mercury Toxicity from Dental Fillings: How to Find Out if Your Dental Fillings Are Poisoning You and What You Can Do About It.* San Diego, CA: Scripps Publishing.

Timbrell, J.A. *Principles of Biochemical Toxicology,* Second Edition. Bristol, PA: Taylor and Francis, 1991.

Upah, G. *Homesick Syndrome: A Guide Book to Residential Environmental Health Hazards,* Second Edition. Dallas, TX, RCI Environmental Institute: November, 1991, (214) 250-6608.

Weissman, J.D., M.D. *Choose to Live.* New York: Grove Press, 1988.

Zamm, A., M.D. *Why Your House May Endanger Your Health.* New York: Simon & Schuster, 1980.

Ziff, S. *Silver Dental Fillings: The Toxic Time Bomb.* Santa Fe, NM: Aurora Press, 1984. Also see, *Bio-Probe Newsletter.*

Ziff, S., and Ziff, M.F., D.D.S. *The Hazards of Silver/Mercury Dental Fillings: Restorative Dentistry without Silver Amalgam Fillings* and *Mercury Detoxification.* Health Information Booklets published by BioProbe, Inc., P.O. Box 580160, Orlando, Florida 32858-0160, (407) 299-4149. Also by these same authors and publisher: *Infertility and Birth Defects: Is Mercury from Silver Dental Fillings a Hidden Cause?*, BioProbe, 1990.

ORGANIZATIONS

ADAM (a dental amalgam mercury syndrome): A non-profit lay organization patient support group. Newsletter. P.O. Box 854, Kirkland, WA 98083-0854.

The American College of Advancement in Medicine (ACAM), 23121 Verdugo Drive, Suite 204, Laguna Hills, CA 92653, (714) 583-7666.

The American Academy of Environmental Medicine, P.O. Box 16016, Denver, CO 80216, (303) 622-9755.

Environmental Defense Fund, 257 Park Ave. S., New York, NY 10010, (212) 505-2100.

Foundation for Advancements in Science and Education (FASE), 4801 Wilshire Blvd., #215, Los Angeles, CA 90010, (213) 937-9911.

Foundation for Toxic-Free Dentistry, P.O. Box 580160, Orlando, FL 32858-0160.

Healthmed Detox, 5501 Power Inn Road, Suite 140, Sacramento, CA 95820, (916) 387-8252.

Human Ecology Action League, 2250 North Druid Hills Road, #236, Atlanta, GA 30329, (404) 248-1898.

International Academy of Oral Medicine and Toxicology, P.O. Box 608531, Orlando, FL 32860-8531, (407) 298-2450.

Natural Resources Defense Council, 122 E. 42nd St., New York, NY 10164.

RCI Environmental, Inc., 17772 Preston Road, Suite 202, Dallas, TX 75252, (214) 250-6608. Provides educational materials to the public and conducts a comprehensive training seminar on residential environment health hazards; provides inspector's certification for residential environmental health hazards.

Toxic Element Research Foundation and Compat Labs, Inc., 5080 List Dr., Colorado Springs, CO 80919, (800) 331-2303.

Washington Toxics Coalition, 4516 University Way NE, Seattle, WA 98105, (206) 632-1545.

NONTOXIC HOUSEHOLD AND/OR PERSONAL PRODUCTS

Baubiologie Hardware Catalog, 207B 16th St., Pacific Grove, CA 93950, (408) 372-8626.

Bi-O-Kleen, 133 S.E. Salmon St., Portland, OR 97214.

The Chronic Fatigue and Immune Dysfunction Syndrome (CFIDS) Buying Club, 1187 Coast Village Rd. #1–280, Santa Barbara, CA 93108-2794, (800) 366-6056.

Flowright, 1495 N.W. Gilman Blvd. #4, Issaquah, WA 98027, (206) 392-8357: Air filters/purifiers, water filters, personal care and household products including carpeting, non-toxic paints and sealants, environmental contamination inspection and evaluation.

Livos, 614 Agua Fria St., Santa Fe, NM 87501, (505) 988-9111.

The Natural Choice (ecologically sound products), 1365 Rufina Circle, Santa Fe, NM 87501, (505) 438-3448.

Nigra Enterprises, 5699 Kanan Rd. (BR), Agoura, CA 91301-3358, (818) 889-6877: Air filters/purifiers, water filters.

Water Star Products and Services, P.O. Box 8375, Kirkland, WA 98034, (206) 821-2555. Reverse Osmosis Water Filtering Systems.

MEDICAL LABORATORIES PERFORMING ENVIRONMENTAL TESTING

Accu-Chem Laboratories, 990 N. Bower, Suite 800, Richardson, TX 75081, (214) 234-5412 (in Texas), (800) 451-0116 (outside Texas).

Antibody Assay Laboratories, 1715 E. Wilshire #715, Santa Ana, CA 92705, (714) 972-9979; (800) 522-2611.

Huggins Diagnostic Laboratory, P.O. Box 2691, 5080 List Drive, Colorado Springs, CO, 80919 (719) 548-1600: Biocompatibility of dental materials and urine mercury excretion.

Immunosciences Laboratory, 8730 Wilshire Blvd., Suite 305, Beverly Hills, CA 90211, (800) 950-4686.

National Medical Services, Inc., 2300 Stratford Ave., Willow Grove, PA 19090, (215) 657-4900.

Pacific Toxicology Laboratory, 1545 Pontius Ave., Los Angeles, CA 90025, (213) 479-4911, (800) 32-TOXIC (in California); (800) 23-TOXIC (outside California).

Serammune Physicians Lab, 1890 Preston White Drive, Suite 201, Reston, VA 22091, (703) 758-0610 or (800) 553-5472.

MEDICAL CENTERS PROVIDING A HUBBARD-TYPE DETOXIFICATION PROGRAM

Healthmed Detox, 5501 Power Inn Road-Suite 140, Sacramento, CA 95820, (916) 387-8252.

Allan Lieberman, M.D., Center for Environmental Medicine, 7510 Northforest Dr., North Charleston, SC, (803) 572-1600.

Northwest Healing Arts Center, 13401 N.E. Bell-Red Road, Suite 4A, Bellevue, WA 98005, (206) 747-9200.

William Rea, M.D., Environmental Health Center, 8345 Walnut Hill Lane, Dallas, TX 75231, (214) 368-4132.

Albert Robbins, D.O., Robbins Environmental Medicine Center, 400 Dixie Highway, Building 2, Boca Raton, FL 33432, (407) 395-3282.

Jeffrey White, M.D. 3715 Azeele, Tampa, FL 33609, (813) 876-6117.

PSYCHONEUROIMMUNOLOGY: THE BODY-MIND CONNECTION

This chapter examines the mind, our psychological and emotional sides, and how they influence our physical health. We will look at many variables—stress, coping skills, personality traits, social connectedness, self-esteem, and more—to see how they correlate with both susceptibility and resistance to physical illness. Case histories and a stress inventory will help you gain some perspective on the patterns influencing your life. I will discuss several therapies and provide self-help guidelines and instructions for various meditation, skilled relaxation, and imagery exercises. In previous chapters, you learned how taking care of the body influences the mind. Here you will learn that the mind and body are inseparable. Improving your level of psychological fitness and emotional health will directly benefit your body.

JACKIE

Jackie is a twenty-five-year-old woman who came to see me in my office recently. She appeared anxious, jittery, depressed, fearful, and feverish. An examination revealed a very red throat, swollen, tender lymph glands in her neck, and a generally tender abdomen. She told me that she had developed an upper respiratory infection and abdominal pain in the last two weeks, as well as a urinary tract infection, a vaginal yeast infection, constipation, headaches, back pain, a stiff neck, poor appetite, and an inability to sleep.

From a conventional medical viewpoint, Jackie's physical complaints marked her as a candidate for antibiotics, antifungal cream, laxatives, aspirin or stronger pain medication, and sleeping pills. I questioned her further.

I learned that in the last four weeks several traumatic and confusing events had taken place. Jackie had quit the job where she had worked for over a year. Although she'd felt well suited to the job, personal differences had become too aggravating for her to continue. However, now that she was in a new position with new people and new responsibilities to learn, she felt quite unsure of herself.

On top of her job shift, she'd just ended a four-year relationship with a man and had gotten herself involved immediately with another man. This new relationship was now presenting problems. To add to her list of woes, she was sharing an apartment with an extremely incompatible roommate and rarely felt at peace in her own home. And finally, Jackie's mother had been recently diagnosed with cancer.

We spoke in some detail about each of these circumstances. Jackie said she felt sexually compatible with her new boyfriend, but she didn't feel that the relationship would be deep or long-term. Nevertheless, she had a strong sense that her boyfriend was becoming very attached to her and possibly interested in marriage. She felt guilty that he was falling in love when she was just seeking companionship and solace from a wounded heart.

The situation with her roommate, whom Jackie considered to be loud and rude, was past the point of tolerance. Jackie needed to live with someone who could respect her need for quiet and solitude. Although the two had been friends for nearly a year before moving in with each other, Jackie hadn't known that the woman would be so inconsiderate. They had previously agreed to move to a larger apartment, but Jackie was now trying to back out of it, giving the excuse that she could not afford it. It was easier for her to lie than to demand respect and consideration.

So here we have a woman, previously in very good health, who in the last four weeks had encountered back-to-back consecutive changes in her life: the loss of a relationship, of a job, and potentially of her mother. In the midst of her depression, grief, and shock, she was struggling with a new job, a new relationship, and an insensitive roommate. There seemed no respite or escape from her difficulties. The two people from whom she could potentially get the most support, her roommate and boyfriend, were the same ones with whom she was not being truthful. She was growing more and more uncomfortable and distant with both of them. In addition to her anger, anxiety, and confusion, she had begun to feel powerless. Jackie's coping mechanisms became overloaded, and it didn't take long for physical symptoms to manifest themselves.

As she described all of these events and their dynamics, looking at them from a different perspective, she began to cry and release some of her tension and anxiety. She began to appear relaxed and relieved. I recommended a number of medications for her various infections, but I also strongly suggested that counseling would be of much benefit to her. I also asked her to let me know within a week how she was feeling.

After three weeks without a word, I phoned her to learn that she was feeling quite herself again, no longer suffering from any of the ailments she'd presented in my office. I also learned she had taken none of the prescribed medications or remedies.

During this phone conversation, Jackie shared with me that she had become aware of her real feelings, of her own inner truth. After talking with me in my office, she had felt a greater sense of balance, centeredness, and relief from her recent experiences as well as an improvement in all her physical ailments. The effects of the visit were so remarkable to her, she told me, that she'd felt no need at first to seek counseling. She decided that she needed to have more frequent heart-to-hearts with close friends who could listen well and be empathetic. But after a time, she'd decided to find a counselor anyway, someone who could help her further explore what she'd begun to discover with me.

Soon thereafter, she began expressing her real feelings to her boyfriend and to her roommate. She'd come to realize that she needed to be more truthful with the people in her life for her own sanity and survival. And this required her to get into the habit of looking carefully at her feelings, needs, desires, and values. She made it a point to have "conversations with herself." These helped her get a clearer picture of what she really wanted and how to go about getting it. She began to understand how important it was to know herself, to know what made her feel good and what threw her off balance.

Being truthful with others required assertiveness and courage, which did not come naturally to Jackie. But being frank about her real feelings began to seem much easier when she remembered how deeply her health and self-esteem depended on it. She said that being so open and truthful with others sometimes got her into trouble because she wasn't yet skillful in the art of communication. But in the end, she knew that being truthful was a vital way to maintain self-respect, generate closeness with others, and stay well physically. Her new approach also helped her feel much more a part of things in general. It also seemed to help her cope much better than she expected with her mother's illness.

Jackie was never taught any of the principles and skills that help one to develop psychological fitness and emotional health. She wasn't even taught how deeply emotional and physical well-being interrelate. In her schooling, she had learned about physical fitness and a little bit about nutrition, but virtually nothing about the skills she needed to put her in touch with herself. She didn't know how to accept herself, how to communicate with others, or how to be balanced and happy. As time went on, she viewed her counseling more as continuing education than as therapy. She began to take courses that helped her to develop self-knowledge, self-confidence, communication skills, and inner peace. These courses filled in the gaps of her previous schooling, and the gaps in her life.

We now come to the story of Sara. While a nutritional program seemed to be the answer to her physical problems, her emotional life began to sabotage all her good efforts.

SARA

Sara is a fifty-six-year-old woman who came to see me in my office for a rheumatoid arthritis condition. With the aid of the pain and anti-inflammatory medications she'd been taking for years, she could walk and perform most routine tasks without much difficulty or limitation. Fortunately, she hadn't developed the joint deformities that sometimes occur with this illness. However, she was severely limited without her medications. She was also taking a diuretic for slightly elevated blood pressure and a sleeping pill every night for "nerves."

Sara was interested in an alternative approach to her arthritis and wondered if there was anything she could do to reduce or eliminate her apparent dependence on medications.

I suggested a comprehensive plan that involved the

elimination of suspected food allergens and common health hazards in her diet and the inclusion of nutritious meals with therapeutic vitamin and mineral supplements specific for her condition and needs. After just a few weeks on her new program, which she followed as best she could, she was experiencing much less pain and stiffness in her joints with much smaller doses of her pain and anti-inflammatory medications.

With this improvement, her motivation and hopes soared, and she decided to follow my suggestions religiously. After three more weeks, she was off her medication entirely and not just the arthritis medication, but her sleeping pill and diuretic as well. Her nerves calmed down. She could fall asleep easily, and her fluid retention and blood pressure normalized. We both felt that our successful efforts merited applause and congratulated each other on a job well done.

Three months later, however, Sara showed up in my office again and told me that despite staying with the program that had been so successful for her, her joints had begun to swell and hurt again. She was back on her arthritis medication, as well as the sleeping and blood pressure pills.

When I asked her how things were going with her family, she suddenly became very tearful, reached for a tissue, and proceeded to tell me through her sobs that "it was her daughter's fault" that her arthritis had returned. Sara had been looking forward to a vacation she'd been planning to take with her husband. She had made elaborate preparations, and her excitement was building to great heights. She was working terribly hard, deserved a break, she felt, and was readying for her tenday getaway.

Then she explained that she'd had to cancel her vacation because of a crisis in her daughter's life. Her daughter would need Sara's support because her son-in-law would be in court facing a felony conviction right in the middle of Sara's planned vacation. When Sara learned about the conflict of dates and began struggling to decide whether to go on the vacation or cancel it on her daughter's account, Sara's symptoms came back with a vengeance. Almost overnight, her joints began to swell and grow painful again. Her blood pressure became elevated, and she couldn't get any sleep. She'd had to start taking her old medications again.

Sara revealed to me that she had blamed herself when her daughter had decided to marry a man who had a history of being in and out of jail. She felt she must have been a very poor mother for her daughter to marry such a loser. In the past, whenever her son-in-law was in some kind of trouble, Sara invariably interrupted her own goals and pursuits to be with her daughter because of the tremendous guilt she felt. But at the same time, she steamed with unexpressed anger at her daugh-

ter. This unresolved conflict constantly made her feel defeated, as if she had betrayed herself.

It became apparent to me that Sara's physical condition was intimately related to her emotional turmoil. I pointed out that while her arthritis was not actually "her daughter's fault," it had quite likely been influenced by her reaction to her daughter's woes as well as by her feelings about herself.

Although the nutritional approach seemed initially to be the cure she sought, her emotional crisis had rendered it ineffective. I suggested that she could regain control of her life and body if she was willing to work on these emotional issues. Resolving her inner conflicts could have a profound effect on her arthritis as well as on the quality of her life in general. From that point on our work together was directed toward helping Sara forgive herself and build her self-esteem.

THE BODY-MIND LINK

Jackie and Sara taught me that as powerful as medicines and nutritional approaches might be in the treatment and prevention of illness, emotional and psychological factors can play an equal if not larger role. My formal medical training had generally ignored the relationship between the psyche and physical illness. Modern medicine considered emotions too intangible to influence the body. So, it confined itself largely to defining and categorizing illness on a purely physical level and finding the most effective pharmaceutical agent or surgical procedure to provide relief.

In recent years, this split between the mind and body has been called more and more into question. As a result, over the last decade, a new field of medicine has been emerging: psychoneuroimmunology, the study of the relationships between the mind/consciousness, the brain/nervous system, and the immune system.[1] By observing changes in the immune system in connection with various stresses, emotional states, and personalities, scientists have begun to document what behavioral scientists have been telling us for centuries and what medicine men, shamans, and faith healers have known for millennia: our minds and emotions—what we think and feel, how we perceive and react, what we believe in—have a profound effect on the health of our bodies.

The more we learn in the field of psychoneuroimmunology (hereafter referred to as PNI), the more apparent it becomes that the dualistic Cartesian distinction between the mind and body is no longer useful or even accurate. Some scientists now feel that the term *bodymind* is far more appropriate. Research has demonstrated unmistakably that functions and substances we previously thought were relegated solely to the functioning of the brain occur throughout the body—even in cells of the immune system. Scientists are both shaken and excited by the realization that what we think of as mind may not necessarily be a brain function, but rather an organizing glue that maintains a balance, a wholeness, among various bodymind components.

The Immune System and Our Emotions

The immune system is composed of cells that originate in the bone marrow and develop into various white blood cells. These white blood cells circulate throughout the bloodstream and lymphatics and serve us by recognizing and destroying foreign invaders. Lymphocytes are key soldiers in this army, as they are responsible for producing both an antibody and killer cell assault on bacteria, viruses, and cancer cells. T lymphocytes are "instructed" in their duties in the thymus gland, while B lymphocytes mature in the spleen and elsewhere.

Macrophages, neutrophils, and monocytes are other white blood cells with specific functions (see Chapter Sixteen for more details). These components and others interact in a finely orchestrated and fascinating manner to defend our bodies from attack. However, when this system is suppressed, it allows infections and cancers to occur. When it is overstimulated, for instance, by continual responses to stress, it will begin to attack the self, producing autoimmune conditions such as systemic lupus erythematosus or rheumatoid arthritis.

In recent years, PNI research[2] has determined that the cells of the immune system contain receptor sites on their membranes for neurotransmitters, or neurohormones—more generally called neuropeptides—which are secreted by the brain. The hypothalamus and amygdala—the emotional centers in the brain—contain forty times more receptor sites for these neuropeptides than other parts of the brain. Neuropeptides, therefore, may be considered the biochemical mediators of emotion.

Moreover, white blood cells also house receptors for adrenal/stress hormones. In effect, your immune cells know when you're scared, depressed, angry, or happy. They know if you're in love or desperately lonely. They can access what you're thinking and feeling not only from the neuropeptides and other biochemicals in the bloodstream, but from nerve fibers that originate in the brain stem and spinal cord that communicate directly to the thymus, spleen, bone marrow, and lymph nodes. What astounds researchers is the recently discovered fact that the cells of the immune system are capable of producing all the brain neuropeptides themselves. This indicates that the immune system not only receives messages *from* the brain, but it can also transmit detailed information back *to* the brain.

STRESS

The Effects of Stress on the Immune System

There is much documentation from both animal and human PNI research that stress impairs immune function and can trigger illness. One well-known piece of research[3] demonstrated that the stress of bereavement in a group of recent widowers significantly reduced lymphocyte proliferation. Such immune impairment may explain the increased mortality of older widowers shortly after the loss of their wives. Another study by Kiecolt-Glaser et al.[4] demonstrated that medical students under the stress of exams suffered several significant immune impairments: diminished lymphocyte count—specifically natural killer and helper cells—and drastically reduced ability to produce interferon (from natural killer cells).

Similar and other adverse effects have been documented from elevated circulating cortisol and adrenaline levels that the adrenal glands and central nervous system produce when stress levels are high[5] (see Chapter Eleven). It is known that macrophages' ability to scavenge lipids from arteries is impaired when cortisol levels are high—which may predispose such a stressed individual to coronary artery disease and other forms of atherosclerosis. Under such stress, it is also known that lymphocytes secrete subnormal levels of interleukin-2 and are less able to set in motion the normal amplification of the immune response. And in terms of localized immune function in all the mucous membranes of our body, elevated cortisol levels from chronic stress will dramatically decrease the production of secretory IgA. With reduced levels of this antibody, we are more susceptible to colds, flu, bronchitis, pneumonia, sinusitis, intestinal, bladder, and vaginal infections, and allergies—particularly food allergies. Researchers and clinicians alike have come to the conclusion that illness and mortality are likely consequences of prolonged stress and the immune impairments it brings on.

Stress, it seems, is detrimental to our immune system and thus to our health. Yet we see from the research done by T. H. Holmes and R. H. Rahe that stress may not necessarily be what we think.[6] They have shown that illness can result from reactions not only to negative events (divorce, marital separation, death or illness of a family member, personal injury, trouble with one's boss or in-laws, foreclosure on a home loan, major fire in the home, and so on), but also to positive events as well. These include marriage, marital reconciliation, retirement, pregnancy, new family member, business promotion, career change, outstanding personal achievement, graduation from school, vacation, Christmas. The degree of change in one's life—whether from a positive or negative occurrence—is what seems to determine the level of stress we feel and therefore the degree of our susceptibility to illness.

Holmes and Rahe developed the social readjustment rating scale, sometimes called the Holmes scale or the stress scale, which lists common changes in our lives in order of severity (see below). The greater the number of significant changes that occur over a certain defined period of time, the higher the stress points we accumulate and the more susceptible we may become to emotional and physical disease. What happened to Jackie is a good example of how an accumulation of changes can overwhelm coping abilities, disturb immune system functioning, and lead to illness. Using the Holmes scale, Jackie's personal and social crises added up to over 192 points in the four weeks before I saw her.

SOCIAL READJUSTMENT RATING SCALE*

Circle yes or no to each life event in this list that happened in the last twelve months. Upon completion, total the score.

LIFE EVENT	ANSWER	POINT VALUE
Death of spouse	yes no	100
Divorce	yes no	73
Marital separation	yes no	65
Jail term	yes no	63
Death of close family member	yes no	63
Personal injury or illness	yes no	53
Marriage	yes no	50
Fired from work	yes no	47
Marital reconciliation	yes no	45
Retirement	yes no	45
Change in family member's health	yes no	44
Pregnancy	yes no	40
Sex difficulties	yes no	39
Addition to family	yes no	39
Business readjustment	yes no	39
Change in financial status	yes no	38
Death of close friend	yes no	37
Change to different line of work	yes no	36
Change in number of marital arguments	yes no	35
Mortgage or loan over $10,000	yes no	31
Foreclosure of mortgage or loan	yes no	30
Change in work responsibilities	yes no	29
Son or daughter leaving home	yes no	29
Trouble with in-laws	yes no	29
Outstanding personal achievement	yes no	28
Spouse begins or stops work	yes no	26
Starting or finishing school	yes no	26
Change in living conditions	yes no	25
Revision of personal habits	yes no	24
Trouble with boss	yes no	23
Change in work hours, conditions	yes no	20
Change in residence	yes no	20
Change in schools	yes no	20

LIFE EVENT	ANSWER	POINT VALUE
Change in recreational habits	yes no	19
Change in church activities	yes no	18
Mortgage or loan under $10,000	yes no	18
Change in sleeping habits	yes no	16
Change in number of family gatherings	yes no	15
Change in eating habits	yes no	15
Vacation	yes no	13
Christmas season	yes no	12
Minor violation of the law	yes no	11

150 or less	37 percent chance of getting sick within the next two years. Roughly one in three.
151–299	50 percent chance of illness within the next two years.
300 or above	80 percent chance of illness within the next two years.

Adapted from T. H. Holmes and R. H. Rahe, "The Social Readjustment Rating Scale," Journal of Psychosomatic Research, vol. 2 (1967), 213–218.

Personality Traits and Varying Responses to Stress

Although many of us succumb to illness shortly after significant change and stress in our lives, many remain well in spite of a large accumulation of stress points. It would be a mistake to consider stress points a surefire predictor of disease. Many other factors account for susceptibility to illness, and conversely, many more factors than the *lack* of stressful changes account for resistance to illness. What may be distressing for one individual may be viewed as stimulating for another. Events that may lead to the breakdown of one individual's immune system may evoke in another a gathering of forces and a heightened immune response. The coping skills we have learned, our basic personalities, and the specific character traits we acquire along the way—all seem to play a major role in how stress affects our immune systems.

Two of the pioneers in this field, O. Carl Simonton, M.D., and Stephanie Matthews Simonton, Ph.D., conducted tests with terminal cancer patients (see *Getting Well Again*, Los Angeles: Jeremy Tarcher, 1978) and found that the fighters, those who had a strong self-image and the will to live, who simply wouldn't give up, had much more of a tendency to recover from their illnesses. These were commonly very independent, sometimes ornery, scrappy, and cantankerous individuals who were often uncooperative and "difficult" patients—people who would not follow medical orders well, people who, perhaps out of their depression and fear, would initially act out, make scenes, and make it hard on others around them. An unusual number of such people

THE BODY HAS NO SECRETS

We all have unique responses to stress. Some of us will get angry or irritable, develop an ulcer or gastritis; some will get diarrhea, a spastic colon or respond with tense muscles. Some develop headache, depression, anxiety, or fatigue. Some exhibit high blood pressure, cancer, arthritis, an allergy or autoimmune disease. Why, however, does one individual respond with stomach cramps and another with a headache?

Many times the organ or body part involved in psychosomatic illness (a physical ailment developed as a response to accumulated stress) can actually symbolize an internal emotional conflict—the "disease specificity model" popularized as early as 1950 by psychiatrist Franz Alexander, M.D.[7] For example, many individuals with stomach ulcers will say that something is "eating" them. Those with asthma or breathing difficulties may be trying to get something "off their chest." Those with difficulties urinating may be "pissed" off. Those with constipation may fear "letting go" of something. Those with arthritis may have very "stiff or rigid" attitudes. Those with acne, herpes, or other skin eruptions may be "sore" at someone, wanting to break out. Those with high blood pressure or night sweats may be "burning up" over something.

In general, we may not be consciously aware of the original emotional conflicts that trigger our ailments. Because of an inability or unwillingness to deal directly with emotional pain when it occurs, we may actually "somaticize" our conflicts—unconsciously transfer them to a specific body part, a part often symbolic of our inner conflict. The physical symptom then replaces the emotional pain, which we then seem to forget, although the body part retains the memory of this emotional pain.

Through appropriate therapy, or sometimes spontaneous realization, we can come to remember the original emotional pain and then deal directly with the original conflict. If this process is successful, we no longer need to express our turmoil through the body, and our physical symptoms subsequently subside.

It's fascinating how the body can give us specific clues to our emotional conflicts. Perhaps not all physical symptoms or ailments are symbolic of an unresolved psychological or emotional conflict. However, appropriate investigation of physical symptoms will often reveal that many are. Think about your physical symptoms and where they are located. Could they perhaps be symbolic representations of some kind of emotional conflict in your life? It can sometimes be difficult to pinpoint the symbology of your specific symptoms, but if you persist, it will become clear how closely the body and mind function together. By contrast, it is fairly easy to relate your ailments to accumulated stress: simply use the social readjustment rating scale.

Sometimes, however, without any therapy or conscious realization, a physical symptom will subside. In such cases, the body is functioning as an automatic stress insulator and even as a stress processor, without your even being aware of what it's doing on your behalf. For example, let's say you develop a sore throat or overwhelming fatigue as a result of too much stress or a particularly difficult emotional conflict. You decide to take a day off and stay in bed. As a result, you become distracted or distanced from the stress in the process of gargling, taking cold medications, or sleeping for extra hours. In this case, your body symptoms have served as a useful mechanism for coping with stress. You've taken care of yourself, gotten some rest, and your body soon heals. Symbolically, this represents the dissipation of your psychological or emotional conflict. Rested and renewed, you can now resume your normal activities.

The real problem is that when such symptoms become chronic, repetitive, or disabling, this stress-relief mechanism no longer works. This is when your conscious awareness of just what's going on in your life and body is required. Only then can you get the help you need to restore your physical and emotional balance.

would subsequently recover from their cancers or out-live their prognoses.

As it turned out, it was the martyrs—those who had always put themselves last and needed to please everyone else—who were less likely to recover from their illnesses. They would carry out every order from their doctors—the "perfect" patients. Yet, these were the people who would relinquish their will and spirit, who often kept their fears and dread and despondency to themselves and lived under a cloud. They were often characterized by the resentment and anger they suppressed inside and by a marked inability to forgive. Also, they had a strong tendency toward self-pity coupled with a poor self-image. Many were unable to develop and maintain meaningful long-term relationships. Others had histories of a lifelong pattern of rejection, self-condemnation, and depression. Although they may have experienced a major loss (death of spouse or child, divorce, retirement) in the six to eighteen months before the onset of their cancer, unlike those who tended to recover, they lacked the character or personality traits that might have enabled them to fight back. In the end, they were the ones who, after being informed that they had eighteen months to live, would die right on time.

The Three C's

William F. Fry, Jr., M.D.,[8] a psychiatrist at Stanford University, and Dr. Suzanne C. Kobasa,[9] a psychologist at the University of Chicago, have observed three personality factors that seem to confer resistance to common stress-related disorders and diseases: commitment, control, and challenge.

COMMITMENT refers to getting involved deeply, investing, giving one's all. Individuals who possess this trait will not give up easily; they are not quitters. They have an unusually high degree of purpose in their activities, jobs, or lives. Their lifestyles are quite active.

CONTROL pertains to the belief that one can maintain a significant influence over many aspects of life, including one's health. While it isn't possible to exercise complete, unfailing control over all matters, nevertheless, the "take control" types feel that through their imagination, knowledge, skill, and choice, they do not have to be at the mercy of events or the passive recipients of fate. They believe that they create much of what occurs in their lives, even their good health.

CHALLENGE, the last trait, is the attitude that the many changes in one's life are normal events. Rather than being oppressed and threatened by change, individuals who react to challenge are stimulated to adapt to and overcome new conditions. Openness and flexibility enable them to face changes boldly and enthusiastically.

According to Dr. Kobasa, these personality traits and attitudes create "hardy" types. Their characteristics seem to confer, if not a resistance to mental and physical deterioration in the face of high levels of stress, at least the ability to recover from such deterioration.

Numerous other examples exist that illustrate the power of one's attitude and character.[10] You may have read Norman Cousins's *Anatomy of an Illness*, which relates the story of the author's recovery from a terminal illness through determination and laughter.

You may also be familiar with the work of Gerald Jampolsky, author of *Love Is Letting Go of Fear* and *Teach Only Love*. At the Center for Attitudinal Healing in Tiburon, California, Jampolsky has taught and inspired children with terminal cancer to heal themselves.

In *Love, Medicine and Miracles* and in *Peace, Love and Healing*, Bernie Siegel, M.D., relates how he teaches his cancer patients to activate their own inner healing mechanisms.

Equally significant are recorded data that verify the ability of experienced meditators and individuals adept at biofeedback, self-hypnosis, and other similar practices, to control pain, blood pressure, bleeding, heart rate, infection, and other "involuntary" functions *at will*.[11]

There is also overwhelming anecdotal evidence and some scientific documentation that through conscious and unconscious means, through our thoughts, emotions, attitudes, beliefs, personalities, imagination, and creativity we can enhance our immune response and resist or overcome illness. Carl and Stephanie Simonton have the following to say on the subject:

I'm reminded of an unusual situation we had recently in one of our group therapy sessions, where we had two patients who had almost identical diseases. They were within a few years of age of each other, and both men had lung cancer that had spread to their brain. One man had had the disease for over a year, but had not missed work other than a few hours each time he had a treatment. Early in the development of his disease he had gotten in touch with a lot of things that were causing life to lose meaning for him. He started to spend more time with his family, taking his family with him on business trips. I remember his saying one day, "You know, I'd forgotten that I didn't look at the trees. I hadn't been looking at the trees and the grass and the flowers for a long time. And now I do that." It was interesting to watch him, every week he improved, getting stronger, healthier.

The other man who had lung cancer which had spread to his brain stopped working practically the day he received his diagnosis. He had gone home to sit in front of the television set all day. His wife said that what he did every day was to watch the clock to make sure she gave him his pain medication on time. He was in constant pain. He could not even bring himself to go fishing, which is something he liked to do. He died in a short period of time. The other man is still getting healthier day after day. This is the kind of thing that we try to show our patients. The treatment for both patients was the same medically, the diagnosis was the same, the patients' ages and physical conditions were almost identical. The difference was in attitude, the way the patients reacted once they knew the diagnosis.[12]

EUSTRESS—DYSTRESS

Stress is not necessarily a negative factor in our lives. In fact, stress can be beneficial, even crucial, to our survival and growth. Dr. Hans Selye, father of the stress theory, has coined the terms *eustress* as the type of stress that benefits us, and *dystress* as the type that causes our deterioration.[13]

For instance, we all know of the benefits of exercise: it strengthens the cardiovascular system, tones muscle, controls weight, and heightens energy and well-being. Yet, exercise can certainly be a stress on the body. However, if done appropriately, exercise is usually good for us—it is eustress. On the other hand, failing to warm up or train adequately can cause injuries. And too much exercise can lead to exhaustion and lower levels of resistance. Here, exercise has not been beneficial—eustress becomes dystress.

Take the example of a woman who decides to open a skin care salon. She is challenged by the responsibilities and the necessity of learning how to manage her own business for the first time. She works diligently and conscientiously for months. As a result of her effort, her business becomes very successful. Her self-esteem increases markedly. She has faced a lot of stress in starting up her business. She has been forced to learn skills and become competent in areas previously unfamiliar to her. This eustress has helped her to develop her potential in several areas.

However, after eighteen months, the late hours, the long drives home, the lack of time to make nutritious meals, and the intensity of her work-related activities all begin to wear on her. She becomes increasingly fatigued, short-tempered, and unhappy. Eustress has turned to dystress.

JERRY

Jerry, a twenty-five-year-old man, came to my office one Friday with severe flu symptoms. He had a fever, chills, achy bones, a headache, congested sinuses, a cough, and was feeling generally lethargic. He had caught this flu a few days before, and it only seemed to be getting worse. I recommended a number of remedies and told him to spend the weekend in bed. The next Monday he told me the following story:

I was suffering in bed on Sunday afternoon with even worse symptoms, when the phone rang. I struggled out of bed and down the stairs to the kitchen where the phone was located. It was my mother.

My parents had recently separated after twenty-eight years of marriage. My father had left my mother for another woman, which had devastated her. For months she'd been calling me and sharing the "truths" about their separation, showing me a dark side of my father I had never known.

My own past resentments of my father were rekindled by these stories. I began to think that my father was truly without strength of character or integrity. My mother seemed like a helpless victim, and I wanted to do anything I could to make her feel better. This became an obsession with me. I grew alternately confused, tormented, and depressed. My girlfriend could hardly stand living with me anymore.

So there I was in my kitchen feeling miserable from the flu and on the phone with my mother. She had just launched into another one of her stories discrediting my father when, suddenly, I exploded with anger, which is very out of character for me. I was yelling wildly into the phone at my mother, demanding that she not tell me another story about my father. That I knew my father had his faults and that she was hurt and embittered, but that she had no right to do what she was doing. That I couldn't stand it anymore. That I loved my father in spite of his flaws, and that she couldn't change that!

When I finished, I hung up the phone and went back up to my bedroom to continue being sick. But when I sat down on the bed I realized that I was no longer weak, chilled, achy, congested, or lethargic. My throat was no longer sore, and I had stopped coughing. My severe flu symptoms had disappeared entirely—in ten minutes. What had happened? I wondered what had occurred during my telephone conversation with my mother that caused such a rapid recovery? That's when I noticed that the heavy, confused, depressed, and tormented feeling that I'd been living with for months had lifted!

For months, Jerry had been obsessed with hating his father. He would use every justification he could find to kindle his hatred. Every thought, word, and action concerning his dad reflected this ill will. Yet below the surface there was great love for his father. Jerry had been so anguished by his mother's suffering and had felt so righteous in his newfound hatred for his dad that he'd lost touch with the deep-rooted love he felt for him. Jerry could only see part of the truth—the anger and disappointment. He fell into the trap of thinking that in order to be loyal to his mother he had to close his heart to his father. But in truth, Jerry loved his father dearly despite his anger and disappointment.

Finally, in the midst of his flu symptoms, while on the telephone with his mother, something snapped inside Jerry. His chronic confusion and torment had reached their limits. In his heart, he knew he could no longer continue to kindle his hatred for his father, nor allow his mother to keep feeding it. He knew that in spite of his anger he could no longer deny his love for his father. Denying it was causing too much pain to himself.

In that telephone conversation, Jerry was truthful with himself and his mother for the first time. Although he didn't know how to reconcile his anger and his love, he knew it was important to let them coexist. In reclaiming his love for his father, he rediscovered an essential part of himself. He felt more whole. These realizations seemed to occur spontaneously and instantaneously, much in the same strange way his flu symptoms disappeared moments after.

Do People Catch Colds?
Does Someone Else Make You Depressed?

Do people catch colds or the flu simply because viruses happen to be around? Or do we come down with the flu because our resistance is down and our immune defenses are in a weakened state? Can strengthening the immune system help prevent or eradicate an existing cold or other ailment? By the same token, do we become unhappy, confused, disturbed, or anguished because of events that occur in our lives, or do we react this way because of the current state of our psyches and our interpretations of the events?

Jerry had been confused and unhappy for months. In his thinking, he had created a chasm between his innermost feelings for his father, and his outer actions and words. The more he felt he hated his father and the more he denied his love, the further he drifted from the truth. The greater this disparity became, the more unhappy and confused he grew, and the more susceptible to illness he seemed to become. But once he realized that he did indeed love his father and communicated this truth to his mother, the disparity dissolved, the gap filled in. He felt much lighter, as if a weight had been taken off his back. He no longer felt tormented. Inside, he felt connected again, balanced, and happy. This all seemed to have affected his immune system in a dramatic way, as his flu symptoms just dissolved.

Communicating the Truth

Jerry learned from this experience that his mental and physical health partly depended on being aware of the truth inside of him and in communicating it appropriately. He vowed never to let a disparity like that develop again. But he also knew that to keep that vow he would need to develop some important skills. This meant he would need to learn how to get in touch with his innermost feelings, and then find a way to communicate them effectively and appropriately.

He could see how a part of his mind had clouded the truth, the part that "attached" to his mother's suffering and felt responsible for her recovery. In response he had judged his father harshly, believing that hatred was a way to take vengeance for past and present crimes. He allowed this part of his mind to run riot and it carried him further and further away from the truth. However, through his emotional and physical stress, Jerry discovered the dangers of becoming attached or giving validity to his every thought and feeling. He realized that the deepest truths are often masked by the mind's incessant and convincing chatter.

In trying to communicate his real feelings to his mother, Jerry learned that he lacked the confidence to express himself effectively. He'd always felt that what he had to share with others wasn't very important, that it wouldn't make much of a difference to anyone. He felt inferior, with little respect for his own opinions, believing that he'd be imposing himself on others if he expressed an opinion without being asked to do so. Judging himself harshly, he feared the judgments of others. His actions were often hampered by self-consciousness. Because, more than anything else, he wanted to be liked and accepted, he would never risk speaking or acting in a way that might displease someone.

Jerry realized that this fear of displeasing others seriously impaired his ability to communicate. Because of the experience on the phone with his mother, he'd experienced the feeling that something in him had "snapped," something had corrected itself at long last deep within him. And this awareness had enabled him to recognize and communicate the truth.

He wasn't quite sure how this had occurred, but he knew he'd better learn more about the process. As a first step, he knew he needed to learn how to raise his self-esteem and how to gain more self-respect. The next step was to begin to express himself more effectively. He knew that he'd also need to develop the courage to risk displeasing people even if it meant getting stern or angry with them. The point was to communicate clearly.

As he began practicing, Jerry soon learned that there was more to effective communication than improved self-esteem and courage. Also involved were the skills of using effective language, listening well, and having compassion for others. Gradually, he began to feel that his thoughts and feelings could be valuable to others, that his value in life and his personal growth was partially related to what he could share with others.

Jerry previously considered his psychological and emotional status to be quite normal and healthy. "Everyone has ups and downs," he said. "I'm no different." Whenever he was depressed, he just lived with it. He felt that a person had to be really nuts before seeing a psychiatrist or psychologist. However, shortly after this painful awakening experience with his parents, Jerry entered psychological counseling. This is when he realized that "a person doesn't have to be crazy to see a therapist. Having an interest in understanding the self, in developing one's potential, and in learning how to be happier are reasons enough."

TAKING AN INVENTORY OF YOUR STRESS LEVEL

If you tend to feel stressed at times or can identify with issues similar to those Jerry faced, it might be useful to look at yourself and your life in several different areas. Read the "Stress Inventory" below and make your own list of all the elements in your life that seem to be positive or beneficial to you (eustress) and those that seem negative, detrimental, or inadequate (dystress). Do this for each area of concern in the Inventory.

We'll use Jerry's case to demonstrate. Examine his list, especially the categories, to help you make up your own.

STRESS INVENTORY

CATEGORY	WHAT ABOUT IT IS BENEFICIAL?	WHAT ABOUT IT IS DETRIMENTAL, IMBALANCED, OR INADEQUATE?
Physical health		Always catching colds; frequently bloated and constipated
Exercise		Don't get enough.
Diet		Too much sugar; think I have hypoglycemia; too much caffeine; too much fried foods
Sleep	Six hrs consistently	Could use seven to eight hours, really, but go to bed too late
Skilled relaxation/ meditation		Do not practice such a technique
Environment	Occasionally go to mountains	Polluted city air, city noises, density of people; don't go to mountains enough
Home	Quiet, roomy, feels like "home"	
What I love to do	Get a massage Garden Be in mountains Make love Eat Hit home runs	Don't make love enough Eat too much Haven't found a ball team
Fun		Sometimes feeling like I have to be an adult gets in the way Don't laugh enough
Commitments and responsibilities	None, except rent	Don't have anything important to commit myself to
Relationships	Great sex with girlfriend— sometimes	Feel like I have to rescue mother. Hate father; hate older brother; hate brother-in-law. Get irritable with girlfriend often and become uncommunicative with her. Can't directly express anger and so it comes out in distorted, destructive ways, like looking for faults in her and getting irritated and feeling superior to her

Self-esteem self-confidence	Good when it comes to sports and mechanical things	Pretty low with people. Afraid of others' judgments of me, need other people's approval too much. Always comparing myself with others, either feeling superior or inferior to them. Self-conscious, can't be myself often, can't assert myself very well. Don't respect myself or my opinions. Don't think I matter much to anyone else
Ability to forgive myself		I'm my own worst enemy, cruel, unrelenting self-punisher and critic; won't ever let myself forget my failings, won't even consider that I have any decent qualities
Communication skills	Express a lot of myself in writing and performing poetry. Can cry easily enough and express sadness	Can't express anger. Can't assert myself. Don't listen well. Usually have to be right. Oftentimes use wrong words or say things inappropriately—stick my foot in my mouth; speak without thinking first
Pleasing self vs. pleasing others		Seem to have a pathological need to please others
The degree emotions govern behavior		At the mercy of my emotions; get fully attached to them—they rule me
The degree that behavior is governed by addictions: foods, tobacco, alcohol, street drugs, prescription drugs, sex, gambling		May make a special trip at midnight just to buy something sweet

Self-knowledge—knowing inner feelings, needs, what is of ultimate importance to me		Pretty much out of touch. Frequently say "I don't know" when asked why I'm feeling bad or why I've done something weird
Integrity-honesty		Tell "white" lies pretty much, to bolster my ego and to keep it and my reputation from being threatened
Ability to have influence over my life, over events, or changes		Fate rules. I have no power to change anything
Gender role (male or female)		Feel like I have to be macho: strong, invulnerable and right. Can't show weakness
Sex		Feel like I have to "perform" and please her to the point that it's not fun for me. Everything is planned and there is no spontaneity. It's a source of frequent arguments and inner discontent
Touching (non-sexual)	Hug and hold hands with girlfriend sometimes. Pet dog a lot	Rarely touch or get touched or hugged by others
Ability to function at or near my capacity		Far from my capacity
Use dreams to try to understand myself	Don't have nightmares	Hardly remember them
Go over events of the day in my mind and see if I can learn anything or draw anything useful (or do creative visualization or imagery)	Replaying over and over in my mind pleasant things that happened	Just try to forget what was unpleasant, try to put it out of my mind, don't want to be reminded

General temperament—positive or negative	More down than up
Connectedness: connection to or part of a group, family, community, couple, pet. Feel responsible or important to above. Feel cared for and loved	Do not belong to community or religious groups. My mom loves me. Don't really feel committed to my girlfriend. Have some friends, but feel lonely a lot

From this list, it is evident just how many areas of Jerry's life are sources of dystress. As many of his difficulties are common to us all, we will examine them one by one and discuss possible ways of changing dystress to eustress.

Dealing with Stress— Changing Our Bodies and Environment

Diet In looking first at dietary factors, we can see how a few positive changes could have a significant impact. Reducing the amount of sugar and caffeine in Jerry's diet, introducing whole foods, stabilizing his blood sugar level, and fortifying his diet with B vitamins, vitamin C, and a few other nutrients would strengthen his nervous system from a biochemical standpoint and raise his tolerance to cope with stress (see Chapters Three and Ten).

Exercise Exercise could have a similar effect as well. Jogging, bicycling, swimming, hiking, walking— any aerobic activity at least three times weekly could help elevate his mood, improve his general level of well-being, and heighten his ability to cope with the stresses in his life.

Environment Perhaps Jerry should spend more weekends out of the city by one of his favorite mountain lakes. He should go where the air is clean; where the sounds of nature are sweet to his ears; where there are no crowds, phones, automobiles, or city lights. Such an environment would certainly soothe his nervous system, provide a rejuvenating effect, and fortify him to handle the stresses of day-to-day life.

Sleep Getting enough sleep is another common-sense change that could make a significant and dramatic difference in the quality of Jerry's life. Inadequate sleep can contribute to depression and irritability, and impair our ability to cope. Too many of us try to get by on too little sleep. Try getting to bed earlier or arranging a nap if possible (see Chapter Seventeen, "Insomnia").

Skilled Relaxation Individuals who meditate or do a skilled relaxation exercise on a regular basis commonly report that such a practice contributes substantially, if not dramatically, to their well-being, both physical and mental. The rejuvenating and balancing effect of such practices on the nervous system enables most people to endure far higher levels of stress without adverse consequences (see pages 303 and 304).

Doing What You Love Doing what you love to do and making regular time for your activities will nurture you and strengthen your coping mechanisms. Playing or writing music, going to the theater, gardening, sailing, woodworking, spending time with a favorite friend, traveling, playing tennis or bridge, reading a novel, playing on a sports team, playing with a child. Doing whatever you enjoy and having fun at it; being inspired or rejuvenated by it can be a powerful and effective health-promoting measure.

Giving Yourself a Treat Many people would do well to break their work and responsibility rhythms at least several times weekly and do something just for themselves. Many of us mistakenly think that giving ourselves such a "treat" is selfish, indulgent, and violating some ethic. We don't seem to realize that it enables us to function at a much higher level in the areas important to us. I've seen so many mothers of young children find themselves on the verge of breakdowns, when all they need is to give themselves "permission" to arrange regular time away from their children. Just a few hours a week has helped some of them regain their balance, as well as be better mothers in the process.

Treat yourself to something you love. Try something especially pleasurable for the body and nerves such as a steam bath, sauna, or therapeutic massage. Such activities relax and fortify your nervous system.

Home If you spend a lot of time at home, your residence should provide the atmosphere and comforts that can nurture and revitalize you. Home life should help you feel centered and peaceful. You may be surprised just how good you can feel from uncluttering table or desk tops, corners, or floors where you have things stacked, closets, doors, or cabinets. Try moving furniture around for a new look, or putting in or removing a rug. Try painting the bedroom, or perhaps making a major purchase. Such changes can transform this very personal and important space in your life in profound ways. Begin with just one room and you may notice an immediate difference in how you feel.

Commitments and Responsibilities Overcommitting oneself is one sure way to accelerate "burnout." Learning to say, "Thank you for considering me, but no, I cannot participate," can be a crucial way to maintain the time for yourself. Are some of your commitments and responsibilities part of your dystress load? If so, make a list of them all. Then see if you can let go of the activities that are least important to you.

On the other hand, some people need to take on additional commitments and responsibilities to generate some vitality or develop their abilities and potentials. Most of us need a certain amount of challenge and stress to keep from stagnating. Where do you fit in this scheme between burnout and stagnation?

Dealing with Stress—
Changing How We Think and Feel

Clearly, even if Jerry took to heart all of the above external measures, his dystresses would still far outweigh his eustresses. Given his imbalances in such important categories as relationships, self-esteem, communication skills, and self-knowledge, he would still have to deal with anxiety, irritability, depression, frustration, inhibition, and self-punishment. Thus, Jerry needs to make internal changes that can help him raise his self-esteem and communicate more effectively. He also needs to get in closer touch with his feelings and his needs. He needs to learn how to let higher ideals rather than raw emotion influence his behavior. And above all, he needs to establish personal goals and engage in activities that give him a sense of purpose in his life.

MAKING CREATIVE CHANGES IN YOUR LIFE

How Personal Crises Stimulate
Change and Growth

Most of us manage to gather the courage and wisdom to save our own necks once we awaken to the fact that we've overstressed our physical and mental health to the point that we're having great difficulties functioning normally in our daily lives. It's just such crises that become the most powerful turning points in our lives.

This is when people like Jerry, Jackie, and Sara begin to realize the importance of being in touch with their inner feelings, of being able to communicate the truth as they see it, of standing up for oneself, of building self-esteem, and of forgiving oneself.

This is when those of us who are experiencing such crises of opportunity start reading books on how to raise self-esteem or communicate more effectively or assertively. This is when we sign up for workshops and personal growth seminars dealing with these issues and with raising consciousness. Many of us find a therapist to help us gain more insight and self-understanding, to release our feelings and emotional blocks, and to practice new behaviors.

It's at times like these that we begin to practice some form of meditation or visualization to get more in touch with our own inner spirit and our higher guidance. This is when we turn to positive affirmations or self-hypnosis to end our old self-sabotaging patterns and to learn new self-affirming behaviors.

During times of personal crisis we gather our deepest forces and commit ourselves to new attitudes and principles of living. This is when we see very clearly what is most important to our health and happiness—to our very existence. And we find the strength and courage to establish new goals in line with our life's true purpose. Our lives begin to move in new directions as we become responsible for ourselves in new ways. We become more genuine and real, and our actions begin to produce healing and growth, not only in our lives but also in the lives of others.

Using Your Stress Inventory for Optimal Wellness

While crisis is a powerful catalyst for change, it isn't necessary to wait for disaster to hit before you take any of these active measures. Complete your stress inventory list if you haven't already done so. Consider how you generally feel and function. Consider the possibility that you may be impaired in the future by accumulated dystresses. Look in the "detriment/imbalance/inadequacy" column and see what you might improve first with simple measures. Make an action plan to help you carry out these improvements. As these easier issues begin to improve, go on to the more complex issues facing you. Try not to do more than one thing at a time. You don't want to overload your system and create new stress with these changes any more than you'd want to change everything in your diet all at once, or start taking five new vitamin and herbal supplements all at once. One day at a time, one step at a time is what keeps your progress even and steady.

For every category in which you have imbalances or inadequacies, ask yourself what the consequences would be if they continued to exert an influence in your life. What will your life be like in six months, in one year, in five years, in ten years, in twenty years, if you do not take any active measures to change?

- What will it mean if you always put yourself last and deny the importance of your own needs?
- What will it mean if you never learn to love or forgive yourself or forgive another?
- What will it mean if you continue to be bitter and angry?

- What will it mean if you continue to suffer from loneliness yet do nothing to alleviate it?
- What will it mean if your fears and emotional blocks are preventing you from developing your potential and from experiencing the fullness of life?

Look hard and honestly at these questions. If you carefully evaluate the consequences, you'll know exactly why it's necessary to make improvements. All these personal, everyday issues, all these unresolved conflicts, all these old responses and ingrained attitudes, add up to a powerful impetus for change: a weakened immune system and an unfulfilled life.

You may think you're fine now, but how well can you stand up to a major crisis should one come your way? While you may intellectually appreciate the fascinating mechanisms involved in psychoneuroimmunology, unless you put its principles to work in your life, you're not going to develop any increased resistance to cancer, arthritis, or heart attack. Nor will it contribute to making your life happier, more authentic, or more fulfilling. What can help in both these areas is taking your courage in your own two hands, taking a good long look at yourself, and getting on with the nitty-gritty work that you know needs to be done.

WORK ON YOURSELF: MY PERSONAL STORY

I'd like to share some of my personal experiences in this area with you as an example of one person's journey. After I did my own stress inventory, I could plainly see a number of major imbalances and corresponding consequences. I was often uncomfortable in situations that shouldn't have had that effect on me. For example, I often felt very self-conscious and simply couldn't relax and just be myself. I considered myself inferior, I tended to put many people on pedestals, judged people too quickly, and generally found that I did not represent myself to others in the authentic way I wanted to be seen and understood.

Much too often I allowed self-sabotaging thoughts to undermine my confidence and thwart my success. Because I was afraid to be a leader, I became accustomed to failing. I needed people's approval so much that I was unable to express anger toward or confront an equal or someone I admired. My relationships with women didn't last. I found myself telling a lot of little white lies, not with any intent to deceive, but because I was so out of touch with my feelings that I couldn't communicate truthfully or responsibly. My self-esteem was so low and my insecurity so high, I thought it was more important to know how someone else was feeling rather than how I was feeling. I would let my emotions rule me. I was periodically depressed for weeks at a time and didn't know why.

As a result, I was functioning far below my capacity and unable to enjoy life fully; and because of this I wasn't able to contribute anywhere near my full potential to my work or my life.

There were so many barriers that I wanted to overcome, but where did I begin? I finally realized that the first place that needed attention was my inner self. Who was I really? What did I think, and want, and need? Once I committed myself to asking these hard questions, I discovered something truly fascinating had begun to happen. I found that I really didn't need a plan or road map. I seemed to be led wherever I needed to go. Some of the things I tried were of enormous benefit. Some only helped slightly. But each one led me to the next step.

I took several popular personal growth seminars, where I learned concepts of self-responsibility and how to create my own reality. I also learned some basic exercises in skilled relaxation, creative visualization, and positive affirmation.

One of my more intense experiences was the year I spent in group psychotherapy that met weekly and used gestalt, transactional analysis, and psychodrama techniques. In working with this group, I recalled a traumatic event from childhood, one in which I made a decision about life and myself. It was a decision that was imprinted so deeply that it formed the basis of many attitudes I still carried in my adult life. I came to realize that these attitudes about how to survive in the world that were formed in my childhood were no longer useful to me as an adult. In fact, they were creating many of my present difficulties, especially my low self-esteem.

In group therapy, I would replay a childhood event, often casting other group members in key roles. This enabled me to relive the event and feel the pain, anger, or fear I had buried since childhood. I was able to reconnect with and release these stored emotions. Then we would restructure the drama to play out different responses. This began an internal process in which I was able to release old pain and undo previous damage. Freeing up this emotional energy made it possible for me to develop new, more appropriate and constructive attitudes and patterns for my life today.

I discovered that many of my present difficulties in relating to people and the world were closely associated with how I had related to my parents as a child. Much of the group work centered on working out these issues. Improving my relationship with my parents was not one of my original goals in entering the group, but it proved to be the most vital aspect of the work. In giving me the understanding necessary to forgive my parents and to relate to them with healthier adult patterns, I have been able to relate to the rest of the world in a healthier and more mature way. This work all starts at home. And it can be done whether your parents are alive or deceased.

A note about forgiveness: In a workshop on unconditional love and forgiveness, I learned that forgiving someone doesn't necessarily equate with condoning someone's actions. "Forgiving cancels the demands, expectations, and conditions that block the attitude of love," writes Edith Stauffer in *Unconditional Love and Forgiveness*.[14] What forgiveness actually does is release you from the destructiveness of anger, bitterness, and hostility.

OTHER PATHS TO BODY-MIND WHOLENESS

Because we are all unique, a therapeutic approach that may be successful for one individual may not be so for another. If you're looking for the help of a professional, you may first need to do some research to find a therapy that suits your specific needs. And then you'll want to interview various therapists until you meet one you feel you can trust and with whom you'll be able to work well.

The following list gives you examples of the many approaches available. All of them offer effective, powerful techniques for increasing self-understanding and overcoming psychological and emotional obstacles. The majority are discussed in Feiss's *Mind Therapies, Body Therapies: A Consumer's Guide*:[15]

Art therapy
Bioenergetics
Creative or guided imagery and visualization
Dance/movement therapy
Dreamwork
Focusing
Gestalt therapy
Hakomi
Hypnotherapy and regression
Intensive journal
Jungian analysis
Lomi work
Neurolinguistic programming (NLP)
Postural integration
Primal therapy
Psychodrama
Psychosynthesis
Rational emotive therapy
Reality therapy
Rebirthing
Reevaluation counseling
Reichian analysis
Strategic therapy
Structural integration
Transactional analysis
Vipassana

Dreamwork

Investigating my dreams is another method I use to understand myself and to further my progress. Dreamwork is an important part of Jungian and other therapies.

Once at a medical meeting I said something to the group that I immediately regretted. I began to criticize myself harshly, judging my statement as ridiculous and unorganized. I tormented myself with these self-degrading thoughts all evening, seriously doubting I'd ever be able to successfully address a group of doctors.

That night as I lay in bed I was in a very tormented state. But before falling asleep, I earnestly asked for a dream to help me understand and eradicate the part of myself that tends to sabotage my efforts to succeed, the part that torments me so endlessly. My request was very specific and made in a ceremonial manner, for I'd discovered that this "priming" of the subconscious is frequently essential to evoke an appropriate dream.

Several hours later, I awoke with the following dream fresh and clear in my mind.

> I was alone behind enemy lines charging the enemy without my rifle. I was yelling at them, taunting them, "Come on and shoot me, you imbeciles, shoot me!" After charging forward valiantly and being apparently immune to their bullets, I was suddenly wounded in the shoulder.
>
> In the next scene, I was being cared for by my compatriots. I felt victorious. The enemy wasn't able to kill me. They could only wound me.

My conclusion from that dream was, "Go ahead and keep charging, Ralph. You won't get killed. And if you get hurt, you'll still recover easily enough." The dream left me with a feeling of confidence and trust. I knew I had nothing to fear anymore. The next day, I eagerly set about to organize a talk I was scheduled to give at the next meeting. That talk turned out to be quite successful, and I was more at ease than I could ever have imagined.

However, that dream represented far more than simply success at the talk. Dreams can provide rich and symbolic material that helps us see and understand ourselves while allowing us to feel more secure and grounded in the world. Why not try asking for a dream for a very specific purpose—this is called "incubating" a dream. Create your own ceremony for priming your subconscious. Also, try keeping a dream journal so you can track your own inner processes. Writing down, dating, and titling your dreams gives you a basis for further dreamwork. For further information on dreamwork techniques, see *Breakthough Dreaming: How to Tap the Power of Your 24-Hour Mind* by Gayle Delaney, Ph.D., or *Dream Work: Techniques for Discovering the Creative Power in Dreams* by Jeremy Taylor.[16] If you want to pursue working with your dreams, find a therapist involved in dreamwork and dream groups.

Meditation

Many years ago I went on a Vipassana meditation retreat. Vipassana is not a religion or cult, nor does it require a guru or master. It is a pure, untainted technique for one and all.[17] During the ten days of instruction and practice, we were in perfect silence, even between sessions and during meals, except when addressing questions to the teacher. It was a rare and special opportunity to discover a kind of consciousness I had not previously experienced.

The technique involved attuning my awareness first to my breath, then in a very orderly fashion to other bodily sensations. The emphasis of the technique is primarily to preserve one's equanimity, to maintain an even, unreactive mind in the face of the many changing, sometimes disturbing and painful sensations of the body. In regularly practicing this meditation, one eventually learns to observe things as they really are and to maintain an even mind through life's changes and experiences. One can thus develop mastery over the mind instead of being a slave of it. Rather than reacting out of old emotional responses, one can develop the ability to act out of wisdom and compassion.

Unlike some of the therapies mentioned above, Vipassana does not involve actively going into the past and working through old emotional traumas. It involves going into the body and accepting what is found and felt there. And yet, through this process, old traumas and destructive patterns can be released indirectly. Like most forms of meditation, Vipassana sharpens the mind, leaves one relaxed and alert, and lessens the need for sleep. (See page 304, "Attuning to the Breath," for the initial Vipassana exercise; and see page 303 for further discussion of meditation.) Vipassana and other similar receptive techniques may not be suitable for everyone. And in fact, depending on my state of mind, it's not always appropriate for me. Sometimes a more active type of meditation serves me more effectively.

One such active, or concentrative, form of meditation, called Kria Shakti, involves the principles of creative visualization and affirmations. In this meditation, I first create a very special, private place in my mind. In each session, I visualize myself in this place, meeting and talking with two spirit beings who serve as my guides. I can bring into this special place any question, any problem, any person, anything I have an interest in or need to know more about. I go there to nurture my spirit, and it is always affirmed that in this place I have access to universal knowledge to use for the greatest good.

Kria Shakti is a sacred practice that I believe enhances my well-being and functioning on many levels. The more regularly I practice this technique that summons the creative energies of my imagination, the more real it becomes for me, and the better it serves me. It has helped me solve many dilemmas, answer difficult questions, and learn how to approach and communicate with difficult people. I've come to know myself better with this technique—all for practical and worthwhile purposes. A session usually leaves me refreshed, alert, and relaxed as well.

There are countless forms and styles of such exercises that use the creative imagination. You should be able to find one that feels very right for you. You will be surprised how, even with an extremely busy life, you can make time for it. With regular practice, it can be a powerful and effective tool.

Some counselors discourage people from going into the "old garbage" of their lives, and urge their clients to focus exclusively on the "here and now." They use meditation practices, imagery techniques, and visualizations of desired goals and affirmations tailored to this approach. These techniques have undoubtedly been helpful for many people, even if they have experienced deep emotional traumas. However, for those of us with deeply ingrained self-sabotaging behavior patterns, it sometimes proves more beneficial to find the right therapist with whom the old emotional traumas can be safely and skillfully explored, worked through, and released.

Whether you need in-depth therapy or not, if you're like most people, you should find much benefit from practicing self-care de-stressing techniques. Just as our heart, lungs, and muscles benefit from regular aerobic exercise, functioning better and with increased resistance to disease, our psyche benefits equally from the right skilled relaxation exercise, meditation, or creative imagery technique done regularly. When the body/mind is stronger and more balanced, your immune system is less susceptible to breakdown.

Whatever healthfully alters your consciousness most effectively, whatever changes your ever-vigilant, worried, or perhaps obsessed mind and relaxes your nerves best, do it! And do it with consistency—once a day at the minimum. Whether you're practicing positive affirmations, watching a comedy program, reading or writing a science fiction book, taking a walk, going for a horseback or bicycle ride, listening to or creating music, weaving, taking a relaxing bath, or any activity you particularly love—do what works best for you. You'll find that you are insulating your immune system, and the quality of your life, from the adverse effects of stresses.

My Experiences in Perspective

Over the years, I have gone to many lectures, workshops, and retreats. I've listened to many tapes and read numerous self-help books in the areas of self-forgiveness, self-knowledge, communication, self-esteem, and overcoming barriers. At times, I've kept a journal that included my dreams and significant experiences. I've learned how nurturing and important it is to touch and be touched. Sharing heart-to-heart feelings with someone I trust is another vital part of my well-being.

All of this has helped me grow beyond my adolescent idea that being tough and independent are the most important qualities of adulthood and manhood. I have recognized my need for others, for a connectedness with them. I need to care for and love and to feel cared for and loved. I need to feel part of a social order, something more than just myself. I believe Patch Adams, M.D., humanist, clown, physician, and founder of the Gesundheit Institute in Arlington, Virginia, when he says that loneliness is one of the most devastating human conditions.

PETS AND THE IMMUNE SYSTEM

Pets can make an extremely important contribution to our emotional and physical well-being. Since pets require attention and care, they foster a sense of responsibility and compassion in their keepers. For many of us, the continual communication, especially since it is non-verbal and tactile, and the emotional bond that develops creates a vital sense of social connectedness and a release from isolation and loneliness.

Kenneth Pelletier, Ph.D., associate clinical professor at the University of California School of Medicine in San Francisco, and Denise Herzing, M.A., also at the University of California School of Medicine in San Francisco, have noted that, since the human/animal bond is specifically emotional in nature, and given that emotions and neuropeptides may be linked, our pets may very well help maintain or enhance the strength of our immune systems.[18]

THE GURU WITHIN

There is much to learn in the world, and few would doubt the value of keeping an open channel to what others may teach. You can benefit profoundly from therapy, from personal growth courses, workshops, tapes, books, and so on. They can provide the inspiration and confidence to create a more fulfilling life and give you tools you need to minimize the risk of premature physical illness and disease. Developing effective coping strategies and hardy attitudes will help you deal with life's stresses. And, yet, perhaps the ultimate goal in your involvement with these external sources of learning is to develop your own personal inner guidance.

With this in mind, remember that your own experiences are often the best teachers. You need not become addicted to seminars, workshops, or even to therapy. I have known individuals who feel that they cannot terminate therapy if there are any stones in their past left unturned. And I've also come across many people who live to go to workshops and trainings. Often they're addicted to these gatherings—to the euphoria they sometimes produce, or to the idea of learning the latest and greatest technique. I have nothing against euphoria or new techniques, of course, but somehow many of these individuals don't seem to become happier or more fulfilled in their real lives. It's as if they consider their normal lives to be void of the richness they find in their seminars and teachers.

But life IS rich. Every seemingly routine day can be a workshop filled with invaluable lessons. You need only stand back and look for them. Some of the simple meditation and visualization exercises in the following section may help you do this. Self-knowledge and genuine growth are most often cultivated by what we learn from our own experiences, by being open to the teacher or guru within. This passage from *Life and Teaching of the Masters of the Far East* by Baird L. Spaulding best illustrates this point:[19]

He recognized that God does not speak in the fire, the earthquake, or the great wind, but in the still, small voice—the still, small voice deep in our own souls.

When man learns this, he will become poised. He will learn to think things through. Old ideas will drop away, new ideas will be adjusted. He will soon find the ease and efficiency of system. He will learn at last to take all the questions that perplex him into this silent hour. There he may not solve them, but he will become familiar with them. Then he will not need to go hurrying and battling through the day and feel that his purpose has been defeated.

If a man would come to know the greater stranger—himself—let him enter his own closet and shut the door. There he will find his most dangerous enemy and there will he learn to master him. He will find his true self. There will he find his truest friend, his wisest teacher, his safest adviser—himself.

TOOLS FOR RELIEVING STRESS

Skilled Relaxation and Visualization

This section offers several exercises that can help you manage stress and be more fit psychologically and emotionally. Some can also lead you to deep spaces that can assist you in other ways. I suggest you try any one that appeals to you and work with it initially for several days at least, if not several weeks. Do it at least once or more times daily. Initially, some of these exercises might be easier to do and more effective if you make a cassette tape recording of the instructions to help guide you through them. (You could also have someone read the instructions and take you through the exercise.) The more regularly you practice a technique, the greater the benefits you will experience.

After you've become familiar with one exercise, experiment with others and see how they affect you. There are a broad range of techniques offered here; one or more of them should suit you. Feel free to modify them. Some exercises may be more useful in certain states of mind than in others. For instance, an exercise that is helpful when you feel vital and energetic may not be as appropriate when you're feeling exhausted—and the reverse is also true. One that helps calm your anxiety and agitation may not be as helpful for depression. Use these techniques with common sense. In certain states of mind, talking with someone or engaging in active physical exercise may sometimes be more appropriate. You can purchase professionally recorded tapes that can lead you through similar relaxation and visualization exercises and positive affirmations. You can find titles to suit nearly any need or interest: stress management, optimum performance, self-confidence, preparing for surgery, weight loss, addictions—many are available.[20] An excellent overview and practical guidebook for meditation is Joel Levey's *The Fine Arts of Relaxation, Concentration, and Meditation: Ancient Skills for Modern Living*.[21]

Skilled Relaxation

Skilled relaxation refers to a variety of exercises designed to help both the mind and body relax. Relaxation calms nerves, encourages creativity, increases energy, promotes circulation, and reduces blood pressure. Biofeedback, autogenics, breathing techniques, relaxation response, and self-hypnosis are a few examples.

Relaxation Response This concept was developed by Herbert Bensen, M.D., in his book with Miriam Klipper, *The Relaxation Response*.[22] The technique is easy. Simply choose a word or short phrase that brings you a feeling of peace, harmony, or joy. While sitting, lying, or standing, preferably with your eyes closed, breathe normally and say your chosen word or phrase silently with each exhalation. Do this for at least five minutes two or three times a day.

Whole-Body Relaxation When the body relaxes, the mind relaxes, so give this method a try. While lying on your back or sitting with eyes closed, lift up one leg as you inhale and hold a very deep breath while tightening every muscle in that foot and leg. Really tense those muscles, more and more—hold about ten seconds. Then release that leg. Now lift up the other leg while inhaling. Hold your breath and tighten the muscles in that leg for five to ten seconds. Hold. Hold. Now release. Repeat the same procedure as you move up the body. Progressively tense and relax the buttocks and pelvis, the abdomen and chest, the arms and hands, the face and scalp. Finally, tense the entire body on your inbreath. Tense it all together, holding your breath. Hold. Hold. Then totally release the tension on the outbreath. Relax your whole body and breathe normally.

Progressive Relaxation for the Mind It is equally true that when the mind relaxes, the body relaxes. With eyes closed, sitting upright comfortably with both feet on the floor and hands on the lap—or while lying down, arms at your sides—take a deep breath, sending it right down into your lower abdomen, filling it like a balloon. Then allow more breath in and fill up your chest. Hold for a moment. Then let the breath go.

Now, take an even deeper breath, deeper, deeper. Fill up your abdomen and your entire chest with it. Now release the breath, letting go of any tightness or tension. Take an even deeper breath, deeper, deeper, and release it, releasing with the breath any tension. Take one more very deep breath and then let it go. Feeling calm and tranquil, breathe normally now.

Feel your jaw relax. Let it open slightly. Let those jaw muscles ease and calm. (Pause.) Let the muscles around your eyes and forehead relax. Feel them smooth and ease. (Pause.) Feel your eyebrows sitting there easy and light and your entire scalp feel calm and light. (Pause.) Now let your neck and shoulder muscles be loose. Feel them relaxing and loosening. (Pause.)

Sense the increased blood flowing down your arms and into your hands and fingertips, warming and soothing them. Feel them tingle and pulsate slightly as they are warmed and eased. (Pause.) Feel this happening now in your forearms (pause), then elbows (pause), then your upper arms and shoulders. (Pause.) Feel the movements of your chest and back and abdomen with each breath. With each exhalation feel these muscles relaxing more and more. (Pause.) Feel the muscles in the pelvis and rectal areas relaxing more and more. (Pause.)

Sense the increased blood flow moving down your legs and into your feet, warming and soothing them.

Feel them tingle and pulsate slightly as they are warmed and eased. Feel the same in your calves (pause), and your knees and thighs. (Pause.) Now feel your whole body eased and soothed and calm. Feel how calm and tranquil your body is. Feel all of your muscles relaxed. (Pause.) Now, eyes still closed, visualize the room you're in. Recall where the furniture is, the windows and doors. Now, gradually and slowly, open your eyes and return.

Slow Deep Breathing This exercise relaxes the mind and body and centers your awareness. Sitting or lying with eyes closed, bring in your breath slowly and fully to the pit of your stomach. Place your hand over your abdomen where you can feel each breath coming in. Do not force or hurry, this is a quiet, deepening and centering practice. Keep your breathing steady, slow and full. Let your exhalation come out of its own accord. Continue for up to five or more minutes.

Vigorous Deep Breathing This approach relaxes the mind and body. Sit upright comfortably, feet on the floor, hands relaxed. Take moderately forceful and deep breaths through both nostrils, first filling the stomach then the lungs. Follow this with a forceful exhalation through the nostrils. Practice for up to one to three minutes.

This technique can be extraordinarily energizing and relaxing. Take the breaths one every four to five seconds at first, then increasing to one full breath every two to three seconds in the last minute. The increase in oxygen brings energy and mental clarity and the decrease in carbon dioxide a lightness and near euphoria.

As this is a type of hyperventilation, you may also experience some tingling sensations in the face and head and hands, as well as a temporary light-headedness. Take precautions not to do this exercise too vigorously or for too long, particularly if you are prone to fainting. As a safeguard, do it while sitting on a sofa. At the end of the intense breathing period, take the last in-breath very deeply and hold it for as long as you are comfortable. Then release it, and let your breathing rhythm find its normal pattern. Continue to sit with your eyes closed, feeling all the sensations in your body, and easing yourself into the stillness and calm you've created.

Attuning to the Breath This is the initial phase of Vipassana meditation. It may be done for five minutes or twenty to thirty minutes, or even for sixty minutes. While sitting upright, eyes closed, draw your attention to your breath, to the sensation your breath makes in your nostrils as it enters and leaves the nose. Just focus on this breath sensation in your nostrils, breathing as you naturally do. (Pause.)

If your mind wanders, just notice that it has drifted. Notice where it has drifted to without any self-judgments or evaluations. Just simply notice where the mind is—whether it's remembering or planning or analyzing or responding to a painful place in your body or to a noise. Then gently and softly bring your awareness back to the sensation of your breath touching your nostrils as it enters and leaves your body. Focus simply on the breath, the sensation of the breath in your nostrils.

When you are ready to end the meditation, gradually, gently, and softly bring your attention back into the room and slowly open your eyes.

A Breathing Exercise[23] Place the tip of your tongue against the ridge behind and above your front teeth. Keep it there through the whole exercise as it keeps the energy within the body and doesn't allow it to dissipate.

Exhale completely through your mouth, making a whooshing sound. Then, with your mouth closed, inhale deeply and quietly through your nose to a count of four. Hold the breath for a count of seven. Hold. Hold. Then exhale through the mouth to a count of eight, making the whooshing sound.

Repeat the inhale, hold, and release for a total of four breaths.

This can be done in any position. If you are seated, keep the back straight. Do this at least twice a day, and whenever you feel stressed, anxious, or off center. Don't do this more than four breaths at one time, but do the exercise as often as you wish.

With practice, this will become a very powerful means of inducing a state of deep relaxation that gets better and better over time. It's a vitamin for the nervous system and will help you gain control over your emotions and cravings.

SUGGESTED READING

Achterberg, Jean. *Imagery in Healing*. Boston: Shambala, 1985.

Advances, The Journal for Mind-Body Health. Quarterly Publication of the Institute for the Advancement of Health, 16 E. 53rd St., New York, NY 10022.

Anderson, Robert, M.D. *Stress Power: How to Turn Tension into Energy*. New York: Human Sciences Press, 1978.

Bandler, Richard, and Grinter, John. *Frogs into Princes— Neuro Linguistic Programming*. Available from Real People Press, Box F, Moab, UT 84532, 1979.

Benson, Herbert, M.D., and Klipper, Miriam. *The Relaxation Response*. New York: Avon, 1976.

Blair, Justice. *Who Gets Sick*. Los Angeles: Tarcher, 1988.

Bloomfield, Harold, M.D., and Felder, Leonard. *Making Peace with Your Parents*. New York: Ballantine, 1984.

Borysenko, Joan. *Minding the Body, Mending the Mind*. New York: Bantam, 1987.

Bradshaw, John. *Bradshaw on the Family: A Revolutionary Way of Self-Discovery*. Deerfield Beach, FL: Health Communications, 1988.

————. *Healing the Shame that Binds You*. Deerfield Beach, FL: Health Communications, 1988.

Bry, Adelaide, and Blair, Marjorie. *Visualization: Directing the Movies of Your Mind*. New York: Harper & Row, 1978.

Caprio, Betsy, and Hedberg, Thomas M., S.D.B. *At a Dream Workshop*. Mahwah, NJ: Paulist Press, 1987.

Cousins, Norman. *Anatomy of an Illness*. New York: Norton, 1979.

————. *Head First: The Biology of Hope*. New York: Dutton, 1989.

Garfield, Patricia, Ph.D. *The Healing Power of Dreams: Techniques for Interpreting and Using Your Dreams to Reveal Hidden Health Problems, Speed Your Recovery, and Promote Lifelong Health*. New York: Simon & Schuster, 1991.

Gawain, Shakti. *Creative Visualization*. New York: Bantam, 1983.

Gendlin, Eugene. *Focusing*. New York: Bantam, 1981.

Goldberg, Herb. *The Hazards of Being a Male: Surviving the Myth of Masculine Privilege*. New York: NAL/Dutton, 1977.

Green, Elmer and Alyce. *Beyond Biofeedback*. New York: Dell, 1977.

Hart, William. *The Art of Living: Vipassana Meditation as Taught by SN Goenka*. New York: Harper & Row, 1987.

Hay, Louise. *Healing Yourself*. Santa Monica, CA: Hay House, 90401.

James, John, and James, Muriel. *Passion for Life: Psychology and the Human Spirit*. New York: Dutton, 1991.

Jampolsky, Gerald, M.D. *Love Is Letting Go of Fear*. Berkeley, CA: Celestial Arts, 1988.

————. *Teach Only Love: The Seven Principles of Attitudinal Healing*. New York: Bantam, 1984.

Janov, Arthur. *The Primal Scream: The Cure for Neurosis*. New York: Dell, 1970.

Jung, Carl G. *Man and His Symbols*. New York: Doubleday, 1964.

The Kripalu Self Health Care Guide—A Personal Program for Wholistic Living, compiled by the staff of the Kripalu Center for Wholistic Living, based on the teachings of Yogi Amrit Desai. Summit Station, PA: Kripalu Publications, 1979.

Leightman, Robert, M.D., and Japikse, Carl. *Active Meditation: The Western Tradition*. Canal Winchester, OH: Ariel Press, 1982.

Levey, Joel. *The Fine Arts of Relaxation, Concentration and Meditation: Ancient Skills for Modern Living*. London: Wisdom Publications, 1987.

Levine, Stephen. *A Gradual Awakening*. New York: Anchor/Doubleday, 1979.

Locke, Steven, M.D., and Colligan, Douglas. *The Healer Within: The New Medicine of Mind and Body*. New York: Mentor/NAL, 1986.

Middleton-Moz, Jane, and Dwinell, Lorie. *After the Tears: Reclaiming the Losses of Childhood*. Deerfield, FL: Health Communications.

Mindell, Arnold. *Dreambody: The Body's Role in Revealing the Self*. Salem, MA: Sigo Press, 1982.

Institute of Noetic Sciences, 475 Gate Five Rd., Suite 300, Sausalito, CA 94965 (newsletter and seminars).

Orr, Leonard, and Rae, Sandra. *Rebirthing in the New Age*. Berkeley, CA: Celestial Arts.

Pelletier, Kenneth, Ph.D. *Mind Is Healer, Mind Is Slayer: A Holistic Approach to Preventing Stress Disorders*. New York: Delta, 1977.

Piero, Ferrucci. *What We May Be*. Los Angeles: Tarcher, 1982.

Rossman, Martin L. *Healing Yourself: A Step-By-Step Program for Better Health Through Imagery*. New York: Walker, 1987.

Roud, Paul C. *Making Miracles: An Exploration into the Dynamics of Self-Healing*. New York: Warner Books, 1990.

Samuels, Mike and Nancy, M.D. *Seeing with the Mind's Eye*. New York: Random House, 1975.

Schaef, Anne Wilson. *Co-Dependence Misunderstood-Mistreated*. New York: Perennial Library/Harper & Row, 1986.

Selye, Hans. *Stress without Distress*. New York: NAL/Dutton, 1975.

Siegel, Alan B., Ph.D. *Dreams that Can Change Your Life*. Los Angeles: Tarcher, 1990.

Siegel, Bernie, M.D. *Love, Medicine and Miracles*. New York: Harper & Row, 1986.

————. *Peace, Love and Healing*. New York: Harper & Row, 1989.

Simonton, Carl, and Mathews-Simonton, Stephanie. *Getting Well Again*. Los Angeles: Tarcher, 1978.

Stauffer, Edith. *Unconditional Love and Forgiveness*. Burbank, CA: Triangle Publishers, 1987.

Taylor, Jeremy. *Dream Work: Techniques for Discovering the Creative Power in Dreams*. Mahwah, NJ: Paulist Press, 1983.

Travis, John, M.D., and Ryan, Regina. *The Wellness Workbook*, 2nd ed. Berkeley, CA: Ten Speed Press, 1986.

Weil, Andrew, M.D. *Spontaneous Healing*. New York: Knopf, 1995.

CHAPTER 16

THE TEN COMMON DENOMINATORS OF ILLNESS AND THE IMMUNE SYSTEM

From the information presented in the previous chapters, you can now understand that chronic illness may be triggered by a number of underlying conditions. In this chapter, you will see more clearly how the ten common denominators of illness contribute to immune breakdown and, conversely, how their recognition and treatment—or their prevention—lay the groundwork for strengthening and maintaining the immune system. Terri's case history below demonstrates that an integrated and broad therapeutic approach, one that encompasses the treatment for many of these ten common denominator conditions, could overcome the recurrent infections that left her debilitated for up to six months a year.

You will see that such a broad-based approach, including "Living by the Laws of Nature," should be implemented for any immune system imbalance, whether the manifestations are cancer, autoimmune disease, or, as in Terri's case, chronic or recurring infections. Next we will identify the cells and structures of the immune system and discuss their individual roles and relationships. The chapter will conclude with a review of specific immune system enhancers.

TERRI G.

Terri was a forty-six-year-old "retired" dental assistant whose episodes of chronic bronchitis forced her to quit her job. Finally, she even had to abandon her weekly volunteer church work. For an entire year, Terri did not feel strong enough to go to a movie theater. Her history of susceptibility to bronchitis began in childhood when she would develop two or three of these chest infections

yearly, characterized by intense coughing, fever, and malaise.

When Terri turned twenty-five, her episodes began to be associated with asthma. She was tested several times for allergies to dust, mold, pollen, and animal dander, but nothing ever showed up. With every bout of bronchitis and asthma, she wondered when modern medicine would finally develop a cure for her lifelong problem. In the meantime, the only approaches offered to her were antibiotics, inhalers, and sometimes, steroids.

Prior to her first visit to me, Terri suffered eight episodes of bronchitis, always complicated by asthma, each requiring two to three weeks of antibiotics in addition to around-the-clock inhalers so she could breathe. She reported that each episode would occur during her premenstrual cycle. Her doctors believed that this was just a coincidence, but Terri felt it was an important clue. She was chronically tired, even between bronchitis episodes, and overweight in spite of constant dieting. In addition, food always seemed to unsettle her stomach, and she was chronically constipated. Although a stressful lawsuit had preceded her most recent pattern of declining health, the major stress was over, and she felt that something else was impairing her resistance.

Laboratory tests revealed that Terri was suffering from intestinal yeast overgrowth, food allergies (to eleven common foods), low adrenal function, low stomach acid, and elevated mercury levels. Her elevated mercury levels were likely caused by years of mercury exposure as a dental assistant as well as the silver-mercury amalgam fillings in her own mouth.

Initially, Terri's treatment consisted of the Ultra Clear cleansing program to eliminate her food allergens and enhance her liver detoxification capacity. Next, she began a hypoallergenic Candida-control diet, took prescription antifungal medication and nutrients for her PMS. She also received an intravenous vitamin/mineral injection every one to two weeks, with an anti-infection, immune-enhancing herbal combination formula. This treatment program seemed to keep her episodes at bay. Terri was also treated for low adrenal function with DHEA (dehydroepiandrosterone) and for hypochlorhydria with supplemental hydrochloric acid. Finally, her mercury overload was addressed. At this point, she no longer required the injections unless she felt the onset of an episode, which was rare.

Terri's wellness program required her total commitment. It could work only with her full participation, and she knew it. She wanted to build her health reserve rather than following a crisis care model and just taking drugs.

Since the treatment program, Terri has not had a single recurrence requiring antibiotics or inhalers. Her weight is down without dieting. Her energy and vitality have been restored and her life no longer feels restricted. She attributes her success not only to specific treatments for underlying conditions and immune boosters, but also to recognizing the importance of "Living by the Laws of Nature."

NURSING YOUR IMMUNE SYSTEM BACK TO HEALTH

Like Terri, you too can make efforts to overcome illness by nourishing your immune system, by releasing it from its burdens, and by allowing it to work in your favor again. Treating the conditions we've been discussing in the previous chapters may enable you to regain your health. Although the resolution of these conditions alone may be inadequate for full recovery, the process may be essential for other treatments to be effective.

Whatever your illness, there is much you can do—in spite of being told otherwise by your doctor—to attempt to reverse its course. From what you've learned thus far in this book, I hope that you realize the phenomenal influence you, your thoughts, and your actions can have upon your immune system and health.

The chart that follows on the next page summarizes immune system hazards that result from the "Ten Common Denominators of Illness," and dietary hazards and excesses discussed in the previous chapters. It will help you recognize at a glance how these conditions interrelate and potentially lead to three endpoints of immune dysregulation—infection, cancer, and autoimmune disease.

A weakened immune system has many hidden faces. So varied are its expressions that it's not surprising modern medicine has failed to find the magic bullet or the white knight cure for so many of our dreaded diseases.

Given all the interwoven systems upon which immune function depends, you can easily see that maintaining it requires caring for nearly the whole body. Resurrecting a damaged immune system necessitates far more than the use of simply a chemotherapeutic agent or a whole-foods diet.

HOW THE IMMUNE SYSTEM WORKS[1]

Just what is this immune system we keep hearing about? What glands, organs, cells, and chemical messengers are involved? And how do they interact? Exactly what does it mean to strengthen or weaken the immune system?

The immune system can be compared to a defending army, always prepared to protect the body against attackers such as viruses, bacteria, fungi, cancer cells, and other foreign invaders. The primary defenders in the immune system are white blood cells. Other troops include lymphokines and monokines, chemical messengers made by the white blood cells; antibodies; the skin; and the epithelial lining of our respiratory, gastrointestinal, and genitourinary systems; and our psyche—our thoughts and feelings, which recent research has demonstrated to be an inherent aspect of immune function. No military battle in the history of mankind can compare to the intricacy, intelligence, and drama of our own immune system in combat. Let's take a closer look.

The "Commanders-in-Chief": The Lymphocytes

Grown in the bone marrow, white blood cells are found in large numbers in the blood system, and in lymphoid tissues such as the thymus, spleen, lymph nodes, and appendix (see Figure 16–1). Red blood cells, also found in the blood system, are busy transporting oxygen, so white blood cells alone must defend the body's health.

If the immune system is the body's army, then the white blood cells are the "Commanders-in-Chief" and the foot soldiers, traveling throughout the bloodstream, lymphatics, and body tissues to fend off invaders. Their job is to recognize the particular infecting agent—whether it be bacteria, a virus, or a cancer cell, for example—and to wage a specific counterstrike.

The body has two main lines of cellular defense: T lymphocytes and B lymphocytes. T cells and B cells both develop from stem cells in our liver and bone marrow when we are fetuses. T lymphocytes are so named because they mature and/or are instructed in their duties in the thymus gland—a small structure located under the upper breastbone. The B lymphocytes remain in the bone marrow until they are mature.

The thymus and bone marrow are considered to be primary organs of the lymphatic system. Both T and B

DIETARY HAZARDS AND THE TEN COMMON DENOMINATORS OF ILLNESS—HOW THEY LEAD TO IMMUNE BREAKDOWN

Cancer = increased cancer risk   Infection = increased infection risk

Autoimmune = increased autoimmune risk

DIETARY HAZARDS

    High Fat ⟶ Cancer, Infection

    Trans-fatty Acids,
    Partially Hydrogenated Oils ⟶ Cancer, Infection, Autoimmune

    Rancid Oils and Fats ⟶ Cancer

    Refined Carbohydrates
    Including Sugar ⟶ Cancer, Infection

    Low Fiber ⟶ Cancer, Autoimmune

    Excess Calories ⟶ Cancer

    Food Additives and
    Chemical Contamination ⟶ Cancer, Infection, Autoimmune

    Excessive Alcohol ⟶ Cancer

NUTRITIONAL DEFICIENCIES ⟶ Cancer, Infection, Autoimmune

POOR DIGESTION AND ASSIMILATION
TOXIC BOWEL ⟶ Cancer, Infection, Autoimmune

SLUGGISH LIVER ⟶ Cancer, Autoimmune

HYPOGLYCEMIA
ADRENAL EXHAUSTION ⟶ Cancer, Infection, Autoimmune

YEAST OVERGROWTH ⟶ Infection, Autoimmune

FOOD ALLERGY ⟶ Infection, Autoimmune

ENVIRONMENTAL ILLNESS ⟶ Cancer, Infection, Autoimmune

PSYCHONEUROIMMUNOLOGY: THE BODY-
MIND CONNECTION ⟶ Cancer, Infection, Autoimmune

FIGURE 16–1. Primary Lymphoid Organs

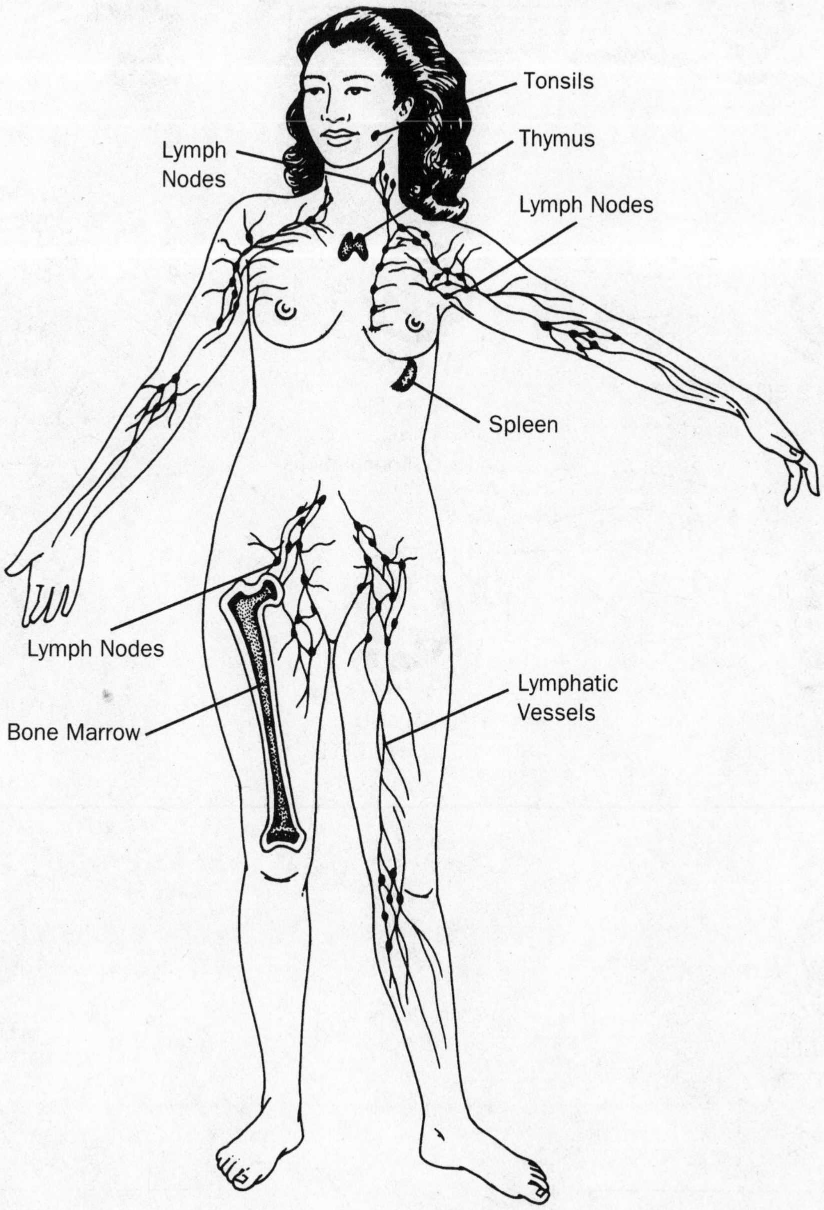

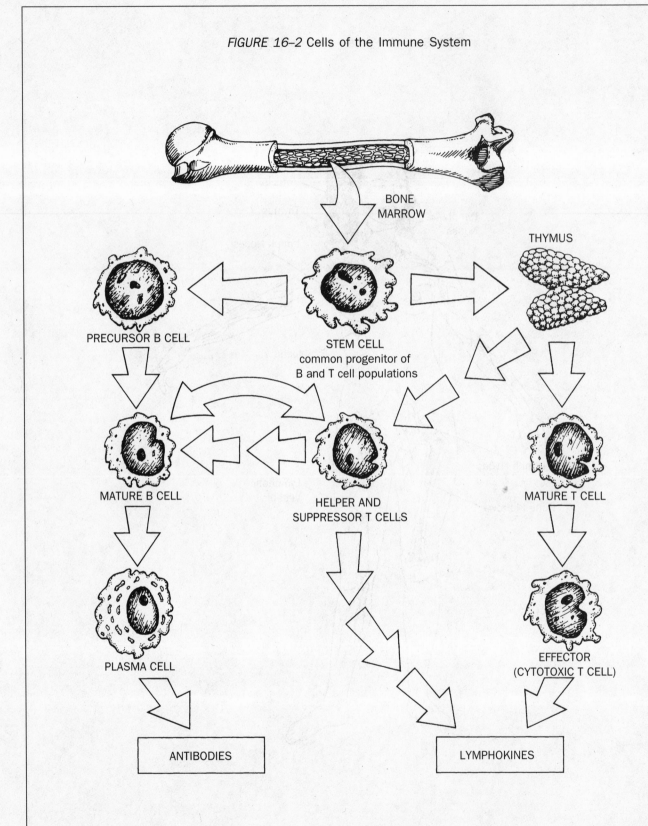

FIGURE 16–2 Cells of the Immune System

cells circulate throughout the bloodstream and lymphatic channels. They can also be found in secondary lymphoid organs such as the spleen, lymph nodes, and other lymph tissues, including tonsils, the Peyer patches in the intestines, the mucus-secreting surfaces of the gut, and the respiratory and urinary tracts. Lymphocytes can also accumulate in the connective and epithelial tissues throughout our bodies.

HELPER-INDUCER T CELLS, also called helper T cells, or simply T cells, are the commanders of the immune army, and serve as the central hub of immune operations. The chief responsibility of the helper T cells is to rouse the other defender cells into motion. They interpret intelligence information and communicate with all other lymphocytes through numerous specific chemical messengers. One line of communication is directed toward B cells.

B CELLS do the "dirty work" of the immune system by producing antibodies, the weapons that help win the war against invaders. Unlike the T cells, which are always on active duty, moving throughout the entire blood route and lympathics on surveillance missions, B cells do much less migrating, and rest inactive in the lymph system until the T cell calls them to the site of attack. When the helper T cells recognize a virus, bacteria, tumor cell, or anything foreign, they stimulate B cells to make antibodies specific for that particular foreign agent. Antibodies then help to destroy the invader. Helper T cells are long-lived and become memory cells: whenever they spot a future exposure to the same agent, they'll initiate an even faster and more vigorous immune response.

After recognizing a foreign agent or antigen, B cells are stimulated by helper T cells that have previously recognized the same antigen, and produce antibodies specific for that foreign agent, or invader. Some of these stimulated B cells will also become memory cells (the T cell can't do all the work alone!). In the future when they recognize the same antigen, or invader, under stimulation by helper T cells they can produce a quicker and more vigorous antibody response than before.

More Troops: The Other Lymphocytes

SUPPRESSOR T CELLS keep B cells in check by inhibiting their antibody production in order to prevent overproduction. Suppressor T cells also accomplish this goal by direct suppression of helper T cells.

CYTOTOXIC T CELLS are instructed/activated by helper T cells to kill invading cells that are, for example, infected with viruses.

NK (NATURAL KILLER) CELLS are also created by helper T cells to kill tumor cells and probably microbial organisms. They perform their work by drilling holes in the membranes of enemy cells. Unlike B cells, for example,

natural killer cells do not need to be stimulated into action. They can recognize foreign agents and act independently; and thus, they are born, or "natural," killers. Their activity is enormously augmented, however, by communication from a helper T cell that has been sensitized by previously recognizing the same specific foreign invader.

K CELLS, like natural killer cells, kill foreign invaders. However, unlike NK cells they require the help of an antibody made by B cells specific for the enemy cell.

Immune Cells Other Than Lymphocytes

The immune system has many weapons in its war against invaders. A brief discussion of some of these weapons follows.

Monocyte/macrophage Monocytes and macrophages are created in the bone marrow, and have the ability to engulf and ingest infecting microbes, tumor cells, any foreign debris, and even old or dead red blood cells and other body matter that needs recycling. Like helper T cells, monocytes circulate throughout the system, whereas macrophages live in tissues or at sites of active immune response. Kuppfer cells in the liver are an example of a macrophage. Activated by sensitized helper T-cells, circulating monocytes are converted to macrophages, which are central in triggering the immune response. The macrophages engulf the foreign agent and highlight their antibodies so the helper T cell can quickly identify the invaders. Once the antibodies are marked by the macrophages as foreign invaders, helper T cells determine the immune response needed to neutralize or destroy the body's invader. Thus, the macrophage serves as a scout, providing the intelligence information with which the helper T cell determines subsequent immune response.

Activated macrophages After marking the enemy cell so the helper T can identify it, the sensitized macrophage releases chemical factors—or lymphokines—that attract still more macrophages and other white cells. The battle then goes into full gear. Macrophages secrete more chemicals, or lymphokines with names like interferon gamma, interleukin-3, and granulocyte macrophage stimulating factor in order to eliminate the invading threat. These substances in turn alter and strengthen the surrounding macrophages, enhancing their ability to unleash a biochemical attack to kill the microorganism.

Granulocytes Additional fighters in the war against invaders are granulocytes, essential components of the white blood cell system.

NEUTROPHILS are summoned to sites of inflammation and infection. Their primary job is to engulf microorganisms, particularly bacteria.

EOSINOPHILS congregate particularly at sites of allergic and parasitic reactions. They release enzymes to relieve the biochemical cause of allergy attacks.

BASOPHILS/MAST CELLS are prime elements in initiating an effective immune response. Basophils are found throughout the bloodstream and at sites of inflammation. Their counterparts, mast cells, reside largely in tissues.

Platelets In addition to their role in clotting, platelets attract white blood cells to sites of injury.

Lymphokines and Monokines

Lymphokines Another integral part of the immune response are lymphokines, the chemical messengers produced by lymphocytes to strengthen and regulate a series of defensive and offensive immune actions. These chemical messengers are created and released by sensitized helper T cells to contain and destroy enemy cells. Some examples of lymphokines are:
- Interleukin-2
- Gamma-interferon
- Interleukin-3
- Granulocyte-macrophage stimulating factor
- Alpha-interferon

Monokines Working in coordination with lymphokines are monokines, biochemical substances produced by macrophages. Interleukin-1 is a monokine, which is needed for the production of interleukin-2 and also to produce a chemical that assists in the destruction of tumor cells.

Lymphokines and Stress Lymphokines are central to amplifying the immune response. However, it should be noted that the production of one important lymphokine, interleukin-2, can be reduced by stress. Chronic stress, therefore, can have a markedly negative effect on a person's immune response.

Antibodies

Needless to say, the immune system would offer feeble resistance to life-threatening infections without the presence of antibodies. Antibodies, or serum proteins known as immunoglobins (Ig), serve as the primary cellular secretions of the humoral branch of the immune system. These B cell lymphocyte products fall into several major categories:

IgG is the main serum protein, which coats microorganisms, leaving them open to destruction.

IgA is the major class of antibody found in secretions such as milk, saliva, tears, and respiratory and intestinal secretions. It works to contain localized infection from spreading throughout the body.

IgM antibodies, the initial immune response to foreign invaders, attack bacteria. Less is known about the role of IgD antibodies, which are found in trace amounts in the serum.

IgE antibodies, which bind tightly to mast cells and basophils, are involved in the body's reaction to allergic conditions such as hay fever, asthma, and hives. IgE antibody levels also become elevated in people suffering from parasitic infections.

The Complement System

All of the antibodies belong to the humoral arm of the immune system, which includes the complement system. The complement system, which is composed of eighteen plasma proteins, is vital to the body's defense. This system has two parts: the classical, which battles autoimmune disease, and the alternative pathway, which fights infection.

The Skin

Nothing serves us as diligently in the war against disease as the skin that covers our bodies. Although our skin is not inherently part of what we consider to be the immune system organs, our outer covering—plus the epithelial linings of the mouth and gastrointestinal tract; the nostrils, sinuses, bronchials, and lungs—the respiratory tract; the genitourinary tract, and the conjunctiva of the eyes serve as primary barriers to infection.

In a state of health, these rapidly replicating cells of our skin and the linings of our various tracts prevent attachment and penetration by infectious agents, primarily by secreting mucus, a protective agent that lines cells; secretory IgA, which helps sequester foreign agents; and lysozymes, enzymes that actually digest foreign organisms.

Laboratory Tests to Assess Immune Function

With this understanding of your immune function, the concept of a *strong* or *weak* immune system should now have a precise meaning for you. A strong immune system will protect you from infectious agents—including latent cancer viruses, newly formed cancer cells, and foreign antigens.

The most common and inexpensive general screening test for immune function includes the white blood cell count and differential (percentages of lymphocytes, neutrophils, eosinophils, monocytes, and basophils).

THE ASTOUNDING INTERRELATIONSHIPS OF THE IMMUNE SYSTEM

By now you are able to truly appreciate the complexity and intelligence of the human immune system.

- The bone marrow and thymus are its main organs.

- Helper T lymphocytes are the hub of operations, serving as both intelligence officers and battle commanders, communicating to and enabling other white cells of the immune system to perform their various combat tasks. Such communications are delivered in the form of the various chemical messengers—lymphokines—interleukin-2, gamma–interferon, colony stimulating factors, and others.

- Macrophages primarily issue the call to battle in their role as scouts; they are then promoted to elite battalions. The helper T cell commanders, armed with the intelligence information gathered by their scouts, can now recognize these foreign antigens and decide what lymphokines to secrete. This determines which branch of the immune system will be engaged and/or enhanced.

- Under helper T cell direction, cytotoxic T cells, NK cells, macrophages, and B cells all perform their various combat tasks.

- Humoral (antibody B cell–mediated) immunity is generally considered a separate arm of the immune system and viewed as separate from cellular/T cell immunity. Technically, however, antibodies are not separate since B cells also depend upon communications from helper T cells to perform their task of producing antigen-specific antibodies. Another factor that diminishes their separateness is the fact that when these antibodies bind to or coat foreign agents they make it possible for some components of the cellular immunity system to function effectively. Antibodies are also able to neutralize bacterial toxins, viruses, and many other allergenic substances on their own.

- It is also very important to keep in mind that our thoughts and emotional reactions exert an enormous influence over our immune system through the network of nerve fibers from the brain and spinal cord as well as the neuropeptides secreted into the bloodstream. The central and autonomic nervous systems communicate directly with the organs and cells of the immune system. Therefore, what we think and feel and believe has a powerful ability to affect the function and size of the thymus gland, lymphocyte counts and ratios, lymphocyte function, and lymphokine and antibody secretions.

Skin tests for delayed hypersensitivity response also demonstrate the level of strength of the cellular immune function.

More sophisticated and expensive tests include absolute total CD_3 lymphocyte counts, helper and suppressor T cell counts and ratios, NK cell counts, lymphokine production, null cell count, lymphocyte proliferation and activation responses, interleukin-2 receptor assay, and others. Humoral immune function can be demonstrated by various immunoglobulin (antibody) levels, their affinity and response, B-lymphocyte counts, complement (C3) levels, and others.

Various autoimmune profiles can detect whether or not your immune system has become overactive and is attacking your body with antinuclear antibodies, antiovarian antibodies, antibrush-border antibodies, antiparietal cell antibodies, and others.[2] A health professional experienced in the use and interpretation of all these immune parameters can guide you through the tests most appropriate for your needs.

IMMUNE-ENHANCING AGENTS AND APPROACHES

In strengthening the immune system, you must consider what will bolster lymphocyte and other white cell counts, and their critical secretions, such as interferons and interleukins, and antibody levels. You must consider what will repair and maintain the integrity of the skin and mucosal epithelial linings, and of course you must also consider what will empower your psyche—the psychoneuroimmunological side of immune competence.

The previous chapters offer information that serves as groundwork for immune maintenance and enhancement. Chapters Three, Four, and Six in particular (covering diet and specific nutrients) address the nutritional foundations for maintenance of immune function. There are many books, review articles, and primary research papers that discuss the relationship between nutrition and immune function. They document the host of nutrients our immune systems require in order to carry out their normal processes.[3] The following table lists the nutrients associated with various aspects of immune function.

NUTRIENTS INVOLVED IN IMMUNE FUNCTION

EPITHELIAL TISSUE BARRIERS

Vitamins A, B-2, B-3, B-6, B-12, folic acid, C
Minerals iron and zinc
Protein
Essential fatty acids

CELL-MEDIATED (T CELL) IMMUNITY

Protein/calorie
Vitamins A, B-6, folic acid, C, E
Minerals zinc, iron, selenium
Essential fatty acids

HUMORAL/B-CELL (ANTIBODY-MEDIATED) IMMUNITY

Protein
Vitamins B-5, B-6, folic acid in addition to A, B-1, B-2, B-3, biotin, C
Essential fatty acids

Supplementing Nutrients Beyond the RDA

Obviously, a broad range of nutrients is required for immune function. Unfortunately, due to food processing and refining and poor food choices, most Americans don't even get the RDA minimums of many nutrients from their diet (see Chapter Six). But even when they do, these levels for many nutrients are considered to be inadequate. A whole-foods diet is basic to maintaining and strengthening our immune function because of its superior nutrients and life energy. But due to chronically depleted soils in the United States, even whole foods grown on chemically fertilized soils may lack the high level and quality of nutrients that many of us need.[4]

Therefore, bolstering our diet with select vitamin and mineral supplementation beyond the RDA—as discussed in Chapter Six—may prove wise for supporting our immune function. Psychological stress, sleep deprivation, environmental pollutants, age, athletics, infection, injury, cancer, and other factors all change our metabolic requirements. These factors often increase our nutrient needs far in excess of the RDA. In their practices, many nutritional and orthomolecular physicians have observed significant improvement from nutrient supplementation in such immune system challenges as the common cold, allergies (food, inhalant, and chemical), infectious mononucleosis, chronic (Epstein-Barr) virus/chronic fatigue syndrome, polysystemic candidiasis, hepatitis, and even cancer and AIDS. Although "observation" of beneficial response is not always synonymous with "proof," it is convincing enough evidence to encourage such physicians to continue incorporating these safe substances into their overall treatments. In some illnesses, these nutrients provide the mainstay of treatment, whereas in others they work to enhance the outcome of and prevent adverse consequences from more conventional therapy.

SUPPORTING THE IMMUNE SYSTEM

In the remainder of this chapter, I list and briefly discuss a variety of substances and approaches generally not in the realm of conventional medical practice, but which can be incorporated into an immune-enhancing program. This covers more nutrients, food and glandular extracts, herbs, and approaches such as biooxidative therapy, bacterial vaccines, homeopathy, etc. Of paramount importance in this discussion, I feel, are the "Laws of Nature," which provide us with a basis for building and maintaining our immune reserves. With so many available immune-enhancing options, you may feel both encouraged and overwhelmed. It is our hope that this summary will help you find a practical context from which to work.

Additional Immune-Enhancing Agents and Modalities

COENZYME Q-10 has been documented in research and clinical practice as having immune-boosting effects (Chapter Six).

LACTOBACILLUS BULGARICUS, a common bacterial culture for yogurt, has a particular strain (LV-51) that has been used in Europe for cancer treatment and other conditions requiring immune fortification. LV-51 is found to stimulate leukocyte production, T lymphocyte production, and antitumor activity of macrophages.[5]

ALGAE (spirulina, blue-green algae, chlorella). These extracts may increase macrophage tumor necrosis factor-alpha and have anti-cancer activity.[6] Although the studies pertain only to the carotene extracts of spirulina, and not to the whole product, the nutrient content of algae (see Chapter Five) and other chlorophyll food supplements like wheat grass or barley grass (juice or powder) make them worthwhile to consider as food supplements.

HERBAL MEDICINES such as ginseng, licorice root, echinacea, astragalus, osha, lomatium, and others have been shown to impart numerous benefits to immune function, particularly the cell-mediated branch. Such benefits include macrophage stimulation, increased phagocytosis, increased NK (natural killer) cell counts, increased interferon, and an enhancement of delayed hypersensitivity response. A number of herbs also have direct antiviral and antitumor activity. However, some herbal medicines, like certain nutrients, can suppress immune function in excessive doses. (See Chapter Twenty-one for more discussion.)

MEDICINAL MUSHROOMS, such as shiitake, reishe, and ganoderma, also stimulate the production of interferon and other well-defined immune parameters.[7] A reputable source of shiitake is *Lentinus edodes* by Eclectic Institute of Sandy, Oregon. You can find capsule combinations of these agents in some health food stores. (Also see page 460, "Immune-enhancing Power Mushrooms and Mycelin 3.")

GLANDULAR EXTRACTS, particularly thymus and spleen, have been considered potentiators of immune function by many naturopathic physicians and other health professionals, and are frequently prescribed.[8] Due to a concern about viral contamination, however, I hesitate to recommend raw glandular tissues (see discussion on page 205). A source of thymus extract that is boiled, yet still retains active fractions, is Thy-Max (by T. E. Neesby of Fresno, CA).

ACUPUNCTURE has been found to enhance many immune parameters. It can increase the numbers of T cells, lymphocytes in general, T cell ratios, NK cell activity, B cells, and phagocytic activity (see Chapter Twenty-one).

HOMEOPATHY has been used effectively to treat infections and immune deficiencies. One investigator has found that this approach increases the helper/suppressor T cell ratio in AIDS patients. (See Chapter Twenty-one.)

STAPHAGE LYSATE, bacterial vaccine—one made from the staphylococcus bacteria—has been shown to increase resistance specifically to staph infections. Even more exciting, it functions as a general immune system booster as well and is used by physicians for conditions benefited by immune enhancement to generally increase resistance to many foreign agents. This effect occurs in part through macrophage activation. (See Chapter Twenty.)

HYDROTHERAPY, one form of which includes alternating hot and cold applications, mobilizes circulating white cells to effectively combat localized infections. If done constitutionally, hydrotherapy accomplishes many goals, one of which is to mobilize and stimulate general resistance and vitality (see Chapter Twenty).

BIOOXIDATIVE THERAPY (ozone and hydrogen peroxide). When used according to accepted protocols—intravenously, orally, or both—this approach has been found, primarily by European physicians and some currently in the United States and Mexico, to be a safe and effective treatment for acute infections (viral, bacterial, and fungal). Several sources report that chronic fatigue and immune dysfunction syndrome, atherosclerotic heart disease, diabetes, and even some cases of AIDS and cancer respond favorably to such treatment. These therapies work by both supersaturating the blood with oxygen, and by oxidizing foreign agents.[9]

MAGNETIC FIELD THERAPY operates on the premise that all cellular functions depend upon specific electromagnetic influences.[10] Magnetic polarities play an essential role in both nerve transmission and the functioning of an immune cell. A growing number of practitioners are treating their patients with applications of unipoled solid-state magnets or electromagnets at specific points on the body. Much positive clinical experience is being amassed for this modality in the treatment of bacterial, viral, and fungal infections, cancer, AIDS, emotional illness, insomnia, headaches, back pain, injuries, and other conditions. Magnetic field therapy is heralded by some as the medicine of the future. Books (including self-help publications) and magnets can be obtained at Enviro-Tech Products, 17171 SE 29th Street, Choctaw, Oklahoma, 73020, (405) 390-3499. Certain electromagnetic frequencies (known as electromagnetic pollution) may have adverse health effects. "Life-Field Polarizers" and other polarizing mechanisms can help counter certain electronics and household emissions. Contact N.E.E.D.S.: Products for the Chemically Sensitive, 572 Charles Ave. #12A, Syracuse, New York 13209, (800) 634-1380.

There are also many practitioners who can favorably affect the bioelectric fields of their patients with their hands and their own bioelectric energy. Two such modalities are known as "*bioenergetic therapy*"[11] and "*therapeutic touch*" (see Chapter Twenty).

FASTING for several days periodically and systematically undereating a whole-foods balanced diet are two treatment modalities believed even by conventional medical investigators to increase immune response and prolong life (see Chapter Eighteen).

LIVING BY THE LAWS OF NATURE: BASIC IMMUNE-ENHANCING APPROACHES

We get so impressed with therapeutic nutrients, herbs, medications, vaccines, homeopathy, acupuncture, and all the various therapies that natural and allopathic medicine offer that we forget the simplest and perhaps most profound healing treatments that we can all provide for ourselves. The basic health maintenance measures listed below not only boost immune response, but also enhance the quality of our lives. They can help offset the stress and tension of our daily lives, recharge our batteries, and rejuvenate our mood and energy. More technical measures will often work more effectively—or even become unnecessary—if we put some of these basic measures to work for us.

EAT WISELY. Use predominantly whole foods, and attempt to individualize your diet according to the principles discussed in Chapter Four. Avoid overeating, and consider doing periodic short fasts to strengthen the immune system and boost your physical and mental energy.

GET ENOUGH SLEEP. Don't shortchange yourself too frequently on this revitalizing nutrient. Your physical energy, mental acuity and stability, the health of your relationships (family, social, professional), and your resistance to infections all depend on your getting enough sleep.

EXERCISE REGULARLY. Your bones, muscles, circulation, physical and mental energy, and your immune system are all assisted by physical exercise. The endorphins and enkephalins alone that are released by exercise make you feel wonderful—enough of a reason to exercise. If you are bedridden, or stuck at a desk for long hours, stretching and isometrics are possible and can be very beneficial if done appropriately. Remember, though, excessive exercise can diminish immune response as well as other health parameters, so don't overdo it!

RESTRICT ALCOHOL CONSUMPTION to the equivalent of one to two ounces or less of hard liquor or one to two glasses or less of wine or beer daily. A small, daily amount of alcohol can be relaxing and may even diminish the incidence of heart disease and prolong life. However, there can also be hazards (addiction, adverse behavioral and cognitive responses, driving risks, and so on) even with small amounts. As a result, some individuals might be better off finding more healthful ways to relax. And even those who can tolerate alcohol should avoid it altogether during periods of illness. Excessive alcohol consumption can increase the risk of cancer and infection and decrease lymphocyte count and NK cell activity.

AVOID THE USE OF STREET DRUGS. Marijuana, for example, diminishes macrophage and NK cell activity, and impairs both interferon production and cytotoxic T cells.

AVOID LOW-FREQUENCY (60 HERTZ) PULSATING ELECTROMAGNETIC FIELDS such as those found in electric blankets and waterbed heaters. They have been linked to miscarriages and low-birth-weight infants. Pregnant women, and perhaps anyone with marginal immune function, should avoid the use of these items. Most computer terminals, particularly if you spend hours directly behind or to the side of someone else's screen, may put you at risk. Electric razors have even been implicated in adverse health effects.

There has been a twofold increase in the incidence of leukemia in those living near high-tension power lines.[12] See Paul Brodeur's *Currents of Death: Powerlines, Computer Terminals, and the Attempt to Cover Up the Threat to Your Health*, New York: Simon & Schuster, 1989.

MINIMIZE THE UNNECESSARY USE OF PHARMACEUTICAL MEDICATIONS. Seek safe and effective alternatives when possible.

FIND TIME TO BE ALONE AND TO RELAX. Skilled relaxation—meditation, imagery/visualization, biofeedback, and self-hypnosis—all help you alter your normal, active, vigilant mental processes and mind chatter. In addition to its accepted use for high blood pressure, high blood cholesterol, angina, cancer, back pain, insomnia, and Raynaud's disease, skilled relaxation is an important way of undoing the harm that anger, fear, grief, and excessive mental concentration or worry can cause to your psyche, immune system, and other parts of your body.

When it isn't possible to resolve the sources of tension in our lives, a skilled relaxation technique can help us boost our tolerance to stress, cope with difficulties better, lower serum cortisol and cholesterol levels, and prevent immune deterioration. Any form of relaxation—whether a bath, a massage, a hobby, a game—is extremely beneficial. Any activity that healthfully alters your consciousness and eases your mind out of its normal train of thought will do. Relaxation is as essential to the health of our psyches and immune systems as aerobic exercise is to the health of the cardiovascular and musculoskeletal systems (see pages 303–304 "The Exercises").

STAY IN TOUCH WITH YOUR FEELINGS AND VALUES. Be honest with yourself and authentic with others. Don't allow anger, fear, or jealousy to fester inside you. Find appropriate ways to express your feelings and satisfy your emotional needs. Make every effort to resolve the conflicts of your daily life, and attempt to practice self-forgiveness. Above all, find time for yourself no matter how busy your life may be. (See Chapter Fifteen.)

CULTIVATE A SENSE OF HUMOR. Laughter has proven antistress effects on our physiology.[13] It can lower serum cortisol and adrenaline and therefore ease the body's stress response and preserve immune function. Norman Cousins's *Anatomy of an Illness* provides an illuminating example of this. Through a self-devised treatment—a main component of which was laughter—the author was able to overcome a "terminal" illness.

MUSIC and sound have been used for centuries by shamans and healers and are being used today to mobilize inner healing capacities. Many well-known present-day authorities are also taking advantage of this modality in their work.

Psychiatrist John Diamond, M.D., author of *The Life Energy in Music* (1986) and *Life Energy Analysis: A Way to Cantillation* (1988), both from Valley Cottage, N.Y.: Archaeus Press, writes prescriptions for specific pieces of classical music for his patients. His knowledge of music and the human psyche is such that he can match the works of specific classical composers to his patients' particular personalities and travails. Taking this music prescription has helped many of his patients manage or resolve difficult issues.[14] Diamond also believes that music affects the thymus gland, the seat of cell-mediated immunity.

Long before his book *Love, Medicine, and Miracles* became popular, surgeon Bernie Siegel, M.D., demonstrated to the surgical department at a Yale University Medical School hospital the benefits of playing the patients' choices of music during their surgical operations.

Pioneering music therapist, musician, and teacher, Helen Bonny, Ph.D., coauthor (with Louis Savary) of *Music and Your Mind: Listening with a New Consciousness*, Barrytown, NY: Station Hill Press, 1990, has used classical music to quicken healing and shorten the stays of hospitalized patients. Even plants benefit from certain kinds of music (see *The Secret Life of Plants* by Peter Tompkins and Christopher Bird, New York: Harper & Row, 1973).

Just how music works to enhance healing is not well understood. It is felt by many current investigators that sound may affect us in the same way as light, electromagnetic energy, cosmic energy, and thermal energy in that they all trigger the pineal gland (once considered the master gland) in the brain to secrete melatonin, a neuropeptide. Melatonin fits into the benzodiazepine (Valium-like) receptors in the hypothalamus and stimulates immune-enhancing neuropeptides, the chemical mediators of emotion. If music can give you chills, make you cry, make you feel wonderful, sublime, relaxed, or charged up for battle, it's highly likely that beneficial neuropeptides will be pouring out of your brain and, among other things, enhance immune function.

Create a special time—just as you do for meals or exercise or meditation—to listen to carefully chosen music. Consider it an essential nutrient for the psyche and heart. Art, nature, and in fact, anything beautiful and inspiring may work in a similar way. Read *Music: Physician for Times to Come* by Don Campbell (Wheaton, IL: Quest Books, The Theosophical Publishing House, 1991), an anthology of essays on music and healing, and contact the Institute for Music, Health, and Education or other organizations for more information.[15]

SUNLIGHT. In the last decade, sunlight has been documented to be important for maintaining a positive mood in a certain percentage of individuals. Those affected with wintertime depression—"seasonal affective disorder" (SAD)—in northern latitudes where winter days can be extremely short and the amount of sunlight is diminished are now being treated with light therapy (see Chapter Seventeen, "Seasonal Affective Disorder"). Both Jacob Liberman, O.D., Ph.D., in *Light: Medicine of the Future* (Santa Fe, NM: Bear and Company, 1991) and Zane R. Kime, M.D., in *Sunlight Can Save Your Life* (Penryn, CA: World Health Publications, 1980) discuss sunlight's health-promoting effects, some of which are decreased serum cholesterol, increased testosterone, increased synthesis of vitamin D, lowered blood pressure, and treatment of psoriasis, neonatal jaundice, tuberculosis, and other conditions.

H. Gordon Ainsleigh, D.C.,[16] in a recent article in the *Townsend Letter for Doctors* strongly correlates sunlight exposure with less incidence of breast,[17] colon,[18] and other cancers.[19] Malignant melanoma (the most feared "sun-induced" skin cancer) has been related specifically to "blister and peel" sunburning, especially if this type of sunburning occurred before the age of twenty.[20] You may be surprised to know that melanoma is less common in those who work outdoors than in those who work indoors.[21] Regular and nonburning exposure to the sun, Ainsleigh concludes, is a good thing—should be sought a few hours, perhaps three times, weekly. He believes it will not increase the incidence of melanoma and, in fact, can decrease the incidence of internal cancers. Although sunlight can increase the risk of skin cancers far less dangerous than melanoma, such as squamous cell carcinoma, that can occur on areas of the body that get regular sun exposure—like the face or hands—a hat, sunblock, and common sense can help protect these areas. With proper protection and moderation, the benefits of sunlight seem to outweigh the risk.

Photobiologist John Ott, author of *Health and Light* and *Light, Radiation and You*, has done much original research on the effects of sunlight and the relationships between light and health. He was also instrumental in developing full-spectrum lighting. You may want to consider installing full-spectrum lighting in your home or office if your time outdoors is limited or if you live in northern latitudes from October through March.

Some people consider the "Ott Light" to be the indoor lighting source closest to natural sunlight (Environmental Lighting Concepts (813) 621-0058). It also shields users from the low-level cathode radiation inherent in fluorescent tube lighting. While "Vitalite" tube lights are more economical than Ott bulbs and are also full spectrum, they do not shield the radiation. There are incandescent bulbs from Europe that are advertised as full spectrum, and although they are superior to regular incandescent bulbs, and do not pose the radiation problem of "Vitalites," to my knowledge they are not as effective simulators of natural light as the Ott light or Vitalite.

There is also dichromatic green light, which, according to one source, is particularly healing for stress disorders and adrenal exhaustion (par 38 dichromatic 150-watt spot or floodlights made by both Sylvania and General Electric).[22]

Since much of the effect of sunlight is thought to be transmitted through the eyes and then to the pineal gland, Ott suggests that eyewear that blocks full-spectrum transmission (this includes most glasses, contact lenses, and sunglasses) may also block some of the health benefits of sun exposure. Because of the risk of sunlight-induced cataracts, UV-radiation-blocking lenses are advisable, especially where sunlight is intense and prolonged. Finding a balance between risks and benefits may have to rest with common sense, personal choice, and professional advice.

In his book, Dr. Liberman suggests getting at least an hour outdoors daily without UV-blocking lenses. (Certain medical conditions or medications may contraindicate such exposure. Check with your doctor.) On days when I spend most of my time indoors, I'll take walks without wearing my glasses, which amounts to around twenty to thirty minutes of sunlight. On days when I spend hours outdoors, particularly between the strongest UV radiation hours of 10 A.M. and 3 P.M., I will be certain to wear UV-radiation-blocking sunglasses. Incidentally, it is not advisable to have sunlight shine directly into your eyes. Many of sunlight's benefits may be derived from indirect exposure.

CULTIVATE A COMMUNITY. Humans are social creatures. We need other people in various essential ways that we may not often realize. Patch Adams, M.D., of the Gesundheit Institute of Arlington, Virginia, believes that loneliness is the most devastating of human illnesses. To feel our best, we need to feel a part of something larger than ourselves. We need intimate connections with others: another person, a family, a neighborhood, a community group, a religious group, a professional association, a social group or sports team, and so on. Even a pet or a plant to care for brings us significant health benefits.

As independent and individualistic as some of us like to think we are, most of us need to feel that we are of worth and importance to others. We need others to bring out the best (and worst) in us, and they need us for the same reasons. Self-imposed alienation and isolation can have devastating effects on our health and emotions. In countries where there is a strong family and community orientation, individuals often live to be over a hundred years old.[23] In these special communities where longevity abounds, one looks forward to being a venerated elder in one's old age. Many health professionals believe that much of the mental and physical deterioration of old age is a culturally induced phenomenon. In a youth-centered society such as ours, few of us look forward to being an elder when our belief systems, conditioned by forced retirements and nursing homes, program us to become debilitated, sexless, useless, and ignored. But you can change this belief system. See *Ageless Body, Timeless Mind* by Deepak Chopra, M.D., New York: Harmony Books, 1993. See also *Longevity: Fulfilling our Biological Potential* by Kenneth Pelletier, Ph.D., New York: Dell, 1982.

And don't underestimate the importance of intimate relationships and a supportive community: your happiness and health depend on them.

TOUCHING AND BEING TOUCHED also bring us significant health benefits, whether it's a handshake, a pat, a hug, even friendly wrestling or other friendly contact sports. Maintaining close relationships and a feeling of community ties in closely with this health concept. Infants who are well fed but who are not held and cuddled regularly fail to thrive—touch is an essential nutrient for them. And animals who are held and "gentled" every day resist infections far better than those who are fed equally well but not touched at all.

Is it any wonder that you feel so good holding a child—if you're not doing it all day long? Is it any wonder that hugging and snuggling and caressing are so wonderful? We would all do well to remember that we are enhancing the psychoneurological phenomena that support our immune function whenever we feel good through touch and whenever we feel less separate from others. While some cultures embrace, kiss on the cheeks, hold hands, or converse with faces inches apart during common social exchanges, our standoffish culture barely condones the custom of shaking hands. Our discomfort with touch puts us at a disadvantage. It separates us from a vital human nutrient. You may feel that some people are going a bit far when they claim they need twelve hugs a day for optimal health and at least three for sheer survival—but they may well be on the right track.

FINDING MEANING AND PURPOSE IN YOUR LIFE, being

dedicated and committed to something you feel is worthwhile, to something you feel uniquely able to contribute to, to something you love to do, can help maintain your immune strength. A physician diagnosed with breast cancer once spoke at a medical conference and confided that staying in touch with her long-cherished intent to see her daughter graduate from college helped her enormously in extending the life expectancy from her life-threatening illness.

I have known several individuals with chronic illnesses who effected "miraculous" recoveries when they quit the type of work that had been "killing" them—work to which they were ill suited, work that did not allow them to be themselves, to develop their uniqueness and creativity, work that prevented them from simply having fun. Finding the right work gave them and their immune systems a new lease on life.

Establish a goal or direction or hobby you can pursue with passion, something that is you, something you love to do. You will be happier, and your immune system may very well begin to rejoice.

SERVICE ACTIVITIES. Helping others, without any expectation of personal gain, can also improve your immune function. When you know that you've really been of help to someone or something, you feel just plain wonderful. Whether service to others distracts you from dwelling on your own negativities, or simply makes you feel good, your immune system thanks you. Some individuals consider service to be part of their spiritual practice. See Ram Dass and Paul Gorman, *How Can I Help? Stories and Reflections on Service* (New York: Knopf, 1987).

DEVELOP A SPIRITUAL PERSPECTIVE. Your goal of enhancing your immune function—and perhaps saving your life—may seem to be the ultimate purpose of your health pursuits. However, from a spiritual perspective, our health is believed to emanate from the soul, which embodies the highest qualities of humanity—love, compassion, integrity, truthfulness, wisdom, enlightenment, courage, nobility, purposefulness, forgiveness, humility, and gratefulness. Thus, whatever helps us develop and manifest these soul qualities is helpful—even if the messenger happens to be an illness or a tragedy.

From this perspective, if your cancer awakens you from complacency, hatred, or greed, and forces you to redefine your values, ideals, goals, your manner of living—if it helps you open to your higher guidance—then the disease can only be considered a gift from the soul. Many of us are fixated on the illusion of health. We insist that we be symptom-free and energized in body and mind. We may even be obsessed with the rules of health, with doing everything "right"—diet, exercise, managing stress, and so on. In *The Art of Living*, Vol. 4, Robert Leichtman, M.D., and Carl Japikse tell us that:

[T]o understand fully the true nature of health and its manifestation, we must realize that the external conditions of illness are often healing events—not real illnesses. Just as a fever is not an illness, but the body's effort to raise its temperature so as to destroy the invading virus that is the illness, so also many conditions of sickness and even death are, from the perspective of the soul, events leading to greater health. Once a cancerous pattern develops in the emotions—for example, bitter resentment—it blocks off the expressiveness of the soul. For the soul to regain the use of the emotions for its own purposes, the pattern must either be neutralized or shoved out. The soul will try to encourage the personality to neutralize the resentment, but if this guidance is ignored, it may have to resort to the only other means available, by jettisoning the pattern into the physical body. When that happens, of course, the body develops a cancer. . . . [I]t would be an error to consider the physical cancer only in terms of "illness." It is the soul's attempt to heal the real illness—the lack of tolerance and forgiveness.

Usually, too much attention is put on illness. We worry about losing our health or succumbing to some horrible disease. The more we understand about the true gifts of health, however, the less illness seems threatening to us. Since true illness is a lack of some spiritual quality, we can neutralize the threat of illness quite easily—by dedicating ourself to expressing as many of the qualities of the soul as we can. By acting as an enlightened, loving, and wise human being, we cultivate an aura of spiritual health that protects us from illness and disability, and helps us to function as we have been designed to.[24]

CREATING AN OPTIMAL WELLNESS PROGRAM FOR YOUR NEEDS

Given this wealth of opportunities to boost your immune function, where do you begin? Start with what you can safely and appropriately do on your own. Look closely at the Laws of Nature and see what is fitting for you and what you are drawn to. See what you can improve upon.

Some of these areas, such as finding meaning or purpose, making more room for humor, or becoming part of a community, are not as easy to come by as beginning a program of dietary supplements. But they're every bit as vital. And you can begin working in these areas while pursuing your vitamin program and other ways of strengthening your immune system.

Look carefully at the chapters that discuss the Ten Common Denominators of Illness. Start with the conditions that seem applicable to you, and follow the commonsense recommendations outlined in each chapter. For further help with these conditions, seek the assistance and guidance of appropriate health care professionals.

If you'd like some help sorting out what extra immune-boosting supplements and agents to use, read the individual discussions in Chapter Six for nutrients and Chapter Nineteen for herbs. See if some of these recommendations fit other ailments or susceptibilities you have. You may discover that what you use to treat specific ailments may also favorably and directly affect your entire immune function. For example, if you have premenstrual symptoms, agents that help here and with immune function as well include vitamins B-6, E, A, and essential fatty acids. If your prostate gland is enlarged, flaxseed oil and zinc would be appropriate for both your prostate and immune function.

Look up the conditions or illnesses you have in Chapter Seventeen, "Common Ailments," or in the index, and you may find specific immune-enhancing recommendations to help guide you. Formulas combining immune-enhancing vitamins, minerals, herbs, mushrooms, and algae commonly recommended by health professionals are sometimes available in health food stores. Herbal immune-enhancing formulas are listed in Chapter Nineteen under "Immune Enhancing." You

may require professional guidance to find the ones most appropriate for you. (See pages 105, 106, where food concentrate powders containing many of these agents are discussed.)

There is only so much you can put in your mouth and swallow. Often, even the best immune-enhancing supplement program will not be effective because there is basic groundwork yet to do—such as a diet to clean up or one or more of the Ten Common Denominators of Illness to work through (see Chapters Three through Fifteen). There could also be other conditions such as diabetes, hypothyroidism, or intestinal parasites that need to be diagnosed by a physician and treated. Sometimes a nutritional or herbal supplement program or any treatment is less effective because too many Laws of Nature are being violated. And the third possibility is that your body may prefer a completely different mode of treatment such as acupuncture, homeopathy, hydrotherapy, or other such modalities discussed in Part V. Naturally, specialized health professionals would need to be consulted for these treatments.

Often the best results and safest outcome will occur with a combination of approaches. Such a program would include conventional medical diagnosis and treatment, when necessary; holistic/nutritional/alternative diagnosis and treatment; various self-care measures; and following the Laws of Nature. Your specific illnesses, goals, and preferences will determine how effective each of these will be in your overall treatment and recovery.

PART FOUR

COMMON AILMENTS, NATURAL REMEDIES, AND PREVENTIVE APPROACHES

COMMON AILMENTS A TO Z

In this section, you will find an alphabetical list of common ailments, an explanation of related or underlying causes of the conditions, and suggested treatments and preventive measures.

Wellness, using natural remedies and preventive methods, goes beyond traditional diagnosis and treatment by prescription medication. The A to Z of common ailments in this section, from abscess to yeast infection, must be viewed as more than a collection of symptoms to be eradicated by a general approach, but rather as an indication of an underlying systemic weakness draining one's health reserve. For some ailments, accepted alternative means of cure are suggested. Although often effective immediately, they may not be effective in the long run. Consequently, for long-term health management and maximum self-care, always go back and carefully review the chapters of this book that discuss each of the Ten Common Denominators in detail. Remember, treating symptoms alone will never create the foundation of health needed to achieve optimal wellness.

Always consult a qualified medical doctor if you have any questions or if symptoms persist.

The following key to the Ten Common Denominators of Illness will help you understand the abbreviations that appear after **Related and Underlying Causes** for each ailment:

ADR   Adrenal Exhaustion

Y   Yeast Overgrowth

CHEM   Chemical Hypersensitivity and Environmental Illness

ND   Nutritional Deficiencies

DietH   Dietary Hazards

B/M   Psychoneuroimmunology: The Body-Mind Connection System

FA   Food Allergies

ToxB   Toxic Bowel

SL   Sluggish Liver

HYP   Hypoglycemia

DIG   Maldigestion and Poor Absorption

Always review the abbreviations that refer to the Ten Common Denominators before you embark on any treatment program.

To access detailed discussions of specific topics referred to in the A to Z section, see the following chapters:

- Where nutritional recommendations are listed, refer to Chapter Six.
- Where herbal remedies are listed, consult Chapter Nineteen for more information.
- Where dietary hazards (sugar, rancid oils, etc.) and whole-foods diets are discussed, see Chapters Three and Four.
- Where stress management, skilled relaxation exercises, and psychological or emotional factors are mentioned, see Chapter Fifteen.

Also note the following:

- Each common ailment is followed by a variety of

treatment options, including: dietary recommendations, detoxification programs, nutritional supplements, and herbal remedies, etc. To institute all of these measures simultaneously could be overwhelming and is not advisable. Frequently, not all measures are necessary. Reviewing the Common Denominators that pertain to the ailment in question can help you to prioritize treatment measures and will alert you to any precautions.

- There are many products and nutritional supplements mentioned in this section. For your convenience, we have listed manufacturers that offer quality products. If you cannot obtain the recommended products or reasonable duplications in a health food store, ask your doctor or pharmacist. Some are available from companies that sell to health food stores or that distribute only to doctors or pharmacies.
- If you are pregnant, consult your doctor about the use of any recommended products or procedures.
- All recommendations are for adults except where specifically stated. Although many remedies are safe for children, consult your physician before administering any treatment.

Abscess or Boil

This infection is characterized by an accumulation of pus in a well-defined sac. Abscesses and boils are most frequently caused by bacteria.

Related or Underlying Causes

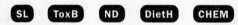

Other factors that can predispose one to such an infection include a poor dietary regime with too high a sugar intake and a general lack of basic nutrients and vitamins. Check especially for heavy metal intoxication.

Treatment and Preventive Measures

Treatment should take a dual approach, both external and internal, since toxins must be released and the system purged.

External

First, increase circulation to the affected area and promote drainage. This can be accomplished by:

SOAKS
- Treat with hot soaks for fifteen to thirty minutes at least twice a day. Soak the affected area directly in water as hot as you can stand without burning, or apply a washcloth soaked in hot water. Adding Epsom salts to the soaking water may have a better drawing effect. Another concept of hydrotherapy, alternating hot and cold water applications, can also be helpful (see Chapter Twenty).
- Prepare an herbal tea soak made from powdered goldenseal (1 part), powdered myrrh (1 part), and ground cayenne pepper (¼ part). Steep 2 to 3 teaspoons of this mixture per cup of water. Use similarly to the Epsom salt soak.

POULTICES
Poultices are effective for drawing out toxins from the skin. They are made of common herbal, vegetable, or clay substances that are sometimes heated and mixed into a pastelike thickness. This mixture is then spread on gauze, linen, or other cotton material and applied to the body.
- A potato poultice can be especially effective in dealing with a troublesome abscess or boil. Simply grate enough raw potato to make half a cup and mash with a little flour to give it more consistency. Fold into a length of cheesecloth and apply to the abscess for at least several hours.
- A chlorophyll poultice can be mixed in a small bowl by blending fresh wheat grass juice with the wheat grass pulp. Apply the wet pulp directly to the boil. Cover it with plastic wrap and leave in place for thirty minutes. Do this three times a day. The juice and pulp of any deep green leafy vegetable can also be used.

PERSONAL HYGIENE
Personal hygiene is very important in the prevention of boils. Be sure to bathe or shower regularly. Dry brush the skin (see Chapter Eighteen).

Internal

DIETARY RECOMMENDATIONS
- Eat whole foods and extra vegetables and fruits (cleansing foods), minimize sweets, and avoid overeating.
- Drink large quantities of water and other fluids. Green juices are especially recommended for their cleansing effect. If fresh wheat grass or other green juice is unavailable, use liquid chlorophyll (1 or 2 tablespoons three times a day mixed in water or juice), available in health food stores.

DETOXIFICATION PROGRAM
- Follow the Liver Flush and Purifying Diet or fast for a few days to speed the healing process.

NUTRITIONAL SUPPLEMENTS

- Take immune-supporting nutrients. A good multiple vitamin and mineral formula may do, but be sure to take vitamin A (25,000 I.U. daily), vitamin E (400 I.U. daily), and extra vitamin C (3,000 to 6,000 milligrams a day).

HERBAL REMEDIES

- Drink echinacea and burdock root teas (at least three or four cups a day) for their anti-infection and purifying effects.
- Silica cell salts (four tablets three times a day) or horsetail tea may enhance the suppurative process (the escape of pus).
- Use goldenseal alone (two or three capsules four times a day) or in an antibacterial herbal combination.

RESISTANT ABSCESSES AND BOILS

- Although the above approaches are usually successful, boils or abscesses that prove resistant to these methods are best treated by incision and drainage by a doctor. Sometimes oral antibiotics are required.
- If all else fails for recurrent staph boil infections, have your doctor try staphage lysate, a bacterial vaccine, and check for intestinal yeast overgrowth.

Acne

A condition that produces skin inflammation and blemishes, often on the face but also affecting the back, shoulders, and chest. Blemishes can include pimples, blackheads, and whiteheads. In the most severe form, cysts may result. Although most common in adolescents, acne can also affect adults.

Related or Underlying Causes

    DietH **SL** **ToxB** **FA** **Y**

A junk food or fast-food diet, especially one high in fat, is often the culprit in acne conditions. Pay particular attention to possible dairy product allergies. Low stomach acid and/or insufficient pancreatic enzymes, along with essential fatty acid deficiency, may be important factors. Nutritional deficiencies of vitamin A, zinc, sometimes vitamin B-6, and chromium can also contribute to the problem.

If acne is triggered during the premenstrual part of your cycle, see PREMENSTRUAL SYNDROME.

Treatment and Preventive Measures

External

Acne is a superficial manifestation of an internal imbalance. Dermatologists can recommend many topical treatments to alleviate symptoms. Also, concentrate on internal treatments and underlying causes.

- Avoid touching your face, since this action may introduce bacteria. Remember, the palm side of your hands and fingers is especially oily.
- Use a gentle glycerin soap daily to wash your face, but excessive washing can dry your skin. Take a wet, warm washcloth (as warm as you can stand) to your face briefly several times a day to remove excess oils. Follow with a brief application of a cold washcloth.
- Dry brush daily. Use a special, softer brush for your face (see Chapter Eighteen).

Internal

DIETARY RECOMMENDATIONS

- Follow a whole-foods diet, emphasizing fresh vegetables and fruit.
- Drink six to eight glasses of water a day.
- Drink green juices for their cleansing effects.

DETOXIFICATION PROGRAMS

- Do an intestinal cleansing program; follow the Liver Flush and Purifying Diet and/or fast for several days periodically.

NUTRITIONAL SUPPLEMENTS

- Vitamin C (1,000 milligrams three times a day).
- Vitamin A (25,000 I.U. daily). Higher doses of vitamin A are frequently required for treating cystic acne, if the underlying causes discussed above do not apply or if other treatments have not helped. In adults, up to 300,000 I.U. daily of vitamin A has been effective. Taking vitamin E (800 I.U. daily) may lessen the required dose of vitamin A to 150,000 I.U. daily. *Warning: Since severe toxicity symptoms may result from this high dose of vitamin A, it must be taken only under medical supervision.*
- Vitamin B-6 (25 to 50 milligrams a day) in a B-complex formula.
- Zinc (30 to 60 milligrams a day).
- Chromium (200 to 500 micrograms a day).
  Note: Some of the items above can be taken as part of a multiple vitamin/mineral.
- Flaxseed oil (1 teaspoon or three capsules a day).
- Borage oil (two or three capsules a day, a key source of gamma linolenic acid).

HERBAL REMEDIES

- Drink several cups daily of blood-purifying teas, such as red clover and burdock root.

Agoraphobia

See ANXIETY.

AIDS (Acquired Immune Deficiency Syndrome)

AIDS is a disease that results in severely lowered counts of helper T lymphocytes and thus in an increased susceptibility to life-threatening infections and certain cancers.

Related or Underlying Causes

 ND **CHEM** **B/M** **DietH**

AIDS is ostensibly caused by HIV (human immunodeficiency virus), which is spread through sexual fluids and blood and blood products. However, some researchers and health professionals believe that the virus is only a cofactor, and that an immune system weakened by drug and chemical exposure, multiple previous infections, nutrient deficiencies, and other factors play an important role in susceptibility.

Treatment and Preventive Measures

Individuals afflicted with HIV, ARC (AIDS-related complex), and AIDS require the crucial support of a broad-based nutritional and herbal program to boost immune function. The sooner such a program is implemented upon learning of HIV-positive status, the better the chances of delaying immune deterioration and prolonging health. Pharmaceutical agents such as antibacterial, antifungal, antiparasite drugs and others are also often required. Consult your doctor.

DIETARY RECOMMENDATIONS
- Follow a whole-foods diet, minimizing sugar, alcohol, excessive fat, and other common health hazards. Identify allergy-triggering foods and avoid them. Tailor the diet according to blood and body type (see Chapter Four). If weight loss and muscle wasting are issues, the diet should include extra protein (perhaps a total of up to 100 grams daily—consult your doctor).
- Drink fresh vegetable juice (at least one large glass daily).

DETOXIFICATION PROGRAMS
- If weight loss and muscle wasting are not issues, try a periodic short fast or the Liver Flush and Purifying Diet for its cleansing effects.

NUTRITIONAL SUPPLEMENTS
- Take a high-potency multiple vitamin and mineral supplement, such as Perque 2 (one or two tablets twice a day), available from Seraphim of Reston, Virginia.
- Take zinc (30 milligrams a day), coenzyme Q-10 (30 milligrams two or three times a day), and cysteine/N-acetylcysteine (500 milligrams two or three times a day).
- Try a free-form amino acid formula without arginine, such as Amino-Virox (two to four capsules twice a day), available from Tyson and Associates of Hawthorne, California; combined essential fatty acids (GLA and EPA), such as Salmon Oil and GLA (from Carlson Laboratories of Arlington Heights, Illinois) or Omegasyn (from Biosyn of Boston), one or two capsules of either twice a day; and vitamin C (1,000 to 2,000 milligrams three times a day). Intravenous vitamin C is recommended if the condition becomes more serious. Consult a nutritionally oriented physician.
- Thymus glandular (one or two capsules up to three times a day), such as Thy-Max by T. E. Neesby of Fresno, California. This is a boiled glandular. (See warning on glandulars, page 205.)
- Spleen glandular, with Siberian ginseng, such as PCM4 (from Emerson's Ecologics of Acton, Massachusetts, and Omega Nutripharm of Birmingham, Alabama). (See warning on glandulars, page 205.)
- DHEA, or dehydroepiandrosterone (5 to 20 milligrams twice a day—consult your doctor about exact dose), if this adrenal hormone is found to be low.
- Hydrochloric acid (one to four 10-grain capsules per main meal—consult your doctor about exact dose) if an HCl deficiency is found.
- Intestinal flora products, such as HMF by Interplexus of Kent, Washington (one capsule twice a day) and *Saccharomyces boulardii*, available from Allergy Research/Nutricology of San Leandro, California. The latter is especially useful for diarrhea (300 to 600 milligrams per meal, up to 2,000 milligrams a day).

HERBAL REMEDIES
- D-Plex (echinacea root, astragalus root, dandelion root, gum benzoin, red raspberry leaf, garlic bulb, jalapeño pepper): up to eight capsules three times daily, acutely, then two to five capsules a day for a maintenance dose. Or take HIV-Plex (Chinese astragalus root, licorice root, Chinese self-heal, Chinese violet leaf): three to seven capsules three times a day. Both of these formulas are available through Herb Technology/Khalsa Health Center, Seattle, Washington.

- Chinese herbal formulas, such as Enhance and Clear Heat from Health Concerns of Oakland, California (consult your doctor for treatment protocol).

OTHER THERAPIES
- Emotional factors play a powerful role in AIDS. Most long-term AIDS survivors have been successful in part because they believe they can survive. This essential attitude also requires social support from friends, families, AIDS activist groups, and practitioners, as well as the assistance of various social services agencies.

Alcoholism

The American Medical Association officially recognized alcoholism as a disease and a serious health problem in 1966. An estimated 8 to 12 percent of the adult population in the United States is physically and psychologically dependent on alcohol. It often takes many years before the consequences of excessive or chronic drinking become evident. Many alcoholics are dual-addicted, often addicted to alcohol and other drugs or prescription medications.

Related or Underlying Causes

   HYP

Alcoholism is a disease with genetic, biochemical/nutritional, and psychosocial roots. Alcoholics, both active and recovering, are almost always hypoglycemic and have multiple nutrient deficiencies and food allergies. In addition to food allergies, also be sure to check for leaky gut syndrome, which may be prevalent in active and recovering alcoholics. Allergies to the ingredients of the preferred alcoholic beverages may perpetuate the alcohol addiction. For example, grapes are the potential allergen in wine, wheat in beer, and corn in bourbon. Brewer's yeast, found in most alcoholic beverages, is another potential allergen.

Treatment and Preventive Measures

DIETARY RECOMMENDATIONS
- Follow the diet for the treatment of hypoglycemia given in Chapter Ten.
- Identify and avoid allergy-triggering foods.

DETOXIFICATION PROGRAMS
- Follow the Ultra Clear Program (Metagenics, San Clemente, California) as outlined in Chapter Nine, to decrease systemic toxicity.

NUTRITIONAL SUPPLEMENTS
- Follow the nutritional supplement program for hypoglycemia outlined in Chapter Ten.
- In addition, take N-acetylcysteine (500 milligrams three times a day) or lipoic acid, available as Thiotic by Ecological Formulas, Concord, California (up to two capsules three times a day), which protect against liver deterioration common in alcoholism, as does L-carnitine (200 to 300 milligrams three times a day).
- Glutamine (500 to 1,000 milligrams three times a day) and niacinamide (500 to 1,000 milligrams three times a day—see Chapter Six for precautions) have been used successfully to lessen both hypoglycemia and alcohol craving.

HERBAL REMEDIES
- See "Liver-Protecting Agents," Chapter Nine, for herbs that are specifically protective to the liver.
- Take milk thistle (one or two 70-milligram capsules three times a day).
- Take Phyllanthus Amarus (one capsule three times a day), available from Allergy Research/Nutricology of San Leandro, California or as Livit 1 from Interplexus of Kent, Washington.

Allergy

A condition of inflammation triggered by the interaction of antibodies and white blood cells with an antigen, a "foreign agent" which has entered the body. After exposure, symptoms can be immediate (within minutes) or delayed (from several hours to several days).

The site of the allergic inflammation determines the symptoms experienced. For example, an inflammation of the skin will produce a rash or hives. An allergic inflammation in the brain will cause depression or fuzzy thinking. Inflammation in the joints and muscles will cause pain in those areas.

Allergic symptoms can occur in nearly any part of the body.

Related or Underlying Causes

Allergies can be triggered by foods, environmental chemicals, heavy metal intoxication, inhalants (see HAY FEVER), parasites (see PARASITES), and stress.

Treatment and Preventive Measures

For preventive measures for allergy management, see Chapter Thirteen.

For immediate relief of acute reactions, try the following.

NUTRITIONAL SUPPLEMENTS
- Buffered vitamin C (2,000 to 3,000 milligrams taken once a day).
- Vitamin B-5 or pantothenic acid (500 to 1,000 milligrams taken once a day).
- Vitamin B-6 (50 to 150 milligrams taken once a day).

HERBAL REMEDIES
- Nettles (three or four capsules taken once a day).
- Quercetin (up to 1,000 milligrams taken once a day).

OTHER THERAPIES
- Alka-Seltzer Gold (two tablets in 16 ounces of water).
- Take a gentle laxative, such as unflavored Milk of Magnesia, for food allergy reactions.

Alzheimer's Disease

Progressive deterioration and dysfunction of brain tissue that leads initially to memory loss and cognitive impairment. Eventually, the disease results in severe speech and behavioral disturbances, an inability to care for oneself, and premature death.

Related or Underlying Causes

Bioecologic and nutritional medicine both view Alzheimer's as a set of brain symptoms caused by a number of potentially treatable conditions resulting from a lack of needed nutrients and elevated chemical residues. Look for heavy metal intoxication, especially aluminum and mercury. Also check for low thyroid function (see HYPOTHYROIDISM).

Treatment and Preventive Measures

Early intervention is essential. It is important to take antioxidants and nutrients that have a direct bearing on neurotransmitter synthesis and brain function in general. Many of these essential nutrients can be found in special formulas designed to aid memory and brain function.

Others can be found in a high-potency multiple vitamin/mineral preparation.

NUTRITIONAL SUPPLEMENTS
- Take the following brain nutrients daily: B complex (with at least 100 milligrams of the various B vitamins and 400 to 800 micrograms of folic acid), extra vitamin B-12 (1,000 micrograms sublingual or injected—see below), niacinamide (500 to 1,500 milligrams), glutamine (500 to 1,000 milligrams), phenylalanine (500 to 2,000 milligrams), tyrosine (500 to 2,000 milligrams), zinc (30 to 60 milligrams), and essential fatty acids (1 teaspoon or three capsules of flaxseed oil and two or three capsules of borage oil).
- Antioxidant support is important to preserve brain tissue from free radical injury. This includes N-acetyl-cysteine (1,500 milligrams), beta-carotene (25,000 to 50,000 I.U.), vitamin E (800 I.U.), vitamin C (3,000 milligrams), and selenium (200 micrograms).
- Take Aminomine (two capsules two to three times a day) from Tyson and Associates of Hawthorne, California, an amino acid supplement formulated for brain function.
- Injectable nutrients, intravenous or intramuscular, may bring faster results, particularly if absorption from the gastrointestinal tract is not quite up to par, which is common in older individuals. Vitamin B-12 may be the most important nutrient to try by injection, as it is the most difficult to absorb. An intramuscular injection of 1,000 micrograms of B-12 (1 milliliter), with the addition of up to 5 milligrams of folic acid (½ milliliter) and B complex, with 100 milligrams of B-1 plus varying amounts of other B vitamins (1 milliliter) can bring results within a day. If an individual is severely deficient, several daily injections may be needed to produce results. Weekly and then bimonthly injections may be necessary indefinitely.
- Some individuals respond much better to intravenous injections of the B vitamins, magnesium and other minerals, and vitamin C (see the formula listed in CHRONIC FATIGUE SYNDROME).

HERBAL REMEDIES
- Use the following herbs, which have well-known positive effects on brain function: ginkgo (40 milligrams, one capsule twice a day), gotu kola (500 milligrams, one capsule twice a day), and Siberian ginseng (100 milligrams, one capsule twice a day). Or use a tincture combination of these herbs (Ginkgo-Centella Compound from Eclectic Institute of Sandy, OR) (up to thirty drops twice a day).

OTHER THERAPIES
- Chiropractic and cranial adjustments, exercise, social

interaction, and intellectual stimulation and challenge may all prove beneficial.

Amenorrhea

Amenorrhea is the absence of menstrual periods in a woman of menstruating age. It can also involve a woman who stops having her period for no apparent reason or a woman who does not resume her normal menstrual period after discontinuing use of birth control pills. Amenorrhea may require a medical workup if it occurs in an adolescent who should have started her period but hasn't.

Related or Underlying Causes

Pituitary gland and ovarian failures, often temporary, are the primary causes. However, hypothyroidism (see HYPOTHYROIDISM) and poor adrenal function may be indicated.

Nutritional deficiencies have been shown to play a key role in this condition, since they affect the entire endocrine system, particularly if dieting and extreme weight loss programs are implemented. Excessive exercise training, especially for competitions such as marathons, can deplete a woman's fat stores, resulting in amenorrhea. Extreme stress and emotional tension can also contribute to this disorder.

Treatment and Preventive Measures

DIETARY RECOMMENDATIONS
- An adequate, nutritious diet with an appropriate fat content is important for a normal menstrual cycle.
  Warning: Insufficient protein intake (beware, vegetarians) and an elevated serum carotene level from too much carrot juice or carotene supplementation can also cause amenorrhea.

NUTRITIONAL SUPPLEMENTS
- Fatty acids. Begin a therapeutic trial of essential fatty acids. Take unrefined flaxseed oil (1 or 2 teaspoons daily) and borage oil (one capsule two or three times a day).
- To promote the metabolism of essential fatty acids, add vitamin E (400 I.U. daily), vitamin B-6 (50 to 100 milligrams a day included in a B-complex formula), zinc (15 to 30 milligrams a day), and magnesium (up to 400 milligrams a day).

- Beta-carotene (50,000 I.U. daily) can be useful if carotene overload is not the case. (A reasonable measure of this is observing a yellowish orange hue to the palms. A blood test can verify.) Beta Plex from Scientific Botanicals of Seattle provides beta plus other carotenes.

HERBAL REMEDIES
- Certain herbs are known to help bring on a menstrual period: false or true unicorn root, squawvine, pasqueflower, and black cohosh. Take a combination formula (one to two capsules three times a day) or strong tea (up to three cups a day).

OTHER THERAPIES
- Treat thyroid and adrenal dysfunction, if found.
- Acupuncture has proven effective for treating amenorrhea.
- If excessive exercise and fat loss are factors, reduce workouts appropriately to help reestablish regular menstrual flow.
- Counseling or therapy may be a very useful adjunct to the other suggested modalities in treating emotional/psychological issues and/or stress.
- Diathermy—ultrasound treatments to the pituitary, thyroid, liver, spleen, adrenal, and ovary areas—can stimulate the pituitary/ovarian axis and help menstrual cycles resume. Consult a naturopathic physician for further information.

Anal Fissure

See FISSURE (ANAL).

Angina Pectoris

Chest pain caused by insufficient blood and oxygen supply to the heart muscle. The pain, which often causes a heavy sensation located in the center of the chest, is brought on by exertion, stress, cold weather, or eating.

Related or Underlying Causes

This condition is caused by arteriosclerotic plaque in the coronary arteries (see ARTERIOSCLEROSIS)

and/or coronary artery spasm. An inefficient or weak heart muscle and high blood pressure can be contributors. Low or high thyroid function can be factors as well (see HYPOTHYROIDISM and HYPERTHYROIDISM).

Treatment and Preventive Measures

CONVENTIONAL MEDICAL TREATMENT
• Prescription medication may be necessary.

DIETARY RECOMMENDATIONS
• Eat a low-fat, high-fiber diet.

NUTRITIONAL SUPPLEMENTS
• Take coenzyme Q-10 (10 to 30 milligrams three times a day), carnitine (250 to 1,000 milligrams four times a day), magnesium (400 to 800 milligrams a day), taurine (500 to 1,000 milligrams three or four times a day), vitamin E (800 I.U. daily), and vitamin B-6 (up to 50 milligrams a day). Start with maximum doses. As consistent improvement is noted, reduce after several months to the lower doses. You may not require all of the nutrients listed. Consult a nutritionally oriented doctor.
• If the oral supplementation program is not effective enough, intramuscular injections of magnesium sulfate (500 milligrams with 100 milligrams of vitamin B-6) once a week may be necessary.

OTHER THERAPIES
• Consider chelation therapy (see ARTERIOSCLEROSIS).
• Get regular exercise (as tolerated).
• Practice stress management and relaxation skills.

Anus, Itchy

Itchiness in the anal area which may or may not be accompanied by rash or irritation.

Related or Underlying Causes

Insufficient bathing; food allergy or intolerance, commonly to milk products, tomatoes, coffee, vinegar, alcoholic drinks, and any repetitive food, beverage, or condiment in the diet. Pinworms can be the culprit. Itchy anus can also be caused by a reaction to laundry soap or fabric softener.

Treatment and Preventive Measures

• Gently clean the anal area with wet tissue or with commercial wipes after every bowel movement. Dry thoroughly. Ointments may be helpful, such as A and D or Desitin from a pharmacy, or calendula from a health food store.

Anxiety and Panic (Also Nervousness, Irritability)

Varying levels of sometimes uncontrollable nervousness, agitation, worry, and fear, which can lead to hyperventilation, body tingling, light-headedness, chest pain, a rapid and pronounced heartbeat, and other symptoms.

Related or Underlying Causes

This ailment may have its roots in psychological and emotional triggers. Also, check for excess caffeine, sugar, and/or food additives in diet.

Anxiety can also be caused by hormonal imbalances that can occur in a woman whose nutritional stores have been depleted by prolonged nursing and whose diet may be deficient in protein and calcium.

See HYPERTHYROIDISM and also PREMENSTRUAL SYNDROME.

Treatment and Preventive Measures

CONVENTIONAL MEDICAL TREATMENT
• Pharmaceutical intervention may be needed when other approaches are inadequate. (See INSOMNIA.)

DIETARY RECOMMENDATIONS
• Reduce your intake of caffeine, sugar, and food additives. Follow the dietary recommendations for hypoglycemia in Chapter Ten. Test for and eliminate allergic foods.

NUTRITIONAL SUPPLEMENTS
• The following nutrients may provide acute relief and offer preventive support: B-complex vitamins (50 to 100 milligrams a day); extra niacinamide (500 to 1,000 milligrams three times a day; see precautions); extra vitamin B-1 (up to 100 milligrams three times a day); calcium (500 to 1,500 milligrams a day); magnesium (500 to 1,500 milligrams a day); and vitamin

B-12, preferably by intramuscular injection (1,000 micrograms a week with 2 or 3 milligrams of folic acid). Sublingual B-12 tablets may be taken (2,000 micrograms a day), but injection is the preferred method.

Note: A very small percentage of the population will become more anxious from taking a B-complex formula. Avoid B complex if you are sensitive to it in this way.

HERBAL REMEDIES

- Calming herbs may be helpful. Take a sedative combination formula containing valerian, chamomile, skullcap, hops, and passionflower (two to four capsules as needed).
- Drink passionflower and/or chamomile tea (brewed up to 4 to 5 teaspoons per cup).

HOMEOPATHIC REMEDIES

- Combination homeopathic remedies are available in most health food stores. Individualizing for the best single remedy may be more effective (see Chapter Twenty-one).

OTHER THERAPIES

- Try aerobic exercise, yoga, tai chi, or some other active form of movement.
- Try visualizations, affirmations, breathing exercises, and meditation. Familiarize yourself with these techniques when you're in a relatively nonanxious state. Find what suits you best and practice regularly. In this way, you will have a ready remedy in time of acute need.
- Cranial electric stimulation can be effective.
- Consult a psychotherapist or professional counselor.

Appetite, Excessive

An inability to be satiated by normal amounts of food. See OVERWEIGHT.

Related or Underlying Causes

Overeating may be due to emotional factors or hypochlorhydria deficient pancreatic enzyme secretion, intestinal parasites or worms (see PARASITES), or anxiety and nervousness (see ANXIETY). It can also be related to processed, nutrient-poor food.

Treatment and Preventive Measures

Identify and treat these causes. See also WEIGHT CONTROL.

Appetite, Poor

Lack of desire to consume food.

Related or Underlying Causes

Chronic disease, acute infections, or inflammatory processes often result in symptoms of poor appetite. Other precipitating causes may be depression (see DEPRESSION), low stomach acid and/or insufficient pancreatic enzymes, vitamin B-complex deficiency, and an excessively sedentary lifestyle. Many older people are susceptible to these factors.

Treatment and Preventive Measures

Identify and treat any of the above-mentioned conditions with professional medical help.

DIETARY RECOMMENDATIONS

- Eat a whole-foods diet.
- Identify and eliminate allergy-triggering foods.

NUTRITIONAL SUPPLEMENTS

- Two vitamin supplements are useful in treating this condition: B-complex vitamins (10 to 100 milligrams twice a day) and vitamin B-12 (1,000 micrograms sublingually once or twice a day). Depending on the severity of the condition and your age, both supplements may be better administered by intramuscular injection.
- If indicated, take betaine hydrochloride capsules with meals (as directed by your physician).
- If indicated, take digestive enzymes (one capsule with each meal).

HERBAL REMEDIES

- Take bitters. Consistently excellent results in appetite improvement have been obtained with Bitters Formula, a combination herbal bitters compound sold by Herb-Pharm of Williams, Oregon. Stir a teaspoonful of bitters into a small glass of water. Sip gradually for thirty minutes before meals.

  An aperitif, such as Campari or Angostura Bit-

ters, if not contraindicated, may also be effective (sip slowly for thirty minutes before meals).
- Try gentian herbal tincture, with or without dandelion root (fifteen to twenty drops in a glass of warm water sipped slowly for thirty minutes before meals).
- Try gingerroot (one or two capsules three times a day) or drink gingerroot tea (three cups a day).

Arrhythmia

See PALPITATIONS.

Arteriosclerosis (Coronary Artery Disease)

Also called hardening of the arteries, this condition involves a thickening of the walls of the arteries resulting in an impairment of the flow of blood. Plaque, which accounts for the arterial congestion, is a combination of cholesterol, protein, calcium, platelets, fibrin, and other substances. Severe plaque formation results in blocked arteries.

When circulation becomes insufficient, the consequences can be serious: the arterial wall is damaged and blood and oxygen flow to vital organs is severely compromised. Heart attacks, for example, occur when a blood clot closes off the artery completely. Plaque formations in arteries can also cause high blood pressure.

The location of arteriosclerotic symptoms within the body depends on where the circulation is impaired. If plaque involves the coronary arteries leading to the heart, the symptoms may be angina or chest pain, a rhythm disturbance, or heart attack. If neck (carotid) or brain arteries are involved, dizziness, senility, or a stroke may result. If the blockage clogs the aorta, or leg arteries are involved, cold feet, muscle cramps, or gangrene can result. Impotence can afflict an individual if circulation in the lower abdomen and pelvis becomes defective. Poor blood flow in the retina of the eye can lead to vision deterioration or blindness. Severe plaque in the renal arteries can lead to kidney failure.

As arteriosclerotic vessels lose their elasticity, high blood pressure often results (see BLOOD PRESSURE, HIGH).

Arteriosclerosis is the most prevalent chronic disease and the number-one killer in the United States. In 1993 alone nearly one million Americans died of complications resulting from arteriosclerosis, with heart attacks accounting for half of those deaths.

Related or Underlying Causes

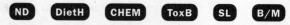

Theories abound about the causes of arterial plaque development. Diets high in saturated fat, elevated LDL cholesterol, and lowered HDL cholesterol serum levels have drawn the most attention (see CHOLESTEROL, HIGH). Other factors, particularly arterial injury from nutritional deficiencies and free radical damage, may be equally, if not more, important.

Arteries consist, in part, of collagen, a network of interconnecting structural fibers maintained by several nutrients, especially vitamin C. Inadequate vitamin C will cause an actual breakdown of arterial walls and blood leakage. Blood leakage in arteries triggers an emergency response in the body—the depositing of more LDL cholesterol and apolipoprotein (a) needed to repair tears. However, these measures also have an adverse effect, creating arteriosclerotic plaque and sticky protein residues.

Heredity greatly influences blood levels of both protein and LDL cholesterol, although diet, nutritional supplementation, exercise, and stress management can significantly reduce them.

Once inside arterial walls, protein and LDL stimulate muscle cells in the wall of the artery to grow, increasing plaque size. For the development of arteriosclerotic plaque, injury to the artery is felt to be the primary cause, while cholesterol and other plaque components are secondary. In addition to vitamin C deficiency, other factors triggering arterial injury include deficiencies of vitamin B-6 and the minerals silicon and, possibly, copper. Of course, cigarette smoking, high blood pressure (see BLOOD PRESSURE, HIGH), and diabetes (see DIABETES) injure arteries, as does excessive vitamin D, iron, lead, and sugar, even in nondiabetics. Xanthine oxidase from homogenized milk products and peanuts and peanut oil may also cause arterial injury. Some of the above injuries occur through deficiencies of antioxidants, the nutrients that help prevent free radical assault, which are now beginning to assume primary importance in both the prevention and treatment of arteriosclerosis.

Environmental pollutants provide another source of free radical attack on arteries. Lead from exhaust fumes and other sources is particularly toxic to blood vessels. Hydrocarbons and numerous other substances polluting the environment contribute to free radical assault. Chlorine, a popular additive to most municipal water supplies, has also been implicated.

Stress, lack of exercise, low thyroid function (see HYPOTHYROIDISM), and deficiencies of chromium, essential fatty acids, and fiber are all related to plaque formation.

Treatment and Preventive Measures

CONVENTIONAL MEDICAL TREATMENT

- Cholesterol-lowering drugs are commonly prescribed for serum cholesterol elevations (see CHOLESTEROL, HIGH).
- Surgery is often recommended for more severe cases of plaque disease. In a bypass procedure, a vein, or preferably, the internal mammary artery, is connected to the diseased artery on both sides of the plaque congestion so that blood flow is rerouted around the blockage and restored. In a balloon angioplasty, a wire with a deflated balloon on the tip is threaded into the blocked artery and inflated to stretch and open the plaque-congested area. In an endarterectomy procedure, the plaque is actually scraped from the artery.

DIETARY RECOMMENDATIONS

- A healthy diet is critical as a preventive and treatment measure when dealing with arteriosclerosis.
- Eat a whole-foods diet, minimizing the following: excess saturated fat, margarine and foods containing partially hydrogenated vegetable oils, processed and refined vegetable oils, heated polyunsaturated oils, refined flours and cereals (which lack many nutrients and fiber and contain added iron), sugar, and peanuts, including peanut butter and peanut oil.
- Regularly include the following protective foods: olive oil for salads and sautéing; flaxseed oil, at least 1 teaspoon four or five days a week; garlic and onions; legumes; and oat bran. If you're not a vegetarian, use cold water omega 3-EPA–rich fish (mackerel, herring, albacore tuna, lake trout, dogfish, sable fish, salmon, lake whitefish, halibut) or wild game.
- Avoid drinking chlorinated water; instead, drink filtered artesian spring or other water free of chlorine and other environmental pollutants.
- One important dietary approach to prevent and reverse plaque formation in the arteries is the low-fat, low-cholesterol regimen pioneered by Dr. Nathan Pritikin and more recently popularized by Dr. Dean Ornish.

Dr. Ornish is assistant clinical professor of medicine at the University of California, San Francisco, School of Medicine, and director of the Preventive Medicine Research Institute in Sausalito, California. His program for reversing heart disease offers an effective approach that is gaining approval in traditional medical circles.

Dr. Ornish recommends a vegetarian diet comprising only 10 percent fat, with more than half of the fat derived from polyunsaturated and essential fatty acids. Only 5 milligrams daily of dietary cholesterol is permitted. Fried foods and processed and rancid oils are excluded, along with refined foods. Only whole foods supplying cardioprotective nutrients and fiber are allowed.

According to the program, a dietary balance needs to be maintained, with the average daily food intake equaling 15 to 20 percent protein and 70 to 75 percent carbohydrate (predominantly complex). Calories are unrestricted. Salt is not limited, except for individuals with high blood pressure. No caffeine is allowed.

Since the Ornish approach prohibits meat, people using the diet are recommended to take vitamin B-12 (1,000 micrograms a day). An hour of daily exercise, including yoga, stretching, and skilled relaxation practices, is crucial to the effectiveness of the program.

If you do not have arteriosclerosis and you want to follow a program to prevent it, a 10 percent fat diet may be stricter than needed and not easy to sustain over the years. You might want to try a more realistic diet allowing 20 to 25 percent fat.

Even with some plaque formation in arteries and some saturated fat in the diet, an individual can remain free from heart attacks, strokes, and other complications of arteriosclerosis. There are many populations with a substantial amount of saturated fat in their diets who rarely get heart attacks or strokes. Although biopsies show plaque in their arteries, their diets, lifestyles, and environments provide protective factors that minimize dietary hazards and render them relatively immune to this disease.

DETOXIFICATION PROGRAMS

- Liver cleansing and building techniques improve cholesterol ratios and general health. Because the liver is so critical to cholesterol synthesis and formation, optimizing liver health can be extremely beneficial. (See LIVER FLUSH and PURIFYING DIET.)

NUTRITIONAL SUPPLEMENTS

Many nutrients can be used to treat and prevent arteriosclerosis. Some preserve the structural integrity of arteries and act as antioxidants, others lower cholesterol and protein levels, while some serve all these functions.

- Vitamin C deficiency, a common condition, can injure the arteries. Vitamin C supplements can inhibit platelet aggregation, increase clot-dissolving activity, and increase HDL cholesterol values. Dosage: Take 500 to 1,000 milligrams of vitamin C two or three times a day.
- Beta-carotene's antioxidant function has protective

value for cardiovascular disease. Dosage: Take up to 50,000 I.U. daily.

- Inadequate intake of vitamin B-6, common in American diets, can lead to injury in arterial walls, setting the stage for plaque development. B-6 deficiency can also weaken the heart muscle and raise serum cholesterol levels. Dosage: Take up to 50 milligrams a day.
- Vitamin E, a potent antioxidant that fights free radical pathology, is the king of cardiovascular nutrients. Vitamin E heightens antioxidant defenses, preventing the oxidation and buildup of LDL cholesterol in the arterial wall. Vitamin E can decrease platelet adherence to damaged artery walls, much like vitamin C. While helping the myocardium (heart muscle) use oxygen more efficiently, vitamin E can even lift HDL cholesterol levels. Dosage: Take up to 800 I.U. daily (see Chapter Six).
- Essential fatty acid deficiency and prostaglandin imbalance are closely linked to high blood pressure, high cholesterol levels, and spasms of the coronary arteries. Another related condition is clot formation, which causes heart attacks and strokes. Dosage: Take 1 or 2 tablespoons a day of unrefined flaxseed oil. Choose other dietary oils and fats wisely.
- Silicon deficiency weakens collagen tissues in arterial walls and renders the arteries susceptible to structural damage. Treatment: Use a multiple vitamin formula that has up to 2 milligrams of silicon, or use rice bran syrup.
- A magnesium deficiency, whether dietary or the result of chronic use of "soft" water, has been linked with cardiovascular disease. Alcohol and most diuretics also induce magnesium loss. Capable of preventing arrhythmias, magnesium has been shown to cut platelet aggregation and avert spasm of the coronary arteries. It also improves the metabolic efficiency of the myocardium and reduces angina when other measures fail. Dosage: Take up to 800 milligrams of magnesium a day.
- Chromium is lost in the refining of grains. Dietary supplements of high-chromium brewer's yeast, if tolerated, have been shown to lower serum cholesterol and triglyceride levels and lift HDL levels. Chromium also boosts glucose tolerance, another important aspect of artery protection. Dosage: Take 200 micrograms of chromium a day, up to 1,000 micrograms, as part of a cholesterol-lowering regimen.
- Selenium is another key element in preventing coronary heart disease. It's a part of the body's antioxidant arsenal. Treatment: Eat whole foods and take up to 250 micrograms a day.
- A copper deficiency causes higher serum cholesterol levels along with the lesions similar to those seen in coronary artery disease. Copper deficiency leads to increased free radical pathology. Dosage: Take up to 3 milligrams of copper a day or 4 milligrams if you suffer from high cholesterol or coronary artery disease. Copper should be taken in conjunction with zinc. However, if you take supplemental zinc that is more than fifteen times the milligram amount of your supplemental copper, you probably need to raise your copper dose. *Warning: Too much zinc can also create or aggravate a copper deficit.*

Some multiple vitamin/mineral preparations are incomplete and contribute to copper deficiency because they contain zinc and leave out copper. If you use a separate copper supplement, take it at least eight hours before or after the zinc dosage. *Warning: Too much copper contributes to increased susceptibility to free radical pathology.*

- Coenzyme Q-10, a well-known cardiac nutrient, is used to treat angina, congestive heart failure, and hypertension. It is also an antioxidant, considered by some more potent than vitamin E. Dosage: Take 10 to 30 milligrams two or three times a day.
- Carnitine can lower both triglyceride and total cholesterol levels. It can also decrease angina and blood pressure, while directly increasing the metabolic efficiency of the liver and the heart. Thus, it is very useful for treating congestive heart failure. Dosage: Take up to 750 milligrams of DL carnitine twice a day.
- Lysine and proline are amino acids involved in the structural repair of damaged collagen in arteriosclerotic blood vessels. Dosage: Take up to 500 milligrams once or twice a day.
- Cysteine/N-acetylcysteine, a potent sulfhydryl antioxidant, is a heavy metal scavenger and liver protector. It is sometimes used to improve cholesterol ratios and to help lessen the risk of coronary artery disease. Take up to 250 milligrams three or four times a day.
- You may find many of the above cardioprotective agents formulated together: Heart Life and Heart Life Plus by Life Services of Neptune, New Jersey; Q-10 Plus by Thorne Research of Sandpoint, Idaho; and Angioguard, by NF Formulas of Wilsonville, Oregon. Other formulas are available in health food stores or use a good multiple vitamin/mineral formula and add the desired extra items. When a combined nutrient approach is used, it may not be necessary to use the higher dose levels recommended above.
- If you are an adult male or a nonmenstruating adult female and are not anemic, make certain your nutritional supplements are iron-free.

HERBAL REMEDIES

Most of the following herbs have multiple functions for treating and preventing cardiovascular diseases and arteriosclerosis. (See "Herbs and Their Medicinal Uses.")

- Hawthorn berry, ginkgo biloba, and catechin all protect arterial walls. Take solid hawthorn berry extract (¼ to ½ teaspoon twice a day), from Scientific Botanicals, Seattle; ginkgo (40 milligrams twice a day); and catechin from gambir from Thorne Research of Sandpoint, Idaho (400 milligrams twice a day).
- Green tea, unroasted, is also high in catechin, which helps maintain connective tissues in arteries and elsewhere. If you do not have high blood pressure and are not caffeine sensitive, the benefits may offset the small amount of caffeine. Drink up to 2 cups a day.
- Take garlic (one 500-milligram capsule or tablet three times a day).
- Gugulipid, an extract from the Indian mukul myrrh tree, used for centuries by Ayurvedic physicians, has excellent cholesterol-lowering properties. One source, combined with vitamin C, niacin, and chromium, is Guguplus, sold by Enzymatic Therapy of Green Bay. Dosage: Take one capsule three times a day.

OTHER THERAPIES

- Aerobic exercise, thirty minutes three times a week or a thirty- to forty-five-minute daily walk, can help prevent arteriosclerosis and even reverse it. It also has many other benefits. The duration and intensity of exercise sessions need to be gauged by individual tolerance. If you have heart disease or are over the age of fifty and do not exercise regularly, consult your doctor for guidance.
- Stress management measures, including skilled relaxation exercises, are as vital to a treatment and prevention program as physical exercise.
- Chelation therapy, a series of intravenous administrations of EDTA (ethylenediamenetetraacetic acid) combined with several nutrients, has been shown to reverse arteriosclerosis blockages. It has been used successfully in cases of severely blocked coronary arteries that would have required bypass surgery. Extreme angina (chest pain), leg cramps, and even threatening gangrene have also been successfully treated with EDTA. It is very safe when administered according to the protocol established by the American Board of Chelation Therapy in Chicago, Illinois, and the American College of Advancement in Medicine in Laguna Hills, California. Some physicians recommend it not only for treatment, but also as a preventive measure.

Arthritis

Painful, swollen, or stiff joints, caused by an underlying condition of degeneration or inflammation. There are two primary types of arthritis: osteoarthritis and rheumatoid arthritis. Osteoarthritis, also known as degenerative joint disease, is caused by the wear and tear of old age, overuse, or injury. Rheumatoid arthritis is an autoimmune inflammatory condition in which one's own antibodies attack the joints, initiating bone deterioration.

Related or Underlying Causes

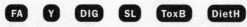

Although osteoarthritis and rheumatoid arthritis are two distinct diseases, some underlying causes, predisposing factors, and treatment modalities apply to both conditions. By identifying and treating these causes and related disorders, joint inflammation can be limited or halted.

Agents and approaches listed for rheumatoid arthritis usually apply to other autoimmune types of joint problems as well, such as psoriatic arthritis.

With any arthritic condition, be sure to test for food allergies and leaky gut syndrome. Look especially for sensitivity to vegetables in the nightshade family (tomato, potato, green or other peppers, eggplant, and tobacco). Parasites may also be another factor to be ruled out (see PARASITES).

Since free radicals are involved in any form of arthritis, look for antioxidant nutrient deficiency.

Treatment and Preventive Measures

CONVENTIONAL MEDICAL TREATMENT

- Steroids such as prednisone.
- Nonsteroidal anti-inflammatory drugs—aspirin, Tolectin, Naprosyn, Motrin/ibuprofen, Indocin, and Feldene—are prescribed. Although they often do a good job of relieving arthritis, they can cause gastrointestinal irritation, inflammation and ulcers, and kidney and other complications. They can also accelerate cartilage deterioration in your joints. Use these medications only when needed.

   If it is necessary for you to take these drugs, protect your intestinal mucosa with deglycerrhizinated licorice root extract (DGL, up to 1,000 milligrams a day). Experiment with safe and effective alternatives so that you can lower the dosages or live without these drugs.

DIETARY RECOMMENDATIONS

- Follow a whole-foods diet that minimizes free radicals and trans-fatty acids. Excess weight exacerbates arthritic symptoms.
- Eat plenty of fresh blueberries and cherries, as they provide beneficial flavonoid molecules.
- A three-month diet that eliminates nightshades may be especially helpful in reducing symptoms.
- A three-week allergy elimination diet that omits any repetitively eaten foods may bring relief.

DETOXIFICATION PROGRAM

- Begin first with a bowel cleansing, then a liver flush. Try a periodic fast for one or more days, as well as daily dry skin brushing.

NUTRITIONAL SUPPLEMENTS

Make sure your routine includes the nutrients and other substances involved in cartilage synthesis and maintenance and antioxidant protection:

- Take supplemental beta-carotene (15,000 to 25,000 I.U. daily), along with vitamins E (400 to 800 I.U. daily), C (2,000 to 3,000 milligrams a day), B complex (25 to 100 milligrams a day), and especially B-6 (50 to 100 milligrams a day. See precautions).
- Also add the following minerals to your daily program: zinc (30 milligrams), selenium (200 micrograms), copper (2 to 3 milligrams), and manganese (up to 100 milligrams for six to twelve months, then 20 milligrams a day). Consult your doctor.
- Methionine (250 milligrams three times a day) nourishes the cartilage and acts as a natural anti-inflammatory.
- Glucosamine sulfate (500 to 1,000 milligrams three times a day) is an actual building block of the cartilage that lines the bone surfaces of joints. More easily absorbed than chondroitin sulfate, this agent stimulates the synthesis of new cartilage and actually inhibits deterioration.
- Shark cartilage capsules (up to 2,200 milligrams three times a day) have also been effective in providing arthritis relief. They are available from Allergy Research/Nutricology of San Leandro, California.
- Try niacinamide (up to 1,000 milligrams three times a day) or the timed-release form (800 milligrams twice a day) (available from Willner Chemists, New York) for effective symptomatic relief of osteoarthritis, especially involving the knees. *Warning: Such high doses can temporarily irritate the liver, so medical supervision is advised.*
- Essential fatty acids can bring relief, particularly in rheumatoid arthritis, but try them for any arthritic condition. Take EPA fish oil (up to 1,000 milligrams three times a day) along with borage oil capsules (two or three times a day, providing an approximate daily dose of 500 milligrams gamma linolenic acid).
- SOD/CAT, wheat sprout–derived enzymes (six tablets taken together every morning at least thirty minutes before breakfast, tapering the dose to three tablets a day after you see results), are free radical fighters and anti-inflammatory agents. Be patient. It may be weeks before you see any results. SOD/CAT is available from BioMed Foods of Honolulu.

HERBAL REMEDIES

- Hawthorn berry (¼ to ½ teaspoon of the solid extract two to three times a day), sold by Scientific Botanicals of Seattle, is extremely useful for maintaining cartilage health.
- Take bilberries (up to 80 milligrams three times a day in capsule form).
- Boswella, an Ayurvedic herb, is used successfully for rheumatoid arthritis (150 milligrams three times a day).
- Try turmeric, yucca, and devil's claw (in combination formulas, three to four capsules as needed, three times a day). Herbal Bromelain from Eclectic Institute, Sandy, Oregon, contains these traditional arthritis herbs plus black cohosh, ginger, celery, onion, and feverfew.
- Cayenne ointment rubbed into the skin of the affected area (up to three or four times a day) increases circulation to the joint and may enhance the outcome of other treatments. Available as Cayenne Ointment from Herbal Technology/Khalsa Health Center of Seattle.
- Sea cucumber extract may provide safe and efficient relief for both osteo and rheumatoid arthritis. (Available from SeaCare, Dept. S-11, P.O. Box 8033, Country Road 687, Hartford, MI 49057, (616) 621-2040.)

OTHER THERAPIES

- DHEA (dehydroepiandrosterone) supplementation is often helpful for autoimmune arthritis (see Chapter Eleven).
- Try hydrotherapy, alternating hot and cold packs on the affected area, or just use cold packs.
- Acupuncture may be effective.
- Shortwave diathermy. (Consult a naturopathic physician.)
- Bee venom injections can be extremely useful for both short- and long-term relief for osteo and rheumatoid arthritis.
- Do appropriate exercise—swimming, isometrics, and other forms of activity that do not cause direct pounding or contribute to deterioration of the joints.
- Treat structural abnormalities (leg length discrepancy, postural problems, etc.) with an appropriate health care professional, such as an osteopath, chiropractor, podiatrist, or bodyworker.

Asthma

Inflammation and swelling of the bronchioles in the lungs, causing partial airway obstruction, may produce wheezing and shortness of breath. Asthma is usually aggravated by respiratory infections. It sometimes becomes apparent only after exertion. Can be life threatening.

Related or Underlying Causes

Chronic sinus infections may also be at play (see SINUS INFECTIONS). Other contributors are allergies to inhalants (see HAY FEVER), and parasites (see PARASITES).

Treatment and Preventive Measures

CONVENTIONAL MEDICAL TREATMENT

- For an acute asthma attack, consult your physician. Common treatments include expectorants, theophylline, antihistamines, inhalers, ephedrine, and bronchodilators. If breathing is not becoming easier or is growing increasingly difficult despite your efforts, emergency medical intervention is indicated.

DIETARY RECOMMENDATIONS

- Avoid sulfites, an asthma-aggravating agent, and other food additives and preservatives, found in processed fruits and vegetables.

NUTRITIONAL SUPPLEMENTS

- Take magnesium (up to 800 milligrams daily), vitamin C (3 to 4 grams a day), vitamin E (400 I.U. daily), beta-carotene (up to 100,000 I.U. daily under medical supervision), selenium (250 micrograms a day), and vitamin B-6 (up to 100 milligrams a day). Some individuals have responded to vitamin D (400 to 800 I.U. daily), vitamin A (25,000 to 50,000 I.U. daily) and calcium (1,000 to 1,500 milligrams daily). (See Chapter Six for precautions.)
- Take molybdenum (500 micrograms twice a day), as a molybdenum deficiency may contribute to sulfite sensitivity. Intravenous injections of molybdenum are sometimes more effective. If you use molybdenum, also take copper (2 to 4 milligrams a day), but *do not* take at the same time as the molybdenum.
- Take hydrochloric acid with pepsin as directed.

INJECTABLE SUPPLEMENTS

- According to the work of Jonathan V. Wright, M.D., of Kent, Washington, regular intramuscular injections of B-12 have been extremely beneficial in many children and sometimes effective in adults. Administer 1,000 micrograms daily until control is achieved. Continue injections weekly or biweekly, according to need. When using B-12 shots daily, add injectable folic acid (up to 5 milligrams) to supplement the B-12 once or twice a week initially. When the shots are administered once a week or less frequently, add the folic acid each time.
- A multiple nutrient intravenous injection of magnesium, along with calcium, vitamins C, B complex, B-6, B-12, and B-5, can relieve an acute asthma attack in minutes (see this formula under CHRONIC FATIGUE SYNDROME).

HERBAL REMEDIES

- Take quercetin (1,000 to 2,000 milligrams a day), a potent anti-inflammatory herb.
- Licorice root extract (¼ teaspoon two or three times a day) increases the half-life of your own cortisone and thereafter indirectly exerts an anti-inflammatory action. (See Chapter Nineteen for precautions.)
- Ephedra (ma huang) (3 cups of tea a day) is useful for providing relief. Or use Ephedra Plus (one or two capsules two or three times a day), a combination herbal formula containing ephedra, ginger, licorice root, marshmallow root, and other synergistic herbs, available from PhytoPharmica, Green Bay, Wisconsin. *Warning: Too much ephedra can increase your heart rate and be too stimulating. Do not use if you have high blood pressure or heart disease.*
- Allerplex I, an anti-allergy herbal combination capsule (one to three capsules two to four times a day), can help diminish and control symptoms. Available from Herb Technology/Khalsa Health Center of Seattle.
- Try an herbal tincture of equal parts lobelia, cayenne, and skunk cabbage (1 teaspoon of the mixture followed by a glass of water every fifteen minutes until breathing improves). Most herb stores will have a similar formula or can mix it for you. *Warning: Too much lobelia can induce vomiting.*

Atherosclerosis

See ARTERIOSCLEROSIS.

Athlete's Foot

See FUNGUS.

Attention Deficit/ Hyperactivity Disorder

An inability to pay attention, concentrate, remember, think clearly, or learn effectively. Often associated with behavioral disturbances. Commonly referred to as hyperactivity disorder.

Related or Underlying Causes

Birth trauma and head injury can alter neurological organization. They can cause cranial bone impingement or locking of cranial joints, a structural problem that can affect learning and behavior. Insufficient or abnormal neurological organization may be a related cause, commonly a result of insufficient creeping and crawling due to the overuse of playpens, walkers, and similar devices. Diminished amounts of serotonin, a neurotransmitter in the brain, may cause hyperactivity due to inadequate vitamin B-6 or a vitamin B-6 dependency. Insufficient dietary tryptophan may also be linked. ADD may also be, in part, a manifestation in the child of marital discord or other dysfunction in the home.

Treatment and Preventive Measures

CONVENTIONAL MEDICAL TREATMENT
- Prescription medications such as methylphenidate (Ritalin) are commonly used, although dextroamphetamine, pemoline, and desipramine are also prescribed.
- Counseling and behavior modification are recommended when appropriate.

DIETARY RECOMMENDATIONS
- Avoid sugar, soft drinks, and all preservatives and additives. Salicylate-containing foods may need to be avoided. Identify and avoid allergy-triggering foods. Follow the diet recommended for hypoglycemia.

NUTRITIONAL SUPPLEMENTS
- Take calcium (300 to 800 milligrams a day) and magnesium (100 to 400 milligrams a day).
- For children five years and older: take B complex (10 to 25 milligrams a day), extra niacinamide (up to 200 milligrams a day), extra vitamin B-6 (up to 15 to 30 milligrams per kilogram of body weight for the 15 percent of children who are B-6 dependent), vitamin C (500 to 1,000 milligrams a day), calcium (300 to 800 milligrams a day, depending on the age and weight of the child), magnesium (100 to 400 milligrams a day, depending on the age and weight of the child), zinc (up to 5 milligrams a day), and iron (5 milligrams a day). Many of these nutrients can be found in a multiple vitamin/mineral. Check with your doctor that these doses are compatible with the child's weight and medical history.
- Amino acid supplementation, particularly those favorably affecting brain metabolism (phenylalanine, glutamine, 5-hydroxytryptophan) may also be helpful. A nutritionally oriented physician can test for deficiencies and/or recommend the appropriate amino acids and doses.

  Note: Although the doses above are generally considered safe for children over five years of age, it is strongly recommended that a physician or other qualified health professional be consulted. Some children may require higher doses than those given above, another reason for professional supervision.

HOMEOPATHIC REMEDIES
- A constitutional prescribed homeopathic remedy can bring dramatic results.

OTHER THERAPIES
- Neurological organization therapy (see Suggested Reading, page 426).

Back Pain

One of the most commonly reported ailments, back pain frequently occurs in the high and low back areas. It can also be located centrally or on either side of the spine. Back pain can range from mild to debilitating.

Related or Underlying Causes

Back pain can be caused by muscle spasm; underdeveloped or weak back or abdominal muscles; and ligament injury or ligaments that are too loose, allowing excessive mobility and instability of spinal vertebrae or the sacroiliac joint. It can also be related to bulging or damaged discs between the vertebrae, locked or misaligned cranial or atlas vertebrae, and temporomandibular joint (TMJ) syndrome in the jaw. Arthritis is another cause of back pain.

Also linked to back pain are: poor posture; improper back support while seated; inappropriate footwear, such as high heels; insufficient arch support; inadequate support from mattresses; lifting heavy objects improperly; discrepancies in leg lengths; and insufficient, excessive, or incorrect types of exercise. Nutritional deficiencies and constipation can also contribute to the condition.

Treatment and Preventive Measures

Read *Healing Back Pain* by John E. Sarno, M.D. Begin with stress management and skilled relaxation techniques, regardless of what other approaches you take.

DIETARY RECOMMENDATIONS
- Include adequate amounts of water and fiber-rich foods to maintain daily bowel evacuations.
- Implement measures to improve digestion and assimilation, if necessary.

NUTRITIONAL SUPPLEMENTS
- Maintain adequate daily supplemental levels of calcium (800 to 1,000 milligrams), magnesium (up to 800 milligrams), iodine (150 micrograms), and manganese (20 milligrams).

EXERCISE
- Practice strengthening or stretching exercises. Active exercise can help you feel more in control and enable you to manage better while preventing the recurrence of the problem.
- Establish a regular walking program.
- Consider starting a supervised, graduated weight-lifting or weight-training program for strengthening specific muscle groups.
- Take a yoga or tai chi class.
- Try a simple calisthenics program of sit-ups and push-ups. Do very slight, very gentle back arches while lying on your stomach. Two or three stretches can be useful, safe, and appropriate. Follow the regimen for ten minutes, perhaps three or more times a week.
- A physical therapist or other health professional can create an appropriate individualized program. This is especially important if your back problem is severe.

BODYWORK
- Try physical therapy and/or appropriate manipulative therapy such as osteopathy, chiropractic, or naprapathy. Consider cranial/sacral adjustments, which can help relieve acute back pain and contribute to prevention as well.
- Acupuncture is often very effective for back pain.
- Remedy leg length discrepancies either through a bodyworker or by using professionally prescribed shoe lifts.
- Investigate Feldenkrais and Alexander techniques or other movement therapies. Certified instructors can teach you how to move, hold, and understand your body. Over time, these techniques may lessen your need for continual bodywork.
- Back swing and gravity guidance devices allow you to hang in an upside-down position, using the force of gravity to keep your spine properly adjusted. *Warning: These devices are not appropriate for everyone, particularly those who have had retinal detachments or other conditions where increased pressure in the head is not advisable. Consult your doctor.* A slantboard has a similar effect on the spine, although the incline is less severe, which may be an advantage for some individuals.

OTHER THERAPIES
- Temporomandibular joint and bite dysfunction may be playing a role in back pain. See a qualified dentist.
- Sleep support: Be sure your bed provides excellent support. Water beds and soft mattresses are generally not advised. Consider the Swedish-made Dux, thought to be the Cadillac of beds. (Contact Dux Interiors of New York for a distributor in your area.)

Bad Breath

Socially offensive breath normally indiscernible to the individual.

Related or Underlying Causes

Check for gum and sinus infections (see PERIODONTAL DISEASE and SINUS INFECTION), poor dental hygiene, tooth problems, lung ailments, cancer, and cigarette smoking.

Treatment and Preventive Measures

Consult your doctor for proper treatment of gum and sinus infections.

DIETARY RECOMMENDATIONS
- Eat fiber-rich foods, especially fresh fruits and vegetables.
- Drink water (six to eight glasses a day) to enhance routes of elimination.
- Gargle and swallow plenty of green juice, or liquid chlorophyll, which cleanses the system and helps neutralize bad breath.
- For a breath freshener, chew on sprigs of parsley.

DETOXIFICATION PROGRAMS
If constipation or bowel toxicity is present, take an intestinal cleansing powder (1 or 2 teaspoons once or twice a day in 6 to 8 ounces of water, followed immediately by an additional 6 to 8 ounces of water).
- Dry brush your skin.

HERBAL REMEDIES
- Take chlorophyll-rich herbs in powder or tablet form, including wheat grass, barley grass, alfalfa, chlorella, or spirulina.

Bed-wetting

The involuntary escape of urine during sleep.

Related or Underlying Causes

Check for nerve compression affecting the bladder from a poorly aligned spinal column. A bladder infection or an illness such as measles or mumps may be linked. Emotional factors must also be considered.

Treatment and Preventive Measures

Structural problems may require chiropractic or osteopathic manipulation. Check for specific food allergies, such as dairy products. Restrict fluids before bedtime. No standard treatment is recommended for bed-wetting before age six.

Homeopathic remedies can be very effective. If self-prescribing is ineffective, consult a homeopathic physician.

Bladder Infection (Cystitis)

An infection, usually bacterial, in the bladder or urethra causing burning or pain while urinating, bloody urine, and frequent and urgent desire to urinate.

Related or Underlying Causes

  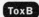

Intestinal bacteria frequently cause this condition in women. These bacteria are introduced into the vaginal and urethral areas, commonly during sexual intercourse and/or from soiled toilet tissue due to the close proximity of the anus and urethra. Pooling of urine in the bladder from resisting the urge to urinate can also be another contributing factor. For women, there may be other complicating causes, such as ill-fitting diaphragms or allergy to spermicidal jellies. Some women who have difficulty experiencing orgasms and suffer from pelvic congestion (blood engorgement and stagnation in the pelvic veins) may be predisposed to bladder infections. Postmenopausal women with atrophic vaginitis and atrophic urethral tissues may be more prone to bladder infections as well.

Emotional and nervous tension cause excessive muscle contraction. If this centers in the urethra, an outflow impairment will occur, causing a residual of urine that can stagnate and trigger an infection.

Also consider hypothyroidism (see HYPOTHYROIDISM).

Treatment and Preventive Measures

CONVENTIONAL MEDICAL TREATMENT
Nonpharmaceutical treatments can be used successfully in uncomplicated cases, thereby averting the need for antibiotics. However, pyelonephritis, an infection in the kidneys, is quite a serious threat to your health and can occur as a complication of a simple bladder infection. *Warning: If the natural treatments for bladder infections do not work within twenty-four to thirty-six hours, or if a fever or back pain develops along with your bladder symptoms, contact your doctor to begin treatment with antibiotics.*
- If a tight urethra is the cause, urologists commonly recommend urethra dilation. Some women are helped by this procedure. Others are helped only temporarily and need to investigate other causes for their recurrences.

DIETARY RECOMMENDATIONS

- Drink at least 2 quarts of water and other healthful fluids daily, mostly away from meals, as a cure and preventive.
- Acidify the urine to discourage bacterial growth. Drink several glasses of unsweetened cranberry juice (not fructose-sweetened cranberry drink) at the first sign of infection, and later reduce to a few cups a day for preventive purposes. Because the unsweetened juice is not very palatable, consider cranberry concentrate capsules (see "Herbal Remedies" below).

DETOXIFICATION PROGRAM

- If you suffer from bowel problems, take acidophilus/bifidus supplements (at least one capsule twice a day).
- An intestinal cleansing program may stop recurrent bladder infections.

NUTRITIONAL SUPPLEMENTS

- Vitamin C (1,000 milligrams per hour) can halt a bladder infection. Reduce dose or stop if loose bowel movements occur. If necessary, implement other measures.

HERBAL REMEDIES

- Uva ursi (250 milligrams containing 25 milligrams of arbutin, every few hours initially) is probably the preferred herb for this condition. Take capsules standardized to at least 10 percent arbutin content. As symptoms improve, use less frequently, changing doses to three to four times a day for up to seven days. Uva Ursi Plus by Scientific Botanicals of Seattle, Washington, is standardized at 18 percent arbutin content. *Warning: Do not use cranberry juice or acidify the urine while on uva ursi.*
- Combination herbal capsules, tinctures, or teas specifically formulated for bladder infections are available in most health food stores. A traditional one includes uva ursi, buchu, juniper berries, parsley, marshmallow root, lobelia, ginger, and goldenseal. Dosage: Take one to three capsules or twenty-five to thirty drops of tincture five to seven times a day when acute. Or drink 4 to 8 cups of the tea every day.
- Or try Arbu-Tone or Aqua-Flow (two or three capsules five to seven times a day), by Phyto-Pharmica/Enzymatic Therapy of Green Bay, Wisconsin, containing uva ursi, lespedeza boldo, hydrangea, vitamin B-6, magnesium, and potassium.

  Sometimes the antiseptic action of these herbal formulas is not sufficient. A stronger antibacterial-acting herb may be needed, such as goldenseal (two to four capsules four to six times a day for a week).
- If the above approaches do not quickly alleviate the burning of cystitis, use marshmallow root (1 or 2 cups of strongly brewed tea every hour, or three or four capsules of the powdered root every one to two hours until symptoms subside). Marshmallow root soothes the lining of the urinary tract, although it has no antibacterial effect. It can be discontinued soon after the burning ceases, but continue other remedies for at least a week.

HOMEOPATHIC REMEDIES

- Classical homeopathy may be curative for recurrent urinary infections. For acute episodes, take cantharis or apis mel (6c or 30c), specific remedies for symptoms of burning. As with all remedies, each has particular characteristics that are best matched to your individual overall symptoms and traits.
- Take combination homeopathic drops specific for bladder infections (ten to fifteen drops every hour until there is some improvement, then gradually reduce dose), available in health food stores.

OTHER THERAPIES

- Try hydrotherapy: take a sitz bath, which involves resting the pelvis and buttocks, not the legs, in a basin of water. Alternate immersions—hot (four to six minutes) and cold (one to two minutes). Sitz baths are particularly helpful if pelvic congestion is present.
- Do not hold urine. If you feel an urge to urinate, find a bathroom quickly.
- Try to make a habit of urinating soon after sexual intercourse. Also use cranberry capsules or the above kidney/bladder herbs prophylactically before and after intercourse.
- Acupuncture can be helpful, even curative.

Blood Pressure (High)

Also known as hypertension, high blood pressure is a condition in which the muscles in the walls of the arteries constrict, causing the heart to pump harder or in which arteries have lost their elasticity due to arteriosclerosis. Consistent blood pressure readings higher than 140/90 indicate the existence of this condition. High blood pressure may be associated with headaches, lightheadedness, ringing in the ears, bloody noses, and other related phenomena. Or no obvious symptoms may be present at all.

Related or Underlying Causes

Key factors include excess weight, a sedentary lifestyle, dietary hazards, nutritional deficiencies, and poorly managed stress. Heavy metal accumulation, especially lead or cadmium, is a common cause. Hypothyroidism can sometimes cause hypertension (see HYPOTHYROIDISM). Also, check with your doctor for the possibility of arteriosclerosis and renal artery stenosis (closing of the major artery to the kidney). Food allergies can also be a factor.

Treatment and Preventive Measures

CONVENTIONAL MEDICAL TREATMENT

- If your high blood pressure is not treated effectively, you may be more susceptible to heart attack, stroke, and congestive heart failure. Consult your doctor if lifestyle and other self-care approaches are not effective in normalizing blood pressure within a reasonable time frame. If blood pressure elevation is extreme (about 200/110), see your doctor immediately.

DIETARY RECOMMENDATIONS

- Avoid the following dietary hazards: caffeine, too much meat or sugar, and alcohol. Salt restriction will help 30 percent of those with high blood pressure, but the condition of the remaining 70 percent will not be affected.
- Dietary deficiencies may be fueling the problem as well. Eat foods rich in potassium, including legumes, fresh vegetables, vegetable soups, broths, and fresh vegetable juices. Eat potassium-rich fruits, such as bananas, apricots, peaches, and prunes.
- If your diet is high in meat and poultry, try switching to a predominantly vegetarian diet. Identify and avoid allergy-triggering foods. Eat fresh garlic regularly.

DETOXIFICATION PROGRAMS

- Do the Liver Flush and Purifying Diet and go on periodic fasts. Identify accumulation of lead, cadmium, or other heavy metals. Treat appropriately.

NUTRITIONAL SUPPLEMENTS

- Magnesium (up to 500 milligrams twice a day), calcium (up to 500 milligrams twice a day), unrefined flaxseed oil (2 teaspoons a day or three to six capsules a day), borage oil (three capsules a day), and choline (up to 1,000 milligrams three to four times a day).
- To lower blood pressure, take carnitine (up to 1,000 milligrams three to four times a day) and coenzyme Q-10 (up to 30 milligrams three times a day).

  Note: You may only need one or two of the nutritional supplements listed above to improve your condition. Consult your nutritionist or physician.

HERBAL REMEDIES

- Garlic supplements (freeze-dried, oil, or aged) can help lower blood pressure (use one or two capsules or tablets three times a day). Garlic may work more effectively combined with other ingredients. Take HYBP (hibiscus flower, strawberry leaf, garlic, and onion: one to three capsules up to three times a day) or, for more severe hypertension, take VHYBP (fumitory, artichoke, persian garlic, onion, strawberry leaf, raspberry leaf, garlic, citrus peel, chicory, pear, olive leaf, fox geranium, and red grape leaf: one to three capsules up to three times a day). Both items are available from Ancient Formulas, Inc., of Wichita, Kansas, (800) 543-3026.
- Hawthorn berry extract (¼ to ½ teaspoon three times a day) may be helpful. Available from Scientific Botanicals of Seattle.

OTHER THERAPIES

- Avoid cigarette smoking.
- Lose weight if you are too heavy (see OVERWEIGHT).
- Begin a regular exercise program.
- Implement stress management techniques and practice skilled relaxation exercises regularly.

Boils

See ABSCESS.

Breast Cysts, Lumps, and Other Breast Ailments

See FIBROCYSTIC BREASTS.

Bronchitis

An infection, usually bacterial, in the bronchi (the air passages of the lungs) that produces cough, phlegm, chest pain, fever, and malaise.

Related or Underlying Causes

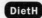

Obesity, cigarette smoking, and secondhand smoke are often linked to bronchitis. For a discussion of predisposing factors, see COLDS, COUGHS, FLU, SORE THROATS.

Treatment and Preventive Measures

CONVENTIONAL MEDICAL TREATMENT

- Contact your doctor if a chest cold does not begin to lessen in a week or if it is associated with severe coughing, persistent fever, or malaise. Antibiotics may be needed. (However, a professionally prescribed homeopathic remedy will often bring quicker relief.)
- Cough suppressant medication is indicated if frequent coughing interrupts sleep and causes chest pain. Excessive coughing can "throw out" a sensitive back, disrupt a recent surgical repair, or impair you in other significant ways. However, coughing serves an important purpose by eliminating the by-products of infection—dead white cells, bacteria, mucus, and other irritants. Use cough suppressants only when necessary.

NUTRITIONAL SUPPLEMENTS

- N-acetylcysteine is a mucus-thinning and immune-enhancing agent used to treat and prevent bronchitis. Take 200 to 500 milligrams up to five times a day for two to three days for acute treatment, then reduce dosage to two to three times a day until the bout is over. Continue this dosage for at least three months if bronchitis is chronic and recurrent to see if any improvement is achieved. During prolonged use, supplement with zinc (15 to 30 milligrams daily) and copper (1 to 2 milligrams daily).

HERBAL REMEDIES

- Herbs such as goldenseal, echinacea, garlic, myrrh, and bee propolis are useful for bronchitis because of their antibacterial and immune-enhancing effects. Take several capsules of one or more of these agents four to five times a day or use combination antibacterial herbal formulas such as OptiBiotic from Eclectic Institute of Sandy, Oregon (two capsules four times a day), or Isatis Gold from Health Concerns of Oakland, California (three tablets every two hours while awake).

    In addition to anti-infection herbs, consider using specific lung and cough herbal combination formulas such as cough and bronchial syrup from NF Formulas of Wilsonville, Oregon. See Chapter Nineteen.
- Bromelain (250 to 500 milligrams three times a day away from meals) may enhance the effect of antibiotics—and presumably herbs—and has an antibiotic as well as anti-inflammatory properties. It also thins mucus and may be useful to supplement other prescribed treatments.
- Gingerroot tea can be helpful and soothing to lungs. Grate 2 or 3 tablespoons of fresh gingerroot. Let it steep in 1½ to 2 cups of water for 15 to 20 minutes. Strain and add a little honey and lemon juice to the tea. Drink several cups daily.

HOMEOPATHIC REMEDIES

- Combination homeopathic preparations specific for bronchitis are available in some health food stores and from homeopathic distributors. Individualizing a remedy may bring the best results.

OTHER THERAPIES

- A castor oil pack or ginger compress can bring relief to the chest.
- Diathermy/magnatherm (ultrasoundlike treatments to the chest) can hasten healing. Contact a naturopathic physician for this therapy.
- A humidifier may provide some comfort.
- Avoid smoking and exposure to secondhand smoke.
- Rest is vital to recovery.

Bruises

Vivid discolorations caused by an accumulation of blood under the skin brought on by the breakage or leaking of small blood vessels.

Related or Underlying Causes

- When bruises are not caused by obvious trauma, consider nutritional deficiencies, such as inadequate vitamin C, bioflavonoids, and rutin. These produce fragile capillaries. Inadequate vitamin K also causes a bleeding tendency. Low vitamin K may be the result of insufficient dark, leafy greens in the diet and/or inadequate acidophilus/bifidus organisms in the intestines due to antibiotic use or yeast overgrowth. Liver and blood diseases can also produce a tendency to bruising and bleeding.

Treatment and Preventive Measures

DIETARY RECOMMENDATIONS

- Eat dark, leafy greens at least four or five days a week (kale, collard, chard, beet, watercress, spinach, turnip, mustard, etc.). Juice the greens.

NUTRITIONAL SUPPLEMENTS

- Vitamin C (1,000 milligrams two or three times a day) and a citrus bioflavonoid complex (1,000 milligrams with rutin twice a day) or quercetin (up to 500 milligrams three times a day). More absorbable forms of bioflavonoids, such as hesperidin, hesperidin methyl chalcone, naringin, grape skin extract, and winter cherry extract may be preferable (FlavoPlex-C by Interplexus of Kent, Washington, two to three capsules once a day).
- Lactobacillus acidophilus and bifidus supplements (at least one capsule of a quality brand twice a day).
- Chlorophyll supplements: Take chlorolipids (one or two capsules two or three times a day) from Biotherapeutics/Enzymatic Therapy of Green Bay, Wisconsin.
- If bruising persists, see a physician.

Burns

The severity of burns can vary. First-degree burns appear red or pink, and sometimes swollen. A minor burn or a painful sunburn is an example. Second-degree burns are a little worse, characterized by the presence of blisters. Third-degree burns are the most serious, appearing deep-red, brown to black, sometimes with underflesh exposed. They require immediate medical help and their discussion is largely omitted from this text.

Treatment and Preventive Measures

For first- and second-degree burns, the best course of action is immediate immersion in cold or icy water to minimize any further thermal injury. Do not break the blisters, but should they break, treat them as any open sore. The goal is to avoid infection. Keep the open blister area clean, washing it gently with soapy water periodically and covering it with a non-stick gauze dressing until healing has begun.

NUTRITIONAL SUPPLEMENTS

For first- or second-degree burns involving more than just a small area, the following may be helpful:

- Take vitamin A (50,000 to 100,000 I.U. daily) for no longer than a week, then 25,000 I.U. daily. Also, take vitamin C (5,000 to 10,000 milligrams a day) initially, along with vitamin E (400 to 800 I.U. daily) and zinc (30 milligrams).

HERBAL REMEDIES

EXTERNAL

- Aloe vera has wonderful antibacterial and healing properties for both first- and second-degree burns. Squeeze the gel straight from the leaf of the plant or purchase the gel. Keep the gel or aloe leaf refrigerated, as the cold applications are more soothing when the burn is still new.
- Cool applications of calendula or chamomile tea can be soothing. Use as many times a day as needed.
- Calendula ointment or a combination calendula/goldenseal/bee propolis ointment can be applied to open blisters.
- Vitamin E spray (Key E Spray by Carlson's Laboratories of Arlington Heights, Illinois) or oil can be applied to acute burns. Store it in the refrigerator. However, for open blisters, wait until skin healing has begun. Topical vitamin E has been known to prevent or minimize scar contractures from serious burns.

INTERNAL

- If infection prevention is needed, use an antibacterial formula (see Chapter Nineteen).

HOMEOPATHIC REMEDIES

- For acute pain from burns, take cantharis as directed if blisters appear.
- Take urtica urens as directed if skin is just red.

Note: Medical attention is recommended for any significant burn.

Bursitis

A common, painful inflammation that occurs in the bursa sac that surrounds major joints, such as the shoulder or hip, sometimes associated with calcium deposits on the adjacent tendon.

Related or Underlying Causes

Bursitis is caused by trauma, overuse, an overly alkaline or acidic diet, systemic toxicity, and possibly nutritional deficiencies.

Treatment and Preventive Measures

DIETARY RECOMMENDATIONS

- If your diet is excessively acidic or alkaline, make the appropriate adjustments (see Chapter Four).

DETOXIFICATION PROGRAMS

- Follow the Liver Flush and Purifying Diet or fast for up to one week.

NUTRITIONAL SUPPLEMENTS

- Take calcium (up to 400 milligrams a day) and chelated magnesium (up to 800 milligrams a day).
- Daily vitamin B-12 intramuscular injections for up to two weeks (then less often) are effective for some sufferers (see ASTHMA).

HERBAL REMEDIES

- Bromelain and turmeric (two or three capsules up to four times a day spaced between meals) may be helpful as anti-inflammatories (available from Scientific Botanicals of Seattle).

OTHER THERAPIES

- Auricular therapy (ear acupuncture) may be useful.
- Try acupressure or shiatsu.
- Try hydrotherapy: alternating hot and cold packs or just cold packs.
- Bee venom injections can also be effective.

Cancer

A general term referring to the uncontrolled growth of cells that, if not arrested, can invade adjacent structures and metastasize (spread) to distant sites. It compromises the functioning of vital organs and steals the body's nutrients and vital energy, often resulting in death.

The four major types of cancer are carcinomas (cancer of the skin, glands, and organs), sarcomas (cancer of the bones, tissues, and muscles), and lymphoma and leukemia (cancer of the bone marrow/blood/lymphatic system). Cancer is on the rise: it is currently estimated that in the United States one person in three will develop cancer, and one will die of it every sixty seconds.

Related or Underlying Causes

   DietH   ND   CHEM   B/M

The causes of cancer are many. While alcohol abuse accounts for a scant 3 percent of cancer cases, tobacco use contributes to 30 percent of the total number of cases. Tobacco use is a major factor in cancer cell growth. A person who smokes two or more packs a day is twenty to twenty-five times more susceptible to lung cancer than is a nonsmoker. Passive, or secondary, smoke may also contribute. However, poor dietary habits, with a 35 percent share, is the most significant cause.

Some of the leading dietary causes that promote cancer are excessive fat (particularly rancid, oxidized fat and altered vegetable oils), insufficient fiber intake, several food additives, excessive sugar intake, and inadequate antioxidant and immune system nutrients.

The underlying environmental causes are numerous carcinogenic agents in the air, food, and water, primarily industrial and agricultural chemicals; excessive ultraviolet radiation, such as overexposure to sun and sunlamps; and iatrogenic causes, such as excessive X rays, excessive estrogens, and chemotherapeutic and other drugs. Certain electromagnetic frequencies have also been linked to cancer, especially those emitted by high-tension power lines, unshielded video and computer display terminals, and possibly electric blankets and electric razors.

Psychological, emotional, and behavioral factors have been related to cancer. Researchers have identified a "cancer personality," characterized by passivity, obedience, martyrdom, and depression. Long, unresolved bitterness may also apply. Chronic, poorly managed stress and tension in themselves may be important factors, as they suppress the immune system by altering adrenal hormone balance.

WARNING SIGNS OF CANCER

Know the warning signs that might indicate cancer: unusual persistent thickening or lumps, bloody stools, change in bowel or bladder habits, bloody urine, unexplained weight loss, unexplained appetite reduction, unexplained fatigue, sores that do not heal, obvious change in a mole or wart, persistent cough or hoarseness, difficulty swallowing or persistent indigestion, and unusual vaginal bleeding. Consult your doctor if any of these signs occur. Ask your doctor for the regular early detection cancer-screening tests recommended for your age and sex.

Treatment and Preventive Measures

CONVENTIONAL MEDICAL TREATMENT

If you have been diagnosed with cancer, you are probably experiencing intense fear and foreboding. Your first treatment is particularly crucial to the outcome. Your initial response may be to give up your power and autonomy to an authoritative white-coated figure who confidently prescribes a course of treatment.

The problem here is that conventional cancer treatments may kill you before your cancer does. Don't allow yourself to be rushed into treatment. Resist the pressure to proceed with your doctor's recommendations until you've had a chance to sit back and look at the situation from a calmer perspective, even if it takes up to three to four weeks to get over your initial shock. It's a rare cancer that will grow significantly worse in a month. Tumors are years in the making.

Insist that your doctor explain the diagnosis and treatments in very plain language. Also, enlist a friend or family member to act as your advocate in the discussion. Be sure to bring a list of questions to ask. Ask your doctor if you can tape the visit so you can listen to the information again at home, where you can concentrate better.

Believing and having confidence in your doctor is not enough. You must also believe in the recommended treatment and feel positive about it. Ask your doctor the precise success rate of the treatment with other patients with the same cancer at the same stage. Find out about the quality of patients' lives during and after treatments. Always get a second or third opinion. You may want to obtain the "Coping with Cancer" videotape, which reviews common questions about cancer, treatments, lifestyles, quality of life during therapy, and the role of the immune system. Send $19.95 to Video Tape, Northwest Oncology Foundation, P.O. Box 3726, Bellevue, Washington 98009.

To improve your treatment success rate, also have your doctor check for low thyroid function (see HYPOTHYROIDISM) and adrenal dysfunction. This adrenal condition, particularly low levels of DHEA (dehydroepiandrosterone), is common among cancer patients. Supplemental DHEA can significantly boost immune function (see Chapter Eleven).

DIETARY RECOMMENDATIONS

Nutritional support is essential to feed your immune system and give you the strength to better tolerate cancer treatments.

- Eating a whole-foods diet with abundant fresh vegetables and fruit will provide important vitamins, minerals, and fiber. Such foods also provide specific cancer-fighting biochemicals, called phytochemicals. Allhyl sulfides from garlic, onions, leeks, and chives; dithiolthiones from broccoli; and isothiocyanates from cabbage, cauliflower, kale, brussels sprouts, collards, and other cruciferous vegetables trigger the formulation of glutathione S-transferase, an important enzyme involved in protecting a cell's DNA (genetic material) from carcinogens. Isoflavones from soybeans and other legumes block estrogen stimulation of cells, which may reduce the risk of breast and ovarian cancer. Indoles from cruciferous vegetables also render estrogen less effective. Ellagic acid from grapes, limonene from citrus fruits, and caffeic acid from many fruits all act as anticarcinogens.
- Limit dietary hazards such as sugar; common, refined, polyunsaturated, and partially hydrogenated oils; and excess fat.
- Avoid fried foods; nitrates, as found in cold cuts and cured meats; peanuts and peanut butters that are not certified as free of aflatoxin; smoked foods; and charcoaled or charred meats.
- See the discussion in Chapter Four concerning macrobiotics and raw foods, which have been used for the prevention and nutritional treatment of cancer.
- Limit or omit alcoholic beverages.
- Avoid overeating.
- Take a fiber supplement if dietary adjustments do not optimize your bowel transit and retention times. Flaxseed powder (1 tablespoon once or twice a day) has particular preventive value for breast and bowel cancers.
- Assure that your digestion and assimilation functions are adequate.

DETOXIFICATION PROGRAMS

- Liver flush, bowel cleansing regimens, and fasting diminish toxicity and are powerful health maintenance measures. *Warning: You must avoid those cleansing techniques that cause excessive weight loss if you cannot afford to lose weight.*

NUTRITIONAL SUPPLEMENTS

The following nutrients have proven cancer-fighting properties:

- Take extra antioxidants: vitamin C (3,000 to 10,000 milligrams a day); vitamin A, preferably mixed carotenes (50,000 to 75,000 I.U. daily); vitamin E (up to 800 I.U. daily); N-acetylcysteine (500 milligrams one to three times a day); and flaxseed oil (1 or 2 teaspoons a day). See Chapter Six for precautions.
- Take a high-potency vitamin/mineral formula (without iron, unless there is anemia, as discussed in Chapter Six). If it does not contain between 10,000 and 15,000 I.U. of vitamin A, supplement this total with extra vitamin A.
- Free-form amino acid supplements (at least 3½ grams a day) are also useful when your appetite is poor or your weight is low, when your immune competence is compromised, or when protein adequacy is questionable. Try Aminoplex from Tyson and Associates of Hawthorne, California.

HERBAL REMEDIES

- Take immune-supporting herbal combinations, such as Echimmune by NF Formulas of Wilsonville, Oregon (one or two capsules three times a day), which contains echinacea, licorice root (see precautions, astragalus, ligustrum, and shiitake mushroom. Other immune-enhancing formulas are listed in Chapter Nineteen.

OTHER THERAPIES

- Seek psychological and emotional support. The will to live is paramount. Thus, giving yourself permission to ask for and take advantage of the proper emotional support is absolutely vital.
- Avoid isolation by seeking the support of appropriate loved ones and friends. Tell them up front what you do and do not need from them.
- Join a support group. Studies document that cancer patients involved in support groups significantly outlive others with identical cancers who are not active in support groups.
- Psychological counseling can be invaluable in helping you get in touch with your true feelings and in enhancing your ability to communicate them. These measures can strengthen your immune function.
- Spiritual counseling can do wonders for helping you maintain your fighting spirit and the will to live. It can also help you learn to forgive.
- Nurture yourself. Don't let the demands and stresses of life prevent you from taking proper care of yourself in the ways you need.
- Practice stress-reduction techniques, such as meditation and visualization.
- Find something to laugh about every day. Laughter is an effective stress reducer and powerful immune enhancer.
- Exercise regularly. It enhances well-being and immune function.
- Live by the laws of nature, as discussed in Chapter Sixteen.

OTHER PREVENTIVE MEASURES

- Minimize exposure to environmental chemicals in the home and workplace. Install a good water purification system. Take proper precautions when exposure is unavoidable.
- Avoid unnecessary X rays.
- Take estrogens only as long as necessary, or find alternatives (see MENOPAUSE).

Carpal Tunnel Syndrome

A swelling or thickening of the ligament that joins the two forearm bones at the wrist, causing pressure on the median nerve. This results in tingling, numbness, weakness, and pain in the wrist and hand.

Related or Underlying Causes

Overuse and injury of the hands and forearms are the most common contributing factors. Improper ergonomics, such as imbalanced chair and table height, can cause intense strain on the wrists.

Vitamin B-6 deficiency is another common cause. Consider hypothyroidism, especially if both wrists are involved.

Treatment and Preventive Measures

NUTRITIONAL SUPPLEMENTS

- Vitamin B-6 (100 milligrams daily up to 200 milligrams three times a day) or pyroxidal-5 phosphate (50 to 100 milligrams three times a day). If there is a B-6 dependency, you may require much higher doses. However, after a successful response, reduce to the lowest effective dose. Use a B-complex formula (25 to 50 milligrams a day), and add magnesium as well (up to 400 milligrams a day).
- Reduce your intake of vitamin B-6 antagonists: hydralazine dyes in the diet (such as yellow #5); hydralazine-treated foods, such as potato chips; and excess dietary protein. Note that hydralazine-containing drugs, such as hydralazine and INH, and medications such as dopamine, penicillamine, and birth control pills increase vitamin B-6 needs.

HERBAL REMEDIES

- Bromelain and Curcumin (available from Scientific Botanicals of Seattle) may help to quiet the inflammation (two or three capsules up to four times a day spaced between meals).

OTHER THERAPIES

- Physical therapy can be quite helpful, especially local pulsed ultrasound.
- Hydrotherapy is also helpful in reducing the inflammation by stimulating circulation throughout the involved area. Use alternating hot and cold applications.
- Exercise that does not involve the wrist, along with techniques for reducing stress and tension, may help the healing process.
- Several topical antitrauma homeopathic agents may be helpful: Arnica Gel (Boiron/Borneman of Norwood, Pennsylvania) and Traumeel cream (BHI of Albuquerque, New Mexico). Apply to affected areas several times a day.

Cervical Dysplasia or Abnormal Pap Smear

Abnormal cells of the uterine cervix ranging from mild, harmless irritation to very severe changes indicating a wide range of cellular mutations representative of cervical cancer. *Note: Before the cervix develops cancer, it goes through several stages of cellular changes, each defined by increasingly abnormal cells.*

Related or Underlying Causes

 ND **DietH**

For well over a decade, the human papilloma virus (HPV) has been implicated in the abnormal cellular changes that can eventually lead to cervical cancer over time. In fact, cervical cancer is sometimes called a venereal disease. Women who begin sexual relations at a young age and who have had multiple sexual partners demonstrate a higher incidence of HPV, abnormal Pap smears, and cervical cancer.

HPV is not the only cause of Pap smear abnormalities. Yeast or bacterial vaginal infections can cause temporary cellular changes. Other factors can contribute, too. Cervical cancer is more prevalent in women who smoke, who take birth control pills, and whose diets are deficient in vitamins A and C, folic acid, beta-carotene, selenium, and possibly zinc.

Treatment and Preventive Measures

CONVENTIONAL MEDICAL TREATMENT

- Regular Pap smears are advised to detect any abnormalities while they are still easily curable—before they progress to an invasive cancerous stage. Consult your physician to determine how often you need to have a routine Pap smear.

  If your Pap smear is just slightly abnormal and you and your doctor are comfortable waiting three months to repeat the Pap, then proceed with the nutritional program given below.
- If your Pap smear is more than just slightly abnormal (Class III, Low-grade SIL, CIN-1) or shows evidence of HPV warts, or if you have repeated Pap abnormalities, then a colposcopy (a procedure in which your doctor examines the area through a magnifying scope) is indicated. Biopsies of suspicious-looking areas can be taken during the colposcopy. If your doctor then suggests a more invasive procedure, ask if waiting three months would put you at any risk. If there is no

significant increased risk and you are not in favor of the procedure, then aggressively follow the nutritional program and make an appointment to be rechecked in three months.

  If your doctor advises you not to wait and a conization or other procedure is warranted, a nutritional program is indicated to enhance your resistance to future recurrences or to prevent other consequences of the nutritional deficiencies. Despite the validity of the viral theory for this disease, many women with varying stages of abnormal Pap smears have been able to reverse their cellular changes through nutrition and immune enhancement.
- Medical treatment for cervical warts may vary according to your findings and your practitioner. Two common treatments are the direct application of trichloroacetic acid and intravaginal 5-fluorouracil. A wart check is also indicated for sexual partners.

NUTRITIONAL SUPPLEMENTS

- Folic acid, part of the B-complex spectrum, is one of the most important nutrients in normalizing and maintaining the health of the cervix. Take 5 milligrams three times a day for at least three months. After a favorable response, use a reduced dose, 5 milligrams a day, for several more months. After this, a daily dose of 400 to 800 micrograms should be sufficient if you're not on any folic acid antagonists, such as birth control pills or Dilantin.

  The highest-dosage folic acid tablet in the United States is 1 milligram, available only by prescription. Health food stores usually carry 800-microgram tablets. In Canada, 5-, 10-, and 25-milligram tablets are available. Scientific Botanicals of Seattle and Thorne Research of Sandpoint, Idaho, carry folic acid liquid, which is convenient for taking in higher doses.

  Note: Birth control pills can cause a folic acid deficiency, especially if the diet is not rich in deep green vegetables. Be sure to include spinach, kale, collards, chard, endive, and turnip greens in your diet. Also eat broccoli, asparagus, lima beans, and black-eyed peas, which contain folic acid.
- Add vitamin B-6 to your diet (50 to 100 milligrams a day). Birth control pills can cause a loss of vitamin B-6, so additional supplements are advised.
- Extra vitamin B-12 is needed as a metabolic partner of high-dose folic acid therapy (1,000 micrograms daily). If oral absorption of B-12 is an issue, use the sublingual, nasal gel, or injected forms. If injected, once every two weeks will suffice.
- Also, take beta-carotene (25,000 to 50,000 I.U. daily), vitamin C (1,000 milligrams three times a day), selenium (200 micrograms daily), vitamin E (400 I.U. daily), zinc (15 to 30 milligrams a day), and

B complex (25 to 50 milligrams one or two times a day).

- High-potency multiple vitamin/mineral formulas contain many of these nutrients and are more convenient to take.
- External applications: Use liquid vitamin A (A Emulsion Forte from Biotics Research Corp. of Houston or Nutrisorb A from Interplexus of Kent, Washington). Apply a generous amount directly to the cervix twice a week with a cotton swab. Or apply it to the tip of a tampon and insert the tampon up against the cervix. Remove within twelve hours.

HERBAL REMEDIES

- A vaginal pack of an herbal-based gel is commonly used by naturopathic physicians. One formula contains anhydrous magnesium sulfate, goldenseal, and essential oils of bitter orange, thuja, vegetable glycerin, VM 120, and tea tree (V.P. Compound from Eclectic Institute of Sandy, Oregon). The pack is placed up against the cervix once a week for approximately twelve hours.
- Apply fresh wheat grass juice to the cervix by taking a retention douche twice a day, in conjunction with a fasting and cleansing program.
- Some naturopathic physicians apply liquid lomatium concentrate (Lomatium Isolate from Eclectic Institute of Sandy, Oregon) directly on the cervix in combination with vitamin A.

OTHER THERAPIES

- Since psychological and emotional issues may sometimes underlie Pap abnormalities, professional counseling may prove very helpful.

Chest Pain

See ANGINA PECTORIS.

Cholesterol (High)

Cholesterol, a fatlike substance synthesized in the liver and found in the brain, nerves, liver, blood, and bile is essential in the production of sex hormones, nerve function, and other vital processes. In excess, it is a cofactor in the development of arteriosclerosis, the hardening of arteries in the body.

Total blood cholesterol levels consist of several cholesterol-protein substances, the two best known being low-density lipoproteins (LDLs), which increase the risk of heart disease and stroke, and high-density lipoproteins (HDLs), which decrease the risk.

It is more effective to assess health risks by calculating the total cholesterol/HDL ratio than to use either measure alone. Dividing total cholesterol by HDL cholesterol gives the ratio. For example, if a man's total cholesterol level is 250 and the HDL is 85, the risk ratio is 250 divided by 85, which equals 2.9. Average risk for a man is 5.0; for a woman, 4.4. A lower risk ratio is synonymous with lower risk of heart and artery disease, so this 2.9 risk ratio is very favorable. Although the 250 total cholesterol is considered high, the very high 85 HDL attenuates the risk.

Other, more complicated ratios calculated from LDL and HDL levels may be more accurate. However, cholesterol levels may not be the single most important factor in assessing cardiac risk (see ARTERIOSCLEROSIS and HEART ATTACK).

Related or Underlying Causes

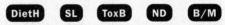

For most individuals, dietary cholesterol has a very small effect on serum cholesterol levels. High levels of total and LDL cholesterol are most commonly caused by a diet rich in saturated fats and sugar and deficient in several essential nutrients (vitamins C, E, and B-6, the minerals chromium, magnesium, and copper, and essential fatty acids). A fiber deficiency, excess caffeine, margarine, and other sources of trans-fatty acids from partially hydrogenated vegetable oils are also significant contributing factors. Lack of exercise and obesity may be equally important to consider, as are sluggish liver metabolism and heredity.

Low thyroid function elevates total cholesterol levels (see HYPOTHYROIDISM). Stress, low levels of DHEA (dehydroepiandrosterone), steroid drugs, some prescribed medications, and cigarette smoking contribute as well.

Treatment and Preventive Measures

CONVENTIONAL MEDICAL TREATMENTS

- Cholesterol-lowering prescription drugs, such as lovastatin, pravastatin, simvastatin, gemfibrozil, probucol, clofibrate, cholestyramine, and colestipol, may be questionable and potentially hazardous. Although studies show improved cholesterol ratios and fewer heart attack deaths in the groups treated with drugs, the benefit of the drugs is sometimes canceled by their risks. Those treated with drugs usually have increased deaths from other causes compared to the nontreated groups. In addition, the first three agents listed above, which block the synthesis of cholesterol by inhibiting the enzyme HMG CoA reductase, also block the synthesis of coenzyme Q-10, one of the most important heart nutrients. Cholesterol is needed in the manufacture of adrenal/stress-combating hormones, nerve sheaths, and sex hormones. It should be noted that chemically tampering with these levels can present documented risks. Many clinicians now feel that currently available pharmaceutical cholesterol-lowering agents should be considered only in the most pronounced cases.

DIETARY RECOMMENDATIONS
- Follow a low-fat (especially low saturated fat), low-sugar, and high-fiber whole-foods diet, as discussed in Chapters Three and Four. Gradually make a transition to a more vegetarian diet. Pay special attention to the use of safe fats and oils, and include essential fatty acids.
- The most effective dietary regimen for lowering cholesterol is that recommended by Dean Ornish, M.D. (see ARTERIOSCLEROSIS). Such a diet and accompanying lifestyle modifications usually normalize cholesterol ratios, reverse plaque buildup, and prevent heart disease.
- Eat cholesterol-lowering and heart and artery–protective foods, such as legumes, oat bran, garlic, and nonfat yogurt.
- Restrict caffeine.
- If you're not a vegetarian, use cold-water omega 3-EPA–rich fish (mackerel, herring, albacore tuna, dogfish, sablefish, lake whitefish, salmon, halibut), or omega 3–rich wild game.

DETOXIFICATION PROGRAM
- Follow the Liver Flush and Purifying Diet and the Ultra Clear cleansing program periodically to decrease systemic toxicity. If bowels are sluggish, continue with an intestinal cleansing program.

NUTRITIONAL SUPPLEMENTS
- Use the following total and LDL cholesterol–lowering nutrients, most of which can be found in a potent daily multiple vitamin/mineral formula: vitamins C (3,000 milligrams), B-3 in the niacin form (50 to 100 milligrams), B-6 (25 to 50 milligrams), and E (400 to 800 I.U.), and the minerals copper (2 or 3 milligrams) and magnesium (400 milligrams).
- Take extra niacin and chromium. Use the no-flush

form of niacin, inositol hexaniacinate (up to 600 milligrams three times a day—see Chapter Six for precautions), and chromium (300 micrograms three times a day).
- The amino acid derivatives N-acetylcysteine (500 milligrams two or three times a day) and L-carnitine (300 milligrams two or three times a day) can also favorably affect cholesterol ratios.
- If you have a history of recurrent or prolonged antibiotics or bowel disturbances related to elevated cholesterols, take acidophilus and bifidus (at least one capsule twice a day). If dietary fiber is lacking, use psyllium husks (1 or 2 teaspoons twice a day in at least 8 ounces of water). In addition, drink six to eight glasses of water daily or incorporate other water-soluble fiber powders.
- Take unrefined flaxseed oil (1 teaspoon or three capsules a day) or fish oil with an EPA/DHA ratio less than 1:1 (three capsules a day).

   Note: Many cases of cholesterol elevation will respond favorably to a combination of the supplements listed above. Taking all of the supplements is usually unnecessary, particularly when following the right diet and exercise program. To help prioritize which supplements to take, choose the cholesterol-lowering nutrients and herbs that directly diminish the risk of heart disease (see ARTERIOSCLEROSIS and HEART ATTACK) or consult a nutritionally oriented medical doctor.

HERBAL REMEDIES
- Garlic (one 500-milligram capsule or tablet three times a day).
- Gugulipid (750 milligrams a day) lowers unfavorable cholesterols. Try Guguplex/Guguplus from Phyto-Pharmica/Enzymatic Therapy of Green Bay, Wisconsin, which contains niacin, vitamin C, ginger, and chromium in addition to the gugulipid. Take one capsule three times a day.
- If sluggish liver metabolism is fueling elevated cholesterol, take a combination herbal formula that stimulates liver cell functioning and contains milk thistle (approximately 350 milligrams), artichoke (250 milligrams), and curcumin/turmeric (150 milligrams). Take one or two capsules three times a day.

OTHER THERAPIES
- Aerobic exercise thirty minutes three times a week, or even a thirty- or forty-five-minute daily walk, can help normalize cholesterol levels and protect your heart and arteries.
- Practice stress management and relaxation techniques regularly.

Chronic Fatigue Syndrome (Chronic Fatigue and Immune Dysfunction Syndrome—CFIDS)

CFIDS is the descriptive name of a syndrome characterized by a myriad of symptoms involving many body systems. The diagnosis is made on the basis of symptoms and the ruling out of other ailments that could cause these conditions.

Many physicians still do not accept the diagnosis of CFIDS and would rather label a patient as depressed or psychoneurotic. If you suspect CFIDS, find a physician who specializes in this condition and will treat you appropriately (see organizations in the resources following).

The symptoms of chronic fatigue syndrome include fatigue, cognitive dysfunction (memory disturbance, mental "fogginess," concentration difficulties, poor analysis or calculation, spatial disorientation), depression, anxiety, mood swings, insomnia, headaches, sleep that does not refresh, muscle and joint aches, low-grade fever or feverishness, painful and swollen lymph glands in the neck and elsewhere, sore throat, and recurrent flulike symptoms. Many of these conditions are made worse by exercise.

Related or Underlying Causes

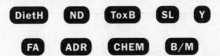

This illness may be, in part, viral in origin (Epstein-Barr and other viruses), and because of other conditions or susceptibilities weakening the immune response, an individual cannot fend off the virus. The following are factors that may predispose an individual to chronic fatigue syndrome: stress; working too hard, too long; excessive demands on your capacity to perform; insufficient sleep; insufficient relaxation; adrenal exhaustion; chemical sensitivity (initial bout or subsequent exacerbation can be triggered by paints, tung and other refinishing oils, or other chemicals); intestinal parasites (see PARASITES); mold and other inhalant allergies; impaired liver detoxification mechanisms; deficiencies or imbalances of amino acids as diagnosed by blood or urine analysis; low thyroid status (see HYPOTHYROIDISM); chronic sinusitis or tonsillitis; poor-quality diet, including too much sugar, fast foods, refined foods, excess caffeine, or alcohol; food allergy; and magnesium deficiency.

Treatment and Preventive Measures

Chronic fatigue syndrome requires a comprehensive effort directed toward enhancing the immune system. By treating underlying conditions, your immune reserve can be strengthened and you can eventually overcome the virus. Often, what seems like chronic fatigue syndrome is actually an unrecognized yeast overgrowth, an intestinal parasite, or chronic sinusitis. Accompanying conditions can respond well to treatment even after a year or more of chronic fatigue syndrome symptoms. Direct immune-enhancing measures and sometimes direct antiviral measures are often implemented.

CONVENTIONAL MEDICAL TREATMENT
- Your doctor should rule out known disorders that could cause symptoms.
- Some doctors prescribe a trial of acyclovir (Zovirax™), an antiviral drug commonly used for herpes and shingles (400 milligrams four times a day for six to eight weeks, with one or two intramuscular injections weekly of 2 milliliters of gamma globulin). Some doctors use gamma globulin only.
- Antidepressants, such as Prozac and Zoloft, are commonly prescribed. Tricyclic antidepressants with sedative effects are often prescribed to help insomnia.

DIETARY RECOMMENDATIONS
- Eat a whole-foods diet. Restrict sugar, caffeine, alcohol, and any junk foods.
- Identify and avoid allergy-triggering foods. Try an elimination diet.
- See dietary recommendations geared toward body and blood types in Chapter Four.

DETOXIFICATION PROGRAM
- If indicated, follow the Ultra Clear program to enhance liver detoxification mechanisms (see Chapter Nine).

NUTRITIONAL SUPPLEMENTS
- Take beta- or mixed carotenes (up to 100,000 I.U. daily), vitamin C (3,000 to 6,000 milligrams a day), zinc (up to 30 milligrams a day), and a high-potency multiple vitamin/mineral. Extra magnesium may be indicated (up to 800 milligrams a day).
- If your doctor is nutritionally oriented, request an intravenous "nutrient cocktail" injection: vitamin C, magnesium, calcium, B complex, vitamins B-12, B-6, and B-5, and a mineral combination of zinc, copper, chromium, manganese, and selenium. Magnesium deficiency has been linked to CFIDS and may be the most important component of this injection (see "In-

travenous Vitamin and Mineral Protocol" on pages 425–426).

- Consult your doctor about intramuscular injections of vitamin B-12 (1,000 micrograms once or twice a week) with folic acid (5 milligrams).
- Take an amino acid replacement supplement (the formula for which is determined by laboratory results of an amino acid blood or urine analysis): MetaMetrix Medical Research Laboratory, Norcross, Georgia, (800) 221-4640; Doctor's Date, Inc., West Chicago, Illinois, (800) 323-2784; or Meridian Valley Laboratory, Kent, Washington, (800) 234-6825. Or use Aminovirox (one or two capsules three times a day), available from Tyson and Associates, Hawthorne, California.

HERBAL REMEDIES

- Take Astra Isatis (three tablets three times a day) or ImmunoPlex 4 (one to five capsules three or four times a day). See Chapter Nineteen for the ingredients and manufacturers of both of these formulas. Also see CHRONIC FATIGUE SYNDROME.
- Additional general immune-enhancing formulas include Echimmune (one to three capsules three or four times a day), Power Mushrooms (three tablets twice a day), and Astra 8 (two or three capsules twice a day). See Chapter Nineteen for these formulas.
- Take lomatium isolate (up to ten drops twice a day) and shiitake mushroom (one or two capsules three times a day), both from Eclectic Institute, Sandy, Oregon.
- Take Siberian ginseng (100 to 200 milligrams once or twice a day).

OTHER THERAPIES

- Small doses of the adrenal hormones dehydroepiandrosterone and hydrocortisone may be necessary (see Chapter Eleven). Treat insomnia (see INSOMNIA); this is vital.
- Stay warm.
- If your liver is affected (enlarged liver with elevated liver enzymes), consult Chapter Nine for information on liver-protective agents.
- Do stretching exercises, yoga, or tai chi, along with slow, deep breathing exercises. Among their many benefits, these activities stimulate lymph flow. Walking and other aerobic exercises are also suggested. However, avoid any exercise that tires you or worsens your symptoms.
- Practice stress management techniques.
- If depression is significant, counseling may be warranted, and possibly antidepressant medications— some of which can boost energy and help insomnia.
- Try constitutional hydrotherapy (as described in Chapter Twenty).

- Try acupuncture.
- Staphage lysate (see "Bacterial Vaccines").

Circulation (Poor)

(See also ARTERIOSCLEROSIS.) Insufficient arterial blood flow, which can result in cold extremities and muscle cramps. Other symptoms include impotence, visual disturbances, senility, gangrene, and diminished kidney function. For poor venous circulation, see VARICOSE VEINS.

Related or Underlying Causes

     ADR Y CHEM ND DietH B/M

Circulatory ailments commonly result from arteriosclerosis (plaque formation), which inhibits the flow of blood. Arterial muscle spasms from low magnesium status, anxiety, cigarette smoking, and Raynaud's disease can also impair circulation with or without arteriosclerosis. Poor circulation can result as well from red blood cell abnormalities. If red blood cells become less elastic or more inclined to clump together, blood flow through constricted arteries will become difficult or impaired. Such red cell disturbances are associated with food allergy, insufficient essential fatty acids and vitamin E, chemical hypersensitivity, and heavy metal toxicity.

Central metabolic or systemic abnormalities may contribute to poor circulation problems, such as low thyroid function, anemia, and congestive heart failure. A sedentary lifestyle also plays a role.

Treatment and Preventive Measures

NUTRITIONAL SUPPLEMENTS

- Try vitamin E (up to 800 I.U. daily; up to 1,600 I.U. daily for muscle cramps in the calves), vitamin B-15 (50 milligrams once or twice a day), niacin (25 to 100 milligrams three times a day), or niacin-inositol hexaniacinate (600 milligrams two or three times daily). This form of niacin does not cause a flush.
- Take unrefined flaxseed oil (1 or 2 teaspoons a day) and borage oil (one capsule with each meal).

HERBAL REMEDIES

- Try ginkgo biloba (40 milligrams twice a day), pycnogenol (20 milligrams twice daily), and cayenne (one or two capsules per meal); include some of the following herbs in your regular diet: ginger, rosemary, garlic, onion, sage, and cinnamon.

OTHER THERAPIES

- Exercise is crucial for effective circulation. Walking or jogging is superb, but any exercise will help. Also, try yoga, tai chi, or stretching.
- Hydrotherapy can enhance the circulation in an extraordinary way. Alternating hot and cold applications of water can be effective (see Chapter Twenty). Try walking in cold water up to your knees for five to ten minutes at least twice a day. Or run cold water from a hose on your legs and feet.
- Several methods of massage therapy can be helpful, including shiatsu, acupressure, and Swedish massage.
- Acupuncture can be effective.
- Stop smoking.
- Skilled relaxation or biofeedback techniques can be effective.

Coated Tongue

A prominent whitish or yellowish film on the tongue obscuring the normal pink color and usually indicating an underlying health imbalance.

Related or Underlying Causes

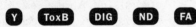

Coated tongue could be caused by overeating, late-night meals and digestive overload, deficiency in hydrochloric acid or pancreatic enzymes, bowel toxicity, food allergies (consider milk products especially), candida overgrowth, and a deficiency of vitamins B-3 and B-12. It could also be a sign of an impending or current cold or flu.

Treatment and Preventive Measures

DIETARY RECOMMENDATIONS

- Eat sensible amounts of food. Refrain from late dinners and nighttime snacks. Minimize snacking between meals. Include high fiber foods: whole grains, legumes, and fresh vegetables and fruit.

DETOXIFICATION PROGRAMS

- Follow the Liver Flush and Purifying Diet, a month-long intestinal cleansing program, or periodic fasting.

NUTRITIONAL SUPPLEMENTS

- Take a B-complex supplement that includes niacin (10 to 25 milligrams), niacinamide (50 milligrams), and

vitamin B-12 (100 to 200 micrograms a day). Also experiment with sublingual vitamin B-12 (up to 1,000 micrograms a day) for one month to see if this addition makes a difference.

Cold, Flu, Sore Throat, and Cough

A viral infection of the respiratory passageways—nasal, sinus, throat, lung—that causes nasal stuffiness or discharge, sneezing, sore throat, or cough. A headache, earache, or fever may also be present. Viruses can also cause chills, body aches and pains, severe headaches, profound malaise, or symptoms characteristic of the flu. Colds and flus are frequently complicated by a bacterial infection leading to a sinus or ear infection, bronchitis, or pneumonia.

Related or Underlying Causes

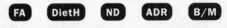

Flu- and cold-causing viruses are ever-present and can infect you whenever the environment within your body becomes weakened and your resistance is lowered. Your resistance may be compromised for many reasons: too much sugar in your diet; chronic overeating and accumulation of mucus; a toxic bowel; a nutrient-poor diet; unrecognized food allergies, especially to dairy or wheat products; yeast overgrowth; air pollution; and inhalant allergies (see HAY FEVER).

Other factors include excessive exposure to cold or eating too many cooling foods in the cold seasons; excessive fasting or cleansing; inadequate intake of vitamins A and C, iron, zinc, or protein; too much activity and not enough sleep; and high stress levels. Other underlying causes are weakened adrenals, a low-functioning thyroid, inadequate physical exercise, and such emotional factors as depression and anxiety.

Note: A persistent sore throat may be caused by streptococcus bacteria and may require immediate medical attention. It should be cultured and treated with antibiotics if "positive."

Take a hard look at the list of possible underlying causes short-circuiting your resistance if you are hit frequently with colds or if they often turn into more serious conditions, such as bronchitis, pneumonia, asthma, sinusitis, or ear infections. Begin a preventive treatment program to lessen your susceptibility.

Treatment and Preventive Measures

If you are beginning to develop a cold, medical and common sense dictate that you get more rest than usual, reduce stress, stop exercising temporarily, stay warm, and eat lightly. Also, consider fasting, nutritional supplements, herbs, and enemas. It is not necessary to use every recommendation discussed for your next cold or sore throat. However, experiment with several combinations to see which methods work best for you—such as fasting on liquids for a day while using extra vitamin C and an herbal combination formula containing echinacea and goldenseal.

DETOXIFICATION PROGRAMS

At the first sign of symptoms, reduce food intake. It is best to fast on liquids so your body can use all of its energy to fight the virus by not having to digest foods. Fasting is one of the more effective and inexpensive remedies to combat a cold or sore throat. One day of fasting may be all you need. (Consult your doctor first if you have diabetes or a seizure disorder.) Drink copious amounts of warm liquids:

- Use herbal teas (see "Teas" below).
- Drink soup broths, vegetable juices, and water. Reduce cold juices and liquids, especially fruit juices, particularly in the cold seasons.
- If fasting on liquids for one day is inappropriate for you, use a hypoallergenic protein powder beverage or meal replacement powder. Avoid the overly sweet ones. Such powders will generally prevent the hypoglycemia or weakness that can accompany fasting on just clear fluids in some individuals. They are usually very easy to assimilate and will allow the body to concentrate most of its energy on immune functioning.

  If a day on powdered beverages is still insufficient, consider a very light diet of fruit and vegetables (see the Liver Flush and Purifying Diet).
- Taking an enema can often accelerate recovery (see Chapter Eighteen). According to the concept of bowel toxicity, a cold can be a manifestation of a toxic colon.

NUTRITIONAL SUPPLEMENTS
COLDS/FLUS

- Take vitamin C (5,000 to 6,000 milligrams a day or up to bowel tolerance levels—too much will cause diarrhea) to cut short a cold or flu. If this is not effective, reduce to normal dose. A serious cold or flu often ends quicker when intravenous vitamin C is given (3,000 to 5,000 milligrams, especially with 5 milliliters of 1:500 diluted hydrochloric acid). See "Intravenous Vitamin and Mineral Protocol" under CHRONIC FATIGUE SYNDROME.

- Vitamin A (100,000 to 200,000 I.U. daily for four to five days) is especially effective in healing mucous membranes (see Chapter Six for dose precautions). Or use beta-carotene (100,000 to 200,000 I.U. daily for four to five days).

SORE THROAT

- Use a liquid form of vitamin A (Nutrisorb A by Interplexus of Kent, Washington) or of beta- (mixed) carotenes (Beta Plex, by Scientific Botanicals of Seattle). The dose for either is up to ten drops twice a day gargled, then swallowed, again, for only four or five days.

- Take zinc lozenges (one tablet every thirty to sixty minutes). Do not take more than 150 milligrams of zinc in a twenty-four-hour period. If this does not help after two days, discontinue. *Note: The chelated zincs designed for superior absorption, such as citrate, picolinate, glycinate, and histidinate, may not work as effectively as the more poorly absorbed gluconate or sulfate forms.*

HERBAL REMEDIES

- Take high-quality echinacea in tincture form or freeze-dried or potency-guaranteed capsules (two or three capsules or 2 teaspoons of tincture four or five times a day). Or use a combination formula containing echinacea, goldenseal, garlic, mullein, ginger, cayenne, and lobelia. Several variations of anti-infection formulas are available (see Chapter Nineteen, "Anti-infection," "Antiviral and Antibacterial"). Use the same dose for these formulas as for echinacea alone.

- Take garlic capsules or tablets (freeze-dried) or garlic oil perles (two or three tablets four to six times a day or eat one clove of garlic three times a day).

- Take cayenne capsules (one or two every hour).

TEAS
FOR GENERAL COLD SYMPTOMS:

- Drink a tea made from a mixture of sage, garlic, and gingerroot. Lightly simmer slices of garlic and gingerroot, then add the sage to steep. Add fresh lemon juice and honey.

- Try drinking a cup of elder flower/peppermint leaf tea (1 teaspoon of each steeped in a cup of hot water). Then take a hot bath and immediately go to bed to "sweat" the cold out.

FOR SORE THROAT RELIEF:

- Gargle a very bitter tea made from goldenseal, combined with myrrh and cayenne (see ABSCESS).

- Gargle and drink a combination tea made of slippery elm, raspberry leaf, and licorice root (steep 1 teaspoon of each ingredient per cup of water).

- Gargle and drink the fresh juice from greens, most particularly wheat grass juice, but other green leafy vegetables will do. Prebottled liquid chlorophyll is also available. Fat-soluble chlorophyll capsules (two capsules four times a day for three or four days), especially with vitamin A, can also be effective for sore throats.

FOR COUGHS:

- To help soothe coughs, drink copious amounts of mullein and chickweed teas (2 or 3 teaspoons of each per cup of water). This is not anti-infective. (See BRONCHITIS.)

HOMEOPATHIC REMEDIES

- Oscillococcinum by Boiron and other homeopathic flu remedies, such as Flu Solution by Dolisos, are available in health food stores. Try using homeopathic remedies as well for colds, sinus symptoms, sore throats, and coughs. Such remedies are most effective when taken at the first sign of symptoms. Combination formulas for specific symptoms are also available.

OTHER THERAPIES

- Lowering stress levels can give a boost to your resistance and hasten your recovery. Talk about bottled-up feelings, such as anger, sadness, loneliness, fear, and frustration, or write them down in a journal. Or express them through music, dance, or other means. Resolving emotional conflicts, even temporarily, can strengthen your immune response.
- Try a steam bath or use a sauna.

Cold Sores (Fever Blisters)

Virally related, these swollen, aching eruptions usually appear on the lips or in the mouth and clear up within three to seven days. An oral form of the herpes simplex virus is often involved. Cold sores unrelated to viruses are sometimes called apthous ulcers.

Related or Underlying Causes

Herpes cold sores often indicate temporarily lowered immune function due to stress, excessive sweets, or other factors (see HERPES). Nonviral cold sores in the mouth may be precipitated by food allergies and overly acidic foods.

Treatment and Preventive Measures

DIETARY RECOMMENDATIONS

- Follow the same recommendations given for herpes (see HERPES), especially paying attention to avoiding foods high in arginine and sugar.

NUTRITIONAL SUPPLEMENTS

- Lysine is an excellent treatment for the herpes virus since it inhibits its growth. Dosage: Take up to 1,000 milligrams three times a day at the first sign of an outbreak. If recurrences are a problem, use 500 to 1,000 milligrams a day as a maintenance and preventive dose.
- Take Isatis Gold (three tablets five to eight times a day), sold by Health Concerns of Oakland, California.
- For a cold sore inside the mouth, use zinc lozenges (5 to 10 milligrams four to five times a day). If outside the mouth, take oral zinc (up to 60 milligrams a day). If recurrences are a problem, take up to 30 milligrams a day as a preventive measure.
- Take vitamin A (up to 50,000 I.U. twice daily for three or four days only). Apply the liquid form of vitamin A (Nutrisorb A from Interplexus of Kent, Washington) directly on the lesion in the mouth, then swallow. For prevention, use up to 20,000 I.U. daily.
- Take vitamin B complex (50 milligrams once or twice a day).
- Calcium, magnesium, and essential fatty acids may also be helpful (see HERPES).
- Rinse your mouth several times a day with liquid acidophilus (1 tablespoon) or acidophilus powder (½ teaspoon).

HERBAL REMEDIES

- Drink hyssop (up to 3 cups a day), which restricts the growth of herpes simplex virus. For sores within the mouth, bathe the lesion with the tea before swallowing. For external sores, use this antiseptic tea as a compress.
- Licorice is also beneficial in fighting herpes eruptions since it boosts the body's production of interferon, an antiviral substance. Dab the powder of its root on sores to promote healing. As a tea, drink up to 3 cups a day. If sores are inside the mouth, bathe the lesion with the tea before swallowing. Licorice root gel (Licrogel by Scientific Botanicals of Seattle) can be applied to external sores several times a day.
- Aloe vera gel can be swished in the mouth as well to bathe internal lesions.

OTHER THERAPIES

- For external sores, see HERPES for other topical remedies.

Colitis

An inflammation of the large bowel that can produce abdominal pain, diarrhea, and/or bleeding. Symptoms can become quite severe, even life threatening, requiring the use of cortisone-type drugs and sometimes surgery.

Related or Underlying Causes

     FA Y DIG ToxB Chem B/M

From a conventional medical viewpoint, colitis is thought to be an autoimmune disease and has no known cause. However, many contributing factors need to be considered: intestinal parasites, leaky gut syndrome, inadequate hydrochloric acid levels, unresolved emotional issues, and poor stress management.

Treatment and Preventive Measures

CONVENTIONAL MEDICAL TREATMENT

- The most common treatment is pharmaceutical: cortisone orally or by enema for more severe symptoms and either sulfasalazine, olsalazine, or other similar medications to help maintain control. Recent studies have demonstrated symptomatic relief from the use of a nicotine transdermal (skin) patch. Consult your doctor.
- Surgical removal of the colon is recommended for those who do not respond adequately to other means.

DIETARY RECOMMENDATIONS

- During an acute episode, avoid raw or rough foods until your bowel quiets down. Running foods through a blender may be useful. Be certain to chew your food well. Take your time and make your mealtime relaxed. Rice cream and vegetable soup are extremely digestible.
- If symptoms do not abate, you may require more extreme measures—a clear fluid diet for several days, vegetable juices and broth, and herbal teas. If you require more calories than a clear fluid diet provides, use a hypoallergenic (no milk, wheat, eggs, or soy products) protein or meal replacement powder beverage (Ultra Clear or Ultra Clear Sustain or Opti by Metagenics of San Clemente, California).
- As a general precaution, even when in remission, avoid sorbitol, a sweetener in gum, foods, and some beverages, as it can cause diarrhea.

NUTRITIONAL SUPPLEMENTS

- Take B complex (25 to 100 milligrams a day) and extra pantothenic acid (up to 1,000 milligrams a day).
- Vitamin E (up to 1,000 I.U. daily) is useful during flare-ups; otherwise, take 400 to 800 I.U. daily.
- Take folic acid (up to 800 micrograms a day), since individuals afflicted with colitis are at risk of developing colon cancer. This is particularly relevant if you are on long-term sulfasalazine or olsalazine medications, which are folic acid antagonists.
- Some patients have successfully taken PABA (para-aminobenzoic acid), a B vitamin (1,000 to 2,000 milligrams three times a day). PABA is molecularly similar to sulfasalazine and olsalazine and is sometimes used successfully in individuals with autoimmune diseases.

HERBAL REMEDIES

- Drink any one or combinations of the following teas to soothe the intestines: flaxseed (well strained), slippery elm, chamomile, and marshmallow root.
- Goldenseal (two or three capsules four to five times a day during flare-ups) is extremely healing to the bowel.
- Take a combination herbal formula recommended for flare-ups that contains goldenseal as well as marshmallow root, wild indigo, geranium, slippery elm, gingerroot, and okra (up to two capsules four to six times a day). Try Roberts Formula or Bastyr B Formula, by Eclectic Institute of Sandy, Oregon, or other similar bowel-healing formulas.
- Licorice root in its deglycyrrhizinated form (up to two or three capsules four to five times a day during flare-ups) is well known for its gastrointestinal healing properties.
- Liquid chlorophyll (1 or 2 teaspoons three or four times a day) can be soothing and healing to the intestines during flare-ups. *Note: Too much chlorophyll may loosen stools.*

OTHER THERAPIES

- Between flare-ups, if you tend toward constipation (test your transit time), find an effective and gentle fiber supplement to use regularly (see Chapter Eight).
- Find a sialic acid concentrate supplement, otherwise known as N-neuraminic acid (mucin). This is directly healing to the intestinal mucosa and may be another of your most valuable supplements. Try Sialex by Cardiovascular Research or Ecologic Formulas of Concorde, California. Take one to three capsules a day.
- One other very effective healing agent is butyric acid (see Chapter Twenty). Take up to three capsules per meal. Because oral use of the capsules does not deliver as much to the large bowel, retention enemas are the preferred route. Use the contents of four to six capsules in four ounces of warm water (Butyrex, by T. E. Neesby of Fresno, California). Depending on the in-

volved area of your colon, once the solution is in your rectum, it may be necessary for you to lie on an incline and massage your abdomen, working the solution up and around to the desired areas. (Tyler Encapsulations of Gresham, Oregon, offers Buty-Col, a complete butyric acid/enema kit.)

- If the use of oral cortisone preparations is sometimes necessary to control your symptoms, ask your doctor to consider prescribing cortisone enemas instead. These are often equally effective but minimize the acute and long-term side effects of oral cortisone.
- Employ enema rescue for flare-ups. In 4 to 6 ounces of warm water, add butyric acid (contents of four to six capsules), deglycerrhizinated licorice root (the contents of 3 or 4 capsules or, if unavailable, add a very strong cup of strained licorice root tea), goldenseal powder (2 teaspoons), Roberts Formula (the contents of three capsules), and liquid chlorophyll (3 tablespoons). Mix well and take as an enema. Retain the mixture as long as possible. Repeat as needed. If you cannot find all of the ingredients, use the ones you can find. Of course, if symptoms persist, consult your doctor.

Convulsions

See SEIZURES.

Cough

See COLD, FLU, SORE THROAT, AND COUGH. See also BRONCHITIS.

Cramps (Intestinal)

Involuntary tightening of intestinal walls, causing mild to severe pain, sometimes associated with vomiting, diarrhea, and/or fever. Can be traced to stomach flu, traveler's diarrhea, overeating, improper food combinations, allergies, intestinal yeast, intestinal parasites (see PARASITES), weak digestion, constipation, adverse effects of antibiotics or other medications, emotional factors, and food poisoning.

Related or Underlying Causes

If severe and unremitting and associated with diarrhea, ask your doctor to test for clostridium difficile, an intestinal bacterial infection.

Treatment and Preventive Measures

NUTRITIONAL SUPPLEMENTS
- If the cramps are related to antibiotics, try acidophilus/bifidus, *Saccharomyces boulardii*, and other antiyeast measures.

HERBAL REMEDIES
- Take 2 or 3 enteric-coated peppermint oil capsules (two or three times a day) or drink a combination of strong catnip, chamomile, and peppermint tea with or without gingerroot.
- For intestinal cramps caused by overeating, try a capsule with equal parts of goldenseal, cayenne, cinnamon, and slippery elm.

HOMEOPATHIC REMEDIES
- Try the homeopathic remedy nux vomica as directed for overeating, or take homeopathic combination drops or tablets for intestinal spasms or cramps as directed. (Spasm-Pain, an effective cramp reliever by Biological Homeopathic Industries, contains aconite, bryonia, colocynthis, atropinum sulphuricum, and cuprum sulphuricum.)

OTHER THERAPIES
- Try a hot water bottle on the abdomen or a castor oil pack.

Cramps (Menstrual)

See MENSTRUAL CRAMPS.

Cramps (Muscle)

Muscle cramps occur during exertion when the oxygen

supply to the muscles is insufficient. They can also happen when an individual is at rest, particularly in bed at night. Cramps can be accompanied by sharp pains and a brief inability to move. Legs, calves, feet, and the back are often target points.

Related or Underlying Causes

In older individuals, a primary cause of cramps during exertion is peripheral vascular disease or arteriosclerosis (see ARTERIOSCLEROSIS and CIRCULATION, POOR).

At any age, cramps can be produced by overexertion, loss of body nutrients through sweat, and buildup of lactic acid in the muscles. Poor posture, arterial disorders, spinal malalignment, leg length discrepancy, and foot problems can also contribute. Common causes of nighttime cramps include poor diet, poor nutrient absorption, chronic diarrhea, diuretics, and calcium, magnesium, and potassium deficiencies (see OSTEOPOROSIS). Insufficient exercise may also be a factor.

Treatment and Preventive Measures

DIETARY RECOMMENDATIONS
- Eat a whole-foods diet to ensure adequate digestion and absorption.
- Drink vegetable juice, a very concentrated source of potassium. Vegetables and fruits, in general, are good potassium sources. (See Chapter Six for a list of calcium- and magnesium-rich foods.)

NUTRITIONAL SUPPLEMENTS
- Take calcium (up to 1,500 milligrams a day), magnesium (up to 1,000 milligrams a day), and potassium (100 to 300 milligrams a day).
- To improve general circulation, take vitamin E (up to 800 I.U. daily).

OTHER THERAPIES
- Apply a heating pad or hot water bottle to the cramped area to increase circulation. Try gently massaging or stretching the muscle.
- An ice pack works well on spasms or cramps, because cold applications reduce swelling. Alternating hot and cold applications may be effective for relieving cramps.
- Massage therapy or shiatsu and acupuncture, as well as spinal manipulation, can help relieve and prevent cramps.

Crohn's Disease

An inflammatory bowel condition usually involving the distal section of the small bowel, producing pain, diarrhea, and bleeding. The discussion and treatment of colitis (see COLITIS) apply as well to Crohn's disease. However, note that colitis therapy recommendations for enemas and butyric acid do not apply to Crohn's disease.

Cystic Breasts or Cystic Mastitis

See FIBROCYSTIC BREAST DISEASE.

Depression

An emotional state characterized by negative thoughts and feelings ranging from chronic low self-esteem to utter despondency. Symptoms include fatigue, loss of interest, indecision, loss of sexual drive, melancholy, futility, flat affect, loss of or excessive appetite, guilt, hopelessness, unusually high use of drugs and alcohol, insomnia or excessive sleep, social withdrawal, and suicidal thoughts.

Related or Underlying Causes

Although legitimate life circumstances or even genetic influences may trigger depression or other forms of mental illness, other contributing conditions are often at work. Such factors could include nutritional deficiencies, inhalant and food allergies, hypoglycemia, and low thyroid function. Chemical hypersensitivity and heavy metal toxicity may also apply.

Some individuals require more sunlight than their environment permits (see SEASONAL AFFECTIVE DISORDER). Others need more full-spectrum lighting than their primarily indoor life permits (see "Sunlight," pages 317–318). Insufficient exercise is another common contributor to depression. Any one of these conditions could imbalance brain chemistry. By identifying and treating the causes, depression can be lessened.

Using this broad-based approach, many individuals have overcome depression without antidepressant medication or have become more functional with a smaller dose. Antidepressant medication and psychotherapy should be prescribed when appropriate, but other options should also be explored.

Treatment and Preventive Measures

DIETARY RECOMMENDATIONS

- Establish a whole-foods diet, reducing sugar, caffeine, alcohol, and altered oils.
- If you have hypoglycemic symptoms, follow the diet and supplement program in Chapter Ten to help stabilize your blood sugar level.
- To see if your depression is related to food allergy, try the elimination diet presented in Chapter Thirteen.

NUTRITIONAL SUPPLEMENTS

- Take the following supplements: B complex (25 to 50 milligrams twice a day), extra B-3, in the niacinamide form (500 to 1,000 milligrams twice a day), vitamin C (up to 1,500 milligrams twice a day), calcium (up to 800 milligrams a day), magnesium (up to 800 milligrams a day), 5-hydroxytryptophan, by prescription only (100 to 400 milligrams at bedtime), and tyrosine (500 to 1,000 milligrams once or twice a day). Phenylalanine, another amino acid used commonly for depression, should be taken (500 to 1,000 milligrams once or twice a day). Also, take lecithin, another useful supplement (up to 20 grams a day).
- Intramuscular injections of vitamin B-12 (1,000 micrograms, combined with up to 5 micrograms folic acid every one to two weeks initially) have proven effective for some depression sufferers. Others require the addition of B complex to the mixture (containing at least 100 milligrams per milliliter of vitamin B-1, along with smaller amounts of B-2, niacinamide, B-5, and B-6). These injections are often needed for seniors and for people whose digestion and absorption are compromised.
- If your depression is PMS-related, take extra vitamin B-6 (200 to 600 milligrams a day) and magnesium (up to 800 milligrams a day, just on the premenstrual days).
- If you are using oral contraceptives, take extra B-6 (25 to 50 milligrams a day) and folic acid (400 to 800 micrograms a day).
- For biological depression (diagnosed by elevated midnight cortisol levels or a positive dexamethasone suppression test—see Chapter Eleven), try phosphatidyl serine (three to six 100- to 200-milligram capsules

daily, before 3:00 P.M.). The product is available as Seriphos by T. E. Neesby of Fresno, California.
- Chronic depression unrelieved by the above treatment can sometimes be helped by a free-form amino acid supplement individually formulated from an amino acid analysis of the blood (see CHRONIC FATIGUE SYNDROME).

HOMEOPATHIC REMEDIES

- Depression, with some of its most severe symptoms, will often respond to constitutional remedies prescribed by a homeopathic physician.

OTHER THERAPIES

- Regular exercise can stave off depression for some sufferers.
- Some sufferers may get relief from a cranial electric stimulator (see Chapter Twenty).

Diabetes Mellitus

Diabetes is a chronic condition characterized by an overabundance of blood sugar due to insufficient insulin production in the pancreas or inability of the body to use insulin. This accumulation of sugar leads to excessive thirst, excessive urination, fatigue, and other symptoms.

At its worst, diabetes can lead to an acute syndrome of lactic acidosis and death, but this complication has become increasingly uncommon due to the use of insulin injections. Known as "sugar diabetes," this condition is far more complex than the term implies. It is an involved metabolic disorder that can promote rapid development of plaque formation in the arteries. Individuals with poorly managed diabetes, consequently, are at least six times more likely to have a heart attack and stroke than are those without diabetes.

The seventh-leading cause of death in the United States, diabetes affects over 4 percent of the population. Its incidence is on the rise, with the estimated number of diabetics doubling every fifteen years. Ninety percent of those affected are non–insulin dependent, termed Type II, adult onset. Diabetics in this category make normal amounts of insulin. However, due to insulin resistance, they often require an oral medication to lower blood sugar levels. Ten percent are insulin dependent, called Type I, juvenile onset. People in this category do not make sufficient insulin and require insulin injections.

Conditions such as kidney failure (diabetic nephropathy), blindness (diabetic retinopathy), peripheral nerve damage (diabetic neuropathy), foot ulcers, and gangrene occur more often in diabetics because of arteriosclerotic problems.

Related or Underlying Causes

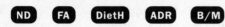

Like arteriosclerosis and other common degenerative diseases of westernized cultures, Type II, adult onset diabetes is largely a disorder of "wrong" living. Excesses of sugar, fat, refined grain products, and calories lacking in specific nutrients and fiber, along with insufficient exercise, stimulate the development of this disease. Chronic stress overload can easily induce insulin resistance and can be the primary trigger for the development of Type II diabetes.

Contrary to popular belief, you are not destined to develop diabetes simply because it runs in your family. You may be able to control or prevent this disease with an adequate understanding of the dietary and lifestyle risks involved.

If you already have Type II diabetes, you may be able to lessen or eradicate it. Even if you have Type I diabetes, you may be able to somewhat decrease your insulin requirement and, more importantly, delay cardiovascular complications.

Blood sugar level control, whether through nutrition, exercise, or medication, is crucial to minimizing such problems. In reversing or preventing this disease, you must relearn or readjust eating preferences and reward systems and habits of physical activity.

Treatment and Preventive Measures

DIETARY RECOMMENDATIONS

- Eat your meals at set times to maintain an even blood sugar level, whether this means three main meals a day or more frequent smaller meals. Follow meal timing and caloric guidelines prescribed by your doctor.
- Eat a fiber-rich, low-fat, low-sugar, whole-foods diet that emphasizes legumes, whole grains, and root and other fresh vegetables (see Chapter Three). Do not overeat. Eliminating sensitizing foods and chemicals may be required for some diabetics whose food allergies and chemical intolerances are affecting their pancreas, causing high blood sugar levels.
- A diet that derives 60 to 75 percent of its calories from complex carbohydrates, 15 to 20 percent from protein, and 10 to 15 percent from fat has proven successful for some diabetics, according to John Anderson, M.D., of the University of Kentucky. Such a diet is also useful in the treatment and prevention of arteriosclerosis, a primary goal of diabetic management.
- Research by Dr. Jukka Karjalainen suggests that cow's milk products may promote diabetes in genetically susceptible individuals. Avoidance of cow's milk products early in life may prevent the later onset of diabetes in such individuals. It may be wise to restrict feeding any cow's milk formula or cow's milk to infants and toddlers, particularly with any family history of diabetes. Older individuals with a family history of diabetes may do well to avoid cow's milk products as well.

NUTRITIONAL SUPPLEMENTS

- Take the following mineral supplements: chromium (200 to 1,000 micrograms a day), zinc (up to 30 milligrams a day), manganese (up to 20 milligrams a day), vanadium (up to 1,000 micrograms a day), and magnesium (up to 800 milligrams a day unless it causes diarrhea).
- Vitamin supplements are also vital for treatment. Take vitamins E (up to 800 I.U. daily), C (up to 3,000 milligrams or more a day—the more vitamin C you take, the less your insulin requirement may be). *Note: Vitamin C can falsely lower blood and urine glucose measurements, particularly if the device or test strips utilize Fehlings reagent. Those utilizing hexose oxidase are less susceptible to alteration by Vitamin C, and those using glucose oxidase are the least susceptible to alteration and are the preferred method.* Also take Vitamin A (up to 25,000 I.U., as well as 10,000 to 25,000 I.U. of beta-carotene), and D-3 (up to 400 I.U. daily). Vitamin D-3 is important if kidney involvement has developed, because the kidneys may not convert vitamin D-2 (ergocalciferol) to D-3 (its active form). Take pyridoxal-5 phosphate, the active form of B-6 (25 to 50 milligrams a day).
- Also take vitamin B-12 orally (up to 1,000 micrograms a day). If there are absorption problems, B-12 may need to be injected intramuscularly at least monthly. Nasal gel and sublingual forms are also available.
- Biotin has successfully reversed symptoms of peripheral neuropathy. Take 10 milligrams intramuscularly daily for six weeks, then three times weekly for six weeks, and 5 milligrams orally daily. A sizable oral dose (2,000 micrograms three times a day) may prevent and alleviate neuropathy without injections.
- Because, as a diabetic, you are a poor metabolic converter of essential fatty acids, you should take gamma linolenic acid (GLA) from borage oil *and* eicosapentaenoic acid (EPA) from fish oil (two capsules of each daily), available from Carlson's Laboratories of Arlington Heights, Illinois, or as Omegasyn from Biosyn of Boston.
- Lipoic acid, found in foods rich in B-complex vitamins, has been shown to prevent glycosylation, one of the primary destructive processes of diabetes. Supplementation with lipoic acid (one capsule three times a

day) may help prevent or slow diabetic complications. Try Thioctic by Cardiovascular Research of Concord, California.

- In addition to insulin, the pancreas produces digestive enzymes and bicarbonate to aid in the digestive process. According to William Philpott, M.D., and Dwight Kalita, Ph.D. (see their book, *Victory over Diabetes*), the digestive function of the pancreas often becomes disordered and depleted in diabetics. In addition to increased digestion and absorption, high blood sugar levels have been corrected, in part, by taking digestive enzymes.
- You might want to take a multiple vitamin/mineral preparation to avoid a nutritional imbalance. If your diabetes is linked to iron overload, you will need an iron-free multiple. A nutritionally oriented health professional may advise you to take extra nutrients beyond those that a multiple can offer.
- Fiber supplementation is also important, particularly if dietary compliance is not optimal. Use guar gum (5 grams per meal), pectin (10 grams per meal), or other fiber powder as an adjunct to a high-fiber diet. *Note: Fiber supplementation does not replace or provide all the benefits of high-complex carbohydrate or high-fiber foods.*

HERBAL REMEDIES
- Of most importance is gymnema sylvestre, an Ayurvedic herb that can significantly lower blood sugar levels. Take Bio Gymnema (up to three capsules three times a day), which contains gymnema sylvestre, pterocarpus marsupium, basil, momardica charantis, and neem, as well as biotin and chromium. Available from Interplexus of Kent, Washington. Monitor blood sugar levels carefully, since this may lower insulin or oral diabetes medication requirements.
- Bilberry, ginkgo biloba, pycnogenol, and hawthorn berry help protect arteries and prevent arteriosclerosis (see Chapter Nineteen). Ginkgo biloba and bilberry are specific to halting diabetic retinopathy and are found combined together with grape pip in Proanthanol by Allergy Research/Nutricology of San Leandro, California.
- Garlic and onions, whether cooked or raw, are known to lower blood sugar levels. (See Chapter Nineteen for information on their remarkable cardiovascular effects and other properties.)
- Quercetin is a flavonoid commonly used in treating diabetes as it inhibits aldose reductase, an enzyme involved in diabetic cataracts, retinopathy, and neuropathy. Dosage: 300 to 500 milligrams two or three times a day. Naringin, another flavonoid, also functions as an aldose reductase inhibitor. Dosage: 300 to 600 milligrams two or three times a day.
- Fenugreek seeds (defatted) can decrease blood sugar as well as insulin levels, total serum cholesterol, and

triglycerides. It can also increase HDL cholesterol. Diabetrol, by Cardiovascular Research of Concord, California, contains fenugreek in addition to several other important antidiabetic, blood sugar–stabilizing, and vascular protection agents.
- Crushed celery seed is an important factor in managing diabetes because of its ability to reduce blood sugar levels. Drink up to three cups of crushed celery seed tea in an infusion or take celery seed tincture as directed.
- Blueberry leaf tea can cut blood sugar levels, increase capillary integrity, inhibit free radicals, and improve venous tone. In France, it is successfully used to treat diabetic retinopathy.
- Bitter melon, also known as balsam pear, is a tropical vegetable with known blood sugar–lowering effects when the juice or the extract of the fruit is used.

OTHER THERAPIES
- Many diabetics are able to improve their glucose intolerance or eliminate the need for medication by reducing their weight (see OVERWEIGHT). Exercise helps control weight while lowering blood sugar levels and decreasing insulin needs. It also lowers cholesterol levels and helps prevent arteriosclerosis and heart attacks.
- Stress management plays an important role in the treatment of diabetes since uncontrolled and poorly managed tension and anxiety contribute to higher than normal levels of hormones (adrenaline, cortisol, growth hormone, and glucagon), which antagonize the effects of insulin. The stress response will cause elevations in blood sugar levels.
- Supplementation with small doses of pharmaceutical thyroid has helped delay many of the cardiovascular complications of diabetes, according to Broda Barnes, M.D., Ph.D. (see HYPOTHYROIDISM).

Diarrhea

Excessive evacuation of loose or watery stools that is more frequent than a person's normal bowel routine. Associated symptoms include fever, cramping, stomach pain, nausea, and thirst.

Related or Underlying Causes

For chronic diarrhea, test for intestinal toxicity and parasites (see PARASITES). Diarrhea may be caused by antibiotics or a sensitivity to a medication or a vitamin supplement even if it was once initially well tolerated. This can also occur if there is too much supplemental magnesium or vitamin C. Folic acid deficiency can cause chronic diarrhea, along with anxiety and other psychological and emotional symptoms. Chronic diarrhea will usually persist until the underlying conditions are remedied.

Acute diarrhea can be caused by bacterial toxins, such as food poisoning, or by a virus, such as stomach flu. Traveler's diarrhea is often triggered by exposure to bacteria and parasites. Though not usually serious, a three- to four-day bout of traveler's diarrhea can be quite uncomfortable and even painful.

Treatment and Preventive Measures

DIETARY RECOMMENDATIONS
- Drink plenty of fluids to avoid dehydration, particularly potassium-rich vegetable broth. If nausea is a problem, drink the water in which barley has been boiled, which is often tolerated when no other fluids will stay down.
- Limit food intake. If you get hungry, try small amounts of rice cream (see recipe in Chapter Five) and/or vegetable soup.
- If your diarrhea is antibiotic-related, try a moderate helping of plain active-culture yogurt once a day.

NUTRITIONAL SUPPLEMENTS
- Not recommended.

HERBAL REMEDIES
- Use cinnamon in tea (1 teaspoon per cup) or on food two or three times a day to slow the diarrhea. Carob powder can provide the same effect (1 teaspoon two or three times a day, in water).
- If you have cramps, try a strong combination tea of catnip, chamomile, and peppermint. Combination antidiarrhea homeopathic drops or tablets (available at health food stores) can also be useful for acute cramps and diarrhea (see CRAMPS, INTESTINAL).
- If you are nauseous, try gingerroot tea. If vomiting is a problem, you may be able to tolerate slippery elm tea.
- If your stomach is not too sensitive, try psyllium husk powder or another gentle bulk agent (1 teaspoon in a glass of water two or three times a day), which will help soak up extra water in the intestines.
- To treat or prevent traveler's diarrhea, try goldenseal, freeze-dried garlic or garlic oil preparations, and/or bitter orange or grapefruit seed extracts (one capsule of each remedy at least three times a day).

OTHER THERAPIES
- Take organisms favorable to the intestines, such as acidophilus/bifidus and/or *Saccharomyces boulardii*

supplements (one capsule of either or both, two or three times a day).
- If the diarrhea is caused by food poisoning or intestinal toxicity, take liquid bentonite (1 or 2 tablespoons). Add to 8 ounces of water. Mix and drink.

Note: Antibiotics or other medical intervention are needed if symptoms are severe or if the illness persists for more than several days.

Ear Infection and Earache

A viral or bacterial infection of either the external ear canal or the eardrum that usually causes pain. Other symptoms of an upper respiratory infection may be present.

Related or Underlying Causes

Recurrent ear infections, especially in children, are frequently caused by food allergies. If ear infections are predominantly one-sided, there may be cranial bone malalignment and pressure on the eustachian tube, the inside passageway that drains fluid from each ear. Consult an osteopathic or chiropractic physician trained in craniosacral therapy. This is especially important if there is a history of previous head injury or forceps or difficult delivery at birth (see COLDS).

Treatment and Preventive Measures

Antibiotics do not have to be the first choice. Many individuals, including children, can heal from an ear infection without medical intervention or complications. However, if the following home treatments do not bring relief in a reasonable amount of time, or if the illness seems severe, contact your doctor.

HERBAL REMEDIES
- Use olive oil with or without garlic, mullein, or calendula oil as ear drops several times daily if you are certain the eardrum is intact. Ear drops often make the pain subside within ten minutes. Herbally medicated ear drops are available from Eclectic Institute of Sandy, Oregon, or as Mullein Oil by Herb Pharm of Williams, Oregon. Before administering the ear drops, heat the bottle of oil in a pan of water until it is warm. Place a few drops on your wrist first to test the mixture's temperature.

OTHER THERAPIES
- Use a heating pad, hot water bottle, or warm wash-

cloth in front of and especially behind the earlobe and under the back of the jaw to bring relief and accelerate healing.

- For further treatment and preventive measures, see COLDS, FLU, SORE THROAT, AND COUGHS.

Eczema (Atopic Dermatitis)

An inflammation of the skin occurring in infants, children, adolescents, and adults, characterized by redness, swelling, and tiny fluid-filled blisters. The blisters may become oozing, scaly, crusting, and can sometimes harden into very thickened skin. Eczema is usually intensely itchy.

Related or Underlying Causes

From a conventional medical standpoint, eczema is generally considered an allergic disease, but it is unclear what triggers the allergy. From the perspective of nutritional medicine, eczema is often a manifestation of a food allergy. It may also be the result of an intestinal yeast overgrowth, intestinal toxicity, or a deficiency of essential fatty acids and zinc. Eczema-like lesions can sometimes be caused by contact with metals such as chrome and nickel. It can also be tied to emotional instability and chemical sensitivity.

Treatment and Preventive Measures

DIETARY RECOMMENDATIONS
- Follow an elimination diet to avoid allergy-triggering foods, and use the Candida-control diet if yeast is a factor.

NUTRITIONAL SUPPLEMENTS
- Take unrefined flaxseed oil (1 or 2 teaspoons a day), borage oil (one capsule two or three times a day), and zinc (30 milligrams a day).

HERBAL REMEDIES
- Take quercetin (300 to 500 milligrams two or three times a day), a bioflavonoid used to relieve many allergic conditions. It helps block the release of histamine.

Edema

See WATER RETENTION.

Endometriosis

Most common in childless women between the ages of thirty and forty, endometriosis occurs when bits of uterus lining grow beyond its usual region into the fallopian tubes, on the ovaries, on uterine ligaments, even on the intestines and other abdominal cavity structures. Complications arise when the abnormal uterine tissues become engorged with blood during a woman's monthly menstrual cycle. Scarring and adhesions can develop.

Although endometriosis can cause discomfort all month long, the worst symptoms usually appear during the menstrual period and can include severe period pain, excessive bleeding, diarrhea, nausea, and vomiting. Painful ovulation can also occur.

Endometriosis can result in painful intercourse and infertility.

Related or Underlying Causes

Controversy continues over the possible cause of this ailment. Some practitioners consider yeast overgrowth to be a contributing factor.

Treatment and Preventive Measures

CONVENTIONAL MEDICAL TREATMENT
- Treatment varies according to severity of condition. Danazol/Danocrine or birth control pills are commonly used to stem menstrual cycles and uterine pain. Danazol is a male hormone and pituitary gland suppressor that simulates menopause. Danocrine simulates pregnancy. Laparoscopic surgery is commonly performed to remove abnormal overgrowths of endometrial tissue.

DIETARY RECOMMENDATIONS
- A whole-foods diet is recommended. There have also been reports of significant improvements achieved with a macrobiotic diet regimen.
- Avoid sugar, fats, salt, caffeine, and dairy products.

NUTRITIONAL SUPPLEMENTS

- Take vitamin E (400 I.U. two or three times a day), vitamin C (up to 3,000 milligrams as directed), calcium (up to 2,000 milligrams a day during painful periods) with magnesium (up to 1,000 milligrams a day, or more if tolerated), flaxseed oil (1 or 2 teaspoons a day), and borage oil (one or two capsules three times a day providing 500 milligrams a day of gamma linolenic acid, the active ingredient).

HERBAL REMEDIES

- Plant estrogens can be used to diminish a woman's own estrogen effect, which may lessen endometriosis symptoms. Try dong quai (three to six capsules a day) or licorice root extract (¼ to ½ teaspoon dissolved in hot water twice a day), or solid extract of alfalfa (¼ to ½ teaspoon dissolved in hot water twice a day). *Note: Avoid alfalfa if there is a history of lupus.*
- Liver-enhancing herbs, which have been used successfully to treat this condition, are beet leaf, dandelion root, and black radish, often found together in lipotropic formulas available in health food stores (see Chapter Nine).

OTHER THERAPIES

- Use deep abdominal massage to increase lymph circulation and to break up tissue adhesion. Alternating hot and cold packs to the abdomen can also boost circulation.
- Castor oil packs to the abdomen should be tried nightly for at least a month.

Epilepsy

See SEIZURES.

Epstein-Barr Virus

See CHRONIC FATIGUE SYNDROME.

Fatigue

A state of abnormally low vitality ranging from mild tiredness to utter exhaustion. Fatigue usually serves as a signal of an underlying physical, mental, or emotional disorder. Contact your doctor for a physical exam and standard blood and other screening tests that may disclose anemia or another common reason for your fatigue.

Related or Underlying Causes

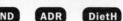

Look further to uncover other causes for your fatigue: excessive use of sugar, caffeine, and alcohol; hypothyroidism (see HYPOTHYROIDISM); poor digestion and assimilation; toxic colon; sluggish liver; heavy metals; hidden and chronic infections such as intestinal parasites (see PARASITES); or sinusitis (see SINUS INFECTION).

Other factors include depression, boredom, poor stress management, insufficient or excessive exercise, structural problems or chronic pain, insufficient or poor-quality sleep (see INSOMNIA), blocked energy or blocked acupuncture meridians, cigarette smoking (see SMOKING CESSATION), and use of marijuana or other illegal drugs. Some prescription drugs may cause fatigue. Consult with your practitioner for any adjustments in medication, if needed.

Fatigue may also result from excessive exposure to fluorescent lighting, video display computer terminal screens, and an excess of positive ions in the atmosphere.

Treatment and Preventive Measures

DIETARY RECOMMENDATIONS

- Avoid overeating and reduce use of sugar, caffeine, and alcohol.

NUTRITIONAL SUPPLEMENTS

- If a standard medical exam and tests fail to uncover the cause of your fatigue, you may need to find a nutritionally oriented doctor to help you uncover and treat any of the conditions discussed above.
- Take a high-potency B-complex formula (50 to 100 milligrams a day) or a daily multiple vitamin/mineral with at least 50 milligrams of the B vitamins.
- If digestive and assimilative capacities are impaired, you may require periodic intramuscular injections of vitamin B-12 (1,000 micrograms) and folic acid (2 milligrams) to help you regain your energy. You may also need injectable B complex (a formula containing 100 milligrams of vitamin B-1 and lesser amounts of the other Bs), or you may require a broader range of intravenous nutrients, as described under CHRONIC FATIGUE SYNDROME.

OTHER THERAPIES
- Get adequate exercise.
- Stop smoking and avoid use of marijuana or any other illegal drug.
- Get sufficient sleep (see INSOMNIA).

Fever Blisters

See COLD SORES.

Fibrocystic Breast Disease

Common among adult females, this disease develops when benign lumps, or fluid-filled cysts, form in the breasts. The cysts cause considerable pain, particularly during menstrual periods, but can be symptomatic any time of the month. Women with this condition were once thought to be more prone to breast cancer, but now this link is uncertain. However, diagnosis of breast cancer from mammograms is more difficult with this condition because of thickening and increased density of the breast tissue.

Related or Underlying Causes

Breast cysts have been linked to excessive caffeine intake, iodine deficiency, low thyroid status (see HYPOTHYROIDISM), and high estrogen state. A high estrogen state is frequently caused by a sluggish liver.

Treatment and Preventive Measures

DIETARY RECOMMENDATIONS
- Reduce or eliminate caffeine and all sources of methylxanthines (theobromine, theophylline): coffee, black tea, caffeinated soft drinks, chocolate, diet pills, and many pain pills (see Chapter 3). If you require some methylxanthine-containing medicine, such as theophylline for asthma, examine any underlying conditions (see ASTHMA) to see if alternative treatments could reduce the need for medication.
- A low-fat diet, particularly minimizing commercial meat and dairy products, will also decrease estrogen levels. Meat from organically raised animals or wild game and nonfat yogurt, organic preferred, will likely not increase estrogen levels.

NUTRITIONAL SUPPLEMENTS
- Take a B-complex supplement (25 to 50 milligrams a day) with extra B-6 (100 to 300 milligrams), especially premenstrually.
- Essential fatty acids can be helpful, such as flaxseed oil (1 or 2 teaspoons a day) and borage oil (one or two capsules three times a day). In addition to their other functions, essential fatty acids make iodine more easily absorbed by the body.
- Take vitamin E (800 I.U. daily).
- Take magnesium (400 to 800 milligrams a day).
- Supplemental iodine (200 to 300 milligrams a day) should be taken under a physician's supervision. Such high doses are available only by prescription (saturated solution of potassium iodide—SSKI) and should be reserved for active disease. After improvement of symptoms, lower doses of SSKI are recommended. For unremitting forms of this condition, intravaginal application of iodine, along with intravenous magnesium, is often effective.
- For preventive purposes, the iodine in a diet rich in seafood and sea vegetables (nori, wakame, kombu, hijiki, etc., available in health food stores) should suffice. Many multiple vitamin/mineral formulas contain 200 micrograms of iodine. Kelp has only 150 micrograms of iodine per tablet, making it useful for preventive purposes but not usually effective for treatment of active disease. Dulse tablets are also a useful source of iodine (use up to three daily).

OTHER THERAPIES
- Work on improving liver function (see PREMENSTRUAL SYNDROME and Chapter Nine).

   Note: All of the above measures used to treat or prevent fibrocystic breast disease may also apply to the prevention of breast cancer.

Fibroids

Fibroid tumors, or benign growths in the wall of the uterus, occur in over 40 percent of American women between the ages of thirty-five and forty-five. The range of symptoms for fibroids can vary with size and location. Many smaller fibroid tumors are often symptomless, while larger ones can cause abdominal pressure, urinary or bowel symptoms, excessive uterine bleeding during or between menses, or painful intercourse. During pregnancy, location of the tumor can become a critical factor if it obstructs delivery or interferes with fetal development.

Related or Underlying Causes

According to the conventional medical view, there is no known cause, although stimulation by estrogen is a major contributing component. (The estrogen content in birth control pills may even be a factor.) Dr. Christine Northrup, a board-certified obstetrician-gynecologist, links a diet high in meat, sugar, and milk products, especially cheese and ice cream, to the development of fibroid tumors. Such a diet is a source of additional estrogen. In addition, dairy products, according to Chinese medicine, are expansive "yin" foods in nature and may contribute to tumor growth.

Treatment and Preventive Measures

CONVENTIONAL MEDICAL TREATMENT

- Surgery, contrary to conventional medicine protocols, may not be the only option. However, significant complications from fibroids may necessitate surgery. Most small fibroids do not need treatment and usually shrink after the onset of menopause, when they are no longer stimulated by estrogen. A sizable number of the larger fibroids contract in size with menopause, and symptoms can lessen greatly.

DIETARY RECOMMENDATIONS

- Avoid milk products and sugar, along with excessive fruit consumption and alcohol. All of these items are very "yin." Steer your diet toward vegetarianism. Following a macrobiotic diet or at least minimizing excesses of extreme "yin" foods (see Chapter Four) may help shrink fibroids.
- To reduce estrogen, restrict dietary saturated fat from commercial meat and poultry. Small amounts of very lean organic meat and poultry can be eaten. A minimal amount of nonfat milk products, organic if possible, may be acceptable.
- Stimulate metabolic breakdown of estrogen by enhancing liver function. Take one tablet of lipotropic factors at each meal. Also, follow the Liver Flush and Purifying Diet and the Ultra Clear program, as discussed in Chapter Nine.
- Avoid frequently eating raw cruciferous vegetables, such as broccoli, cauliflower, kale, cabbage, and brussels sprouts, as they antagonize the thyroid. Thyroid function enhances the metabolic functioning of the liver and has somewhat antagonistic effects itself on estrogen. Test your thyroid function (see HYPOTHY-ROIDISM). Substitute kelp or dulse as sources of iodine for thyroid support.

HERBAL REMEDIES

- To help with excessive bleeding, a combination trillium and viburnum tincture (fifteen to twenty-five drops three or four times a day) is often very effective.
- Drinking shepherd's purse tea (up to three or four cups a day) may also help to curtail bleeding.

OTHER THERAPIES

- Vaginal drawing packs, often prescribed by naturopathic physicians, may help reduce the size of the fibroid if the growth is on the inner aspect of the uterine cavity. A constitutional homeopathic remedy should also be tried for a fibroid in any location.
- Dr. Northrup feels that, in addition to diet, fibroids may be related to psychological ambivalence, anger, or other emotions that may be creating energy blockages in the area of the uterus. Therefore, counseling, hypnosis, or other approaches that may uncover and help you resolve emotional blocks may be required.

Note: Excessive vaginal bleeding can be from other causes, such as uterine or other cancers. Periodic gynecological exams are important whether or not you have abnormal bleeding.

If you need to have surgery, see if your doctor can remove only the fibroids and leave the uterus. Also, depending on the location and size of the fibroids, a laparoscopic or vaginal procedure can be done, avoiding a major abdominal incision.

Fibromyalgia (Fibrositis)

A condition characterized primarily by widespread musculoskeletal pain with specific tender points, fatigue, and sleep disturbance. Other symptoms include irritability, poor memory and concentration, headaches, dizziness, depression, tingling of the extremities, and irritable bowel complaints. It occurs in women ten times more often than in men and affects individuals most frequently between the ages of twenty and fifty-five.

Blood tests and X rays normally do not reveal any specific abnormality. The exclusion of rheumatoid arthritis, lupus, and other conditions that can cause similar pain and fatigue is also part of the diagnostic process. The diagnosis is made on the basis of symptoms (pain in all four quadrants of the body that has lasted three or more months, and tenderness in at least eleven of the eighteen specified "tender points"). Your local Arthritis Foundation chapter can send you a free booklet.

Some practitioners consider fibromyalgia a variant of chronic fatigue syndrome (see CHRONIC FATIGUE SYNDROME). Only in recent years have doctors gained familiarity with this syndrome. It is not unusual for individuals to go from doctor to doctor for years, eluding a correct diagnosis of their symptoms.

Related or Underlying Causes

Although there is no known cause, as with chronic fatigue syndrome, it is useful to assess fibromyalgia patients for food allergy, intestinal yeast overgrowth, nutritional deficiencies, and adrenal exhaustion. Such a comprehensive perspective usually brings the best results. Inadequate amounts of magnesium, malic acid, and other nutrients fueling energy production may also be a factor.

Treatment and Preventive Measures

CONVENTIONAL MEDICAL TREATMENT

- Conventional medical treatment usually includes antidepressant medications, which reduce pain and improve sleep.
- Several promising theories have surfaced that have led to new treatments and encouraging results for this illness. One theory suggests that fibromyalgia pain and fatigue are caused by metabolic shutdown in muscle cells in localized areas. An offshoot of this theory suggests that the metabolic shutdown is caused by phosphate or uric acid accumulations. Treatment with standard gout medications and other drugs that increase output of uric acid and phosphate (Probenecid, Sulfinpyrazone, and Robinul) have brought significant improvement in some individuals. Guaifenesin, a drug commonly used for its mucus thinning and expectorant effect, is one of the more recent medications found to boost urinary uric acid levels and help fibromyalgia patients.

NUTRITIONAL SUPPLEMENTS

- The following key nutritional components have lessened pain and increased energy for fibromyalgia patients: malic acid (1,200 to 2,400 milligrams) with magnesium (300 to 600 milligrams a day), available in a combination formula, with vitamin B-1 and other synergistic factors, as Fibroplex from Metagenics of San Clemente, California, or as Optimox of Torrance, California.
- Periodic intravenous vitamin and mineral injections often bring significant relief (see CHRONIC FATIGUE SYNDROME). You may require three or four injections over a period of two weeks before improvement is seen.

OTHER THERAPIES

- Walking, yoga, tai chi, and other forms of exercise have been extremely helpful.
- Some patients have found relief from trigger point injections, hydrotherapy, massage therapy, and electrostimulation.
- Measures to improve sleep are paramount (see INSOMNIA).

Fissure (Anal)

A split that occurs in the skin of the rectum near the anal sphincter. In many cases, the split may be aggravated and start to bleed during a bowel movement. Sharp pain may sometimes result. Stools may be hard and streaked with blood. This condition is most common after age thirty-five.

Related and Underlying Causes

Anal fissures are often caused by straining to expel hardened, difficult stools. A fiber-poor diet with excesses of white flour, white rice, cheese, junk foods, sugar, dairy products, and meat and other flesh foods is a contributing factor that promotes constipation and painful elimination. Constipation and straining can also be a result of food allergy, intestinal yeast overgrowth, intestinal parasites such as *Giardia*, insufficient hydrochloric acid secretion from the stomach, and low thyroid status.

Treatment and Preventive Measures

DIETARY RECOMMENDATIONS

- Change your diet to include fresh fruits, vegetables, whole grains, and legumes. Add fiber supplements, such as psyllium husk, oat bran, pectin, and/or flaxseed powder, to keep stools soft and to minimize straining during elimination. Drink plenty of water (four to six large glasses daily).

DETOXIFICATION PROGRAM

- A fluid fast, from seven to ten days, may be needed to allow fissures time to heal. Passage of even normal stools can stretch injured tissues, causing pain and bleeding. Use daily enemas or saltwater purges with the fast (see Chapter Eighteen).

NUTRITIONAL SUPPLEMENTS

- Adequate protein is essential for tissue healing. A free-form amino acid supplement such as Aminoplex, by Tyson and Associates of Hawthorne, California, will be supportive. Take a B-complex vitamin (up to 50 milligrams a day) or a multiple vitamin/mineral with this amount of Bs. Add zinc citrate (up to 30 milligrams a day) if your multiple has less than this amount. Take extra vitamin C (up to 1,000 milligrams two or three times a day).

OTHER THERAPIES

- Use a rectal suppository every twelve hours (Calendula and vitamin A by Earth's Harvest of Gresham, Oregon).

Flu

See COLD, FLU, SORE THROAT, AND COUGH.

Flu (Chronic)

See CHRONIC FATIGUE SYNDROME.

Flu (Stomach)

See CRAMPS, INTESTINAL, and DIARRHEA.

Folliculitis

A skin eruption that appears as large pimples or small boils.

Related or Underlying Causes

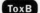

Usually considered to be a bacterial infection, folliculitis can be viewed as toxins attempting to exit the body through the skin. Occasionally, a yeast condition, a food allergy/intolerance, or heavy metals may be contributing factors.

Treatment and Preventive Measures

Treatment is focused on enhancing elimination routes and purifying the blood.

DIETARY RECOMMENDATIONS

- Reduce consumption of junk foods and other dietary hazards, particularly sugar.
- Cleanse the bowels and liver. Switch to a high-fiber diet.
- Drink plenty of liquids between meals, particularly water.

NUTRITIONAL SUPPLEMENTS

- Take vitamin C (1,000 milligrams three times a day) and zinc (30 milligrams a day).

HERBAL REMEDIES

- Include some blood-purifying teas, such as echinacea, burdock root, and red clover (up to three or four cups a day), or take in capsule form (one or two capsules three or four times a day).
- Drink green juice or some other form of chlorophyll.

OTHER THERAPIES

- Skin brush regularly (see Chapter Eighteen). Take Epsom salt baths and saunas.

Fungus

Fungal growths most often appear on the feet (athlete's foot), in the groin, under breasts, and in abdominal folds. Although fungi prefer these dark, warm, and generally moist areas, they can grow on the scalp, arms, or under finger- or toenails. Fungus or yeast infections are commonly seen as red spots, red circles (ringworm), or as a generally inflamed area. They are frequently itchy and sometimes painful. A bacterial infection can occur if scratched excessively.

Related or Underlying Causes

Fungal infections of the skin may be related to intestinal yeast overgrowth. They may appear without apparent cause or in persons with depressed immune systems, particularly following extended use of antibiotics.

Treatment and Preventive Measures

DIETARY RECOMMENDATIONS

- For any skin fungus, reduce sweets. This makes the environment less favorable for the yeast.
- Eat a whole-foods diet to provide the nutrients necessary for maintaining immune function and healing.

NUTRITIONAL SUPPLEMENTS

- Take vitamin C (1,000 milligrams up to three times a day) and zinc (30 milligrams a day).

HERBAL REMEDIES

- Use a tea tree oil or meleluca topical preparation as directed, with a cineole level well below 15 percent so it is not caustic and a terpienne 4-OL level above 30 percent to ensure its effectiveness.
- Use topical preparations of grapefruit or citrus seed extract for skin fungus twice a day. The liquid preparations can be applied under the nails for fungi in this location (two or three times a day).
- Garlic (a clove eaten raw or one or two garlic tablets or capsules with meals) provides an internal antifungal effect that may deter skin fungi.
- See Chapter Twelve for more antifungal herbs.

OTHER THERAPIES

- For athlete's foot, avoid prolonged wear of gym shoes and other footgear that does not breathe well. Wear open-toed shoes or sandals when possible or no shoes at all. Use 100 percent cotton socks. Be sure to dry feet thoroughly after bathing and before putting on socks and shoes. Expose the affected area to the air and sunlight when possible. Walking in hot, dry sand is very helpful.
- For a skin fungus, apply a vinegar solution several times a day. Dilute with water for more sensitive areas.
- If symptoms persist or if none of the above treatments work effectively, use an over-the-counter or prescription antifungal agent. Consult your doctor.

Gallstones

Gallstones consist of pebble-like masses, usually formed from cholesterol and other components of bile. They can remain "silent" in the gallbladder, or they can cause severe pain and illness when they obstruct one of the bile ducts or the pancreatic duct. Such attacks occur characteristically several hours after a fatty meal.

Related or Underlying Causes

Gallstones are caused by chemical imbalances in the bile due to faulty liver metabolism. Such abnormalities are often triggered by a high-fat, low-fiber, high-sugar, refined diet. Interestingly, prolonged crash low-fat diets, especially those medically supervised programs where one consumes only liquid meal replacements, can cause gallstones. Gallstones can be related to food allergy as well, particularly egg intolerance. Obesity may also play a role.

Treatment and Preventive Measures

CONVENTIONAL MEDICAL TREATMENT

- If a nutritional approach is inadequate, ask your doctor about Actigall, a pharmaceutical medication that can dissolve some types of gallstones.
- If tests do not indicate a diseased gallbladder, ask your doctor about lithotripsy, a shockwave procedure that shatters gallstones without a surgical incision. Consider this as an alternative to conventional surgery to remove the gallbladder. With the shockwave method, stones may recur.
- If this procedure is not feasible, ask if laparoscopic gallbladder removal can be performed instead of a major abdominal incision.

DIETARY RECOMMENDATIONS

- Follow a high-complex, high-fiber, low-fat, low-sugar diet.

DETOXIFICATION PROGRAM

- Periodically use the Liver Flush and Purifying Diet.

NUTRITIONAL SUPPLEMENTS

- Take a moderate or high-potency multiple vitamin/ mineral daily.
- Take choline (250 to 350 milligrams), methionine (250 to 350 milligrams), and inositol (25 to 100 milligrams) three times a day with meals. These are often combined in a lipotropic factors supplement.

HERBAL REMEDIES

- For an acute attack, take wild yam tincture (fifteen drops every twenty minutes in a glass of warm water). Lobelia tincture (three or four drops orally with wild yam) may also be helpful. *Note: Excessive lobelia may cause nausea and vomiting.*
- Use a castor oil pack over the liver.

- To help normalize liver metabolism to produce more balanced bile, use beet leaves, dandelion root, black radish, fringe tree, celandine, and other herbs that are often combined in a lipotropic factors supplement (one tablet three times a day with meals).

OTHER THERAPIES

- For an acute attack, a coffee enema can often relax the bile duct and ease pain. Use a strong cup of fresh brewed or dripped (not instant) caffeinated coffee. Dilute to at least 1 pint and retain for twenty to thirty minutes. Whether this measure is effective or not, notify your doctor.

Gastritis

See ULCERS.

Gingivitis

See PERIODONTAL DISEASE.

Gum Problems

See PERIODONTAL DISEASE.

Hay Fever

Hay fever, an allergic reaction to pollens, usually consists of itchy, watery eyes, sneezing, and a runny nose. Although it commonly strikes in the spring and summer months, some sufferers are also afflicted in the fall when mold counts are higher.

Related or Underlying Causes

 FA **DietH** **ND** **ToxB**

Hay fever occurs when the body reacts excessively to grass, pollen, molds, spores, and fumes. Other hay fever–type triggers include cigarette smoke, dust, dust mites, fur, and feathers. Heredity can also play a role, since there can be a predisposition to hay fever among family members.

Treatment and Preventive Measures

DIETARY RECOMMENDATIONS

- Eliminate foods to which you may be allergic or intolerant. Avoid milk products for several weeks. By decreasing some of your total allergic load, your tolerance for inhalants may be heightened and hay fever symptoms reduced without necessarily reducing exposure to pollens or using antiallergy remedies.

DETOXIFICATION PROGRAMS

- Fasting brings relief to some hay fever sufferers, and the benefits can last even after normal eating resumes.

NUTRITIONAL SUPPLEMENTS

- Buffered vitamin C (1,000 to 2,000 milligrams three times a day).
- Vitamin A (up to 25,000 I.U. daily).
- Vitamin B-5, or pantothenic acid (500 to 1,000 milligrams two or three times a day).

HERBAL REMEDIES

- Take Allerplex I (one to three capsules three or four times a day), made with celandine, dandelion root, fenugreek seed, capsicum, thyme leaf, and violet leaf. Available from Herb Technology, Khalsa Center, Seattle.
- Take freeze-dried nettles tablets (one or two tablets three or four times a day). Available as Urtica Dioca from Eclectic Institute of Sandy, Oregon, and as Pollenase from Ecological Formulas of Concord, California.
- Antiallergy herbal combination formulas containing ephedra may also be effective.
- Take quercetin (one or two 300- to 500-milligram capsules three or four times a day). Some preparations of quercetin contain bromelain and vitamin C.
- For eye symptoms, a tincture of eyebright (five to fifteen drops three or four times a day), especially mixed with belladonna tincture, may bring dramatic relief. The mixture should be four parts eyebright to one part belladonna. *Warning: Belladonna tincture can be toxic in large doses, so use only under the supervision of a naturopathic or nutritionally oriented physician.*

HOMEOPATHIC REMEDIES

- Try combination homeopathic tablets or drops specific for hay fever, available in many health food stores. Individualizing your remedy may bring the best results (see Chapter Twenty-one).

Headaches

The simple tension headache is pain associated with constricted muscles in the head and neck, and congested blood vessels. It can be felt in the temples, the forehead, the crown, or the base of the skull. As the most common health complaint, it may last a few hours or a whole day. The migraine headache, far more debilitating, is associated with dilation of cerebral blood vessels, causing throbbing or sharp pain, usually on one side of the head. It is often associated with nausea, vomiting, increased sensitivity to light, noise, and movement. A migraine is usually preceded by visual disturbances and may last four to seventy-two hours. Cluster headaches can often trigger intense pain behind one eye, last an entire day, and occur daily for a period of several weeks. There may be a several-month interval of relief before the next cluster strikes.

Your headaches may not fall exactly in these or other official headache classifications. They may have features of several types.

Related or Underlying Causes

Although the headaches described above may seem to be distinct entities, they often share many common contributing causes: stress, anxiety, depression, generalized fatigue, eyestrain, lack of sleep, insufficient or excessive exercise, and overwork. Check for sinus allergies (see HAY FEVER), sinus infection, ear infection, and tooth abscess, even a "successful" root canal. Check also for structural causes: dental stress (temporomandibular joint dysfunction), spinal, cranial, and first rib malalignments; muscle tension; poor digestion; constipation; hypoglycemia; low adrenal function; and heavy metals and chemical hypersensitivity. Also look for hypothyroidism (see HYPOTHYROIDISM); premenstrual syndrome (if headaches are at that time of the month— see PREMENSTRUAL SYNDROME); vitamin A overdosing; and medication side effects, overdoses, or interactions. High blood pressure, carbon monoxide exposure, cerebral aneurysm, and brain tumor are other causes. Fifty percent of headaches are related to stress.

Migraine headaches are commonly triggered by food allergy/intolerance, preservatives and additives, and Candida overgrowth, although other types of headaches

could be related to these causes. Sensitivity specifically to tyramine-containing foods needs to be considered (see "Dietary Recommendations" below).

Treatment and Preventive Measures

CONVENTIONAL MEDICAL TREATMENT
- Over-the-counter remedies such as aspirin, acetaminophen, and ibuprofen are often temporarily effective for relieving simple or tension headaches. Over-the-counter decongestants combined with analgesics will often be temporarily effective for sinus headaches. For migraines, vasoconstrictor medications or over-the-counter or prescription analgesics may be helpful if taken immediately at onset of attack. A relatively new vasoconstrictor, sumatriptan (Imitrex™), is gaining recognition for giving sufferers acute relief when most other drugs have failed. It is administered by self-injection. Antidepressants, beta-blockers, and blood pressure medications are often prescribed to help prevent migraines.

DIETARY RECOMMENDATIONS
- Follow the whole-foods diet outlined for hypoglycemia. Depending on whether or not you have food allergies, you may need to modify this diet. Follow the elimination diet to identify food allergies.
- Avoid tyramine-containing foods, such as aged cheeses; pickled herring; fermented sausages, such as pepperoni, salami, summer sausage, and bologna; overripe fruits and vegetables, especially avocados and canned figs; any meat, fish, or dairy products left unrefrigerated (causing fermentation); red wine, particularly Chianti; sherry; and vinegar, especially red wine vinegar.

NUTRITIONAL SUPPLEMENTS
- Because most headaches have a stress component, the following nutrients may be beneficial: vitamin C (1,000 milligrams two or three times a day), B complex (50 milligrams one or two times a day), extra B-5 (pantothenic acid, 500 milligrams twice a day), extra B-3 (the niacinamide form, 500 to 1,000 milligrams twice a day—see Chapter Three for precautions), calcium (up to 800 milligrams a day), and magnesium (up to 800 milligrams a day). For more discussion, as well as a list of helpful amino acids, see Chapter Ten.

HERBAL REMEDIES
- Take feverfew to prevent migraines (one or two capsules three times a day).
- Valerian, a well-known herbal sedative, can relieve simple or tension headaches. Take alone or combined with such synergistic-acting herbs as pas-

sionflower, skullcap, and hops (three or four capsules taken together). If no relief occurs within one hour, repeat the dose.

- White willow bark, one of the original plant sources for aspirin before it was chemically synthesized, can be taken as a strong tea (up to 3 cups a day) or in capsule form (two or three capsules three or four times a day). Discontinue use if not helpful within a day. As with aspirin, this herb can be toxic with excessive or prolonged use. Consult a naturopathic physician or qualified herbalist.

HOMEOPATHIC REMEDIES

- Take combination homeopathic medicines formulated for headaches; these are available in health food stores. Individualizing your remedy may bring the best results.

OTHER THERAPIES

- Headaches of all varieties can often be treated successfully with acupressure or shiatsu. While you are seated, have a friend apply pressure with a thumb under the base of your skull on the outside of the muscle that runs along the left side of the spinal column. You can feel a slight indentation. Apply enough thumb pressure to cause some discomfort. This pressure point is generally very tender anyway. Your friend's other hand should be placed gently on your forehead. After five or six slow, deep breaths, have your friend switch hands and apply pressure to the same point on the other side of the neck, with the other hand gently on the forehead. If possible, lie down and have someone cradle your neck and head in their hands while you take slow, deep breaths. This may bring headache relief as well.
- Follow some of the breathing and relaxation exercises outlined in Chapter Fifteen.
- For temporary relief, take a hot water footbath while applying a cold compress to your head and/or to the back of your neck.
- Massage therapy and acupuncture can both be extremely helpful for headache relief and prevention.

Heart Attack (Myocardial Infarction)

A condition in which the heart muscle suffers an acute starvation of oxygen from a sudden blockage of blood flow through one or more of the coronary arteries.

It is usually associated with chest pain, often heavy in nature, sometimes radiating to the neck and shoulders or down the arm, often on the left side. Shortness of breath, sweating, nausea, light-headedness, and severe weakness are also common. Frequently, the only symptom is sudden collapse and death from ventricular fibrillation, an associated heart rhythm disturbance.

Heart attacks claimed the lives of nearly 500,000 Americans in 1993. They have been the number one killer in this country for over a half century.

Related or Underlying Causes

(DietH) (ND) (B/M) (ToxB) (SL) (ADR)

The traditional risk factors for heart attack are cigarette smoking, high blood pressure, obesity, diabetes, being male and over forty years of age, a family history of heart disease, a diet high in saturated fat, and elevated LDL cholesterol and lowered HDL cholesterol blood levels. A fast pace of living, a lack of exercise, and a "Type A" personality characterized by frequent anger, hostility, and time pressures have also been correlated to an increased incidence of heart attack. The more of these factors present, the higher the risk.

There is a general consensus that arteriosclerosis (plaque-congested arteries) is a primary culprit for heart attack risk. Although arteriosclerosis causes diminished blood flow and oxygen to the heart muscle, plaque alone rarely precipitates a heart attack. In fact, plaque development is a gradual process that often triggers the development of new arteries that are stimulated to grow and bypass the diseased sections. A blood clot (a coronary thrombosis) or a coronary artery spasm is most often the final event closing off a coronary artery, whether or not it is diseased with plaque. Heart attacks occur more often in an individual with significant coronary artery plaque. However, they occur also in those without much plaque or even in those without high cholesterol levels.

Other uncommonly publicized causes of heart attacks or related conditions include inefficient heart muscle metabolism, an abnormal heart rhythm coupled with poor oxygen-carrying capacity of the blood.

An abnormal tendency to form blood clots in the arteries occurs from factors that make platelets (specific white blood cells) too sticky, increasing their ability to aggregate. Consuming large amounts of processed, damaged vegetable oils will cause the formation of chemicals unfavorable to healthy platelet creation. (See "Dietary Fats," Chapter Three.) Deficiencies of vitamin C, vitamin E, and magnesium directly increase platelet adhesiveness, as does the consumption of excess sugar and the lack of physical exercise.

Magnesium deficiency alone can render an individual more susceptible to coronary artery spasm. It may be the single most important nutrient deficiency responsible for abnormal heart rhythms. It will also render the heart much more susceptible to dangerous rhythms brought on by stress or exercise-induced adrenaline level increases. Magnesium deficiency relates to inefficient heart muscle metabolism. Deficiencies of copper, selenium, coenzyme Q-10, L-carnitine, and vitamin B-6 will also impair function and metabolism of the heart muscle. The less efficient its metabolism, the less resistant it will be to injury and to temporary decreases in oxygen. Inefficient heart metabolism also increases the chances for symptoms of angina (chest pain) or a more severe heart attack.

Insufficient vitamin E levels decrease the oxygen-carrying capacity of the blood (so does iron deficiency, which is not as common). Low vitamin E status correlates more strongly with death from heart attack than any of the traditional risk factors. Low beta-carotene and vitamin C levels make this correlation even stronger.

Treatment and Preventive Measures

CONVENTIONAL MEDICAL TREATMENT

- For symptoms suggestive of a heart attack, particularly with multiple risk factors or a previous history of heart attack, seek immediate medical care. The sooner treatment is started, the better the chances for survival. In fact, a coronary thrombosis can be dissolved and blood flow and vitality restored to the affected section of heart muscle, especially if treated within six hours of the onset, although advantages have been documented up to twenty-four hours. Special clot-dissolving enzymes can be injected right at the site of the clot through X ray–guided wire tubes (angiographically threaded catheters).
- Treat high blood pressure, diabetes, obesity, and hypothyroidism, if indicated. Eliminate cigarette smoking. If arteriosclerosis is a primary cause of a heart attack, consider chelation therapy (see ARTERIOSCLEROSIS).

DIETARY RECOMMENDATIONS

- For prevention and maintenance, follow the recommendations given under ARTERIOSCLEROSIS and CHOLESTEROL, HIGH.

DETOXIFICATION PROGRAMS

- Follow the recommendations given under CHOLESTEROL, HIGH.

NUTRITIONAL SUPPLEMENTS

- Take vitamins C, E, B-3, B-6, and beta-carotene, the minerals magnesium, copper, and selenium, and flaxseed oil, as recommended under ARTERIOSCLEROSIS.
- Coenzyme Q-10 (30 to 60 milligrams twice a day),

taurine (up to 1,000 milligrams a day), and L-carnitine (up to 1,000 milligrams a day) can provide additional protection. Heart failure, angina pectoris, and high blood pressure may require higher doses.

As soon as possible after a heart attack, during the acute phase, intravenous magnesium (500 to 1,000 milligrams daily for at least five days) and L-carnitine (1,000 milligrams four times a day taken orally for six to twelve months) have been shown to significantly reduce mortality. L-carnitine strengthens the heartbeat, lowers blood pressure, and favorably affects cholesterol ratios.

HERBAL REMEDIES

- Use hawthorn berry, ginkgo biloba, garlic, onions, catechin, and quercetin, as discussed in ARTERIOSCLEROSIS and Chapter Nineteen.

OTHER THERAPIES

- Follow a regular exercise program and develop relaxation and stress management skills, as discussed under ARTERIOSCLEROSIS.

Heartburn

A hot, burning, or acid sensation in the upper abdomen or lower chest usually occurring shortly after a meal. It can last up to several hours.

Related or Underlying Causes

Heartburn can be caused by both insufficient and excessive amounts of stomach acid. Improper food combining or eating excessive amounts can be a cause. Also, check for yeast overgrowth and possible bacterial infection, helicobacter pylori (see Chapter Seven). Anxiety and excessive fatigue can contribute to this ailment. Although the discomfort of a peptic ulcer is usually improved by eating, an ulcer can still trigger heartburn after meals. A defect or weakness in the diaphragm may allow a portion of the stomach to slip up into the chest cavity (a hiatal hernia), where its acid can easily flow back into the esophagus, causing heartburn.

Treatment and Preventive Measures

DIETARY RECOMMENDATIONS

- Restrict acidic, irritating, and difficult-to-digest foods:

fried foods, red meat, citrus fruits and juices, spicy foods, tomatoes and tomato sauce, and coffee.

- Follow the food-combining recommendations discussed in Chapter Seven.
- At the onset of an attack, drink a glass of warm water with the juice of half a lemon. (Although lemon is citrus and initially acidic, it is classified as an alkaline ash food.)

NUTRITIONAL SUPPLEMENTS

- Over-the-counter calcium carbonate tablets are usually very effective (chew one to four as needed). Be certain there is no aluminum in the ingredient list.
- Hydrochloric acid with pepsin may be an effective supplement if low stomach acid is the underlying cause.

HERBAL REMEDIES

- Soothe the stomach using aloe vera juice (1 or 2 ounces) or gel (1 or 2 tablespoons three or four times a day or as needed).
- Deglycerrhizinated licorice root (DGL) can also be an effective choice for combating heartburn. Gastro Relief (one to four tablets chewed as needed) by Phyto Pharmica/Enzymatic Therapy of Green Bay, Wisconsin, has DGL mixed with calcium carbonate.
- Try a combination tea brewed strongly (1 teaspoon of each of the following herbs steeped in 1 cup of water): slippery elm, plantain, and marshmallow root. Or take two to four capsules containing these herbs as needed. GI Encap from Thorne Research of Sandpoint, Idaho.
- Try a combination mixture, Glyconda from Eclectic Institute of Sandy, Oregon, which contains goldenseal, rhubarb, cinnamon, potassium bicarbonate, and peppermint oil.
- Try peppermint or other mint tea brewed strongly or a combination herbal tea or capsule formulated for stomachache or digestion. (See the herbal combination formulas for stomachache at the end of Chapter Nineteen.)

HOMEOPATHIC REMEDIES

- Try over-the-counter combinations specific for heartburn, or individualize with single remedies.

Heart Failure (Congestive Heart Failure)

A weakening of the heart muscle, decreasing its ability to pump blood effectively, resulting in an insufficient blood flow to vital organs. Symptoms include: shortness of breath, edema (water retention), fatigue, enlarged heart, and diminished kidney function.

Related or Underlying Causes

 ND DietH

The causes of heart failure are many: high blood pressure, clogged coronary (heart) arteries (see ARTERIOSCLEROSIS), previous damage to the heart muscle from a heart attack or viral infection, and insufficient nutrients for optimal heart function.

According to Mathias Rath, M.D., former Director of Cardiovascular Research at the Linus Pauling Institute, this condition is currently on the rise, striking three times more people than just twenty years ago. One patient out of every two dies from this condition five years after diagnosis, and eight to nine out of ten die ten years after diagnosis. This occurs despite new medical advances in heart medicines and bypass and transplant surgeries.

Treatment and Preventive Measures

CONVENTIONAL MEDICAL TREATMENT

The following pharmaceuticals are often prescribed:

- Digitalis, to strengthen the heartbeat (Digoxin, Lanoxin).
- Angiotension-converting enzyme inhibitors to lower blood pressure (Accupril, Capoten, Prinivil, Vasotec, Zestril).
- Diuretics to lower blood pressure.

DIETARY RECOMMENDATIONS

- Follow a low-fat, high-fiber, predominantly vegetarian diet, as discussed under ARTERIOSCLEROSIS.

NUTRITIONAL SUPPLEMENTS

With such a poor prognosis, standard drug treatment is obviously inadequate, leading many researchers to believe that nutrient deficiency is an important factor and nutrient supplementation an effective treatment.

- The most important nutrients are carnitine (up to 1,000 milligrams three or four times a day), coenzyme Q-10 (10 to 30 milligrams two or three times a day), magnesium (400 to 800 milligrams a day), vitamin C (1,000 milligrams two or three times a day), selenium (200 micrograms a day), B complex (50 milligrams a day), taurine (up to 3,000 milligrams a day), and vitamin E (800 I.U. daily). *Note: It may not be necessary to use the highest doses recommended for each nutrient listed above if they are used together. A combined nutrient approach may reduce the requirement for any one nutrient.*

HERBAL REMEDIES

- Take hawthorn berry (¼ teaspoon of solid extract two or three times a day), which has a centuries-old reputation as one of the foremost tonics for the heart. It strengthens the heartbeat and has a normalizing effect on the rhythm (see Chapter Nineteen).
- Take cactus grandiflora (up to thirty drops of the tincture three or four times a day), which also has a reputation as a heart tonic.
- Ginkgo (one capsule twice a day), although not a direct heart tonic, can improve heart function by boosting blood flow to the heart.

Hemorrhoids

A condition of dilated, inflamed, and sometimes thrombosed or clotted rectal veins causing itching, bleeding, and pain. It can be internal or external.

Related or Underlying Causes

  SL

Hemorrhoids are most often caused by constipation and straining, two common consequences of insufficient dietary fiber. Vitamin C and bioflavonoid deficiencies may cause diminished integrity of collagen tissues and reduced strength of vein walls. Cirrhosis of the liver and a sluggish liver may increase the pressure in hemorrhoidal veins.

Treatment and Preventive Measures

DIETARY RECOMMENDATIONS

- A whole-foods diet, containing fiber-rich foods (whole grains, legumes, fruits, and vegetables) is essential to maintaining effective bowel function.
- Psyllium husk or flaxseed powder (1 or 2 teaspoons once or twice a day) is a worthy addition to diets lacking needed fiber. In a jar, add the powder to 6 to 8 ounces of water. Screw on lid and shake vigorously. Drink immediately. Other options for supplementing fiber are oat bran, guar gum, and pectin. Normalizing bowel transit time and stool consistency is a must.
- Drink water (six to eight glasses a day), primarily between meals.

DETOXIFICATION PROGRAM

- Periodically do the following: the Liver Flush and Purifying Diet or an intestinal cleansing program.

NUTRITIONAL SUPPLEMENTS

- Use vitamin C (up to 1,000 milligrams three times a day) and bioflavonoids, such as hesperidin, hesperidin methyl chalcone, and naringin (600 to 900 milligrams a day combined).
- Zinc (30 milligrams a day) is important for tissue healing.

OTHER THERAPIES

Natural internal treatments for hemorrhoids can be effective.

- Try an herbal suppository made from aesculus, hamamelis, collinsonia, achillea, mullein, and hypericum. (Herbal Astringent Suppositories can be obtained from Earth's Harvest of Gresham, Oregon.)
- Try inserting rectally a capsule each of vitamin A, vitamin E, and garlic twice a day. Lubricate with vegetable oil if needed.
- For acute relief, an old naturopathic remedy is to insert a piece of raw peeled potato carved to size. Eating boiled onions has provided acute relief for some hemorrhoid sufferers.
- Try direct application with several cotton balls of witch hazel tea or lemon juice.
- Acupuncture can also be effective.
- Sitz baths may bring acute relief (see information on hydrotherapy in Chapter Twenty).
- If an inflamed hemorrhoid is not responding to natural measures or the bleeding is excessive, see your doctor.

    Warning: Rectal bleeding may be a sign of more serious illness. See your doctor for any new or unusual rectal bleeding.

Hepatitis (Viral)

A viral infection of the liver often causing flulike symptoms, such as fatigue, malaise, fever, poor appetite, nausea, muscle and joint pains, and abdominal discomfort. Dark urine, light, clay-colored stools, and jaundice or yellowing of the skin and the whites of the eyes may also occur. The three most common forms of hepatitis are A, B, and C.

The diagnosis is indicated by blood tests that show elevations on a standard liver function panel. Specific blood screening tests for hepatitis A, B, and C confirm the diagnosis.

Acute hepatitis A may last three to six weeks. There are usually no long-term complications. Acute hepatitis B may be similar to hepatitis A in duration and severity or it may be much less severe. In fact, two thirds of all persons diagnosed with hepatitis B have no symptoms or report unrecognized symptoms. These individuals become carriers and transmitters of the virus without knowing it. The worldwide alarm concerning hepatitis B is its widespread prevalence and its association with the eventual development of cirrhosis and cancer of the liver.

Acute hepatitis C is similar to hepatitis B in its long-term complications. However, at this time, the incidence of hepatitis C complications is considered to be less than that of hepatitis B.

Related or Underlying Causes

DietH

The hepatitis A virus is spread through contaminated food and water. It can be transmitted from person to person through oral, anal, or fecal contact.

The hepatitis B virus is spread through blood (transfusions, used hypodermic needles, etc.), sexual fluids, saliva, the birth canal, and mother's milk. High-risk individuals are health care workers, ethnic groups with a high incidence of hepatitis in their native countries (Indochinese, Alaskan Eskimos, Haitians, and others), individuals with multiple sex partners and especially those with a repeated history of sexually transmitted diseases, intravenous drug abusers, individuals who receive certain blood products, hemodialysis patients, fetuses and newborns of mothers who are hepatitis B carriers, and household contacts and sexual partners of hepatitis B carriers.

Hepatitis C, a relatively new virus, is thought to be spread primarily through blood contact (transfusions, used hypodermic needles, etc.) and is the subject of ongoing research.

Treatment and Preventive Measures

CONVENTIONAL MEDICAL TREATMENT

For acute hepatitis, there is no specific conventional medical treatment. The recommended treatment is rest, bland diet, and medications directed toward symptomatic relief. Sanitary guidelines to prevent oral or anal transmission of the virus to others must be strictly followed.

Modern medicine has more to offer in the area of prevention. Gamma globulin injections are given to those traveling to areas where hepatitis A is common (nations where sanitation standards are low) or to those who have been recently exposed to hepatitis A but are not yet ill.

The treatment offered for chronic hepatitis (alpha interferon) has potential side effects and a low success rate. Current research may bring forth new drugs that are more effective. Again, prevention is where modern medicine prevails. Widespread screening and hepatitis B vaccinations hold much promise for slowing the spread of this disease.

DIETARY RECOMMENDATIONS

- For acute hepatitis, as in most infections, there initially is a reduction in appetite. Drink plenty of fluids (six to eight glasses of water a day), including carrot and green juices.
- As the appetite returns, eat light, nourishing wholefoods meals. Avoid excessive calories, fats, and sweets.

DETOXIFICATION PROGRAM

- During the initial phases of acute hepatitis, a short two- to three-day fast may be helpful, including fresh carrot and green juices, herbal teas, and water. Do not do any prolonged fasting.
- Once a normal, healthy eating pattern is resumed, and weight is back to normal, a periodic short cleansing diet (the Liver Flush and Purifying Diet) or short fast is recommended.

NUTRITIONAL SUPPLEMENTS

- Vitamin C in high doses can be extremely useful to speed recovery for any form of acute viral hepatitis. A better result is achieved the sooner high-dose vitamin C is started. Use buffered, powdered vitamin C in doses up to bowel tolerance. Raise the dose until the stool is abnormally loose, then reduce the dose only enough until the stool firms up. This may be 10 to 20 grams a day or more. The bowel tolerance dose diminishes as the body's need for extra vitamin C lessens. As the weeks go by, the vitamin C dose needs to be reduced accordingly. Intravenous vitamin C (up to 50 grams several times a week) is usually even more helpful, as greater amounts of vitamin C can generally be given by this route than orally. High-dose vitamin C is used as well to treat chronic hepatitis.
- Take lipoic acid (100 to 200 milligrams three times a day) available as Thioctic from Ecological Formulas of Concord, California. It is a vitamin cofactor that enhances liver protective mechanisms.
- Thymus glandular tablets, which are meant to enhance immune function, have also been used successfully for both acute and chronic hepatitis (see precautions about raw glandular extracts on page 315). Thymax by T. E. Neesby of Fresno, California, is a boiled glandular. Take two tablets three times a day.

HERBAL REMEDIES

- A ginger compress or castor oil pack applied to the liver area is recommended.

- One of the most effective herbal agents for the treatment of both acute and chronic hepatitis is phyllanthus amarus, an Ayurvedic herb used extensively in India. Take Livit 1 (one tablet three times a day), along with Livit 2, a blend of eighteen other Ayurvedic liver herbs (one tablet three times a day). Both are available from Interplexus of Kent, Washington.
- Take milk thistle (100 to 200 milligrams three times a day).
- Another Ayurvedic formula used for liver disease is Liv. 52, containing capers, chicory, wonderberry, senna, myrobalan, yarrow, manna, and organically complexed iron (three or four tablets three times a day), available from Probiologic of Bellevue, Washington.

Herpes (Herpes Simplex and Herpes Zoster)

Genital herpes (herpes simplex II), one of the more common social diseases, is a virus usually transmitted by sexual intercourse, causing painful lesions on the genitals, the groin or buttocks, in the vagina, on the cervix, or in or around the rectum. Lesions can also appear on the lower abdomen or back. A primary infection usually occurs one to two weeks after exposure. It is often accompanied by fever, malaise, and lymphatic swelling and tenderness in the groin. The lesions normally heal in one to three weeks.

The stigma of herpes can be quite devastating psychologically and emotionally. Some infected individuals feel like sexual and social outcasts. Self-education concerning the management and prevention of herpes, along with open and responsible conversation with your partner, can help you to approach this ailment without guilt, fear, or self-recrimination.

Recurrent infections are usually not as painful or symptomatic as the primary lesions and heal in less time. Lesions can appear as tiny multiple blisters in clusters or as larger ulcerated single lesions.

Herpes can be transmitted to a partner when lesions are present or during the few days before an outbreak when symptoms of tingling or burning are experienced. The virus is not considered contagious at other times. However, it's important to note that active lesions may be present where you can't see them, such as on the cervix or in the rectum. People attuned to their bodies often recognize when they are developing a recurrence.

Once introduced, the virus lives dormant in the nerves. Some people develop one recurrence a month and others one a year. Yet some who are exposed to active lesions do not acquire the disease at all. Research is revealing that the strength of the immune system may determine the severity of the herpes outbreak.

Herpes can serve as a monitor of the body's ability to handle daily stress. Reducing stress and maintaining an immune-strengthening diet are essential to minimizing and preventing recurrences.

HERPES ZOSTER (SHINGLES)

Unlike herpes simplex II, herpes zoster, or shingles, is not sexually transmitted and usually does not recur. It causes very painful lesions on the trunk, neck, head, and face. Lesions occur along sensory nerve pathways and involve usually just one side of the body.

Related or Underlying Causes

DietH **ND** **ADR** **B/M**

Herpes zoster commonly strikes when the immune system is overloaded by fatigue, insufficient sleep, injury, illness, or stress. However, it can sometimes occur for no apparent reason.

Treatment and Preventive Measures

CONVENTIONAL MEDICAL TREATMENT

- For any lesions suggestive of genital herpes or shingles, consult your doctor immediately to verify the diagnosis and discuss treatment options. Learn how to prevent transmitting the virus. If shingles involves the face, vision can be threatened if an eye is affected and treatment is not implemented immediately.

  The prescription drug Zovirax (acyclovir) is often very effective for shortening the course of the outbreak and reducing the severity of shingles. It is also effective and recommended for genital herpes. Because of its effectiveness for both the treatment and prevention of genital herpes recurrences, this medication may incorrectly defer a person from starting a vital immune-strengthening program. Many individuals are able to minimize and even treat recurrences without Zovirax. If possible, use it only as a last resort.

DIETARY RECOMMENDATIONS

- Eat a whole-foods diet and get adequate protein.
- Avoid sugar, caffeine, and other substances that weaken the nervous system, adrenals, and the immune system. Reduce other common dietary health hazards, particularly trans-fatty acids from foods such as margarine and other sources of partially hydrogenated vegetable oils.

ARGININE AND LYSINE IN FOOD

| | Gm/100 Gm | | |
	LYSINE	ARGININE	PROTEIN
Milk	0.3	0.1	3.5
Cheese (all)	1.5	0.7	17
Eggs	0.8	0.8	12
Meat (all)	1.6	1.2	17
Chitterlings	0.7	1.4	8
Gelatin	4.0	8.0**	85
Beans	1.7	1.4	23
Peanuts	1.1	3.3**	27
Peas	2.0	2.0	24
Soybeans	1.6	1.4	35
Almonds	0.6	2.7**	18
Cashews	0.8	2.0**	18
Coconut	0.2	0.5*	3
Acorns	0.6	0.7	10
Chocolate	2.0	4.0**	38
Cottonseed	2.0	5.0**	42
Grains			
Barley	0.4	0.6*	12
Bread	0.2	0.3	8
Field corn	0.3	0.8**	10
Cornflakes	0.1	0.2*	8
Corn germ	0.8	1.2*	14
Gluten	0.2	0.2	10
Zein	0.0	0.3*	16
Oats	0.5	0.9**	14
Rice	0.3	0.4	7
Puffed rice	0	0.1	6
Wheat	0.4	0.7*	14
Bran	0.5	0.7*	12
Germ	1.5	1.8*	25
Gluten	1.5	3.4*	80
Macaroni	0.4	0.6*	13
Vegetables			
Brussels sprouts	0.2	0.3*	4
Cabbage	0.1	0.1	1
Asparagus	0.1	0.1	2
Snap beans	0.1	0.1	2
Beets	<0.1	0	1
Broccoli	0.2	0.2	3
Carrots	<0.1	<0.1	1
Cauliflower	0.1	0.1	2
Mushrooms	0	0.2	
Onions	<0.1	0.2	1.9
Pumpkin	<0.1	<0.1	1
Tomatoes	0.1	0.1	1
Potatoes	0.2	0.1	1.7
Yeast			
Bakers	0.9	0.5	13
Brewer's	3.3	2.2	46

*Relatively high arginine-to-lysine ratio (beneficial for the herpes virus): minimize.
**Exceptionally high arginine-to-lysine ratio (very beneficial for the herpes virus): avoid.
Reprinted with permission from Jonathan V. Wright, M.D., Tahoma Clinic, Kent, Washington.

- The amino acid arginine favors the growth of herpes, whereas lysine-rich foods inhibit it. Avoid foods rich in arginine and lacking in lysine, such as peanuts, most nuts, chocolate, and even some grains. They can contribute to recurrences. (See the table on page 378.) You may be able to handle certain relatively high-arginine foods but be unable to tolerate others. Your tolerances may vary depending on stress levels, allergies, menstrual cycle, and other factors.

NUTRITIONAL SUPPLEMENTS

The following supplements will help improve your ability to shorten or avoid herpes outbreaks:

- Lysine (500 to 1,000 milligrams a day for maintenance or 1,000 milligrams three times a day at the initial signs of acute recurrence), an amino acid that inhibits the growth of herpes virus. Brewer's yeast and milk products contain lysine. Aminovirox (Tyson and Associates of Hawthorne, California), a broad-spectrum multiple amino acid/lysine–rich supplement without arginine, can be used in viral infections and immune-support programs.
- Take B complex (25 to 100 milligrams a day), extra vitamin B-5 (100 to 500 milligrams two or three times a day), and vitamin C (1,000 to 3,000 milligrams a day).
- High-dose buffered vitamin C powder (up to 10 grams a day), given during the course of the initial occurrence, has in some individuals knocked the virus out of their system or rendered them resistant to recurrences. Take the highest dose that your bowel can tolerate without causing diarrhea.
- Vitamin A (up to 20,000 I.U. daily) and beta-carotene (up to 50,000 I.U. daily) can also be effective. Zinc (15 to 30 milligrams a day) is another powerful immune system enhancer.
- Also, take calcium (up to 800 milligrams a day) and magnesium (up to 800 milligrams a day).
- Take essential fatty acids, unrefined flaxseed oil (1 or 2 teaspoons a day), and borage oil (two or three capsules a day). Also, take vitamin E (200 to 400 I.U. daily) whenever using supplemental oils.
- Take immune-strengthening thymus extract or thymus glandular tablets. Raw glandulars may pose a risk (see page 315). One boiled thymus product is Thymax, available from T. E. Neesby of Fresno, California (take two capsules three times a day).
- For the pain of shingles, even after the lesions are gone (postherpetic neuralgia), vitamin B-12 shots can be helpful (1,000 micrograms with 2.5 to 5 milligrams folic acid daily for one week, then tapering eventually to once or twice a month or more as needed).

HERBAL REMEDIES

- Take combination herbal tablets with antiviral and immune-enhancing effects. Two very successful Chinese formulas are produced by Health Concerns of Alameda, California: take Astra Isatis (three tablets three times a day) as a maintenance dose to prevent recurrences and Isatis Gold (three tablets up to eight times a day) for acute recurrences. These and other general antiviral immune-enhancing formulas are listed in Chapter Nineteen.

HOMEOPATHIC REMEDIES

- Homeopathic combination drops or tablets for herpes can be effective. Heparsulph, a single homeopathic remedy, has been helpful in some cases, but an individually constitutional remedy prescribed by a homeopath is always best. Homeopathic remedies have also been used successfully in treating postherpetic neuralgia, the pain that persists after the lesions have healed.

OTHER THERAPIES

- Topical applications for genital herpes lesions are often beneficial. Although many health professionals suggest keeping the lesions open to the air and as dry as possible, several creams and ointments have been shown to decrease pain and healing time of genital herpes lesions: LSO cream, Lysine Plus cream, licorice root cream (Licrogel by Scientific Botanicals of Seattle), glycol thymoline, and goldenseal and myrrh powders (mixed 50:50).
- Other local applications can be extremely soothing. Aloe vera or a clay poultice can be placed on lesions. Apple cider vinegar soaks may be helpful. Or try a thin past application made from vitamin C powder and water. Ice applications can be used to relieve pain.
- For chronic pain, see a practitioner of auricular therapy, a form of ear acupuncture.

High Blood Pressure

See BLOOD PRESSURE (HIGH).

HIV

See AIDS.

Hives

Itchy, red, raised, weltlike skin disorder that can occur individually or in clusters anywhere on the body.

Related or Underlying Causes

   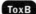

Hives can be caused by allergies to foods, food coloring agents such as salicylates, and food preservatives and other chemical additives. Even prescription medications can be related. Hives can be initiated by an allergy to the sun, heat, contactants (substances that come in contact with the skin) and bug bites. An intestinal yeast or parasite infection (see PARASITES) or other cause of a leaky gut may be at work. An allergy to one's own intestinal bacteria can precipitate hives. Even psychological and emotional factors can be contributing mechanisms, triggering an allergic or hive outbreak.

Treatment and Preventive Measures

CONVENTIONAL MEDICAL TREATMENT
- Take specific over-the-counter antihistamines and prescription medications to relieve symptoms. The prescription drug Benadryl may work well as a temporary measure when taken orally or topically. Take an antiparasite medication if indicated.

DIETARY RECOMMENDATIONS
- Avoid foods with any additives. Follow a food allergy elimination diet, or be tested for food allergies by your doctor. Eliminate all sources of salicylates.

NUTRITIONAL SUPPLEMENTS
- There are quite a few effective natural remedies with antihistamine activity, such as buffered, powdered vitamin C (5,000 to 10,000 milligrams a day, less if any diarrhea occurs) and pantothenic acid (500 to 1,000 milligrams three times a day).
- If imbalanced intestinal flora is related, do an intestinal cleansing, and use lactobacillus sporogenes (from Thorne Research of Sandpoint, Idaho) or an acidophilus/bifidus supplement. (1 capsule of either or both two or three times daily).

HERBAL REMEDIES
- Take quercetin (up to 1,000 milligrams three times a day).

OTHER THERAPIES
- If a leaky gut is at cause, try oral cromalyn sodium

(up to 400 milligrams) to minimize symptoms until underlying causes are addressed.
- If an allergy to one's own bacteria is suspected, an autogenous vaccine, a vaccine made from one's own intestinal bacteria or urine, may provide relief.

Hot Flashes

See MENOPAUSE.

Hyperactivity

See ATTENTION DEFICIT/HYPERACTIVITY DISORDER.

Hypertension

See BLOOD PRESSURE (HIGH).

Hyperthyroidism

Overactivity of the thyroid gland. Symptoms include a racing or jumpy heart, a hot and sweaty feeling, abnormally frequent or loose bowel movements, anxiety, restlessness, insomnia, weight loss, and sometimes goiters. Bulging eyeballs can be a symptom of Graves' disease, a particular form of hyperthyroidism. Your doctor must establish the severity of the condition.

Related or Underlying Causes

CHEM

From a conventional medical standpoint, hyperthyroidism is an autoimmune condition with no known cause. Nutritionally oriented physicians, however, have linked heavy metal toxicity, particularly from mercury, to hyperthyroidism. Food allergy, according to some doctors, may also play a role. Abnormalities in the hypothalamus and pituitary glands have also been related to this condition by practitioners of auricular medicine, a form of ear acupuncture developed by Paul Nogier, M.D., in France.

Treatment and Preventive Measures

CONVENTIONAL MEDICAL TREATMENT

- Severe hyperthyroidism is a serious medical condition and not to be dealt with lightly. Standard treatments include propylthirouracil, a medication that blocks thyroxine production; radioactive iodine, which destroys the thyroid gland; and surgery to remove the thyroid gland.
- Propranolol (Inderal™) is often prescribed to slow the heartbeat until other approaches are taken.
- Occasionally, lithium, used in manic-depressive illness, is prescribed because of its ability to block thyroxine production.
- If your doctor recommends radioactive treatment or surgery, which is irreversible and invasive, ask that he or she first prescribe some of the other potentially beneficial medications. These will, at least, subdue your symptoms and allow you time to be evaluated and treated for the related conditions mentioned above. Further evaluation may eliminate the need for radical treatment. *Note: Have your doctor clearly outline how long it would be safe to stay on propylthirouracil and other medicines and how long radioactive treatment or surgery can be delayed.*

DIETARY RECOMMENDATIONS

- Some cases of hyperthyroidism are mild and can be somewhat improved, in part, by eating generous quantities of raw cruciferous vegetables, such as broccoli, cauliflower, cabbage, kale, collard, brussels sprouts, and mustard greens. These vegetables contain a natural thyroid blocker.

HERBAL AND HOMEOPATHIC REMEDIES

- Using a botanical tincture of lycopus and cactus (twenty-five to thirty drops three times a day) and homeopathic thyroid (200c) has been helpful for mild cases. A constitutionally prescribed homeopathic remedy may offer the greatest hope, even in severe cases.

Hypothyroidism

The thyroid gland, located in the neck under the Adam's apple, produces a primary hormone, thyroxine. This hormone is converted, primarily outside the thyroid gland, to the more active triiodothyronine (T-3), which stimulates every one of the trillion cells in your body. Nearly every system and function depends on receiving adequate amounts of this hormone. Consequently, insufficient thyroxine (hypothyroidism) can trigger a potential myriad of symptoms.

A person with hypothyroidism may experience only some of these symptoms.

Related or Underlying Causes

 ND   Y   CHEM   ADR

Insufficient production of thyroxine is often caused by primary thyroid failure. To confirm the diagnosis, simple blood tests measuring low levels of thyroxine or high levels of thyroid-stimulating hormone can be obtained. A small or inadequate thyroid gland can be inherited. It is likely to occur if a sibling and particularly a parent or grandparent has been diagnosed with hypothyroidism.

Nutrient deficiencies, such as iodine, zinc, copper, iron, selenium, and tyrosine, will also cause the thyroid to underfunction. Some of these nutrients are involved in thyroxine production and others help convert thyroxine to the active T-3. Excessive cortisol levels from chronic stress will also block conversion to T-3.

Frequently, the blood tests above will be normal when an individual is actually suffering from low thyroid status, a circumstance that many physicians do not recognize. A more involved and expensive testing protocol, TRH (thyrotropin-releasing hormone) stimulation test, can identify one cause of this defect in the pituitary gland. Tests to demonstrate an autoimmune inflammation in the thyroid (Hashimoto's thyroiditis) can also be obtained.

All tests may come back normal. However, low thyroid status may still be a possibility due to thyroid hormone resistance.

Heavy metal toxicity from mercury, lead, cadmium, and others and chemical contamination may be important resistance factors disrupting the thyroid hormone's effect on cells (see Chapter Fourteen).

BARNES BASAL TEMPERATURE TEST

Use the Barnes basal temperature test to help identify low thyroid status, whether from thyroid resistance or other causes:

- Take your armpit temperature for ten minutes before getting out of bed in the morning.
- Shake down an oral or rectal thermometer the night before and keep it at your bedside. Do not use a digital or electronic thermometer.
- In the morning, place the thermometer deep in your bare armpit and close your arm on it firmly for ten minutes before arising.
- Keep a record for three or four days.

HOW LOW THYROID STATUS AFFECTS THE WHOLE BODY

BRAIN

Depression   Poor memory and concentration
Mental fatigue   Insomnia
Irritability   Headaches
Anxiety   Difficulty coping

NEUROLOGICAL

Vertigo (dizziness)   Ménière's disease
Hearing loss   Poor vision, night blindness
Neuropathy: burning, tingling, or numb   Carpal tunnel syndrome
  sensations

SPEECH/THROAT

Slow sluggish speech, slurred speech, thick tongue, coarse or hoarse voice

GASTROINTESTINAL

Constipation   Poor appetite
Gas/bloating   Poor digestion

MENSTRUAL/FEMALE

Premenstrual syndrome   Multiple miscarriages
Menstrual cramps   Infertility
Periods that are irregular   Premature cessation of periods
  too heavy   Breast pain
  too light   Fibrocystic breasts

MALE AND FEMALE

Diminished libido   Sensations less pleasurable to genitals
Diminished ability to be aroused sexually   Less interest in sex

MEN

Inability to achieve or maintain erection

Infertility: decreased motility and numbers of sperm

GENERAL METABOLISM

Fatigue, exhaustion, poor stamina
Weight gain, difficulty losing weight
Hypoglycemia
Sluggish liver, high blood cholesterol

Water retention—puffy hands, feet, face
Feel cold, cold hands and feet
Decreased sweating

CARDIOVASCULAR

Slow heartbeat
Weakened heartbeat
Tendency to congestive heart failure and
    enlarged heart

Abnormal heart rhythm, palpitation
Tendency toward arteriosclerosis
Bluish color to skin

IMMUNE SYSTEM

Increased susceptibility to colds, flu, sinus,
    lung infections—any infections

Prolonged bouts of infections
Decreased white blood cell count

MUSCULOSKELETAL

Muscular weakness
Muscle cramps
Muscle pains
Stiff or painful joints

Ligaments that are too lax
Low back pain
Carpal tunnel syndrome

SKIN, HAIR, NAILS

Coarse or dry skin or hair
Easy bruising, bleeding
Hair loss
Eyebrow loss
Pale skin or lips

Cool skin
Adult acne
Slow wound healing
Nail ridges
Decreased sweating

- If you are a menstruating female, start taking your temperature the first day of the menstrual period. This is the time of the month when your temperatures are lowest.
- Postmenopausal women and all males may take their temperatures at any time of the month (including those on estrogen replacement therapy and not having periods).
- If your menstrual periods have become irregular, and you are not quite sure when your next one will come, take your temperature at any time—it could still be diagnostic—and again whenever your period arrives.
- If you have had a hysterectomy and still have your ovaries, or if for some reason your period has stopped temporarily and you still have premenstrual symptoms, begin a temperature test just after the premenstrual symptoms subside—when you would normally expect to have your period. If you do not have premenstrual symptoms, take your temperature any time of the month.
- If you have a cold or flu or any other condition that would raise your temperature, wait until it subsides. Temperatures averaging below 97.8° F may reflect low thyroid status, and those above 98.2° F may reflect hyperthyroidism, or elevated thyroid function (see HYPERTHYROIDISM). The lower the temperature (especially 97.0° F or below), the more suspicious one should be (particularly if there are significant low thyroid symptoms). The Barnes treatment calls for a prescription of natural thyroid hormone. Although this simple temperature test is not foolproof (other conditions such as disturbed adrenal function can cause low temperatures), it can indicate the need for thyroid or metabolic assistance.

  Warning: If thyroid hormone is indicated solely on the basis of low temperatures and hypothyroid symptoms—that is, all thyroid blood tests are normal—it is critical to first assess free cortisol levels (see Chapter Eleven). These levels will often be abnormally high, and correcting them will often improve thyroid function, raise temperatures, and relieve symptoms. To add thyroid hormone to a hypercortisol state may initially relieve symptoms, but in the long run, it will usually lead to health deterioration.

Treatment and Preventive Measures

CONVENTIONAL MEDICAL TREATMENT

- An appropriately prescribed dose of thyroid hormone can effectively reverse hypothyroidism and enable sufferers of this condition to regain full health. Close clinical and blood test monitoring initially help establish the correct dose. This treatment is safe and without adverse side effects if the correct dose is given. Because this treatment may be long-term, even life long, periodic monitoring by your doctor is essential.

DIETARY RECOMMENDATIONS

Holistic approaches to nourishing the thyroid and detoxifying the body have not usually improved thyroid status. Using foods and supplements specific for enhancing thyroid status can produce significant results in some individuals. (If after three months, however, there is not much improvement, strongly consider, if indicated, prescription thyroid.) The following foods can nourish and enhance thyroid function:

- *Iodine*: from fish, sea vegetables like kelp, dulse, arame, hijiki, nori, wakame, kombu, and sea salt. Iodized salt is a source, but not the best, as it usually contains aluminum. Cod liver oil also contains traces of iodine.
- *Zinc*: from beef, oatmeal, chicken, seafood (especially oysters), liver, dried beans, bran, tuna, spinach, seeds, and nuts.
- *Copper*: from liver and other organ meats, eggs, yeast, legumes, nuts, raisins.
- *Tyrosine* (from phenylalanine): found in soy products, beef, chicken, fish.

NUTRITIONAL SUPPLEMENTS

- To enhance thyroid status, include iodine (225 to 1,000 micrograms a day) in your diet. Sometimes more iodine is required and is available in higher concentrations by prescription. Lower doses are available as kelp or dulse supplements or as a part of a mineral or vitamin/mineral supplement.
- Other nutrients include zinc (15 to 30 milligrams a day), copper (2 or 3 milligrams a day), selenium (up to 250 micrograms a day), tyrosine (300 to 1,000 milligrams a day), and iron (for menstruating females, 18 milligrams a day). Other individuals may need iron supplementation for anemia or low iron stores. B complex (25 to 50 milligrams a day) and magnesium (up to 400 milligrams a day) are added as general metabolic enhancers.

  These nutrients, with the exception of tyrosine, can usually be found together in a high-potency vitamin/mineral. Tyrosine can be found separately or in some combination thyroid-enhancing supplements.
- Naturopathic physicians have long prescribed a thyroid glandular extract and sometimes a pituitary extract to treat hypothyroidism. These supplements are usually available in most health food stores. There is little scientific proof that taking an animal glandular tablet can strengthen the same gland in your body (or provide some of the same benefits derived from the gland). They are certainly a concentrated source of gland nutrients. Critics stress that these glandular products work only because they still contain some of the active hormones that supposedly have been removed. Proponents swear by their efficacy and their intended mechanism of action. Efficacy concerns aside, there are safety issues to be addressed (see page 205).

OTHER THERAPIES

- Constitutional homeopathy works subtly and dramatically to reverse imbalances and blocks, and may effectively reverse low thyroid status. Acupuncture may be considered as well.
- Identify and treat yeast overgrowth and heavy metal toxicity.
- Although there is not much evidence in medical literature linking exercise with thyroid status, my clinical observations have shown that aerobic exercise appears to elevate thyroid status in some people, possibly by enhancing circulation and greater cellular uptake of thyroxine. Some patients have experienced a quick recurrence of low thyroid symptoms after stopping the aerobic exercise program, despite maintaining their nutritional program. Aerobic exercise done regularly thirty or more minutes at least three or four times a week may enhance a nutritional program to strengthen the thyroid.

Indigestion

See HEARTBURN.

Infertility

An inability to conceive children by either sexual partner.

Related or Underlying Causes

Common causes of female infertility are varied, ranging from malnutrition to structural abnormalities in the female reproductive system. Other factors include scarred fallopian tubes from pelvic inflammatory disease due either to sexually transmitted diseases or an IUD (intrauterine device)–related infection, hormone imbalances or deficiencies, inability to ovulate, excessive radiation or X-ray exposure, and advanced age. Emotional blocks may also contribute.

Infertility in men can be linked to several causes: abnormally low sperm count, motility, and penetration; abnormally shaped sperm; insufficient seminal fluid; undescended testicles; injured testicles; childhood diseases, such as mumps; viral infections; varicocele (a type of varicose vein in the scrotum); excessive radiation and X-ray exposure; and prostate disorders.

Nutrient deficiencies and heavy metal and chemical toxicity may also contribute to sperm or semen abnormalities and ovarian dysfunction.

Treatment and Preventive Measures

CONVENTIONAL MEDICAL TREATMENT

- Consult your doctor if you have been trying unsuccessfully to get pregnant for twelve months or longer. Preliminary screening for women includes a pelvic exam; a body temperature test; pituitary, ovarian, and thyroid hormone blood tests; and a general blood screening test. A semen and sperm analysis is performed on the man. A fertility specialist may be consulted to order more specific tests, prescribe fertility medication, and possibly resort to in vitro fertilization or other high-tech procedures.

  Consider the possibility of low thyroid status if the tests and examinations show no abnormalities, or even if tests identify a failure to ovulate, an ovarian hormone imbalance, or another nonstructural abnormality. If thyroid blood tests are normal, a trial of thyroid hormone may be warranted (see HYPOTHYROIDISM) and may be the answer to getting pregnant. If you do get pregnant with thyroid supplementation, you should continue the dosage with periodic medical monitoring during your pregnancy. Hypothyroidism can cause miscarriages. Thyroid supplementation should also be considered after pregnancy. Consult with your doctor about this.

DIETARY RECOMMENDATIONS

  Fertility specialists rarely emphasize nutrition. Conventional medicine seems quick to prescribe fertility drugs and perform procedures, and appears less interested in investigating the nutritional foundation upon which fertility depends.

- Eat a whole-foods diet.
- Avoid highly processed and refined foods. Eliminate excessive caffeine, which can contribute to infertility.

DETOXIFICATION PROGRAMS

- Since the best diet and supplements cannot provide their full benefits in a toxic body, identify and treat heavy metal and chemical toxicity. It may also be useful to do bowel and liver cleansing programs. Additional detoxification measures such as fasting may also be warranted.

NUTRITIONAL SUPPLEMENTS

- For women, the following nutrients can be beneficial: vitamin C (1,000 milligrams at least three times a day); zinc (15 to 30 milligrams a day); magnesium (at least 400 milligrams a day); B complex (25 to 50 milligrams a day); B-6 (up to 50 milligrams a day); beta-carotene (at least 50,000 I.U. daily), preferably as a part of mixed carotenes, available as Beta Plex from Scientific Botanicals of Seattle; essential fatty acids (1 or 2 teaspoons of flaxseed oil daily) and borage oil (two or three capsules providing 200 to 300 milligrams of gamma linolenic acid daily); and vitamin E (400 I.U. daily).

- For men whose sperm count, motility, and penetration and other parameters are compromised for no apparently known or treatable cause, try the women's supplementation program above with the following exceptions: omit the extra B-6 and take zinc (up to 50 milligrams a day). If herpes is not an issue, take the amino acid arginine (up to 1,000 milligrams four times a day), which is known to boost sperm count.

HERBAL REMEDIES

FOR MEN:

- Take Siberian ginseng (100 milligrams two or three times a day before 4:00 P.M.).

FOR WOMEN:

- The following herbs and other substances promote fertility in women, and should be taken after the menstrual period stops until it starts again, but not during the period:

   False unicorn root (helonias) and vitex (equal combinations as a tincture (1 teaspoon three times a day).

   Siberian ginseng (up to 100 milligrams twice a day before 4:00 P.M.).

   Royal jelly (1,000 to 2,000 milligrams a day).

   Fertile Garden, a Chinese formula by Health Concerns of Alameda, California (three tablets three times a day). (Use the helonias/vitex or Fertile Garden, not both concurrently.)

- Try the following combination herb program. For the first half of your menstrual cycle (from the end of your period until ovulation) take the following estrogenic herbal tincture: licorice root, vitex, yarrow, and dong quai, mixed in a ratio of four parts to one part to one part to two parts, respectively (1½ teaspoons three times a day). The second half of your cycle, from ovulation to the onset of your period, switch to a progesterone-aiding tincture: blessed thistle, milk thistle, sarsaparilla, and vitex mixed in a ratio of three parts to three parts to one part to one part, respectively (1 teaspoon three times a day). An herb store or naturopathic physician can mix or obtain this formula. Discontinue this mixture during the days of your menstrual flow. Coordinate this treatment with the biorhythm and light program outlined below.

OTHER THERAPIES

FOR WOMEN:

- To normalize inner body cycles, it may be necessary to reestablish proper internal biorhythms with the aid of light. Begin your light therapy program by sleeping eight hours a night in a completely darkened room (not even light from outdoors coming through the windows) during the days from the end of your menstrual cycle to the beginning of your menstrual cycle (the days you will be taking the tinctures). During the three to five days of your period, sleep with a bright light on. If possible, let the moonlight shine through your windows. If your periods are irregular or have stopped temporarily, time this portion of the program so that the middle of the three- to five-day stretch when you are sleeping with the light coincides with the full moon. *Note: This regimen may require several months of application before results are seen.*

Insomnia

An inability to sleep; a pattern of broken or restless sleep.

Related or Underlying Causes

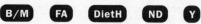

B/M FA DietH ND Y HYP ADR

Insomnia is often caused by anxiety and depression. Substances such as caffeinated coffee, tea, and soft drinks, as well as any chocolate-containing foods and beverages, may contribute. Many over-the-counter and prescription aspirin- and acetaminophen-containing pain medications incorporate caffeine, as do diet pills. Stimulating herbs, such as ginseng, ephedra/ma huang, guarana, kola nut, and ginger, may be related. For some individuals, sugar and alcoholic beverages disturb sleep. For a very small percentage of the population, B vitamins can cause agitation and insomnia. Any of the above stimulants can disturb sleep even if ingested only in the morning. Additional causes of insomnia include calcium, magnesium, and B-vitamin deficiencies; hypothyroidism and hyperthyroidism; chemical hypersensitivity; adrenal overactivity; and insufficient exercise. The pineal gland in the brain regulates the circadian rhythm, the body's built-in clock. Disturbances in the output of the hormone melatonin have been linked to insomnia.

Treatment and Preventive Measures

CONVENTIONAL MEDICAL TREATMENT

- Sedatives, antianxiety agents, antidepressants, and psychotherapy are often prescribed.

DIETARY RECOMMENDATIONS

- Avoid the above sources of caffeine and chocolate. Read labels carefully. Even drinking caffeine in the morning can cause insomnia in some individuals.
- Follow a diet that helps stabilize hypoglycemia.
- Try drinking a glass of scalded milk at bedtime if you are not milk allergic.
- Eating tryptophan-rich foods for the evening meal or an evening snack may help induce sleep: milk products, turkey, chicken, beef, soy products, nuts and nut butters, bananas, papaya, and figs.
- An excessively high animal protein diet, although tryptophan rich, is also plentiful in the other amino acids that compete with tryptophan. Moderate to low animal protein in the diet, or even vegetarianism, will allow more tryptophan into the brain.

NUTRITIONAL SUPPLEMENTS

- Vitamins B-6 (up to 50 milligrams) and niacinamide/B-3 (up to 100 milligrams at bedtime) are often added to combination vitamin/mineral/herbal sedative formulas. Niacinamide alone (1,000 mg three times daily) is often used to lessen anxiety (see precautions).
- Calcium (up to 200 milligrams) is often added to combination vitamin/mineral herbal sedative formulas. Or take calcium alone (500 to 1,000 milligrams at bedtime). Magnesium (500 to 1,000 milligrams) taken with the calcium or alone in the morning may be helpful.
- Take vitamin B complex (25 to 50 milligrams a day with meals). *Note: A very small percentage of the population will develop agitation and worse insomnia with B-complex supplementation.*
- If adrenal-pituitary abnormalities are related (see Chapter Eleven), try phosphatidyl serine, a combination of the amino acid serine and the mineral phosphorus (Seriphos, by T. E. Neesby of Fresno, California) (up to 300 milligrams a day).
- Melatonin (up to 3 or 4 milligrams) may be taken one hour before bedtime. The synthetic form with no added brain tissue is recommended.
- Take 5-hydroxytryptophan (100 to 400 milligrams) near bedtime and at least 1½ hours after any protein is eaten. A biochemical derivation of tryptophan, it is available by prescription only.

HERBAL REMEDIES

- Chamomile tea has a mild sedative effect. It can be effective, especially for children. For adults, brew as strong as seven teaspoons of herb per cup of water.
- Take sedative herbs: valerian, passionflower, hops, and skullcap. Use any alone or in combination as a strong tea. Drink up to several cups as needed. Capsules and tinctures (combination and single herbs) are available in health food stores. Use one to four capsules or up to thirty drops.

HOMEOPATHIC REMEDIES

- Take combination homeopathic sleep or calming remedies, available at health food stores. Use as directed.

OTHER THERAPIES

- Get adequate exercise during the day. Take a warm, not hot, bath before retiring. A foot or body massage can be extremely restful.
- Practice meditation, visualization, or another skilled relaxation or breathing exercise in the evening or just before bedtime (see "Exercises" in Chapter Fifteen). Finish your incomplete business of the day in a visualization exercise, conversation, or journal.
- See a therapist to work out issues you are unable to manage alone.
- Acupuncture can be extremely effective for insomnia.
- Consider cranial electric stimulation (see Chapter Twenty).

Irritable Bowel/ Spastic Colon

A condition common in twenty- to forty-year-olds and characterized by one or more of the following symptoms: abdominal pain or cramps, excessive gas and bloating, alternating diarrhea and constipation, nausea, and the passing of mucus. Painful episodes are commonly associated with frequent bowel movements, which provide temporary relief. In contrast to colitis, there is no inflammation of the bowel in this condition. *Note: These symptoms may also indicate a more serious health condition. See your doctor.*

Related or Underlying Causes

 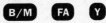   DIG B/M FA Y ToxB

This condition is most commonly attributed to stress and insufficient fiber. Food allergies, especially to milk or wheat, can be a cause, along with parasites and disturbed intestinal flora.

Treatment and Preventive Measures

CONVENTIONAL MEDICAL TREATMENT

- Antispasmodic medications, such as Levsin, Bentyl,

and Donnatal, are often recommended for symptomatic relief.
- Fiber supplements are also suggested.

DIETARY RECOMMENDATIONS
- Increase the fiber content of your diet with vegetables, fruit, whole grains, and legumes. Adding a fiber supplement may help significantly.
- Identify and avoid allergy-triggering foods.

NUTRITIONAL SUPPLEMENTS
- Take acidophilus as directed to normalize intestinal flora and digestive enzymes or hydrochloric acid, as indicated.

OTHER THERAPIES
- Use relaxation techniques to manage stress more effectively.
- See also CRAMPS (INTESTINAL) for suggestions for herbal and other remedies.

Kidney Stones

A stone within the kidney that is usually composed of solidified calcium and oxalate. As the stone moves into and migrates down the ureter to the bladder, waves of extreme back, abdominal, and groin pain occur, sometimes associated with fever and with urinary abnormalities (blood, pus, increased frequency). Although stones often will pass out of the body through the urine, surgery or ultrasonic destruction of the stone is sometimes needed.

Related or Underlying Causes

DietH　ND　Y

Nutritional literature has long linked kidney stones to a high-fat and -protein (meat and dairy), high-sugar, low-fiber diet, particularly when stones are the calcium oxalate type.

Treatment and Preventive Measures

CONVENTIONAL MEDICAL TREATMENT
- Contact your doctor for any symptoms suggestive of a stone. Have your doctor determine the content of the stone. Obtain the specimen by urinating through a strainer to retrieve the stone. If it is a typical calcium oxalate stone, your doctor may recommend restriction of calcium to lower your urinary calcium and prevent recurrences. Although avoiding extra calcium may have merits, eliminating common dietary ex-

cesses (see below) may prove more beneficial. When the acute episode is over, your doctor may suggest the measurement of your twenty-four-hour urinary excretion of oxalate and calcium. If either test is high, it should be repeated several months after implementing the following nutritional recommendations.

DIETARY RECOMMENDATIONS
- Avoid repetitive or excessive ingestion of foods high in protein, fat, and sugar; caffeine, alcohol, phosphoric acid–containing soft drinks; and aluminum. All of these items cause your body to lose calcium in the urine. Repetitive or excessive ingestion of high oxalate-containing foods should be minimized: beets, spinach, parsley, nuts, cabbage, almonds, rhubarb, and sesame seed products that contain the hull.
- Drink plenty of fluids. Restrict intake of salt.

NUTRITIONAL SUPPLEMENTS
- Take vitamin A (50,000 I.U. daily for one week then 25,000 I.U. daily for healing of urinary tissues), along with vitamin C (up to 1,000 milligrams a day). (See Chapter Six for a discussion of vitamin C and oxalate excretion and necessary precautions.)
- Take vitamin B-6 (up to 50 milligrams a day) and magnesium (up to 400 milligrams a day), which, if taken regularly on a long-term basis, can lower urinary oxalate and help prevent recurrences.
- Intravenous magnesium (1,000 milligrams periodically) may aid the passage of stones.

HERBAL REMEDIES
- During an acute episode take lobelia tincture (three or four drops every ten to twenty minutes) and wild yam tincture (fifteen drops every twenty minutes) in a glass of warm water. This may help relax the ureter, reduce pain, and speed the elimination of stones.
- Take cleavers and uva ursi leaf teas, both diuretics, as directed.
- Take wood betony as directed for treatment of kidney stones.

OTHER THERAPIES
- During an acute episode apply a castor oil pack on the abdomen or back (wherever the pain is most severe) for one hour several times a day (see Chapter Twenty).

Learning Disorder

(See ATTENTION DEFICIT/HYPERACTIVITY DISORDER.)

Macular Degeneration

An age-related deterioration of the macula, an oval depression on the retina, leading to blindness.

Related or Underlying Causes

Caused by arteriosclerotic disease in the small arteries of the retina.

Treatment and Preventive Measures

CONVENTIONAL MEDICAL TREATMENT

Monitoring, watchful waiting, and supportive care are offered by ophthalmologists. Generally no specific treatments to prevent or reverse the disease are offered.

DIETARY RECOMMENDATIONS
- Follow the low-fat, whole-foods diet suggested under ARTERIOSCLEROSIS.

NUTRITIONAL SUPPLEMENTS
- Aggressive antioxidant support can slow vision deterioration and has improved vision in some individuals.
- Twice-weekly intravenous infusions of selenium (400 micrograms) and zinc (10 milligrams for one month, then weekly), according to the protocol of the Tahoma Clinic in Kent, Washington, have shown significant results. When not available, these and other trace minerals (pharmaceutical grade) in DMSO (¼ teaspoon applied twice a day topically to the skin) can achieve similar if not equal results. DMSO with trace minerals is available by prescription in Washington State only, from the dispensary of the Tahoma Clinic in Kent, Washington. With either therapy, take the amino acid taurine orally (up to 1 gram three times a day).
- Also, take zinc (up to 50 milligrams a day), vitamin E (up to 800 I.U. daily), beta-carotene (up to 100,000 I.U. daily), selenium (up to 250 milligrams a day), and vitamin C (up to 3,000 milligrams a day).
- Most of the above and other nutrients for eye health, as well as the herb bilberry, can be found in Ocudyne by Allergy Research/Nutricology of San Leandro, California. Extra natural vitamin E is recommended with this supplement.

HERBAL SUPPLEMENTS
- Take bilberry (up to 160 milligrams three times a day) and ginkgo (up to 40 milligrams three times a day). Both herbs can be found combined in Proanthonol by Allergy Research/Nutricology of San Leandro, California.
- Pycnogenol (20 milligrams twice daily) is also recommended as it works not only as an antioxidant but also as a flavonoid to protect and maintain artery walls.

Manic-Depressive Syndrome

Also called bipolar disorder, this condition is a mental illness characterized by alternating periods of mania and depression. Sufferers of this syndrome oscillate between depression and a state of endless energy, agitation, sleeplessness, and sometimes psychosis. The illness may manifest primarily with only one of the extremes (unipolar).

Related and Underlying Causes

B/M **CHEM** **FA**

In this condition, genetic, biochemical, psychological, and emotional factors may play a role. This disorder may also be aggravated by nutritional deficiencies, and yeast overgrowth. It can be worsened by sugar, caffeine, and food allergies.

Treatment and Preventive Measures

CONVENTIONAL MEDICAL TREATMENT
- Drug therapy is commonly needed, and lithium is most often prescribed. In such cases, thyroid blood tests (T4 and TSH) need to be done periodically, as lithium depresses thyroid function.

DIETARY RECOMMENDATIONS
- Eat a whole-foods diet, minimizing alcohol, soft drinks, caffeine, sugar, refined foods, and allergy-triggering foods.

NUTRITIONAL SUPPLEMENTS
- Take vitamin B complex (up to 100 milligrams a day) and zinc (up to 50 milligrams a day). A combination of calcium and magnesium (up to 800 milligrams of each daily) may be helpful. Amino acid testing and appropriate supplementation are recommended (see CHRONIC FATIGUE SYNDROME).
- Take phosphatidylcholine (up to 4,000 milligrams a day) or lecithin (up to 15 grams a day), which may help lessen or prevent the manic phase.
- See DEPRESSION.

Memory Impairment

Inability to remember recent or past details, lack of concentration, and poor mental focus.

Related or Underlying Causes

Memory impairment does not occur automatically with advancing age. It can be caused by hypoglycemia, adrenal exhaustion, low thyroid status (see HYPOTHYROIDISM), chemical hypersensitivity, and heavy metal toxicity. Stress and fatigue alone could be factors. A toxic bowel or liver may also contribute. It can also be linked to arteriosclerosis (see ARTERIOSCLEROSIS) or cerebral insufficiency (see also ALZHEIMER'S DISEASE).

Treatment and Preventive Measures

DIETARY RECOMMENDATIONS
- Eat a whole-foods, anti-hypoglycemic diet. Identify and avoid allergy-triggering foods.

NUTRITIONAL SUPPLEMENTS
- Take vitamin B complex (up to 100 milligrams a day, with up to 800 micrograms of folic acid), vitamin C (up to 3,000 milligrams a day), and phosphatidylcholine (up to 1,000 milligrams three or four times a day).

  The vitamin B-complex supplements, particularly B-12, may need to be injected intramuscularly due to poor gastrointestinal absorption. This is especially important for anyone over the age of fifty experiencing memory problems, fatigue, irritability, or depression. Intravenous injections may be worth trying as well (see ALZHEIMER'S DISEASE).
- Amino acid supplementation is also worthwhile, along with glutamine, phenylalanine, and tyrosine (up to 500 milligrams of each three times a day).

HERBAL REMEDIES
- Take ginkgo (up to 40 milligrams three times a day), ginseng (100 to 200 milligrams a day before 4:00 P.M.), and gotu kola (up to 500 milligrams three times a day), which are particularly useful for treating and preventing senility. Ginkgo and ginseng are also helpful for the treatment and prevention of arteriosclerosis. These three herbs are combined together in a tincture, Ginkgo-Centella Compound by Eclectic Institute of Sandy, Oregon (25 drops two or three times daily).

OTHER THERAPIES
- Regular aerobic exercise, walking, or other movement enhances circulation and may be supportive.
- Chiropractic and cranial adjustments, if indicated, can also be supportive.
- Intellectual stimulation and challenge can aid and boost brain and memory function.
- Include a skilled relaxation exercise as part of a stress management program.

Menopause

Commonly referred to as "the change of life," menopause marks the physiologic end of a woman's reproductive years. This natural part of a woman's life cycle normally starts near the age of fifty, but can begin in the early forties. Menopause is not a health disorder, but many related complaints can occur with its onset. During menopause, production of ovarian hormones, particularly estrogen, drops considerably. As a result, a number of acute symptoms may occur: hot flashes, mild to severe sweats, dryness of the vagina, more frequent urination, sleeplessness, mood swings, headaches, memory impairment, and fatigue. An abnormally elevated follicular-stimulating hormone (FSH) blood level can verify the condition. After menopause, with less circulating estrogen, a woman assumes about the same risk as a man of developing a heart attack. Before menopause, the protection from estrogen decreases the risk of heart attack for women. Also, following menopause, a woman faces a greater risk of developing osteoporosis due to less circulating estrogen and progesterone.

Related or Underlying Causes

Although menopause is a part of a woman's natural maturation process, accompanying symptoms may be aggravated when the adrenal glands are weak. The adrenal hormone dehydroepiandrosterone (DHEA) can be converted to estrogen. In menopause, this DHEA-derived estrogen can help reduce the acute symptoms of lowered ovarian-derived estrogen levels. Menopause symptoms may be worse if DHEA levels are lower.

Treatment and Preventive Measures

CONVENTIONAL MEDICAL TREATMENT
- Research has shown that taking supplemental prescription estrogen maintains bone density, prevents osteoporosis, and reduces acute menopausal symp-

toms. It also lowers the risk of heart attack and stroke with its favorable effects on blood cholesterol levels.

Supplemental estrogen can trigger uterine cancer, but this risk has been nearly removed by adding supplemental progesterone when estrogen therapy is started.

It is also generally believed that an increased risk of breast cancer exists in postmenopausal women taking estrogen for ten or more years, whether or not progesterone is added. Using estrogen less than ten years is generally considered safe if there are no specific contraindications, such as clotting disorders, undiagnosed vaginal bleeding, uterine cancer, acute liver disease, breast cancer or a history of breast cancer, fibrocystic breast disease, high blood pressure, obesity, and diabetes. Some physicians believe that a history of premenopausal breast cancer in a woman's mother, sister, or grandmother should be considered a contributing risk factor and contraindication to taking supplemented estrogen.

Estrogen is routinely recommended for menopausal women unless there are specific contraindications. Many doctors feel that the cancer risks are small. In fact, four times as many American women die of coronary heart disease than of uterine and breast cancers combined. Estrogen can help prevent many of these coronary artery disease deaths. Women are encouraged to start estrogen near menopause, as bone loss in susceptible women is most accelerated in the first several years following menopause.

A growing number of physicians, however, seriously question the widespread prescription of estrogen replacement therapy, even for less than ten years, because many breast cancers are sensitive to and stimulated by estrogen.

There are very effective alternatives for the treatment of acute menopausal symptoms and the prevention of osteoporosis and heart disease. Why subject women to risks from estrogen when its benefits can be achieved without risks?

NUTRITIONAL SUPPLEMENTS

- Vitamin E (800 I.U. daily) and inositol (1,000 milligrams two or three times a day) are specific for acute menopausal symptoms. A multiple vitamin/mineral preparation and vitamin C (up to 3,000 milligrams a day) would be generally supportive.

HERBAL REMEDIES

The following herbal remedies contain plant estrogens that can often relieve acute menopausal symptoms. Even though their estrogen effect is four hundred times weaker than prescription estrogen, they should generally not be used for any conditions for which estrogen is contraindicated, such as estrogen-sensitive breast cancer.

- Take dong quai (up to two 500-milligram capsules two to four times a day) or a dong quai–containing combination herbal formula (see at the end of Chapter Nineteen, "Menopause").
- Solid extract of alfalfa can help alleviate symptoms (¼ teaspoon two or three times a day), available from Scientific Botanicals of Seattle. *Note: Avoid alfalfa if there is a history of systemic lupus erythematosus.*
- Take licorice root capsules (up to six a day) or the solid extract of licorice root (¼ teaspoon two or three times a day), available from Scientific Botanicals of Seattle. *Note: Excessive licorice root can cause fluid retention, elevated blood pressure, and abnormally low potassium levels. Have your doctor monitor you periodically for these potentially dangerous side effects.*
- Siberian ginseng (up to 200 milligrams a day) can also relieve acute menopausal symptoms, due either to effects on the adrenal glands or to estrogenic properties. Some reports suggest avoiding herbal estrogens if there are contraindications to taking prescription estrogen (see above).
- Three percent natural progesterone cream derived from wild yam may provide dramatic relief. Apply topically, rubbing it into clean skin (chest, stomach, inner arm, or inner thighs are best). If you are still menstruating, use ¼ teaspoon twice a day, beginning approximately seven days after the period begins, up until day 21 of the cycle. At this point, use ½ teaspoon twice a day until the period begins. Discontinue this cream during the period until day 7. If you are no longer menstruating, use ¼ teaspoon a day on days 8 to 21 of the calendar month, and ½ teaspoon twice a day on days 22 to 31 of the month. Use none the first seven days of the month. If symptoms warrant, the cream may still be used at this time. The cream can be used for severe hot flashes (¼ to ½ teaspoon every fifteen minutes for four doses). Eventually, use the smallest and least frequent dose that brings relief. Too much cream may cause temporary vaginal spotting. Any persistent postmenopausal spotting or bleeding should always be checked by a physician. Tender breasts and premenstrual-like symptoms may occur from this cream, but are rare. Progesterone cream may increase thyroid activity. If you are taking thyroid hormone, a lower dose may possibly be required (see HYPERTHYROIDISM). Natural progesterone cream is available as Progest Moisturizing Cream from Professional and Technical Specialties of Portland, Oregon.
- When the above approaches are not effective, try EsGen (rub ¼ teaspoon into the skin once or twice a day, as described above for progesterone cream), a natural estrogen cream derived from soybeans. It may be used with progesterone cream to relieve symptoms if there are no contraindications to using supplemental estrogen (see "Conventional Medical Treatment").

Es-Gen is available from Professional and Technical Services, Inc. of Portland, Oregon.

Use both the estrogen and progesterone creams on days 1 through 25 of the month. No hormone cream should be used the last five or six days of each month. Menopausal women generally do not experience water retention, breast soreness, and weight gain on plant-derived estrogen. They often do not have menstrual periods, even when also using progesterone cream.

Although Es-gen is natural, it should be used under medical supervision. Determine the smallest dose that controls acute menopausal symptoms. You may find that you no longer require it after several months. Discontinue use while maintaining treatment with progesterone cream (see OSTEOPOROSIS).

If plant estrogen is ineffective and prescription estrogen is needed (and there are no contraindications), consult your doctor for a prescription of tri-estrogen, a unique combination of estradiol, estrone, and estriol, which will have the same effectiveness as standard prescription estrogen, but fewer risks. The estriol has protective, anti-carcinogenic properties and may reduce the cancer risks from the other estrogens. A pharmacist can compound this blend with a doctor's prescription.

HOMEOPATHIC REMEDIES

- Try combination homeopathic drops (ten to fifteen drops orally as needed) for menopause. Available in health food stores.

Menstrual Bleeding, Excessive (Menorrhagia)

Heavy and/or frequent bleeding that occurs during or extends beyond the normal period interval. It can be accompanied by abdominal discomfort and cramping.

Related or Underlying Causes

Initially, ask your doctor to determine if your bleeding is caused by uterine fibroids, polyps, polycystic ovaries, infection, cancer, or other conditions. Once these are ruled out, consider other causes, such as a yeast overgrowth (yeast toxins can imbalance menstrual hormones) or hypothyroidism (see HYPOTHYROIDISM).

Stress, anxiety, overexertion, and illness can also be factors.

Treatment and Preventive Measures

DIETARY RECOMMENDATIONS

- Avoid processed and particularly partially hydrogenated vegetable oils, sweets, alcohol, caffeine, and nicotine.
- Identify and avoid allergy-triggering foods.
- Eat bioflavonoid-rich foods, such as grapefruit. Especially include those with white pulp.

DETOXIFICATION PROGRAMS

- Follow the Liver Flush and Purifying Diet periodically.

NUTRITIONAL SUPPLEMENTS

- Take vitamin A for several months (75,000 I.U. daily, then taper to 10,000 to 25,000 I.U. daily). Also take vitamin E (400 I.U. daily) and zinc (15 to 30 milligrams a day). Zinc will aid vitamin A absorption (see zinc and vitamin A precautions).
- In some cases, bioflavonoid deficiency may cause excessive bleeding. Take the highly absorbable mixed bioflavonoids naringin, hesperidin, and hesperidin methyl chalcone (two or three 100-milligram capsules once or twice a day), available in a combination formula, Flavoplex-C, from Interplexus of Kent, Washington. Also, take vitamin C (1,000 milligrams three times a day), as vitamin C and bioflavonoids work well together.
- Vitamin K, known for its ability to prevent abnormal bleeding, is very helpful in normalizing menstrual flow. Eat regular portions of dark green, leafy vitamin K–rich vegetables, such as broccoli, brussels sprouts, spinach, and cabbage. Vitamin K levels can be increased as well by taking an acidophilus/bifidus supplement.
- Take Chlorolipids, a fat-soluble chlorophyll extract (1 capsule three times a day), as an alternate source of vitamin K. Available from Biotherapeutics-Enzymatic Therapy of Green Bay, Wisconsin. Or supplement with vitamin K-1 (300 to 500 micrograms a day) for two months.
- Essential fatty acid deficiency may also relate to menorrhagia. Take unrefined flaxseed oil (1 or 2 teaspoons a day) and borage oil capsules (200 to 300 milligrams a day of gamma linolenic acid).
- A potent multiple vitamin/mineral supplement with magnesium (at least 300 to 400 milligrams) will contain the nutrients necessary for the metabolism of the fatty acids, along with vitamin E, which is vital when taking flaxseed and borage oils.
- Sometimes an iron deficiency is both a cause and an effect of menorrhagia. Unfortunately, a simple hemat-

ocrit or hemoglobin blood test may find nothing wrong when iron stores are actually low. A low serum ferritin level may be more accurate and demonstrate the need for taking supplemental iron. *Note: Your physician should monitor the amount and duration of iron supplementation, as well as the cause of low iron stores.*

HERBAL REMEDIES

- To help with symptomatic acute relief of excess menstrual bleeding, take a combination shepherd's purse, geranium, and trillium tincture, or a combination trillium and viburnum tincture (½ teaspoon every fifteen to thirty minutes during waking hours for either combination). If not effective within six doses, discontinue the remedy. Shepherd's purse tea is effective only if the tincture is made from the fresh herb.

Menstrual Cramps

Cramps that occur before, during, and sometimes after a menstrual period. They can cause lower abdominal pain, along with referred pain to the lower back and thighs. Painful cramping can be accompanied by overall fatigue, bloating, irritability, diarrhea, and other symptoms.

Related or Underlying Causes

Menstrual cramps are often caused by abnormally elevated amounts of unfavorable prostaglandin hormones. This imbalance triggers excessive, painful contractions of smooth muscles in the uterus, lower stomach, and other areas. Other common causes of menstrual cramps include hypothyroidism (see HYPOTHYROIDISM); food allergy (especially dairy allergy); structural abnormalities, such as malalignments of the lumbar vertebrae or sacrum; and energy imbalances (see Chapter Twenty-one). Endometriosis (see ENDOMETRIOSIS) can also cause extreme menstrual pain.

Treatment and Preventive Measures

CONVENTIONAL MEDICAL TREATMENT

- Ibuprofen, Naprosyn, and other anti-inflammatory medicines are commonly prescribed for normal menstrual cramps.
- If menstrual pain becomes severe and debilitating, you should be checked for endometriosis.

DIETARY RECOMMENDATIONS

- Reduce the unfavorable prostaglandin levels in your body by avoiding refined, partially hydrogenated, and other unhealthful oils. Do not eat excessive amounts of animal protein. Also, restrict peanut butter, peanut oil, and peanuts.
- Eat omega 3-EPA–rich cold-water fish: herring, mackerel, sablefish, dogfish, salmon, halibut, and others.
- Avoid all cow's milk products for one to two months.

NUTRITIONAL SUPPLEMENTS

- To prevent cramps and encourage synthesis of favorable prostaglandin hormones, take flaxseed oil (1 or 2 teaspoons a day) and borage oil (two capsules or at least 300 milligrams a day of gamma linolenic acid).
- Take vitamin B-6 (25 milligrams a day), zinc (15 to 30 milligrams a day), vitamin C (1,000 to 2,000 milligrams a day), and magnesium (400 milligrams a day), all of which promote favorable prostaglandin hormone metabolism. Vitamin E (400 I.U. daily) should also be taken to provide antioxidant protection while on oil supplements. A good multiple vitamin/mineral supplement may provide most of the above.
- Take calcium (up to 1,500 milligrams) and magnesium (up to 1,000 milligrams a day). Both may be very helpful in relieving acute cramps (see Chapter Six for dose precautions). The glycinate form of magnesium is highly absorbable. Less than half the above dose can be effective and is less likely to cause diarrhea.

HERBAL REMEDIES

- Several herbs offer effective acute symptomatic relief for menstrual cramps. Try any one. Take it beginning a day or so before the onset of your period (one to three capsules two or three times a day). During your period, increase the frequency to three or four times a day as needed. Discontinue when symptoms end. Several of these combination herbal formulas are available from health food stores:
- Equal parts of cramp bark, black cohosh, and piscidia (Jamaican dogwood).
- Piscidia (Jamaican dogwood), available from Scientific Botanicals of Seattle.
- Dong quai root, peony, cramp bark, blue cohosh, false unicorn, and black cohosh, sold commercially as Utero-tone/Fem-Trol by Phytopharmica/Enzymatic Therapy of Green Bay, Wisconsin.

OTHER THERAPIES

- Chiropractic or osteopathic adjustments may bring relief. An exercise program specific for your back may help alignment. You may not be aware of any apparent back problems. However, menstrual cramps may suggest that some structural work may still be in order.

- A hot water bottle, heating pad, or castor oil pack on the lower abdomen over your uterus area will usually bring significant relief.
- Consider acupuncture.

Mitral Valve Prolapse

A congenital abnormality of the mitral valve triggered by excessive valvular tissue, causing parts of the valve to intrude into one of the chambers of the heart. A "click and murmur" is often detected by listening to the patient's heart. The valvular abnormality can be visualized in an ultrasound study (echocardiogram). Those with mitral valve prolapse often experience palpitations, chest pain, dizziness, weakness, and anxiety. The valvular defect does not cause the symptoms, since a fair percentage of individuals with a prolapsed valve do not experience any symptoms. An electrical conductivity impairment may be at work. It is also uncertain why the symptoms first appear in the third and fourth decades of life. It is a benign condition that usually presents no major risks to health.

Treatment and Preventive Measures

CONVENTIONAL MEDICAL TREATMENT

- Treated primarily with beta-blocker medications such as propranolol (Inderal).
- Prophylactic antibiotics should be taken before dental work or other procedures that might introduce bacteria into the blood if any mitral regurgitation, or backward flow of blood, is discovered by an echocardiogram. This prevents an infection of the valve.

DIETARY RECOMMENDATIONS

- Follow the diet for the treatment of hypoglycemia. Identify and avoid allergy-triggering foods.
- Avoid caffeine, chocolate, sugar, and other stimulants.
- Restrict alcohol.

NUTRITIONAL SUPPLEMENTS

- Take magnesium (400 to 800 milligrams a day), coenzyme Q-10 (10 to 30 milligrams three times a day), carnitine (250 to 1,000 milligrams three times a day), and vitamin B-6 (25 to 50 milligrams a day). Such a program may lessen or eliminate the need for beta blockers.

HERBAL REMEDIES

- Hawthorn berry solid extract (¼ teaspoon two or three times a day), from Scientific Botanicals of Seattle, and cactus grandiflora tincture (15 to 25 drops two or three times a day) can help stabilize heart rhythm.

Warning: Do not use hawthorn berry concurrently with beta blockers.

Mononucleosis

Very common among children and young adults, its symptoms include chills, fever, sore throat, painful, swollen lymph nodes in the neck, malaise, and severe fatigue. A blood test may show elevations of abnormal lymphocytes. Also, the "mono-spot" test will be positive. The spleen and liver can become enlarged and an individual can become jaundiced. The usual incubation period is five to twelve days. Contagion may be possible until the fever has subsided.

Related or Underlying Causes

     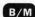

Mononucleosis is caused by the Epstein-Barr virus. Increased susceptibility and lowered resistance to the virus may be brought on by many of the Ten Common Denominators of Illness.

Treatment and Preventive Measures

CONVENTIONAL MEDICAL TREATMENT

- Conventional medicine recommends bed rest until the most acute phase has subsided. Antibiotics for associated strep or other bacterial infections are common, and steroids are sometimes needed to reduce throat swelling, if extreme. Full recovery is generally completed in three to six weeks. Some individuals do not return fully to their normal state of health, while others relapse within a year after apparent recovery. Both groups complain primarily of fatigue and low stamina, and are often diagnosed with chronic Epstein-Barr virus syndrome (see CHRONIC FATIGUE SYNDROME).

DIETARY RECOMMENDATIONS

- If appetite is reduced, as in most acute infections, drink plenty of fluids (six to eight glasses of water a day), including fresh juices, especially carrot and greens, some fruit juice, and vegetable or other broth. As the appetite returns, eat light, nourishing, wholefoods meals, avoiding excesses of calories, sweets, fats, and caffeine. Avoid alcoholic beverages.

NUTRITIONAL SUPPLEMENTS

- Take vitamin C (5,000 to 10,000 milligrams three times a day or the highest dose that does not cause diarrhea). Intravenous vitamin C (see HEPATITIS) will be even more helpful.
- Vitamin A (15,000 to 25,000 I.U. daily), beta-carotene (up to 100,000 I.U. daily), and zinc (30 to 50 milligrams a day) are effective in combating infections. Because other nutrients are also involved in strengthening the immune response, a multiple vitamin/mineral supplement may be useful in this treatment.

HERBAL REMEDIES

Antiviral and immune-stimulating herbal combination formulas can play a vital role in recovering from a mononucleosis infection.

- Take Super-Immuno Tone/Super-Immuno Comp (three or four capsules three or four times a day), which contains echinacea, goldenseal, astragalus, licorice root, and shiitake mushroom, with beta-carotene and small amounts of zinc and vitamins B and C. Available from Phytopharmic/Enzymatic Therapy of Green Bay, Wisconsin.
- Take Echimmune (two or three capsules up to four times a day), which contains echinacea, astragalus, ligustrum, shiitake mushroom, and licorice root. Available from NF Formulas of Wilsonville, Oregon.
- Take Mycelin 3 (one or two capsules three times a day), which contains reishi, shiitake mushroom, and cordyceps. Available from Allergy Research/Nutricology of San Leandro, California.

OTHER THERAPIES

- If your liver is involved, see HEPATITIS for specific liver remedies.
- Glandular tablets have always been a part of naturopathic treatments for mono: spleen, lymph, and thymus concentrates as directed. *Note: Raw glandulars may have safety concerns (see page 315). Use Thy-Max, a boiled thymus glandular (one to three capsules three times a day), available from T. E. Neesby of Fresno, California.*

Multiple Sclerosis

An autoimmune disease of the nervous system in which the myelin sheath surrounding nerve tissue in the brain and spinal cord deteriorates. Nerve transmission is impaired, resulting in a variety of symptoms: visual disturbances; tingling, numbness, and weakness in the extremities; loss of balance; loss of bladder or bowel control; and paralysis. Symptoms may be mild at first, then subside, or they may become severe. They can be intermittent, stable, or progressive and lead to pronounced disabilities and sometimes death.

Related or Underlying Causes

Because multiple sclerosis (MS) is defined as an autoimmune disease, there is currently no known cause. However, many aggravating factors have been observed that lead to active intervention and improved symptom control. Individuals with MS commonly have one or more of the following: food allergy, a high-fat diet; heavy metal toxicity, including mercury from dental fillings; root canals; chemical and inhalant allergies; common bacterial infections (sore throat, bladder infection, etc.); impaired detoxification capacity of the liver.

Treatment and Preventive Measures

Contrary to the conventional medical viewpoint, many treatment options exist and can lead to improved management of the disease, or even alter its course.

CONVENTIONAL MEDICAL TREATMENT

- Adrenocorticotrophic hormone (ACTH) or prednisone (cortisone) administration are the primary treatments. Beta interferon has recently shown some promise.
- Common sore throats and bladder infections must be treated aggressively since these minor infections can trigger severe setbacks of MS symptoms. Because there may be no obvious symptoms of a bladder infection, exacerbation of MS symptoms warrants checking for a bladder infection.
- Identify and treat food allergy, a toxic bowel, heavy metal toxicity, adrenal exhaustion, yeast overgrowth, a sluggish liver, and any associated condition.

DIETARY RECOMMENDATIONS

- Eat a diet low in saturated fat. (See guidelines in Chapters Three and Four.)
- Identify and avoid food allergens.

NUTRITIONAL SUPPLEMENTS

- Take N-acetylcysteine (500 milligrams four times every other day), using 30 milligrams of zinc and 2 milligrams of copper on the days in between; gamma linolenic acid (GLA) from borage oil capsules (up to 500 milligrams a day) and fish oil capsules, or EPA (up to 3,000 milligrams a day).

OTHER THERAPIES
- See bee venom therapy (Chapter Twenty).
- Physical therapy, dance therapy, or other movement or exercise therapy may be vital.

Muscle Cramps

See CRAMPS (MUSCLE).

Nausea

Stomach and digestive discomfort, sometimes followed by vomiting. Depending on the cause, other symptoms may accompany nausea, including abdominal pain, fever, chills, dizziness, and headache.

Related or Underlying Causes

 DietH ToxB SL DIG

Nausea can also be caused by *Giardia* and other parasites (see PARASITES), food poisoning, overeating, environmental illness, stomach flu, and chronic illnesses. It can also be linked to an adverse reaction to a prescription medication or vitamin supplements.

Treatment and Preventive Measures

Address the underlying causes and treat appropriately. Consult a physician if persistent. Consider the following options for symptomatic relief.

CONVENTIONAL MEDICAL TREATMENT
- Antinausea medications, such as Compazine and Tigan, are commonly prescribed.

HERBAL REMEDIES
- Drink gingerroot tea, full strength (four or five thin slices of the fresh root lightly simmered for twenty minutes in 2 cups of water). Steep peppermint with it for its favorable effect on the digestive system. Licorice root can be used to help the flavor.
- Goldenseal root (one or two capsules three or four times a day) may be helpful. Or use Bitters Formula (1 teaspoon mixed in 2 or 3 ounces of water and sipped over twenty minutes), which contains gentian, calamus, angelica, wormwood, and turmeric. The formula, which may enhance appetite, is available from Herb-Pharm of Williams, Oregon.

HOMEOPATHIC REMEDIES
- Try ipecac for effective relief, as directed.
- Nux vomica is often used when nausea is a result of overeating or drinking.

Neuritis/Neuropathy (Peripheral)

Inflammation of a nerve, resulting in pain, tingling, or numbness.

Related or Underlying Causes

 ND CHEM

Neuritis is caused by trauma, virus, heavy metal poisoning, vitamin and mineral deficiencies, spinal malalignment, and diabetes.

Treatment and Preventive Measures

Note: For chronic cases, up to six months may be needed for improvement of the condition.

NUTRITIONAL SUPPLEMENTS
- Take vitamin B complex (25 to 50 milligrams twice a day), vitamin B-1 (100 to 200 milligrams a day), and folic acid (800 micrograms a day).
- Take Allithiamine (providing 50 milligrams of fat-soluble vitamin B-1 per capsule) and Thiotic (providing 100 milligrams of lipoic acid per capsule), both by Cardiovascular Research of Concord, California. Take one capsule three times a day with meals.
- Take calcium (800 milligrams a day) and magnesium (800 milligrams a day).
- Biotin (up to 2,000 micrograms three times a day) may help neuropathy, particularly if diabetes-related (see DIABETES).
- Vitamin B-12 intramuscular injections should be tried (1,000 micrograms twice a week, with 2 or 3 milligrams of folic acid).

HERBAL REMEDIES
- Take kelp (two or three tablets twice a day) to supply nerve nutrients, and skullcap (up to twelve capsules a day) to soothe inflammation of nerves.

OTHER THERAPIES
- Acupuncture and auricular therapy may bring relief.
- Consider bee venom therapy.

- See an osteopathic or chiropractic physician if neuritis is related to structural malalignment.

Neuropathy

See NEURITIS.

Nosebleeds

Unexplained recurrent bleeding of the nose. They are very common among young children, adolescents, and middle-aged adults.

Related or Underlying Causes

Nosebleeds may be caused by capillary fragility stemming from a deficiency of vitamin C and bioflavonoids. Vitamin K deficiency also leads to easy bleeding. Also, consider high blood pressure, a bleeding disorder, inadequate humidity, and drying of the mucous membranes.

Treatment and Preventive Measures

DIETARY RECOMMENDATIONS
- Eat plenty of dark green, leafy vegetables as a source of vitamin K, or take a chlorophyll supplement.

NUTRITIONAL SUPPLEMENTS
- For prevention, take vitamin C (up to 1,000 milligrams three times a day) and highly absorbable mixed bioflavonoids. Take both in a combination formula, (Flavoplex-C, two or three capsules once a day), which contains 100 milligrams each of naringin, hesperidin, hesperidin methyl chalcone, winter cherry, and grapeskin. Available from Interplexus of Kent, Washington.
  Also for prevention, take *Lactobacillus acidophilus*/bifidus supplements (one capsule of a potent brand twice a day), which will indirectly help increase vitamin K levels, a nutrient necessary for the clotting of blood.

HERBAL REMEDIES
- For acute relief, take cayenne capsules (two to four capsules three or four times a day).

OTHER THERAPIES
- For an acute nosebleed, bend your head forward slightly with mouth open to prevent choking on your blood, then pinch your nose firmly. Place a cold, wet cloth across the bridge of your nose while pinching. Stuff your nose with cotton. Also, place a cold cloth on the back of your neck. Continue pinching for another five minutes.
- For prevention, use a humidifier in your bedroom.
  Note: If condition persists, consult a physician.

Obesity

See OVERWEIGHT.

Osteoporosis

A state of diminished bone mass that can result in fractures, especially of the hip. Collapse of spinal vertebrae is also very common, leading to loss of height, "dowager's hump," and spinal pain. Thinning of the bones is a natural occurrence, with bone loss seen in both men and women of advanced age. Postmenopausal women are most at risk since women's bones are inherently less dense than men's and because diminished estrogen and progesterone levels after menopause increase the rate of bone loss.

Related or Underlying Causes

DietH **ND** **DIG** **ADR** **B/M**

Although diminished levels of estrogen after menopause are purported to be key in accelerating bone loss, the natural state of postmenopause should not lead to osteoporosis. This ailment is brought on by multiple factors. Low estrogen levels are only one contributing element and likely not the most important. Although estrogen helps delay bone loss, inadequate amounts of ovarian and adrenal hormones, which actually help build bone, progesterone, and dehydroepiandrosterone (DHEA), may be more significant risk factors. Studies have shown a reversal in osteoporosis, an actual increase in bone density, in postmenopausal women taking natural progesterone, whether or not it was accompanied by supplemental estrogen.

One of the main causes of osteoporosis is lack of weight-bearing exercise, since this type of exercise is crucial in the maintaining of bone density. Excessive exercise can also lead to thinning of the bones.

Inadequate consumption of calcium and other nutrients important to bone metabolism (magnesium, manganese, zinc, copper, boron, silicon, and vitamins C, B-6, D, and K) can lead to osteoporosis. Diminished gastrointestinal absorption of bone nutrients, especially the minerals, can also contribute. Inadequate stomach acid (hydrochloric acid) production, common in those over fifty, often related to poor mineral absorption, is also a cause.

Dietary and lifestyle factors that cause the urinary excretion of calcium are frequently far more important in osteoporosis than outright calcium deficiency. Increased urinary excretion of bone nutrients, particularly calcium, is stimulated by dietary excesses of protein (flesh foods and milk products), fat, caffeine, sugar, alcohol, phosphorus (from flesh foods and phosphoric acid–containing soft drinks), and aluminum (from aluminum-containing antacids, coffeepots, cookware, cans, and bottle tops). Such mineral loss can lead to osteoporosis. Tobacco use also stimulates urinary calcium loss.

Certain hormone excesses, such as hyperparathyroidism, in which excessive amounts of the hormone parathormone are produced by the parathyroid glands in the neck, can stimulate bone loss. Hyperthyroidism or excessive supplemental thyroid hormone will do the same. An additional risk for developing osteoporosis is present for those who are small-boned, slender, Caucasian, or Asian.

Adrenal dysfunction can also play a role in osteoporosis. If your cortisol levels are too high and your DHEA (dehydroepiandrosterone) levels too low, you may be at risk for osteoporosis. Cortisol, a catabolic adrenal hormone, causes tissue or bone breakdown, whereas DHEA, an anabolic adrenal hormone, stimulates tissue and bone building.

Treatment and Preventive Measures

CONVENTIONAL MEDICAL TREATMENT

- X rays will not disclose this condition until the disease is well advanced. Blood level tests of calcium generally are not helpful. The most effective early diagnostic testing to determine present bone density includes dual photon or dual X-ray absorptiometry. Periodontal bone loss may be an early indicator.
- A repeat absorptiometry given approximately two or three years later can determine if diet and treatment regimens have been effective in halting or reversing bone loss. If significant bone deterioration is noted, more aggressive measures will be required.
- Most physicians currently recommend at menopause supplemental estrogen (see MENOPAUSE), low-fat

milk products, calcium (up to 1,500 milligrams a day), and weight-bearing exercise for preventing osteoporosis in the postmenopausal years. Before menopause, calcium (up to 1,000 milligrams a day) is recommended.
- If your serum calcium level is high, consult your doctor to rule out primary hyperparathyroidism, a common, treatable cause of osteoporosis.

DIETARY RECOMMENDATIONS

- Eating a vegetarian or semivegetarian whole-foods diet can substantially reduce the risk. However, be sure to consume adequate amounts of protein.
- Avoid the dietary excesses listed above. It is significant to note that countries with the highest consumption of milk products have the highest incidence of osteoporosis.

NUTRITIONAL SUPPLEMENTS

- The American diet is often rich in calories but poor in vitamins and minerals, many of which are required either directly or indirectly to make bone.
- Take a "bone nutrients" or multiple vitamin/mineral formula daily, providing calcium (up to 800 milligrams), magnesium (up to 800 milligrams), zinc (up to 30 milligrams), copper (up to 3 milligrams), manganese (up to 20 milligrams), silicon (up to 1 milligram), and boron (up to 3 milligrams). Boron can help increase serum estrogen levels. The formula should also include vitamin K (up to 300 micrograms a day), vitamin D (100 to 600 I.U.), folic acid (up to 400 micrograms), B complex (25 to 50 milligrams), and vitamin C (up to 1,000 milligrams).
- Osteoprime Forte (two capsules twice a day), distributed by Biotherapeutics of Green Bay, Wisconsin, and Osteoporosis Formula (three capsules three times a day), by Tyler Encapsulations of Gresham, Oregon, are "bone formulas" containing all of the above nutrients.
- Although up to 1,500 milligrams a day of calcium is recommended from a conventional medical standpoint, it is suspected that this much calcium can interfere with the utilization of the bone nutrients magnesium, manganese, and zinc. Excessive calcium supplementation may have additional adverse effects in combination with inadequate magnesium and excessive vitamin D levels. Smaller amounts of calcium (500 to 800 milligrams) should be adequate if the other bone nutrients are included and a calcium-losing diet and lifestyle are avoided. Using equal amounts of supplemental calcium and magnesium is an emerging concept in nutritional medicine, replacing the previous practice of using twice as much calcium as magnesium. Experimentation may be necessary to find the type of magnesium that does not

cause diarrhea in higher doses. (Try the glycinate form.)

Note: *Avoid the most common and inexpensive kinds of calcium and magnesium supplements—calcium carbonate, oyster shell calcium, and magnesium oxide. These products are not efficiently absorbed into the bloodstream of many older individuals. Use citrate, malate, fumarate, or other absorbable forms.*

- Supplemental vitamin D (100 to 200 I.U. daily) may be sufficient for men and women who consume vitamin D–fortified foods and for premenopausal women who regularly go outdoors. It may be adequate for those who live in climates where there is regular sunlight. A 400 I.U. dosage of vitamin D may be indicated for those under sixty-five who do not fit these requirements, for men over the age of sixty-five, and up to 600 I.U. for postmenopausal women. (See Chapter Six for more discussion of "Calcium," "Magnesium," and "Vitamin D.")

HERBAL REMEDIES

- For postmenopausal women concerned with preserving and building bone mass, use a natural progesterone cream derived from wild yam (approximately ⅛ to ¼ teaspoon twice a day for the first twenty-four days of the month, then none for the last seven days). For the use of progesterone cream before menopause, see PREMENSTRUAL SYNDROME.

  Occasional vaginal spotting may occur with the use of this cream, but it is usually only temporary and may be dose related. Consult a doctor familiar with its use. For persistent vaginal spotting or bleeding, see a doctor. Very rarely, progesterone cream may increase thyroid activity. If you are taking thyroid hormone, your doctor may need to decrease your dose slightly if hyperthyroid symptoms occur (see HYPERTHYROIDISM). Your doctor or pharmacist can order Pro-Gest moisturizing cream from Professional and Technical Services of Portland, Oregon (see MENOPAUSE for more complete instructions). Use under medical supervision.
- If estrogen supplementation is necessary and there are no contraindications, try Es-Gen, an herbal estrogen cream derived from soybeans, along with Pro-Gest Cream (as described for MENOPAUSE).
- If herbal estrogen is ineffective and estrogen is needed, consult your doctor for a prescription of tri-estrogen, a unique combination of estradiol, estrone, and estriol, which will have the same effectiveness as standard prescription estrogen. The estriol is thought to have protective, anticarcinogenic properties. It may reduce the cancer risks from the other estrogens. A pharmacist can compound this blend with a doctor's prescription (Clark's Prescriptions in Bellevue, Washington).

OTHER THERAPIES

- Do weight-bearing exercises, at least four or five days a week for thirty to sixty minutes: walking, jogging, stair climbing, bicycling, skiing, dancing, weight lifting, and so on.
- Stress management and DHEA supplementation may be needed to rebalance adrenal hormone levels and to reverse or prevent an osteoporotic process (see Chapter Eleven).
- Avoid tobacco use.

Ovarian Cysts

Fluid-filled, usually benign growths on the ovaries.

Related or Underlying Causes

Ovarian cysts are often follicular cysts, caused by a failure of an ovarian follicle to rupture and release its egg. The follicle subsequently swells with fluid. A corpus luteum cyst is also a functional cyst and is caused by an unexplained increase in fluid secretion in the ovary after ovulation (egg release). It is often associated with pain, menstrual changes, and hemorrhage. Infrequently, an ovarian cyst is malignant.

An excessively yin diet may lead to cyst growth. Yin foods include sugar, alcohol, milk products, and fruit.

Treatment and Preventive Measures

CONVENTIONAL MEDICAL TREATMENT

- Once diagnosed by pelvic exam and pelvic ultrasound, ovarian cysts should be monitored periodically by your doctor. An operation need not be a first option unless the findings are suspicious for malignancy or there are other clear indications for surgery. Many ovarian cysts shrink completely and spontaneously without medication. Others can be remedied by the use of oral contraceptives.

  Natural remedies can alleviate cysts: try a one- to two-month treatment period, then get rechecked by your doctor. If the cyst is still present and symptomatic, conventional medical treatment may be the wisest choice.

DIETARY RECOMMENDATIONS

- Eat a whole-foods diet.
- Avoid refined, processed foods. Lean toward a macrobiotic diet. Avoiding excesses of yin foods listed above may prove useful (see Chapter Four). Eliminate all

sources of caffeine, such as coffee, soft drinks, black tea, chocolate, and caffeine-containing medications.

NUTRITIONAL SUPPLEMENTS
- Take vitamin E (800 to 1,200 I.U. daily) in addition to a daily multiple vitamin/mineral formula.

HERBAL REMEDIES
- Take Turska's Formula (up to 25 drops three times a day), an herbal tincture formula consisting of gelsemium, phytolacca, bryonia, and aconite. Available by prescription at the Natural Health Clinic of Bastyr University in Seattle.

HOMEOPATHIC REMEDIES
- Take specific homeopathic agents, such as apis mel for right-sided cysts and colocinthus for left-sided cysts.

OTHER THERAPIES
- Use localized diathermy treatments and vaginal drawing packs, as administered by a naturopathic doctor.
- Apply castor oil packs one hour daily for up to one month or more.

Overweight

A condition in which an individual carries an excess of 10 to 20 percent body fat above standard weight limits for normal frame types. An overweight condition predisposes an individual to high blood pressure, elevated blood cholesterol levels, diabetes, stroke, heart attack, gallbladder disease, several cancers, and musculoskeletal problems.

Related or Underlying Causes

(DietH) (ND) (DIG) (FA)

(CHEM) (SL) (HYP) (B/M)

Contributing factors include one or more of the following: excessive calories (especially fat calories), too much refined food and sugar, vitamin and mineral deficiencies, maldigestion, insufficient exercise, hypothyroidism (see HYPOTHYROIDISM), insulin insensitivity (see DIABETES), yeast overgrowth, and hereditary factors. Also consider emotionally triggered eating; poor body image; ineffective metabolism due to age or low caloric intake; brain chemistry deficiencies, often affecting levels of serotonin or beta endorphins; poor food

combining; or eating foods ill-suited to your body type. Weight problems can also stem from a sedentary lifestyle and lack of exercise.

Treatment and Preventive Measures

Successful weight loss should be gradual and occur over a period of many months to years. It is maintained by implementing new lifestyle habits that alter body metabolism, such as diet, exercise, and stress management, to increase vitality and overall health. Weight loss in this manner is not a result of dieting; it occurs as a byproduct of improved health and fitness. Crash diets and temporary weight loss programs or techniques do facilitate dramatic weight loss initially. However, since they do not increase overall health and well-being, they cannot be sustained for any length of time and are doomed to fail. As soon as they are discontinued, the lost weight will almost always return, along with additional pounds.

Use the Master Symptom Survey on pages 17–29 to identify problem areas that must be addressed in order to regain overall health. Successfully treating just one common denominator of illness can encourage you to begin taking additional steps toward weight loss. For example, eliminating sugar craving by treating a yeast overgrowth can begin a series of cascading benefits. Eating less sugar and treating yeast usually means weight loss and increased vitality. This leads to exercise, which takes off more weight and increases energy even more. With more energy, you might be ready to then try a food allergy elimination diet.

DIETARY RECOMMENDATIONS

Many doctors and weight loss centers prescribe basically the same weight loss diets to all their patients and clients. These diets may be effective for some, but fail to provide lasting results for many. A successful weight loss regimen requires a diet tailored to individual needs. For example, one person may need a diet that excludes allergy-triggering foods, while another may benefit from a program treating hypoglycemia or yeast overgrowth. Some people lose weight and thrive on a high-protein, low-carbohydrate diet, whereas others get results on a high-complex-carbohydrate, low-protein diet. Experimentation, trial and error, and professional advice are needed to create the proper weight regimen for you. The diet may need to be individualized for body type (see Chapter Four).

Although every diet must be individualized, there are some basic principles that are applicable to any weight loss program.
- Eat a whole-foods diet, with generous amounts of fresh vegetables. Fresh fruit is recommended, although hypoglycemia and yeast overgrowth diets may

limit amounts. Start with a basic diet incorporating the sound nutritional principles discussed in Chapters Three and Four.

- Drink at least six glasses of water every day, preferably between meals.
- Minimize white flour and other refined and processed foods, junk foods, and excess fat.
- Avoid unhealthy fats, such as fried foods and partially hydrogenated and other refined vegetable oils.
- Avoid eating late-night dinners and snacks.
- Try a food allergy elimination diet.
- Experiment with food-combining principles, as discussed in Chapter Seven.
- Avoid skipping meals or consuming too few calories. Erratic eating habits may cause hypoglycemic symptoms or other adverse conditions. Irregular eating times also defeat the goal of losing weight, because they slow the metabolic rate. The body may switch to a "famine" mode, in which it will vigorously mobilize its energies to store calories as fat. All of this will make it more difficult to lose weight and cause you to gain even more pounds upon resuming normal caloric intake. Eat sensibly and regularly throughout the day.
- Plan occasional indulgences to avoid feelings of self-deprivation. However, restrict the foods that carry a potential for triggering an addictive cycle of eating.

DETOXIFICATION PROGRAMS

- Although not a weight loss program, many individuals lose significant weight on a cleansing program, such as Ultra Clear, as a result of decreased systemic toxicity and food allergy reduction.

NUTRITIONAL SUPPLEMENTS

- Unless there is an intolerance to or appetite-increasing effect from B vitamins, take a multiple vitamin/mineral formula that provides vitamin B complex (up to 50 milligrams a day).
- Take 5-hydroxytryptophan (100 milligrams twice a day) to help block starch/carbohydrate craving. This pharmaceutical derivative of tryptophan is available by prescription only.
- Take chromium (1,000 micrograms a day) and biotin (3,000 micrograms a day) to reduce sugar craving. Glutamine (500 milligrams three times a day) may also help.
- Take borage oil (one capsule two or three times a day) and flaxseed oil (1 teaspoon a day) to block the tendency toward increased fat storage that can occur with some low-fat diets.

HERBAL REMEDIES

- Ephedra and camellia, along with the nutritional supplements N-acetylated glucosamine and L-cysteine (one or two capsules two or three times a day) have been used successfully in weight loss programs. Both are available from Scientific Botanicals of Seattle.

OTHER THERAPIES

- Weight loss and improved health are achieved and maintained partially by regular exercise. Exercise at least four to six times a week. For the beginner, a forty-five- to sixty-minute walk will suffice.
- Acupuncture can help control food cravings and favorably alter the body's metabolism.
- It is sometimes useful to incorporate a protein or meal replacement powder once a day, such as Ultra Meal or Ultra Balance by Metagenics of San Clemente, California. Your doctor or pharmacist can order it for you. Twice daily use merits monitoring by a physician.
- Commitment is essential to sustained weight loss. It must be maintained through a combination of internal and external support. Internal support includes inner guidance, goal setting, self-motivation, and self-love. Build positive external support involving your spouse, your family, close friends, a support group, and others. Additional encouragement may come from your exercise or fitness coach, nutritionist, therapist, and physician.

Palpitations of the Heart

An abrupt change in the regular beating rhythm of the heart that can last moments or hours. Palpitations often recur episodically. They can be associated with a momentary flutter in the chest or light-headedness and chest pain.

Related or Underlying Causes

Palpitations are commonly linked to low body stores of magnesium and potassium. The decreased magnesium and potassium levels often exist despite "normal" blood serum test results. Diuretics (water pills) often precipitate these deficiencies, although low magnesium stores are common without diuretic use. Excessive caffeine intake can reduce magnesium levels through urinary loss, and add a directly unstabilizing effect on heart rhythm. Hyperthyroid function (see HYPERTHYROIDISM) may be a factor. Fear and anxiety, which increase adrenaline levels, can also contribute.

Palpitations can be an early indicator of heart disease (see ARTERIOSCLEROSIS). Consult your doctor to rule out this possibility, particularly if chest pain, dizziness, or malaise are associated. Mitral valve prolapse can also trigger palpitations (see MITRAL VALVE PROLAPSE). Rule out obesity as a possible cause (see OVERWEIGHT). Malalignments of spinal vertebrae may relate.

Treatment and Preventive Measures

DIETARY RECOMMENDATIONS

- Implement sound nutritional principles with a whole-foods diet, emphasizing fresh produce. Eat magnesium-rich foods, such as dark green, leafy vegetables, raw or dry-roasted nuts, whole grains, and soybeans (see Chapter Three).
- Restrict excessive fats, sweets, refined flours, and other common dietary hazards (see ARTERIOSCLEROSIS).
- Drink potassium-rich fresh vegetable juice or eat bananas and other potassium rich foods.
- Restrict or eliminate all sources of caffeine (coffee, tea, and soft drinks, as well as chocolate). Find effective alternatives for caffeine-based pain and theophylline medications.

NUTRITIONAL SUPPLEMENTS

- For general support, take vitamin E (up to 400 I.U. daily), vitamin B complex (50 milligrams a day), and vitamin C with bioflavonoids (up to 1,000 milligrams three times a day).
- To prevent palpitations, take magnesium (up to 800 milligrams a day) to increase magnesium stores and intracellular potassium levels. Intravenous magnesium chloride (1 gram) or intramuscular magnesium sulfate (500 to 1,000 milligrams) can work exceptionally well to normalize heart rhythm. (Oral magnesium is usually insufficient for acute treatment.)
- Take carnitine (300 to 1,000 milligrams three times a day) to strengthen the heartbeat and normalize rhythm.

HERBAL REMEDIES

- Take hawthorn berry solid extract (¼ teaspoon two or three times a day) or capsules (one or two capsules two or three times a day) to stabilize heart rhythm.
- Cactus grandiflora tincture (fifteen to twenty-five drops two or three times a day) can be used with hawthorn berry.
- Take arjuna, an Ayurvedic herb sold by Herb Technology/Khalsa Health Center of Seattle (one or two capsules two or three times a day).

OTHER THERAPIES

- Practice skilled relaxation exercises.
- Consult a chiropractic or osteopathic physician.

Panic Attacks

See ANXIETY and PANIC.

Paranoia

See ANXIETY and DEPRESSION.

Parasites (Intestinal)

Organisms that live in the intestines and cause common gastrointestinal complaints and numerous symptoms outside the intestinal tract. *Entamoeba histolytica, Giardia lambdia, Blastocystis hominis, Dientamoeba fragilis,* and *cryptosporidium* are the most common parasites. Parasites can cause the following acute and chronic symptoms: severe and sometimes explosive diarrhea; bloody, greasy, or foul-smelling stools; abdominal pain and cramps; bloating; constipation; nausea; fever; malaise and weakness; weight loss; chronic fatigue; food allergies; milk and/or gluten intolerance; hives; yeast overgrowth; vitamin B-12 deficiency; irritability; chemical hypersensitivity; arthritis; asthma; and immune dysfunction. Suspecting an intestinal parasite infection is not unusual after returning from a visit to a foreign country with acute diarrhea. It is more of a challenge, however, for patients and doctors alike to implicate parasites as a possible cause of chronic symptoms such as constipation, bloating, nausea, and other common complaints that many individuals learn to live with.

Related or Underlying Causes

Parasites are commonly transmitted from infected feces to the mouth, most often where sanitary and water treatment standards are poor. In such conditions, food and water, even ice, may be contaminated. Although you do not have to travel to an exotic locale to pick up these bugs, the likelihood of contracting them is much higher there. If you develop an intestinal illness while there or shortly after returning home, suspect a parasitic infection.

You can be an asymptomatic parasite carrier for some time before symptoms arise. Illness or significant stress months later can allow the parasitic infection to become active and symptomatic. Even if you have been diagnosed and treated for parasites, chronic symptoms can still recur after treatment. Insufficient treatment and drug resistance are causes of recurring symptoms. When they recur, the symptoms may be different from those in the initial outbreak. I have diagnosed intestinal parasites in individuals who contracted them more than ten years previously.

Food handlers may unwittingly pass on parasites, particularly if they have lived or traveled in other countries where parasitic infections are endemic. Whether in a restaurant or in a home, anyone plagued with intestinal parasites and using poor sanitary habits can infect your food, glassware, and utensils. Anyone living with an individual diagnosed with parasites should be tested, along with sexual partners of that person. Testing a patient's household and intimate contacts for exposure will prevent reinfection after treatment if a family member or sexual partner has unwittingly contracted parasites.

Parasites are a common contaminant of many lakes and streams in the United States. You do not necessarily have to drink the water to become infected. Brushing your teeth with the water, even just swimming and splashing in it, may be enough to cause an infection if the water is heavily infested and gets in your mouth.

Treatment and Preventive Measures

CONVENTIONAL MEDICAL TREATMENT

The routine stool test for detecting intestinal ova and parasites is notoriously inaccurate, particularly when the infection is chronic and when it involves *Giardia* and *Dientamoeba fragilis*. Their cysts will often rupture and evade detection by standard microscopic examination. Even three or more consecutive daily stool samples may not disclose these parasites.

Fortunately, the fecal *Giardia* antigen assay technique that detects "fragments" of ruptured cysts will rarely miss this infection. Immunologic techniques, such as measuring levels of amoeba-specific intestinal or salivary secretory IgA antibodies, also provide improved diagnostic sensitivity. Diagnos-Techs Laboratory in Seattle, Washington, offers these tests. Meridian Valley Clinical Laboratory in Kent, Washington, Great Smokies Diagnostic Laboratory in Asheville, North Carolina, and some hospital laboratories also provide this service.

For the treatment of intestinal parasites, pharmaceutical medicine is usually the most reliable method.

Metronidazole, furazolidone, diiodohydroxycin, and quinacrine are frequently prescribed. One of the more effective agents with the fewest side effects is tinidazole, available through several compounding pharmacists. One very effective treatment recommended for *Giardia* in adults is 2,000 milligrams of tinidazole taken with a meal, repeated a second time in two weeks, and a third time two weeks after the second dose.

NUTRITIONAL SUPPLEMENTS

- Vitamin C (3,000 milligrams a day), vitamin A (25,000 I.U. daily), zinc (15 to 30 milligrams a day), and B complex (25 milligrams a day) are important for resistance to infections.
- Take acidophilus/bifidus supplements (one or two capsules twice a day) to correct the imbalance in intestinal flora usually associated with parasitic infections.
- For a chronic *Giardia* or *Dientamoeba fragilis* infection, take vitamin B-12 (1,000 micrograms) and folic acid (two or three milligrams) intramuscularly once a week for two months.
- As intestinal parasites are often associated with a "leaky gut," take Permeability Factors from Tyler Encapsulations of Gresham, Oregon (one or two capsules three times a day) and see Chapter Thirteen for more discussion on healing the gut.

HERBAL REMEDIES

- Herbal antiparasite preparations may provide a good option for individuals who cannot tolerate the drugs or for cases when drug therapy has failed repeatedly. Generally, the herbs can be taken safely over several months of daily use, unlike many of the antiparasite prescription drugs. The efficacy of these herbal remedies has been validated mostly from clinical experience and not controlled studies. They work well for some individuals and not for others.
- Take grapefruit seed extract and artemisia annua (Chinese wormwood) from Allergy Research/Nutricology of San Leandro, California (available as Para Microcidin: up to 250 milligrams three times a day with food, and as Artemisia: up to 1,000 milligrams three times a day with food).

Health Concerns of Alameda, California, makes two combination Chinese herbal antiparasite formulas: Aquilaria 22 and Artestatin (for both, take three capsules three times a day). Another formula is Intestinalis (one or two capsules three times a day) by Life Center Inc. of New York.

Note: Whatever treatment is used, a repeat stool exam should be obtained approximately one month after the last dose of medication. Immunologic tests should be repeated in three or four months.

Goldenseal (one capsule with meals) can act as an

antibacterial and antiparasitic. Garlic (raw, freeze-dried, capsules, or oil) also acts as both an antibacterial and antiparasitic agent (one capsule or tablet with meals). Take with another antibacterial/antiparasitic herbal medication, such as grapefruit seed extract or Intestinalis (one capsule per meal for either of these).

TRAVEL PRECAUTIONS

To minimize chances of ingesting parasites (or pathogenic bacteria and hepatitis virus) when traveling to areas with questionable sanitary standards, drink only bottled and purified water. This restriction applies as well to ice. Drink juice or other bottled beverages when purified water is not available. Do not eat raw vegetables or unpeeled fruit unless they are thoroughly washed with bottled purified water and soap. If your stay is relatively short, it may be preferable to avoid these foods. It may be wise to use these precautions as well on your return flight.

Up to three weeks before traveling and during the trip once or twice daily (if refrigeration is accessible), use a high-quality lactobacillus acidophilus and bifidus supplement. As an additional preventive during the trip, take grapefruit seed extract or Intestinalis (one capsule of either per meal) or use goldenseal and garlic (one capsule of each per meal). By strengthening your intestinal flora, you can reduce intestinal complaints to a minimum.

If you do get an intestinal illness, you can double the dose of your remedies and add *Saccharomyces boulardii* (up to two capsules per meal), available from Allergy Research/Nutricology of San Leandro, California. Realize that many forms of traveler's diarrhea are minor and will subside on their own in three days. Homeopathic combination tablets or drops specific for dysentery and intestinal spasms and cramps can also be useful. Lomotil™ and other standard diarrhea suppressants provide rapid relief. If you are traveling for more than a few weeks, it would be wise to pack vitamin C, milk thistle, and Livit 1/Livit 2 (available from Interplexus of Kent, Washington) in the event of hepatitis (see HEPATITIS). *Note: For any persistent or serious gastrointestinal symptoms, consult a local health professional for diagnosis and treatment.*

Parkinson's Disease

A disorder affecting the brain, causing the loss of dopamine, a neurotransmitter, and resulting in loss of muscle control. Symptoms include tremors, stiffness, slowness of movement, gait disturbance, and rigid muscles in the face.

Related or Underlying Causes

Recent studies suggest that this disease may be linked to chemical overload, with neurotoxic chemicals in the central system. Such overload may be due to damaged detoxification mechanisms in the liver. Nutritional deficiencies may impair the production of dopamine from the amino acid phenylalanine. Antioxidant deficiencies may also relate to this condition.

Treatment and Preventive Measures

CONVENTIONAL MEDICAL TREATMENT
- This disease is treated symptomatically with the drug L-Dopa.
- More recently, the drug Deprenyl has shown some success.

DIETARY RECOMMENDATIONS
- Eat a whole-foods diet.
- Restrict sweets, refined foods, and junk foods.
- Drink six to eight glasses of water every day.

DETOXIFICATION PROGRAM
- Chemical detoxification and liver-enhancing regimens, such as the Ultra Clear program, may retard or halt deterioration caused by the disease and stabilize the condition. They may or may not reverse symptoms of existing disease.

NUTRITIONAL SUPPLEMENTS
- Take vitamin B (up to 50 milligrams three times a day), vitamin B-6 (up to 100 milligrams a day), vitamin C (up to 3,000 milligrams a day), and vitamin E (up to 3,200 I.U. daily—see Chapter Six for contraindications). If red blood cell copper levels are low, add copper sebecate (4 milligrams a day). Tyrosine (500 to 1,000 milligrams once or twice a day) may also help in the production of dopamine. Also, take a daily multivitamin/mineral supplement. High doses of L-methionine (up to 5,000 milligrams a day) have produced a favorable response.
- Perque 1 (one or two tablets thirty to sixty minutes before meals) is a combination antioxidant and amino acid formula that supports liver detoxification mechanisms. It is available from Seraphim of Reston, Virginia.

OTHER THERAPIES
- Avoid exposure to toxic chemicals in the home and workplace. When use of chemicals is necessary, take

precautions to reduce exposure: protective gloves, proper handling of contaminated clothes, ventilation, vapor mask, proper storage, and so on. See Chapter Fourteen.

Pelvic Inflammatory Disease (PID)

An acute infection of the uterus and fallopian tubes that can sometimes become chronic and recur over months and years.

Related or Underlying Causes

PID is brought on by an inadequately treated primary infection, such as chlamydia. An IUD, or intrauterine device, can also be a precipitating cause. Given the risk of infection and subsequent sterility, IUDs should not be chosen as a form of birth control for women who intend to become pregnant in the future. However, copper-containing IUDs, such as the ParaGard, are regarded as safe by some sources. If you have never had PID and develop unexplained pelvic pain or vaginal discharge, see your doctor immediately.

Treatment and Preventive Measures

CONVENTIONAL MEDICAL TREATMENT
- If PID is diagnosed, antibiotics should be taken as prescribed. Both doxycycline or eiprofloxacin and metronidazole are commonly prescribed together. Chronic or recurring symptoms may be treated with antibiotics as well.

DIETARY RECOMMENDATIONS
- Eat a whole-foods diet, including plenty of fresh vegetables and fruits. Juicing fresh vegetables can also be a very effective way of consuming vitamins, minerals, and live enzymes.
- Avoid cigarettes, alcohol, caffeine, sugar, soft drinks, processed foods, and junk foods.

DETOXIFICATION PROGRAMS
- Liver and colon cleansing and other detoxification programs, such as fasting, can allow your immune system to work more successfully. They can also serve as preventive measures.

NUTRITIONAL SUPPLEMENTS
- Take vitamin A (30,000 to 50,000 I.U. daily—see Chapter Six for dose precautions), vitamin B complex (50 milligrams a day if that amount doesn't cause diarrhea), vitamin C with bioflavonoids (up to 10,000 milligrams a day if that amount doesn't cause diarrhea), and vitamin E (up to 800 I.U. daily). All of these supplements can help decrease internal scarring. Use these extra nutrients with a multiple vitamin/mineral formula to provide the above doses.
- Beta-carotene (up to 50,000 I.U. daily) will provide additional immune and antioxidant support.

HERBAL REMEDIES
- Take echinacea (two or three capsules four times a day), and goldenseal (two or three capsules four times a day) for their anti-infection and immune-enhancing effects, red clover (two capsules three times a day or 2 or 3 cups of the tea) for its cleansing effects, and Siberian ginseng (100 to 200 milligrams once or twice a day). Other than goldenseal, which can be used up to three or four weeks at a time, these herbs can be used for up to six months.
- Also, see the combination herbal formulas listed under "Antibacterial" in Chapter Nineteen.
- Take chlorophyll (10 to 20 milligrams of the fat-soluble variety three or four times a day) available as Chlorolipids from Biotherapeutics of Green Bay, Wisconsin (one or two perles three or four times a day).
- If antibiotics are prescribed, bromelain (one or two 250-milligram or 2,000 m.c.u. [milk-clotting units] per gram capsules/tablets) should be taken with each antibiotic dose to improve absorption. This may exert an additional antimicrobial action and reduce the potential for scarring and infertility.

OTHER THERAPIES
- Take sitz baths and chlorophyll douches. Both are very helpful.
- A naturopathic physician can provide vaginal drawing packs, pelvic diathermy treatments, and constitutional hydrotherapy. All of these therapies are very powerful and effective natural healing modalities.
- Castor oil packs placed daily on the lower abdomen for one hour may bring some healing. Continue for at least one month, then use periodically as needed.
- Exercise moderately, get adequate sleep, and implement stress management measures.

   Note: Yeast overgrowth is often a side effect of lengthy and repetitive courses of antibiotics. Treat appropriately.

Periodontal Disease (Periodontitis) and Inflamed Gums

A disease of the gums and jawbones that can undermine the support of the teeth in their sockets. Gums become irritated and inflamed (gingivitis), then swell and exude pus and can then recede from the teeth. If untreated, the inflammation and infection spread and destroy the connective fibers lining the teeth sockets and the underlying supporting bone. Periodontitis is the primary cause of tooth loss for those over thirty-five.

Related or Underlying Causes

 ND **DietH**

Periodontal disease often starts with gingivitis, or inflammation of the gums. This condition has multiple causes: dental plaque, poor dental hygiene, poor diet, drugs, smoking, alcohol abuse, diabetes, prediabetes, chronic stress, and possibly abnormal electrical currents generated by the interreaction of mixed dental metals (gold, silver, mercury, nickel, etc.).

Periodontal disease may be an early indicator of osteoporosis (see OSTEOPOROSIS).

Treatment and Preventive Measures

CONVENTIONAL MEDICAL TREATMENT

The stage of disease (I-V) determines the extent of treatment, which might include proper hygiene procedures, root planing, and/or gum surgery.

DIETARY RECOMMENDATIONS
- Eat a whole-foods diet with plenty of fresh produce.
- Avoid sweets, soft drinks, and other refined, processed, and devitalized foods.

NUTRITIONAL SUPPLEMENTS
- Take vitamin C (up to 10,000 milligrams a day); a bioflavonoid complex containing naringin, hesperidin, and hesperidin methyl chalcone, such as Flavoplex-C by Interplexus of Kent, Washington (two or three capsules one time a day); vitamin A (up to 25,000 I.U. a day); vitamin B complex (50 milligrams a day); and zinc (up to 50 milligrams a day).
- Brush gums directly and gently with vitamin E oil.
- Take a bone nutrient formula (see OSTEOPOROSIS).
- Rinse your mouth with liquid folic acid (two or three times a day). Available as Folic Acid Liquid from Thorne Research of Sandpoint, Idaho, and Folirinse from Scientific Botanicals of Seattle.
- Take coenzyme Q-10 (10 to 30 milligrams orally two or three times a day).

HERBAL REMEDIES
- For inflamed gums, rinse your mouth with aloe vera gel or juice several times a day. Rinse and drink calendula leaf tea. Rinse and drink fresh wheat grass juice or other fresh green juice. Or rinse with strong tea of myrrh and goldenseal with a touch of cayenne. These are all antibacterial herbs.

OTHER THERAPIES
- Maintain dental hygiene with proper brushing, flossing, and periodic visits to your dentist.

Pharyngitis (Sore Throat)

See COLD, FLU, SORE THROAT, AND COUGH.

Phlebitis

See THROMBOPHLEBITIS.

Pneumonia

See BRONCHITIS.

Premenstrual Syndrome (PMS)

Premenstrual syndrome is a condition characterized by a constellation of symptoms that usually occur up to ten days before the beginning of a menstrual cycle. Any one symptom or combination of symptoms may be present, in either minor or moderate form, or even incapacitating in intensity. Symptoms include fluid retention in hands, feet, and face; abdominal bloating; painful, swollen breasts; weight gain; depression; anxiety; mood swings; irritability; dizziness; insomnia; cravings for sweets and salt; bowel disturbances; acne; headaches; memory impairment and fatigue. PMS may also appear for a few days around ovulation, disappear, and return just before menses.

Related or Underlying Causes

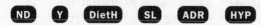

Excess animal fat, dietary sugar, salt, and caffeine are common triggers for PMS, along with insufficient exercise.

Another common cause of PMS is a deficiency of both vitamin B-6 and the mineral magnesium. A B-6 deficiency can contribute to elevated levels of prolactin, a hormone shown in some studies to be present and elevated in women with PMS. A B-6 deficiency can impair the liver's ability to metabolize estrogen, leading to elevated levels of estrogen. This results in an elevated estrogen/progesterone ratio, a very common finding in PMS. Such a ratio is associated with fluid retention, bloating, tender breasts, and weight gain.

A lack of vitamin B-6 or magnesium can also decrease brain dopamine and gamma aminobutyric acid levels. Deficiencies of these brain neurotransmitters are associated with several of the mental/emotional symptoms seen in PMS. Vitamin B-6 deficiency has been linked with edema and depression. B-6 is also necessary for magnesium to function effectively. Finally, a deficiency of either nutrient will block production of an important hormone, prostaglandin E-1 (PGE-1), often linked in low levels to PMS.

Low levels of PGE-1 are also caused by excessive dietary margarine and other sources of partially hydrogenated oils, excessive saturated fat, insufficient unrefined omega 6 and omega 3 fatty acids, especially gamma linolenic acid (see Chapter Three). Additionally, too much dairy and calcium can decrease magnesium absorption, while sugar, stress, and caffeine can increase urinary excretion of magnesium.

Deficiencies of vitamins E and A have also been implicated in PMS. Heavy metal toxicity is a less common cause of PMS.

Treatment and Preventive Measures

CONVENTIONAL MEDICAL TREATMENT
- Diuretics and antidepressants are commonly prescribed.

DIETARY RECOMMENDATIONS
- Eat a whole-foods diet.
- Minimize caffeine, alcohol, salt, sugar, and refined foods.
- Avoid excess animal fat and partially hydrogenated and refined vegetable oils and fried foods.

DETOXIFICATION PROGRAM
- Do the Ultra Clear metabolic cleansing program to increase the liver's ability to metabolize estrogen.

NUTRITIONAL SUPPLEMENTS
- Take extra vitamin B-6 (100 to 600 milligrams a day) or pyridoxal-5 phosphate, the active form of vitamin B-6 (50 to 200 milligrams a day) during the premenstrual phase. Take B complex (25 to 50 milligrams a day) throughout the month, as well as magnesium (300 to 400 milligrams a day). An extra dose of magnesium (300 to 400 milligrams) premenstrually may be helpful.
- Also take vitamin E (400 I.U. a day) and vitamin A (10,000 to 25,000 I.U. a day). Extra vitamin A (50,000 to 75,000 I.U. a day) during the premenstrual cycle is sometimes helpful. *Warning: Too much vitamin A is toxic. See Chapter Six.*
- Take borage oil capsules (providing up to 250 milligrams a day of gamma linolenic acid).
- To improve liver function, use lipotropic factors in a tablet containing a combination of inositol, choline, vitamins B-6 and B-12, methionine, and magnesium.

HERBAL REMEDIES
- Take cholagogue herbs for the liver, including beet, radish, dandelion, chelidonium, and chionanthus. The lipotropic factors (see above) and milk thistle are also included in some formulas (SLF by NF formulations of Wilsonville, Oregon, or Optilipotropic by Eclectic Institute of Sandy, Oregon). Take one tablet of either three times a day throughout the month for several months to help improve liver function.
- Several herbal combination formulas are effective (see "Premenstrual Syndrome," Chapter Nineteen).
- Use the solid extract of alfalfa (available from Scientific Botanicals of Seattle), which contains phytoestrogens, agents that block the effects of elevated estrogen states (¼ teaspoon two or three times a day). *Warning: Alfalfa has been known to exacerbate lupus.*
- A topical cream formulated from the wild yam, possessing progesteronelike activity, has been one of the best solutions for PMS symptoms resistant to all other measures. Your doctor or pharmacist can order Progest Cream, distributed by Professional and Technical Services of Portland, Oregon. There are several ways to use the cream. One treatment is to rub ⅛ tea-

spoon twice a day into the clean skin of your chest, abdomen, inner arms, or inner thighs immediately after ovulation (approximately fourteen days after the beginning of a menstrual period). At day 18 of the cycle, increase the dose to ¼ teaspoon twice a day. At about day 23 of the cycle, and up until your period begins, use up to ½ teaspoon twice a day. More frequent doses are sometimes necessary for severe symptoms. In general, use the smallest dose possible to control symptoms. After several months of use, dose requirements should lessen. Use none during the menstrual period and do not use it again until ovulation. Too much progesterone can sometimes cause acne and breast tenderness, but this is rare. Progesterone cream may potentially incite thyroid activity, and if you are taking thyroid hormone, you may need to lower your dose if you experience hyperthyroid symptoms (contact your doctor and see HYPERTHYROIDISM).

OTHER THERAPIES

- Treat yeast overgrowth, if indicated.
- Treat adrenal exhaustion, if indicated.
- Progesterone allergy may be the cause of premenstrual symptoms in some women. Work with a doctor who can determine the neutralizing dose of progesterone that can bring nearly instant relief. Physicians specializing in environmental medicine (see Chapter Fourteen) are often familiar with this treatment.

Prostate Hypertrophy

A benign enlargement of the prostate gland that occurs in 50 to 60 percent of men over the age of forty, although symptoms usually become more apparent after the age of fifty. Prostate enlargement can impair the flow of urine, since a part of the urethra runs through the prostate, causing a variety of urinary symptoms: urinary frequency (particularly causing nighttime awakenings), reduced urine flow, difficult urination, and excessive dribbling after urinating. The diagnosis is usually made by a digital rectal exam although ultrasound is sometimes used.

Related or Underlying Causes

Prostate enlargement is thought to be caused by an excessive conversion of testosterone to dihydrotestosterone (DHT) in the gland. DHT causes cells to multiply exces-

sively, eventually causing the prostate to swell. The reason for this excessive conversion has not been defined, but a deficiency of zinc and essential fatty acids is thought to play a role.

Treatment and Preventive Measures

CONVENTIONAL MEDICAL TREATMENT

- After the age of fifty, it is recommended that men have a yearly rectal exam to check for prostate enlargement, along with a prostate-specific antigen blood test for prostate cancer screening. Until recently, conventional medical treatment for benign prostate enlargement consisted of waiting until the enlargement and symptoms were serious enough to warrant surgery. Now the pharmaceutical drug Proscar™ is given to block the conversion of testosterone to DHT.

DIETARY RECOMMENDATIONS

- Eat a whole-foods diet.
- Avoid refined and processed foods, especially partially hydrogenated vegetable oils, such as margarine and mayonnaise.

NUTRITIONAL SUPPLEMENTS

- Take a multiple vitamin/mineral formula with at least 400 I.U. of vitamin E. Take extra zinc if necessary, to provide a daily total of 30 to 50 milligrams.
- Take unrefined flaxseed oil or unrefined pumpkin oil (1 or 2 teaspoons a day).
- The amino acids glycine, alanine, and glutamic acid are also useful for this condition. They are often found in combination prostate formulas that contain zinc and the herbs discussed below.

HERBAL REMEDIES

- For decades, naturopathic and European physicians have been prescribing the herb saw palmetto for prostate hypertrophy with impressive clinical results and no significant side effects. Saw palmetto berries, which are rich in fatty acids, can prevent the formation of DHT and inhibit its binding to cells, thus increasing its breakdown and excretion. Recommended doses of the herb would contain between 85 and 95 percent fatty acids and sterols. Take 80 to 160 milligrams in capsule form twice daily.
- Another herb used to successfully treat this disorder is *Pygeum africanum*, containing at least 13 percent sterols. Take 30 to 75 milligrams a day. Some combination formulas contain both saw palmetto and pygeum.

Psoriasis

A skin condition that covers the body with thick, red, raised patches and silvery white scales. Elbows and knees are the most frequent sites of these lesions, but they may appear anywhere. It is very uncommon after middle age.

Related or Underlying Causes

There is no known cause for this ailment. It is felt to be partially linked to an imbalance in natural biochemicals in the body that regulate cell division. Such imbalances can stimulate abnormally fast division of skin cells. Up to twelve times the normal rate has been observed in psoriatic skin lesions. Circulating toxins from a toxic bowel and free radicals have also been implicated. Psoriasis may have an autoimmune component, as psoriatic arthritis, a form of arthritis sometimes accompanying psoriasis, believed to be an autoimmune disease.

Treatment and Preventive Measures

CONVENTIONAL MEDICAL TREATMENT
- Sunlight or ultraviolet light treatments.
- Topical creams or ointments, sometimes containing cortisone.
- Vitamin D cream (Dovonex).

DETOXIFICATION PROGRAM
- Cleansing the colon is essential. Follow the program outlined in Chapter Eight.

NUTRITIONAL SUPPLEMENTS
- Try unrefined flaxseed oil (1 or 2 teaspoons a day) or fish oil (EPA) (one or two capsules three times a day). Also use borage oil capsules (two or three a day) providing at least 240 milligrams daily of gamma linolenic acid. A multiple vitamin/mineral will ensure the proper absorption of these essential fatty acids. Some people have reported success rubbing these oils into skin lesions.
- Take vitamin A (up to 25,000 I.U. a day) and zinc (up to 30 milligrams a day), which may improve the skin tone.
- Antioxidants should be used to treat psoriasis. Take beta-carotene (up to 50,000 I.U. daily); vitamin E (400 I.U. daily); selenium (up to 225 micrograms a day); and quercetin (up to 500 milligrams two or three times a day). Vitamin C is an important antioxidant, but some reports suggest that using over 1,000 milligrams a day may worsen the condition.

HERBAL REMEDIES
- Solid extract of sarsaparilla, an herb that binds bacterial endotoxins, is highly suggested (¼ teaspoon two or three times a day), available from Scientific Botanicals of Seattle.
- Milk thistle (two or three capsules a day) is also useful, as improving liver function has helped in some cases of psoriasis (it slows the breakdown of cyclic AMP and decreases inflammation).
- Ampex by Scientific Botanicals of Seattle is a topical cream that can be applied directly to lesions several times a day.
- Fumaric acid has been used effectively as a topical agent (Psorex by Cardiovascular Research/Ecological Formulas of Concord, California). Apply the cream directly to lesions several times a day.

Recurrent Infections

See COLD, FLU, SORE THROAT, AND COUGH. See also EAR INFECTION and SINUS INFECTION.

Rheumatoid Arthritis

See ARTHRITIS.

Ringworm

See FUNGUS.

Scarring Prevention

A scar is a pale or light-colored fibrous tissue that is the natural result of the body's healing response to a cut, scrape, incision, or lesion. If scars are large or positioned in sites where joints or muscles are located, they can cause problems with mobility. For instance, a burn on the palm side of the hand can result in a "claw" hand.

Related and Underlying Causes

Scar formation is initiated by cells called fibroblasts, which form collagen or connective tissue to heal gaps.

Treatment and Preventive Measures

NUTRITIONAL SUPPLEMENTS

- Use vitamin E (400 to 2,000 I.U. daily orally), for three to six months. After skin lesions are no longer open and susceptible to infection, apply vitamin E oil topically, twice daily. (See Chapter Six for vitamin E warnings.)

HERBAL REMEDIES

- Oatstraw and horsetail teas, which are high in silica, may be useful for wound healing and minimization of scars.

OTHER THERAPIES

- To lessen the contrast between a scar and adjacent skin, it is suggested to use sunscreen on scar areas exposed to the sun.
- Anecdotal reports have suggested that daily applications of raw honey to burn areas prevents scar contractures.
- Unrefined sesame oil topical applications have been used to minimize "stretch mark" scars.

Sciatica

An irritation of the sciatic nerve, located in the lower spinal area, which radiates pain along the nerve pathway to the corresponding leg or foot.

Related or Underlying Causes

This condition is usually caused by low back and sacral problems, including bulging intervertebral discs, which place mechanical pressure on the nerve. It may also be caused by muscle spasm in the pyriformis muscle.

Treatment and Preventive Measures

CONVENTIONAL MEDICAL TREATMENT

- Anti-inflammatory and pain medications, rest, and physical therapy are often prescribed.
- Walking is recommended as a preventive.
- Traction devices are sometimes indicated.
- In more extreme cases, nerve blocks and surgery are also used.

NUTRITIONAL SUPPLEMENTS

- The following agents provide nutritional support to the discs, spinal vertebrae, and surrounding ligaments. Take vitamin C (1,000 milligrams three times a day), vitamin D (200 to 400 I.U. daily), manganese (up to 50 milligrams a day), calcium (up to 800 milligrams a day), magnesium (up to 800 milligrams a day), and chondroitin sulfate (up to 1,500 milligrams a day) or glycosamine sulfate (up to 1,500 milligrams a day). Find a multiple or a back/disc formula that provides most of these nutrients.
- Proteolytic (protein-digesting) enzymes can be used acutely for their anti-inflammatory effect (one or two capsules three or four times a day between meals and at bedtime).
- Try intramuscular injections of vitamin B-12 (1,000 micrograms a day for one to two weeks), with folic acid (2 or 3 milligrams) added in the syringe at least three times a week. After the initial two weeks, lessen the frequency of the injections to two or three injections a week for a month, then one to four injections a month as needed.

HERBAL REMEDIES

- Bromelain and turmeric (200 to 600 milligrams of both three or four times a day) provide a potent anti-inflammatory effect. Take Bromelain and Curcumin (two or three capsules four times a day between meals and at bedtime) by Scientific Botanicals of Seattle.
- Apply these herbs externally to the affected area as poultices or ointments: buckthorn bark, oat, twin leaf, cayenne, white mustard, and blue gentian.

OTHER THERAPIES

- Competent chiropractic or osteopathic adjustments can be extremely effective.
- Stretching and strengthening exercises are useful to prevent recurrences. Consult your physician or physical therapist for instruction.
- Acupuncture or auricular therapy can also be valuable in managing pain.
- Such devices as Gravity Guidance, Back Swing, and slantboard are sometimes recommended by physicians to help reverse normal gravitational influences on the spine.

Seasonal Affective Disorder (SAD)

Depression produced by a lack of sunlight, which occurs especially in climates that are often cloudy. It is also prevalent in northern latitudes where winter days are extremely short. Associated symptoms may be lack of concentration, poor appetite, fatigue, overappetite, weight gain, insomnia, and excessive sleep.

Related or Underlying Causes

CHEM **B/M**

This form of depression occurs in certain predisposed individuals who have a biologic need for more sunlight than their environment provides.

Treatment and Preventive Measures

- Seasonal affective disorder is best treated by light therapy. One protocol suggests sitting at least 3 feet away from a 2,500 lux light box, four 8-foot cool white fluorescent tubes, initially for up to two hours a day. Exposure to the light may be decreased as your depression lessens. You need not look directly into the light.

  For those who arise at 3:00 or 4:00 A.M. and cannot get back to sleep, evening light therapy may be indicated to push their inner clock forward. For those who sleep excessively and cannot get up in the morning, early morning light therapy is best to push their inner clock back.

  Too much light has its risks. Excessive light exposure can produce eyestrain and headache and worsen depression and insomnia. It can even trigger manic episodes. Professional guidance is best. Some proponents suggest the use of cool white fluorescent bulbs, while others suggest a full-spectrum light source.

  Without formal light therapy, some people have achieved success using a light device in their bedroom that simulates sunrise. It comes on automatically at a preset time at a very low intensity and gradually becomes brighter. Available from Pi Square of Redmond, Washington, (206) 881-5478. SunBox of Gaithersburg, Maryland, distributes both the light therapy box (SunBox) and the dawn simulator (SunUp); (800) 548-3968. Also see DEPRESSION.

Seborrheic Dermatitis

A skin and scalp condition that creates oily, scaly, reddened, irritated areas. It can cause itching and burning.

Related or Underlying Causes

 ND

This condition is thought to be caused by a yeast, *Pityrosporum ovale*. It may also be related to deficiencies of vitamins A and B, as well as a lack of essential fatty acids. Food allergies can also be a factor.

Treatment and Preventive Measures

CONVENTIONAL MEDICAL TREATMENT
- Consult your doctor at the onset of the symptoms. The current treatment is Nizoral shampoo or cream, although sulfur-containing medications are still prescribed.

DIETARY RECOMMENDATIONS
- Eat a whole-foods diet with more fresh fruit and vegetables.
- Identify and avoid allergy-triggering foods.

NUTRITIONAL SUPPLEMENTS
- Take vitamin A (up to 50,000 I.U. daily—see warning in Chapter Six), vitamin B complex (up to 50 milligrams a day), vitamin B-6 (up to 100 milligrams a day), and PABA, or para-aminobenzoic acid (up to 500 milligrams a day).
- Take flaxseed oil (1 or 2 teaspoons a day) and borage oil (three capsules a day) for an increase of dietary essential fatty acid.

OTHER THERAPIES
- For external application, try a topical cream made with vitamin B-6 (pyridoxine) as an active ingredient. Two such products are Doxigel from Scientific Botanicals of Seattle and Vitamin B-6 cream from Clark's Prescriptions of Bellevue, Washington. Both may require a prescription.

Seizures

Also known as convulsions, these abnormal and uncontrolled nerve transmissions in the brain can trigger either minor, localized muscle jerks or full-body, uncontrolled muscle contractions with loss of consciousness (grand mal seizures). Temporal lobe seizures can cause loss of awareness, disorientation, and perceptual distortions without any abnormal muscular activity.

Related or Underlying Causes

Seizures can be caused by brain injury, brain tumor or other expanding lesions, insufficient oxygen to the brain, and low blood sugar. Many individuals have seizures with no known underlying cause.

Other contributing factors are abnormal electric currents from mercury and other metal dental materials, stress, and poor neurological organization (see ATTENTION DEFICIT/HYPERACTIVITY DISORDER). The seizures can also be linked to structural abnormalities or malalignments of the cranial, spinal, or temporomandibular joints.

DIETARY RECOMMENDATIONS
- Follow the hypoglycemia diet, which calls for restriction of sugar, caffeine, and alcohol.
- Eliminate aspartame-sweetened food and beverages.
- Find alternatives to theophylline-containing drugs, which inhibit adenosine, a natural anticonvulsant.

NUTRITIONAL SUPPLEMENTS
- Take vitamin B complex (up to 50 milligrams a day), vitamin B-15, or pangamic acid (50 milligrams twice a day), calcium (up to 800 milligrams a day), magnesium (up to 800 milligrams a day), manganese (up to 20 milligrams a day), and zinc (up to 30 milligrams a day).
- Amino acids, taurine, and gamma aminobutyric acid (1,000 milligrams two or three times a day) have been used with some success.
- Vitamin B-6 (up to 50 milligrams a day) or pyridoxal-5 phosphate (10 to 25 milligrams a day) is needed for amino acids to work. Alpha ketoglutaric acid (600 milligrams two or three times a day) is a helpful synergist.

OTHER THERAPIES
- Stress reduction/relaxation techniques can help in the management of seizures. (See Suggested Reading.)

Senility

See ALZHEIMER'S DISEASE.

Shingles

See HERPES ZOSTER.

Sinus Infection (Sinusitis)

An acute or chronic recurring infection in the respiratory sinuses of the face, usually causing sinus and nasal congestion. There is often a thick yellow-green nasal discharge. Symptoms may include pain in the forehead or behind the eyes or upper cheeks, general aching in the upper molar teeth, malaise, fatigue, and fever. In some individuals, the sole symptoms may be fatigue and malaise.

Related or Underlying Causes

The infections are caused by bacteria. Other precipitating factors are air pollution and inhalant allergies. Inflammation in the sinuses leads to swollen tissues, which block the outflow of sinus secretions. Fluid stagnates in the sinus cavities, causing infection. Sinus infections often follow a viral cold, flu, or sore throat. The reasons for being susceptible to acute or recurrent viral infections are many (see COLD, FLU, SORE THROAT, AND COUGH).

Treatment and Preventive Measures
CONVENTIONAL MEDICAL TREATMENT
- Antibiotics and a mucus thinner, such as guaifenesin, are first-line treatments. Cortisone nasal sprays are also used. For the most severe and recurrent cases, sinus surgery may be required. Sinus X rays will commonly demonstrate a sinus infection. However, X rays sometimes will be ineffective, and a CAT scan may be necessary to identify the infection.

DETOXIFICATION PROGRAMS

- Take an enema to speed recovery if a toxic colon is linked to a sinus infection.

NUTRITIONAL SUPPLEMENTS

- For an acute infection, take buffered vitamin C powder or crystals (10,000 milligrams a day or whatever amount can be tolerated without developing diarrhea).
- Take vitamin A (up to 200,000 I.U. daily for up to one week, then no more than 25,000 to 50,000 I.U. daily), which also has anti-infection properties. *Warning: High doses of vitamin A can be toxic; see Chapter Six.* Vitamin A taken nasally can be useful in reducing inflammation of sinus membranes. Mix seven drops, or about 70,000 I.U., of liquid vitamin A (best if it is micelized, which is the most absorbable form—available as Nutrisorb A by Interplexus of Kent, Washington) into fifteen to twenty drops of water or saline (see "Other Therapies"), either from a squeeze spray container or a medicine dropper. Sniff deep into nostrils/sinuses three times a day and swallow the residual that comes into your throat.
- Take N-acetylcysteine (up to 500 milligrams four or five times a day) to thin mucus. After one week, reduce dose to three times a day. It can be used several months at a time for prevention of symptoms if 30 milligrams of zinc and 2 milligrams of copper are used daily.
- Take bee propolis (500 to 1,000 milligrams three times a day).

HERBAL REMEDIES

- Take goldenseal (two to four capsules four times a day), echinacea (two to four capsules four times a day), and cayenne (one capsule every hour while awake).
- For combination herbal formulas, see "Antibacterial" in Chapter Nineteen.
- Bromelain (250 to 500 milligrams three or four times a day) may help improve the absorption of herbal agents and thin mucus.
- A ginger compress can be useful and soothing. The effect of the herb boosts the circulation stimulated by the heat (see Chapter Twenty).

OTHER THERAPIES

Try breathing in any one or a combination of the following for relief:

- Sniff warm salt water (saline) (½ teaspoon sea salt dissolved in 1 cup warm water or salt water with a pinch of baking soda). Use a saline squeeze spray bottle, which is available over the counter, or try a medicine dropper. While pressing one nostril closed, sniff water into the other nostril and allow it to come into your throat, then spit it out. Alternate nostrils with this process several times and repeat three or four times a day.

  For recurrent sinus infections, daily sniffing may prevent inflammation. The saltwater sniff also removes debris from the mucous membranes.
- Strong goldenseal tea (3 or 4 teaspoons goldenseal root powder steeped in 1 cup water for twenty minutes) is also an effective therapeutic sniff. Strain and let it cool to warm, then sniff several times into each nostril.
- Try sniffing steam. Drape a towel over your head then carefully bend over a pot of boiling water, creating a steam tent. Breathe the steam. A few drops of eucalyptus oil in the water will make the steam more penetrating. Chamomile tea vapors also work. For recurrent sinus problems, try the Steam Inhaler, an electric steam unit from Bernard Industries, Inc. (305) 861-2536.
- A steam bath or a sauna can relieve sinus congestion. Hot steam can also prevent a nasty head cold or sore throat from worsening.
- A hot shower can relieve the pain and pressure of sinusitis. You may prefer alternating hot and cold packs to the face (see "Hydrotherapy" in Chapter Twenty).
- Diathermy, performed by a naturopathic physician, will hasten recovery.
- Craniosacral therapy, administered by an osteopathic or chiropractic physician, may lessen sinusitis recurrences by manipulating locked cranial bones.
- Get plenty of rest, drink lots of fluids, and minimize stress.

Skin Cancer

Skin cancer has three categories: squamous cell carcinoma, basal cell carcinoma, and melanoma. The most serious skin cancer, melanoma, is the least common. Watch for the following warning signs of skin cancer:

1. An open sore that bleeds and fails to heal completely.

2. A growing lesion on the face, on or in the ears, or anywhere on the body.

3. A reddish spot on the body that may itch or be painful. Sometimes it appears harmless.

4. A spot with a smooth surface and ridges around its borders. It may be yellow or white in color.

5. A mole that changes in appearance.

Related or Underlying Causes

Excessive sun exposure can cause cancerous changes in the skin. In fact, repeated and prolonged sunlight triggers the majority of skin cancers. On the other hand, sunlight is an important nutrient. Moderate sun exposure and the use of protective clothing and sunblock are essential (see Chapter Sixteen).

Treatment and Preventive Measures

CONVENTIONAL MEDICAL TREATMENT

- Consult a doctor if you notice any skin growths or changes. In many cases, a biopsy of the affected area can determine if further treatment is needed. More serious measures may be necessary if skin cancers are not caught in time. With skin cancer, early diagnosis is crucial. More serious measures may be needed if skin cancers are not caught in time.

DIETARY RECOMMENDATIONS

- Avoid trans-fatty acids (partially hydrogenated vegetable oils) and dietary free radicals.

NUTRITIONAL SUPPLEMENTS

- Take vitamin A (up to 50,000 I.U. daily). *Warning: Excessive vitamin A can be toxic.*
- Take beta-carotene (up to 50,000 I.U. daily), but reduce dosage if your skin becomes orange.
- Take vitamin E (400 I.U. daily) and vitamin C (up to 3,000 I.U. daily).

Smoking Addiction

Nearly 400,000 people die each year in the United States from complications arising from smoking, according to the National Institutes of Health. Nonsmokers who breathe secondhand smoke are also very susceptible to cigarette-induced illness.

Related or Underlying Causes

Cigarette smoking causes a significant number of all deaths in the United States, either by cancer, chronic obstructive lung disease, or heart disease. The smoking addiction is maintained by a chemical dependence on the ingredients of cigarettes, primarily nicotine. Smoking of-

ten satisfies an oral fixation or a need to be doing something with the hands. For many, smoking serves to camouflage unmet emotional and social needs.

Cessation of smoking often produces withdrawal symptoms, such as headaches, body aches, depression, anxiety, and irritability.

Treatment and Preventive Measures

Successful cessation of cigarette smoking requires intelligent planning:

1. Reducing physiologic craving and withdrawal.
2. Managing stress more effectively.
3. Satisfying emotional and social needs, as well as oral fixations, in healthy ways.
4. Avoiding the foods, beverages, people, and situations that trigger smoking.
5. Seeking the support and company of nonsmoking friends.
6. Rewarding yourself regularly for your good efforts.
7. Doing breathing, relaxation, affirmation/imagery, and physical exercises.

Several of the above measures may be needed to end smoking addiction. Paramount to your success is your awareness, commitment, and willpower. A smoke-free work environment will also help.

DIETARY RECOMMENDATIONS

- Eat a whole-foods diet with a special emphasis on maintaining stable blood sugar levels.
- Avoid the foods and beverages that trigger the impulse to smoke, such as coffee, alcohol, and desserts.

NUTRITIONAL SUPPLEMENTS

- To ease withdrawal symptoms and craving, take high-dose buffered vitamin C powder (5 to 10 grams a day). *Note: Reduce dose if this causes diarrhea.* Also, take vitamin B complex (100 milligrams a day), vitamin B-5, or pantothenic acid (up to 1,500 milligrams a day), niacinamide (up to 1,500 milligrams a day), and calcium and magnesium (up to 800 milligrams of each a day). These supplements will strengthen your nervous system and adrenal glands.
- Take sodium bicarbonate (baking soda) no more than 1 teaspoon three times a day in a large glass of water. Alkalinizing the system will both reduce cravings and ease withdrawal symptoms.
- If you still smoke, protect yourself from some of the damage of cigarette smoking with antioxidant nutrients: vitamin C (3,000 to 6,000 milligrams a day), beta-carotene (25,000 to 35,000 I.U. daily), vitamin B-1 (100 milligrams a day), vitamin B-6 (50 milli-

grams a day), vitamin E (400 I.U. daily), selenium (200 micrograms a day), cysteine (500 milligrams a day), and other antioxidant nutrients. All of these can be found in combination formulas at health food stores.

HERBAL REMEDIES
- Take a lobelia- and oatstraw-containing herbal formula designed to aid in smoking cessation, such as Nicoril by Biotherapeutics/Enzymatic Therapy of Green Bay, Wisconsin.
- Nerve-soothing, sedative formulas containing hops, skullcap, and passionflower may be helpful for treating anxiety (take one or two capsules three or four times a day).

OTHER THERAPIES
- One extremely effective method of reducing cravings and withdrawal involves acupuncture and auricular therapy, which involves the injection of a small amount of sterile fluid into specific acupuncture points in the ear and near the nostrils.
- Practice breathing techniques, skilled relaxation exercises, and/or imagery exercises that suit you. They can provide a powerful reinforcement for your goals and help you to maintain commitment.

Spastic Colon

See IRRITABLE BOWEL.

Sprains

A tear of a ligament causing pain, swelling, sometimes bruising, and, if severe, joint instability. Whiplash injury to the neck and a twisted ankle are examples of sprains.

Related or Underlying Causes

A sprain can be caused by excessive force applied to a joint, stretching a ligament beyond its capacity. Common sprain areas include the knee, ankle, back, and wrist. Sports activities, falls, collisions, and overuse are often precipitating factors.

Treatment and Preventive Measures

NUTRITIONAL SUPPLEMENTS
- To help ligaments heal and strengthen, take manganese (50 milligrams a day), vitamin C (3,000 milligrams a day), bioflavonoids (up to 1,000 milligrams a day), zinc (30 milligrams a day), and glucosamine sulfate or chondroitin sulfate (up to 1,500 milligrams a day). Health food stores generally carry these supplements in combination formulas.
- Rub vitamin C cream into the skin of the sprained joint several times a day (Derma C by Interplexus of Seattle, Washington).
- Take proteolytic (protein-digesting) enzymes (1 or 2 between meals and at bedtime).

HERBAL REMEDIES
- Take Bromelain and Curcumin, available from Scientific Botanicals of Seattle, Washington, or Curcumax/Curcuzyme by Phytopharmica/Enzymatic Therapy of Green Bay, Wisconsin (two to three capsules three or four times a day between meals).
- After four or five days, when the acute phase has passed and swelling has diminished considerably, rub cayenne ointment into the skin of the sprained joint (three or four times a day), available from Herb Technology/Khalsa Health Center of Seattle.

HOMEOPATHIC REMEDIES
- Use the following homeopathic remedies immediately: arnica (four pellets dissolved in mouth every ten to fifteen minutes, if using a 6x or 12x strength; less often for 6c or higher strength). Use arnica gel or ointment topically (Boiron/Borneman of Simi Valley, California) or Traumeel cream (Biological Homeopathic Industries of Albuquerque, New Mexico).

OTHER THERAPIES
- Ice and elevation are effective first-aid measures. Adequate immobilization, sometimes including casting, is crucial to allow for effective healing. An inadequately immobilized sprain may result in poor healing and a weak ligament, making it susceptible to recurrent sprains.

Staph Infections

See ABSCESSES. See also "Staphage Lysate" in Chapter Twenty.

Stomach Flu

See DIARRHEA and INTESTINAL CRAMPS.

Stroke (Cerebrovascular Disease)

The sudden blockage of blood flow to the brain, resulting in destruction of vital areas within the organ. The severity of symptoms depends on which area and how much of the brain is affected. Strokes commonly lead to loss of consciousness, loss of speech, paralysis, and death.

Stroke is the leading cause of serious disability and the third-largest cause of death in the United States, ranking behind heart disease and cancer. Approximately 500,000 individuals a year suffer a new or recurrent stroke, 78 percent of whom are over the age of sixty-five. The incidence of stroke in males is 19 percent higher than in females, and is approximately twice as common in blacks as in whites.

Related and Underlying Causes

Stroke is most often related to high blood pressure (see BLOOD PRESSURE, HIGH) and arteriosclerosis (see ARTERIOSCLEROSIS).

Three primary mechanisms can stop the flow of blood to the brain: a thrombosis (blood clot), a hemorrhage (rupture of a blood vessel), and an embolism (obstruction of a blood vessel by a solid body, such as a tumor, blood clot, air bubble, or fat globule).

Treatment and Preventive Measures

CONVENTIONAL MEDICAL TREATMENT
- Life support, and eventual physical and speech therapy.
- Treatment of high blood pressure is vital in preventing strokes.

DIETARY RECOMMENDATIONS
See ARTERIOSCLEROSIS and BLOOD PRESSURE, HIGH.

NUTRITIONAL SUPPLEMENTS
See ARTERIOSCLEROSIS and BLOOD PRESSURE, HIGH.

HERBAL REMEDIES
- Take ginkgo, which has special use in both the prevention of arteriosclerosis in arteries of the brain (40 milligrams twice a day) and in the treatment of a stroke (80 milligrams twice a day). See also ARTERIOSCLEROSIS, and BLOOD PRESSURE, HIGH.

Sty

An infection in the follicle of an eyelash or in a gland in the eyelid, resulting in localized redness and swelling. It often itches at the onset of symptoms.

Related or Underlying Causes

The cause is usually bacterial. It may also indicate a lowered immune system or a nutritional deficiency.

Treatment and Preventive Measures

The most effective measure is the application of a warm compress. However, vitamin, mineral, herbal, and homeopathic supports may be helpful.

NUTRITIONAL SUPPLEMENTS
- Take vitamin A (up to 25,000 I.U. daily), vitamin C (up to 5,000 milligrams a day—or less if this causes diarrhea), and zinc (50 milligrams a day).

HERBAL REMEDIES
- Take goldenseal (two or three capsules four times a day). Use warm goldenseal tea to dampen a compress and apply to affected area for twenty minutes three or four times a day.

HOMEOPATHIC REMEDIES
- Silica cell salts may speed healing.

OTHER THERAPIES
- Use warm, wet compresses (a facecloth immersed in hot water) applied directly to the infected area for twenty to thirty minutes three or four times a day. This may be the easiest and most effective measure.

Surgery

Surgical procedures are commonplace in conventional American medicine. Other than for emergency situations, if you are considering surgery, get a second or third opinion. Ask about effective alternative approaches to treating the problem. Study literature about your ailment. If surgery is the best option, several measures can be taken to prepare yourself for the procedure and to ensure optimal healing and recovery.

Related or Underlying Causes

Common surgical interventions include joint replacement, tumor removal, hysterectomy, cesarean section, vascular repair, biopsy, organ repair and transplant, and trauma.

Treatment and Preventive Measures

NUTRITIONAL SUPPLEMENTS
- Take vitamin C (2,000 to 3,000 milligrams a day). Do not take vitamin C the day before your surgery, but resume taking it right afterward. Request that vitamin C be added to your postsurgery IV fluids.
- Certain nutritional approaches can prepare you for surgery and ensure quicker healing following surgery. Use them for several weeks or more before coming to the hospital. If you are pregnant or nursing, consult with your doctor before using these or any supplements. Tell your doctor that you would like to use your supplements while recovering in the hospital.
- Take bioflavonoids (up to 1,000 milligrams a day).
- Take vitamin A (up to 25,000 I.U. daily—see Chapter Six for warnings), vitamin E (400 to 800 I.U. daily), and zinc (up to 50 milligrams a day).
- Include a free-form multiple amino acid supplement, beginning two weeks before the operation and continuing for two or more weeks after surgery (available as Aminoplex from Tyson and Associates of Hawthorne, California). Such formulas accelerate tissue repair and recovery and maintain nitrogen balance. Or use a protein powder several times a day, such as Ultra Balance or Ultra Meal by Metagenics of San Clemente, California.
- A high-potency multiple vitamin/mineral will also be helpful.
- To prevent postoperative blood clots in the veins take the blood thinning supplements discussed in THROMBOPHLEBITIS. Take these as soon as you are able to eat after surgery. They are less important once you are no longer confined to bed.

HERBAL REMEDIES
- Take Bromelain and Curcumin (Scientific Botanicals of Seattle) or Curcumax/Curcuzyme (Phytopharmica/Enzymatic Therapy of Green Bay, Wisconsin). Both are formulated to reduce tissue inflammation due to surgical trauma while lessening pain and healing time. Take two or three capsules three or four times a day spaced between meals.

HOMEOPATHIC REMEDIES
- Take arnica (up to 6 c.) the night before surgery. Take every one to two hours after surgery. Alternate doses of arnica with hypericum (up to 6 c.) during waking hours. These remedies can diminish pain and reduce the need for medication.

OTHER THERAPIES
- The use of affirmations, imagery, and self-hypnosis can aid recovery and accelerate healing. Several cassette tapes and books are available to help prepare you mentally for the entire surgical process. Bring these tapes and a portable cassette player with you to the hospital and listen to them while you're recovering.
- Transform your "sick room" into a healing environment. Bring your favorite music to play while recovering. Surround yourself with photographs, paintings, or anything that contributes to a healing mood.

Tendonitis

Inflammation of a tendon resulting in pain.

Related or Underlying Causes

This inflammation is usually linked to overuse or injury. It is very common in athletes, dancers, painters, hairstylists, and computer operators. Due to repeated aggravations of the initial injury, the inflammation can become chronic and can last for years.

Treatment and Preventive Measures

CONVENTIONAL MEDICAL TREATMENT
- Anti-inflammatory medications and cortisone injections are standard operations for treating tendonitis.

NUTRITIONAL SUPPLEMENTS
- Take vitamin B complex (50 milligrams a day), manganese (50 milligrams a day), and vitamin C (3,000 milligrams a day) to aid healing. Supplement this reg-

imen with glucosamine sulfate or chondroitin sulfate capsules (500 to 1,000 milligrams three or four times a day), and pycnogenol (25 milligrams three times a day). Health food stores often carry combination cartilage/tendon/ligament formulas containing many of the above nutrients.

HERBAL REMEDIES

- Take Bromelain and Curcumin (two or three capsules three times a day between meals), natural anti-inflammatory agents, available from Scientific Botanicals of Seattle, Washington.
- For chronic tendonitis, apply Zheng Gu Shui liniment, which is very effective and is available from most massage therapy supply stores, as well as some pharmacies and Chinese pharmacies in the United States. It is also sold by Superior Trading Company/Overseas Factory of San Francisco. Topical application of Fu Sho oil (essential oil) is also useful. It is sold by Emerson's Ecologics of Acton, Massachusetts.
- Another treatment for chronic tendonitis is to rub cayenne ointment over the affected area once daily (Herb Technology/Khalsa Health Center of Seattle, Washington).

OTHER THERAPIES

- Acupuncture and acupressure are also successful treatments.
- Alternating hot and cold applications of water on the affected area can accelerate healing (see "Hydrotherapy" in Chapter Twenty).
- Bee venom injections (see Chapter Twenty) have been one of the most effective treatments, particularly for chronic tendonitis.
- Rest the tendon, if possible.

Thrombophlebitis

A blood clot within a vein, resulting in inflammation, swelling, and pain in the affected extremity.

Related or Underlying Causes

 ND **DietH**

The condition is caused by trauma, prolonged bed rest, and poor venous circulation. Standing for long periods of time or a lack of exercise can cause blood to pool in the large veins of the legs, thus becoming more prone to clotting. Blood that clots too easily can greatly increase one's chances of developing thrombophlebitis. Blood platelets become too "sticky" and clot easily if there is a deficiency of essential fatty acids, vitamin E, magnesium, and other nutrients.

Treatment and Preventive Measures

CONVENTIONAL MEDICAL TREATMENT

- Most doctors will prescribe anticoagulant medicines and bed rest, along with support bandages or hose for the treatment of varicose veins. Recovery time varies according to severity of the disease.

DIETARY RECOMMENDATIONS

- Avoid processed and partially hydrogenated vegetable oils.
- Take unrefined flaxseed oil (1 teaspoon a day).

NUTRITIONAL SUPPLEMENTS

- Take vitamin E orally (up to 1,600 I.U. daily. See precautions). If planning on surgery, take 400 I.U. the weeks before; after surgery, use the higher doses to prevent this disorder.
- If your doctor has not prescribed blood thinners and there is no contraindication for them, take fish oil (up to 1,000 milligrams three times a day), garlic (one or two pills three times a day with meals), and magnesium (up to 800 milligrams a day). The natural blood thinners reduce the stickiness of platelets and make them less likely to clot abnormally.

OTHER THERAPIES

- Apply a castor oil pack to the affected area (see Chapter Twenty). Elevate and rest affected area.
- Walking, swimming, jogging, and other exercise can help prevent stagnation of blood in veins and minimize the tendency to clot.
- Slantboarding can help reverse the pooling of blood in the veins. This technique can be particularly useful for those who stand on their feet for many hours. It involves lying on a padded board that is slanted so that the feet are somewhat higher than the head.

Thyroid Problems

See HYPERTHYROIDISM and HYPOTHYROIDISM.

Tinnitus

A ringing, buzzing, or hissing in the ears.

Related or Underlying Causes

It may be caused by wax or some other object in the ear, fever, ear infection, fluid retention, deafness, or a prescribed medication. It can often be caused by conditions that can lead to inflammation and swelling in the head, such as hay fever and inhalant allergies. The problem may also be linked to spinal, cranial, or temporomandibular joint malalignments (TMJ). Reduced circulation and atherosclerosis can also cause tinnitus.

Treatment and Preventive Measures

CONVENTIONAL MEDICAL TREATMENT
- Removing wax from the ear can often relieve tinnitus.

NUTRITIONAL SUPPLEMENTS
- Vitamin B complex (50 milligrams a day) and extra B-6 (50 milligrams) may be useful if fluid retention is diagnosed.

HERBAL REMEDIES
- Take ginkgo (40 milligrams twice a day), which may take up to four months of use to be effective.

Ulcerative Colitis

See COLITIS.

Ulcer (Duodenal, Gastric, Peptic)

An erosion in the mucosal lining of the upper intestinal tract, causing pain or burning. Hemorrhaging is often associated with the condition. Gastric ulcers are sometimes linked with stomach cancer.

Related or Underlying Causes

Ulcers are often caused by excessive hydrochloric acid burning the stomach's mucosal lining. Even when normal levels of hydrochloric acid are present, damage to the lining can occur if the mucosa's protective ability is impaired. The presence of unhealthy bacteria, Helicobacter pylori, is the most common cause of this impairment and is associated with the majority of ulcers. Aspirin, cortisone, and nonsteroidal anti-inflammatory drugs such as ibuprofen can disrupt mucosal function and also cause ulcers.

Other factors that can precipitate or aggravate ulcers include stress, cigarette smoking, caffeine, decaffeinated coffee, soft drinks, alcohol, spices (i.e., black pepper and chili powder), junk foods, fried foods, and highly refined foods. Eating on the run and when stressed can also contribute to the development of ulcers.

Treatment and Preventive Measures

CONVENTIONAL MEDICAL TREATMENT
- Definitive diagnostic tests include an upper gastrointestinal barium X ray or gastroscope (a fiberoptic tube inserted into the stomach and duodenum).
- The diagnosis of unhealthy bacteria, a helicobacter pylori infection, can be made through a blood test or through a gastroscopic biopsy and culture. Successful treatment often requires triple therapy, two antibiotics and bismuth (see Chapter Seven).
- Medications such as Zantac, Tagamet, and Prilosec that block the production of acid are usually prescribed.

DIETARY RECOMMENDATIONS
- Avoid hot spices, caffeinated beverages, alcohol, and soft drinks. Also eliminate fried and junk foods.
- In acute cases, avoid raw vegetables, fruits, and rough cereals, such as nuts and granola. Eat easily digestible foods, such as rice cream, vegetable soup, steamed zucchini, and taro root. Chew food well before swallowing. As symptoms improve, gradually resume a normal, healthy diet.
- If digestion is sensitive, follow food-combining principles.
- Drink fresh, raw cabbage juice (one or two glasses a day for up to ten days) for its direct healing effect. Prolonged use may slow thyroid function.

NUTRITIONAL SUPPLEMENTS

- Take vitamin A (up to 50,000 I.U. daily—see warnings in Chapter Six), vitamin E (up to 800 I.U. daily), zinc (up to 30 milligrams a day), and buffered vitamin C (500 to 1,000 milligrams twice a day, if tolerated).

HERBAL REMEDIES

- To help an ulcer heal, take DGL (deglycerrhizinated licorice root—two capsules or, preferably, chewable tablets three or four times a day). Studies have demonstrated equal healing time comparing DGL and prescription acid blockers. However, DGL retards the recurrence of ulcers more effectively. It is a superior agent because it directly repairs and strengthens the mucous membrane cells.
- Slippery elm powder and goldenseal powder, mixed in a ratio of 2 to 1, is quite effective (two capsules three or four times a day). Slippery elm and marshmallow root teas can be taken liberally, as they coat and soothe the stomach and duodenum lining.
- Take combination herbal capsule formulas to promote gastrointestinal mucosal healing. Try Roberts Formula or Bastyr B by Eclectic Institute of Sandy, Oregon, or GI Encap by Thorne Research of Sandpoint, Idaho.
- Aloe vera juice or gel can also be healing and soothing (1 or 2 ounces of the juice or 1 tablespoon of the gel three or four times a day).

OTHER THERAPIES

- Stress management is key for many people with ulcers.

Ulcer (Venous Stasis)

An erosion of the skin, usually below the knee, which may start as a harmless abrasion and deteriorate into a large, deep chronic ulcer. Healing is very difficult and slow, due to venous blood stagnation. Another factor can be pressure from surrounding swollen, waterlogged tissue, which impairs oxygen supply, nutrients, and disposal of waste and toxins.

Related or Underlying Causes

DietH   **ND**   **ToxB**   **SL**

These ulcers can be caused by multiple factors: chronic varicose veins, long hours standing in one position, constipation, heart failure, liver disease, insufficient dietary vitamin C and bioflavonoids, and lack of exercise (see VARICOSE VEINS).

Treatment and Preventive Measures

CONVENTIONAL MEDICAL TREATMENT

For this condition, doctors generally recommend venous support hose and standard wound treatment.

NUTRITIONAL SUPPLEMENTS

- Take vitamin C (1,000 milligrams three times a day), bioflavonoids (up to 1,000 milligrams a day), and vitamin A (25,000 I.U. daily—see Chapter Six for precautions).
- Take zinc (30 milligrams a day).

OTHER THERAPIES

Aggressive therapies are needed to help the ulcer heal and to avoid further complications. Try several of the following:

- Freshly juiced wheat grass—mix the juice with the pulp and apply directly to the ulcer. This treatment encourages healing and prevents infection. Cover with plastic wrap. Secure it in place with an Ace bandage, but do not wrap too tightly. Remove in approximately thirty minutes. Do this up to three times a day if needed. Contact a health food store to obtain a wheat grass juicer. If there isn't a local source of wheat grass, see directions in Chapter Five for growing it. It is usually worth the effort to grow and juice wheat grass. Drink some as well.
- Grate and mash a raw potato. Apply it to the ulcer for up to one and a half hours, covering it with plastic wrap. Secure it in place loosely with an Ace wrap.
- Alternate very warm compresses with cold compresses (see directions under "Hydrotherapy" in Chapter Twenty).
- Use compresses soaked with goldenseal, myrrh, and cayenne if the area is infected (see ABSCESSES).
- If infection is chronic, ask your doctor to prescribe Silvadene™ cream. Mix 2 teaspoons of the cream with white sugar until it feels gritty. Then apply it generously to the ulcer. Dress with appropriate gauze and wrap gently. Sleep with this kind of wrapping at night for a week or as long as needed. If not using other measures described above during the day, use a fresh wrap in the morning.
- Elevate the affected leg as often as you can during the application of compresses, soaks, and poultices. Continue this as you sleep. Lie down with your calf and foot propped up on a few large pillows above the level of your heart.
- Capable home care is indispensable to maintaining a healing regimen.

- Consult your doctor periodically to monitor your condition.

Underweight

Weight below standard for height and frame size.

Related or Underlying Causes

Underweight can be caused by cancer, hyperthyroidism, a chronic infection, or other serious illness. Other factors include malnutrition, poor appetite (see APPETITE, POOR), an eating disorder, digestive secretion deficiencies (especially pancreatic enzymes), parasites (see PARASITES, INTESTINAL), and chronic diarrhea (see DIARRHEA).

Treatment and Preventive Measures

CONVENTIONAL MEDICAL TREATMENT

Consult your doctor for a complete physical examination and laboratory tests to rule out any underlying illness.

DIETARY RECOMMENDATIONS

- Identify and avoid allergy-triggering foods.
- Eat a well-balanced, whole-foods diet.
- Eat meals slowly and in a relaxed environment.
- If needed, supplement the diet with additional calories from a "Fortified Health Drink" (see Chapter Five) and from hypoallergenic meal replacement powders, such as Ultra Clear Sustain or Opti from Metagenics of San Clemente, California.

NUTRITIONAL SUPPLEMENTS

- Take a multiple vitamin/mineral with B complex (at least 25 to 50 milligrams a day), as well as zinc (up to 30 milligrams a day).

Urinary Tract Infections

See BLADDER INFECTION (CYSTITIS).

Vaginitis

Inflammation of the vagina, accompanied by discharge, burning, itching, and irritation.

Related or Underlying Causes

Often caused by infectious agents: trichomonas, or hemophilus/gardinerella. Antibiotics and steroids alter the balance of natural bacteria in the vagina, predisposing it to infections, especially yeast. Oral contraceptives, diabetes (see DIABETES), and pregnancy can also lead to yeast infections. A toxic bowel can be linked to chronic vaginitis as well. Until the bowel is properly treated, vaginitis will usually recur. Reduced estrogen levels can increase susceptibility. Sensitivity to soaps and fabric softeners may induce the condition as well. Vaginitis is also linked to excessive dietary sugar and mucus-forming foods, such as milk products.

Treatment and Preventive Measures

CONVENTIONAL MEDICAL TREATMENT

- Some infections may require oral antibiotics.
- Antibacterial or antifungal vaginal suppositories are usually prescribed upon identification of organisms from the vaginal discharge.

DIETARY RECOMMENDATIONS

- Eat a whole-foods diet, reducing sweets and other refined foods.
- Identify and avoid allergy-triggering foods.

NUTRITIONAL SUPPLEMENTS

- Take vitamin A (25,000 to 50,000 I.U. daily—see Chapter Six for warnings), beta-carotene (25,000 to 50,000 I.U. daily), zinc (15 to 30 milligrams a day), vitamin C (3,000 milligrams a day), vitamin E (400 I.U. daily), and B complex (25 to 50 milligrams a day). Vitamin A vaginal suppositories are often very helpful (use one vaginally every twelve to twenty-four hours). Available as Calendula–Vitamin A suppositories from Earth's Harvest of Gresham, Oregon.

HERBAL REMEDIES

- Tea tree oil vaginal suppositories have been very successful for vaginal infections, especially yeast. Or try Hydrastis (goldenseal) vaginal suppositories for all vaginal infections. Combination herbal suppositories are also useful: try Calendula–Vitamin A suppositories or

Essential Oil Plus suppositories containing tea tree oil, thuja oil, bitter orange oil, vitamin A, hydrastis (golden seal), lomatium, grapefruit seed extract, and vitamin E. Use one suppository vaginally every twelve to twenty-four hours for up to fourteen days. Longer or recurrent treatments are sometimes needed. Consult your doctor. All of the vaginal suppositories above are available from Earth's Harvest of Gresham, Oregon.

- Try garlic suppositories. Peel a clove of garlic, being careful not to nick it. Wrap it in a piece of gauze. Lubricate with vegetable oil. Insert as a tampon/suppository, leaving a tail of gauze externally. Change every twelve hours for three to five days or more. It may be used for all infectious agents.

- Take pau d'arco (taheebo) tea douche (see Chapter Nineteen for dose instructions), which is useful for yeast, trichomonas, and gardinerella (see douching instructions below).

- Take a goldenseal tea douche (3 or 4 teaspoons of powder per 1 cup of water). Mix the tea in 1 quart of warm water. This may be helpful for infectious vaginitis (see douching instructions below).

- Take echinacea orally (one or two capsules three times a day). Other immune-strengthening herbs may also be used orally (see the herbal combination formulas at the end of Chapter Nineteen). If gardinerella is diagnosed, also consider the antibacterial formulas.

OTHER THERAPIES

- Place boric acid powder in a 00 gelatin capsule and insert one into the vagina every twelve hours for acute infections. If less severe, use every twenty-four hours for seven days. At the same time, insert one or two acidophilus or acidophilus/bifidus capsules in the vagina. Continue this treatment for seven to fourteen days (see caution below). Another round of treatment may be needed several weeks later. This approach is especially helpful for yeast, occasionally for gardinerella, but rarely for trichomonas.

- Acidophilus or acidophilus/bifidus capsules (nonenteric coated) can be used (two capsules twice a day) as a vaginal suppository. Or try a yogurt implant using 2 tablespoons of natural, unsweetened yogurt with active cultures, inserted gently with a vaginal applicator twice a day (see caution below).

- If you are on birth control pills and your yeast infection is not responding to treatment, consider discontinuing the medication, if possible. It may be necessary to use condoms or abstain altogether from sexual intercourse until sufficient healing of vaginal infections has occurred.

- Douching is an effective remedy for many vaginal complaints. Always observe the following guidelines: the bag should be no more than 2 feet above the level of your pelvis, and you should control the inflow so that it is slow and gentle. If you are pregnant be especially gentle, and always consult your doctor first. Do not attempt to hold the water in. Let it flow out of your vagina freely. If your waters have broken, do not insert anything into the vagina.

- For a yogurt douche, add 4 tablespoons of yogurt or a high-potency acidophilus or acidophilus/bifidus powder (2 teaspoons) to 1 quart of warm water and use once or twice a day. Such intensive acidophilus treatments may be sufficient to remedy an acute yeast infection. An herbal or pharmaceutical antifungal agent may be added.

- Less intensive acidophilus treatments may be useful as a preventive measure after other remedies have restored the vaginal ecology. If you are susceptible to yeast infections when taking antibiotics, these treatments should serve as an effective preventive measure.

  Caution: Prolonged or excessive use of vaginal acidophilus douches can become irritating and contribute to inflammation. As helpful as acidophilus is for many women, these organisms produce lactic acid. Excessive amounts can make the vagina too acidic for other favorable bacteria. Acidophilus could therefore aggravate vaginitis and should be discontinued if symptoms worsen.

- For a vinegar and water douche, add 1 tablespoon of white vinegar to 1 quart of warm water. This is effective, especially for yeast, and sometimes helpful for the gardinerella and trichomonas, although not generally as first-line treatment. With the weakly acidifying quality of vinegar, this remedy may be useful as a preventive in keeping vaginal flora in balance.

- Wheat grass juice is a potent and effective douche for any vaginitis. Use it full strength with a dose of at least 1 ounce. Retain juice for fifteen to twenty minutes. Administer at least twice a day if possible. Commercial liquid chlorophyll may also be used, but fresh is always better.

- For a green clay douche, use 1 tablespoon mixed in 2 cups of warm water with ½ to 1 teaspoon of white vinegar. As a retention douche, this green clay mixture may be useful for all forms of infectious vaginitis.

Varicose Veins

Abnormally swollen, prominent veins in which the valves are weakened and therefore allow the backflow of blood. They are most often found in the legs and the rectum. Varicose veins cause serious circulatory problems due to their inability to return blood to the heart. Hemorrhoids are another example of varicose veins.

Related and Underlying Causes

 DietH ND ToxB SL

Health complications arise when venous blood flow is impaired. Pressure is created that causes the veins to distend, pulling the valves apart and allowing blood to back up, stretching and distending the veins even more. As the condition worsens, physical discomfort and reduced mobility can occur.

Several factors contribute to this impaired circulation: standing long hours in the same position, heart failure, liver disease, abdominal tumors, and pregnancy. Constipation can also be an important factor, particularly frequent straining.

Insufficient vitamin C and bioflavonoids can contribute to a weakened collagen structure in the vein walls, causing the veins to be more susceptible to distension and varicosities.

Treatment and Preventive Measures

DIETARY RECOMMENDATIONS
- Follow a high-fiber, whole-foods diet with plenty of raw vegetables and fruits.

DETOXIFICATION PROGRAMS
- Do periodic bowel and liver cleansing programs (see Chapters Eight and Nine).

NUTRITIONAL SUPPLEMENTS
- Take vitamin C (1,000 milligrams two or three times a day), vitamin E (800 I.U. daily), and zinc (up to 30 milligrams a day).

HERBAL REMEDIES
- Add bioflavonoids, including hesperidin, naringin, and hesperidin methyl chalcone (2 or 3 capsules once or twice a day). Available as FlavoPlex-C from Interplexus of Kent, Washington. Other potent flavonoids include bilberry and ginkgo (Proanthonol, from Allergy Research of San Leandro, California: one capsule twice a day).
- Take herbs specific for proper vein elasticity: escin concentrate (from horse chestnut) and hamamelis. Try Venocap (one capsule three times a day) from Thorne Research of Sandpoint, Idaho.

OTHER THERAPIES
- Rub castor oil directly over the varicose veins, especially after a bath or shower. Massage your legs from your feet up toward your groin.

- Get adequate exercise for your legs, especially by walking.
- Use a slantboard ten minutes or more twice a day to reverse the gravitational pooling of blood in the legs. This involves lying on a padded board that is on an incline so that the feet are slightly higher than the head.

    Warning: Avoid slantboarding if you have had retinal detachments, glaucoma, or other conditions where increased pressure in the head is contraindicated.
- Avoid crossing your legs when sitting (it increases pressure in the veins of your calves and feet).
- Cold-water leg soaks (Kneipp baths) have been used successfully in European health spas (popularized in the United States by Bernard Jenson, D.C., N.D., of Escondido, California). Walking in cold water for five to ten minutes a day can have positive results. Or fill a deep basin or tub with cold water, then stand in the water and simulate walking. Also, use a hose to run cold water on your legs. The cold water is tonifying.

Wart

A raised, solid growth on the skin, usually painless. Warts are most common on hands, feet, and face.

Related or Underlying Causes

A wart is usually caused by a virus.

Treatment and Preventive Measures

Most of the following self-care treatments involve topical applications. Some of the treatments may irritate surrounding normal skin. Consult your doctor if the treatments are too irritating or if the skin is very sensitive.

CONVENTIONAL MEDICAL TREATMENT
- A wart is usually removed with liquid nitrogen, salicylic acid, or other irritants.

DIETARY RECOMMENDATIONS
- Eat a whole-foods diet.
- Restrict sweets.

NUTRITIONAL SUPPLEMENTS
- Take vitamin C (3,000 to 8,000 milligrams a day, less if diarrhea) and vitamin A (100,000 I.U. for one week only, then 25,000 to 35,000 I.U.) for their systemic

immune-enhancing and antiviral effects. (See Chapter Six for vitamin A precautions.)

- Try local applications: vitamin C crystals or powder (ascorbic acid) mixed into a paste with water, which can be applied to the wart for several hours once or twice a day. Or try soaking a bandage with liquid vitamin A (available as Nutrisorb by Interplexus of Kent, Washington) and applying it to the wart. Keep it on the wart continuously for three to five days. Change the bandage every twelve hours. Topical vitamin E oil may also be effective.

HERBAL REMEDIES

- A fresh garlic slice can be applied to the wart with tape if the surrounding skin is not sensitive. Put on a fresh slice daily. Cut the garlic only slightly larger than the wart to prevent irritating the surrounding skin.
- Wet a bandage with lomatium isolate (Eclectic Institute, Sandy, Oregon). Keep it on the wart continuously for several days, reapplying a new bandage every twelve to twenty-four hours.

OTHER THERAPIES

- Saturate a bandage with castor oil. Keep it on the wart continuously for three to five days, changing it every one or two days. After several days, it should cause an irritation and inflammation, which should make the wart fall off. Or, the wart may shrink gradually.
- For multiple warts, where bandages may be impractical, apply castor oil like a lotion several times a day.

Water Retention

An abnormal accumulation of watery fluid in tissues, often causing visible swelling. The ankles, hands, face, and abdomen are usually affected.

Related or Underlying Causes

It may be caused by hypothyroidism (see HYPOTHYROIDISM), premenstrual syndrome (see PREMENSTRUAL SYNDROME), excessive salt intake, monosodium glutamate, and depression. Other common factors are potassium deficiency, poor venous circulation, congestive heart failure (see HEART FAILURE), liver disease, and kidney disease.

Treatment and Preventive Measures

CONVENTIONAL MEDICAL TREATMENT

- Consult your doctor to rule out any underlying disease.
- Diuretics may be prescribed to reduce the water level in body tissues.

DIETARY RECOMMENDATIONS

- Identify and avoid allergy-triggering foods. Try an elimination diet.
- Restrict salt or any packaged food with sodium as an ingredient. If this does not help after several weeks, excess sodium may not be the cause of your water retention problem.

NUTRITIONAL SUPPLEMENTS

- Take vitamin B-6 (up to 100 milligrams a day—see Chapter Six for precautions) to increase loss of extra fluid. Also take B complex (up to 25 milligrams a day).
- If prescription diuretics are taken, take magnesium (up to 800 milligrams a day), as diuretics often cause urinary magnesium loss.

HERBAL REMEDIES

- Diuretic herbs are helpful for excreting excess fluids. Health food or herb stores usually have a kidney formula containing such herbs as uva ursi, horsetail, and buchu. Take one or two capsules two to four times a day.

OTHER THERAPIES

- Water retention can be related to the emotions of helplessness, depression, and "holding it all inside." Expressing stored-up feelings, especially anger, can help release excess water. Believing that you can influence your life, instead of being a victim, can also aid the healing process.

Wound Healing

See SURGERY. See also ULCER (VENOUS STASIS).

Yeast Infections

See VAGINITIS.

INTRAVENOUS VITAMIN AND MINERAL PROTOCOL
Adapted from Alan R. Gaby, M.D., of Baltimore, Maryland

INDICATIONS

Chronic fatigue, including Epstein-Barr virus syndrome

Chronic depression

Acute or chronic muscle spasm

Fibrositis (fibromyalgia)

Acute or chronic asthma

Acute or chronic urticaria (hives)

Seasonal allergic rhinitis (hay fever)

Congestive heart failure

Angina

Ischemic vascular disease

Acute infections

Senile dementia

MATERIALS*

Magnesium chloride hexahydrate (20%)
2–5 cc

Calcium gluconate (10%)
1–4 cc

Hydroxycobalamin (1,000 mcg/cc)
1 cc

Pyridoxine hydrochyloride (100 mg/cc)
1 cc

Dexpanthenol (250 mg/cc)
1 cc

B complex 100
1 cc

Vitamin C (222 mg/cc)
1–30 cc

Optional: Multi-Trace Elements-5 or MULTE-Pak-5 providing per 1 cc: zinc (1 mg), copper (0.4 mg), selenium (20 mcg), manganese (0.1 mg), and chromium (4 mcg).

Add 1 cc of sterile water for every 1 cc of calcium gluconate, because the solution is hypertonic. In general, use 1 cc of calcium gluconate for every 2 cc of magnesium chloride. However, for anxiety or migraines, increase the ratio to 1:1. Draw up all nutrients into one syringe and inject slowly over five to fifteen minutes, through a 25-gauge butterfly needle.

PRECAUTIONS

This solution is hypertonic and occasionally causes pain at the site of injection. This can be avoided by diluting the injection by 25% to 50% with sterile water (beyond the dilution of calcium gluconate described above). Most patients experience warmth during the injection. Too rapid administration of magnesium can cause hypotension, which can be severe. Patients with low blood pressure tend to tolerate less magnesium. When administering this treatment to a patient for the first time, it is best to give 0.5 to 1.0 cc, then wait thirty seconds or so before proceeding with the rest of the injection. Start with lower doses for elderly or frail individuals. In patients at risk for hypokalemia, such as those taking certain diuretics, beta-antagonists, or corticosteroids, or patients with diarrhea, serum potassium should be measured and hypokalemia should be corrected before administering this treatment. When in doubt, give 20 to 25 mEq of potassium orally at the time of the injection, and repeat four to six hours later.

*Injectable nutrients available from McGuff Pharmaceuticals of Santa Ana, California, (800) 854-7220 and Merit Pharmaceuticals of Los Angeles, California, (800) 696-3748.

INTRAVENOUS VITAMIN AND MINERAL PROTOCOL
Adapted from Alan R. Gaby, M.D., of Baltimore, Maryland

NOTES

1. In patients with cardiac arrhythmias, calcium should probably not be included, and the maximum tolerated amount of magnesium should be used.

2. For asthma or urticaria, 6 to 30 cc of vitamin C and double doses of pyridoxine, dexpanthenol, and vitamin B-12 may be necessary.

3. For infections and allergic rhinitis, 10 to 30 cc of vitamin C should be used.

4. In some patients, the treatment works better if vitamin B-12 is given intramuscularly in a separate syringe. It is not clear whether this is due to the short half-life of intravenously administered B-12 or whether vitamin B-12 interacts with some other component of the injection.

Adapted by permission of Dr. Alan Gaby.

SUGGESTED READING

AIDS (ACQUIRED IMMUNE DEFICIENCY SYNDROME)

Badgley, Lawrence, M.D. *Healing AIDS Naturally.* San Bruno, CA: Human Energy Press, 1990.

Bauforth, Nick. *Aids and the Healer Within.* Woodstock, NY: Amethyst, 1988.

Gregory, Scott J., M.D. *A Holistic Protocol for the Immune System HIV/ARC/AIDS.* Joshua Tree, CA: Tree of Life Publications, 1989.

Jaffe, Russel, M.D., Ph.D. "Protocols for Host Immune Enhancement." Publication #127, Reston, VA: Health Studies Collegium, 1993.

Kidd, Paris, and Huber, Wolfgang. *Learning to Live with the AIDS Virus: A Strategy for Long-Term Survival.* Berkeley, CA: HK Biomedical-Educator, 1991.

Konlee, Mark. *AIDS Control Diet.* West Allis, WI: Keep Hope Alive, 1993.

Lands, Lark, Ph.D. *Positively Well: Living with HIV as a Chronic, Manageable, Survivable Disease.* Manchester, NH: Irvington Publisher, 1995.

Lauritsen, John. *The AIDS War: Propaganda, Profiteering, and Genocide from the Medical Industrial Complex.* New York: Pagan Press, 1993.

Serinus, Jason, ed. *Psychoimmunity and the Healing Process: A Holistic Approach to Immunity and AIDS.* Berkeley, CA: Celestial Arts, 1986.

The Carl Vogel Foundation provides a discount buying club for nutritional supplements, in addition to printed information, AIDS seminars, and other HIV-related concerns. Carl Vogel Foundation, Inc., 1413 K Street N.W., Washington, DC 20005-3405, (202) 289-4898.

ALCOHOLISM

Bradshaw, John. *Bradshaw on the Family: A Revolutionary Way of Self-Discovery.* Pompano Beach, FL: Health Communications, 1988.

Larson, John Mathews, Ph.D. *Alcohol—The Biochemical Connection.* New York: Villard Books/Random House, 1992.

Moz, Jane Middleton, and Dwinnel, Lorie. *After the Tears: Reclaiming the Personal Losses of Childhood.* Pompano Beach, FL: Health Communications, 1986.

Phelps, Janice Keller, M.D. *Hooked: Hidden Addictions and How to Get Free.* Boston: Little, Brown, 1986.

Schaef, Ann. *Co-Dependence: Misunderstood, Mistreated.* New York: Harper & Row, 1986.

Williams, Roger, M.D. *The Prevention of Alcoholism through Nutrition.* New York: Bantam, 1981.

ALZHEIMER'S DISEASE

Dean, Ward, M.D., and Morganthaler, John. *Smart Drugs and Nutrients: How to Improve Your Memory and Increase Your Intelligence Using the Latest Discoveries in Neuroscience.* Santa Cruz, CA: B&J Publishing, 1990.

Ward, Dean, M.D., Morgenthaler, John, and Fowkes, Steven Wm. *Smart Drugs II The Next Generation: New Drugs and Nutrients to Improve Your Memory and Increase Your Intelligence.* Menlo Park, CA: Health Freedom Publications, 1993.

Warren, Tom. *Beating Alzheimer's: A Step toward Unlocking the Mysteries of Brain Disease.* Garden City Park, NY: Avery, 1991.

ARTERIOSCLEROSIS

Agarwal, R. C., et al. "Clinical Trial of Gugulipid, a New Hypolipidemic Agent of Plant Origin in Primary Hyperlipidemia." *India Journal of Medical Research* 84 (1986): 626–634.

Brunzell, J. D., et al. "Apoproteins B and A, and Coronary Artery Disease in Humans." *Arteriosclerosis* 4 (1984): 79–83.

Budwig, Johanna, M.D. *Flax Oil as a True Aid against Heart Infarction, Cancer, and Other Diseases.* Vancouver, Canada: Apple Publishing, 1992.

Childs, M.D., et al. "Divergent Lipoprotein Responses to Fish Oils with Various Ratios of Eicosapentaenoic Acid and Docosahexaenoic Acid." *American Journal of Clinical Nutrition* 59 (1990): 632–639.

Christakis, G. *The Effect of Dietary Cholesterol on Serum Cholesterol: An Interpretive Review.* Washington, DC: AEP/UEP Egg Nutrition Center.

Cranton, E. M., and Brecher, A. *Bypassing Bypass.* Troutdale, VA: Medex, 1990.

Gey, K. F., et al. "Inverse Correlation between Plasma Vitamin E and Mortality from Ischemic Heart Disease in Cross-cultural Epidemiology." *American Journal of Clinical Nutrition* 53 (1991): 3265–3345.

Herling, I. M. "Lipids and Atherosclerosis: A Perspective." *Practical Cardiology* 16 (December 1990): 33–35.

Ilyia, E. *Free Radical, Oxidative Stress Markers.* Seattle, WA: Diagnos-Techs (1991): 4c-1–4c-5.

Mann, George, ScD., M.D. (ed.) *Coronary Heart Disease: The Dietary Sense and Nonsense.* New York: Paul and Co. c/o PCS Data Processing, Inc., 1993.

McGee, Charles T., M.D. *Heart Frauds: The Misapplication of High Technology in Heart Disease.* Coeur d'Alene, ID: Medipress, 1993.

Ornish, Dean, M.D. *Dr. Dean Ornish's Program for Reversing Heart Disease.* New York: Random House, 1990.

Ornish, D., et al. "Can Lifestyle Changes Reverse Coronary Heart Disease?" *Lancet* 336 (1990): 129–133.

Politzer, Brianna. "Lipid Lowering May Entail Risk." *Medical Tribune* (September 6, 1990): 9.

Rath, Matthias, M.D. *Eradicating Heart Disease.* San Francisco: Health Now, 1993.

Rimm, E. B., et al. "Vitamin E Consumption and the Risk of Coronary Heart Disease in Men." *New England Journal of Medicine* 20 (1993): 1450–1456.

Stampfer, M. J., et al. "Vitamin E Consumption and the Risk of Coronary Heart Disease in Women." *New England Journal of Medicine* 20 (1993): 1444–1449.

Stocker, R., et al. "Ubiquinol-10 Protects Human Low Density Lipoprotein More Efficiently against Lipid Peroxidation than Does Alpha Tocopherol." *Proceedings of the National Academy of Sciences* 88 (1991): 1646–1650.

Strandberg, T. E., et al. "Long-Term Mortality after Five-Year Multifactorial Primary Prevention of Cardiovascular Disease in Middle-aged Men." *Journal of the American Medical Association* 266 (1991): 1225–1229.

For a referral list of physicians who perform chelation therapy, contact the American College of Advancement in Medicine, 23121 Verdugo Dr., Suite 204, Laguna Hills, CA 92653 (714) 583-7666.

ATTENTION DEFICIT/HYPERACTIVITY DISORDER

For neurological organization evaluation and treatment, contact Developmental Movement Center, 10303 Meridian Ave., N., Suite 201, Seattle, WA 98133, (206) 364-1473; Oregon Hope and Help Center, P.O. Box 406, Woodburn, OR 97071, (503) 981-0635; Institutes for the Achievement of Human Potential, 8801 Stenton Ave., Philadelphia, PA 19118, (215) 233-2051; and ARE

Medical Clinic, 4018 North 40th St. Phoenix, AZ 85018, (602) 955-0551

Delacato, Carl. *A New Start for the Child with Reading Problems*. New York: McKay, 1977.

Doman, Glen. *What to Do about Your Brain-Injured Child*. New York: M. Evans, 1990.

LeWinn, Edward B., M.D. *The Human Neurological Organization*. Springfield, IL: Charles C. Thomas, 1977.

Melton, David. *When Children Need Help*. New York: Crowell, 1972.

———. *Todd*. Englewood Cliffs, NJ: Prentice Hall, 1968.

For books on the nutritional treatment of ADD, see:

Cott, Alan, M.D., Agel, J., and Boe, E. *Dr. Cott's Help for Your Learning Disabled Child: The Orthomolecular Treatment*. New York: Times Books, 1985.

Crook, William G., M.D. *Help for the Hyperactive Child*. Jackson, TN: Professional Books, 1991.

Rapp, Doris J., M.D. *Allergies and the Hyperactive Child*. New York: Cornerstone Library/Simon & Schuster, 1979.

For more information, contact the Learning Disabilities Association of America National Office, 4156 Library Rd., Pittsburgh, PA 15234.

See also suggested reading for DEPRESSION.

See also Levinson, Harold N., M.D. *Smart But Feeling Dumb: A Breakthrough Theory on the Diagnosis and Treatment of Dyslexia and How It May Help You and Your Child*. New York: Warner Books, 1984.

BACK PAIN

Sarno, John E., M.D. *Healing Back Pain: The Mind–Body Connection*. New York: Warner Books, 1991.

CANCER

Obtain the "Coping with Cancer" videotape, which reviews common questions about cancer, treatments, lifestyles, quality of life during therapy, and the role of the immune system. Send $19.95 to Northwest Oncology Foundation, P.O. Box 3726, Bellevue, WA 98009. Also obtain the videos "What Your Doctor Won't Tell You about Cancer," "Cancer and Vitamin C: An Interview with Linus Pauling, Ph.D.," and "Self-Healing: An Interview with Norman Cousins," from Malibu Video, 6955 Fernhill Dr., Malibu, CA 90265, (310) 457-0833.

Self-Help Retreats and Seminars

- Cancer Support and Education Center, Menlo Park, CA (415) 327-6166.
- Commonweal Cancer Help Program, P.O. Box 316, 451 Mesa Road, Bolinas, CA 94924, (415) 868-0970.
- William Collinge, Ph.D., M.D.H., (707) 829-6813 or (800) 745-1837.

Budwig, Johanna, M.D. *Flax Oil as a True Aid against Heart Infarction, Cancer, and Other Disease*. Vancouver, Canada: Apple Publishing, 1992.

Dolinger, Malin, et al. *Everyone's Guide to Cancer Therapy: How Cancer Is Diagnosed, Treated and Managed Day to Day*. Kansas City, MO: Andrews and McMeel, 1991.

Exceptional Cancer Patients, 300 Plaza Middlesex, Middletown, CT 06457, (203) 343-5930.

Fink, John M. *Third Opinion: An International Directory to Alternative Therapy Centers for the Treatment and Prevention of Cancer and Other Degenerative Diseases*. Garden City, NY: Avery, 1992.

Fischer, William L. *How to Fight Cancer and Win*. Burnaby, Canada: Fischer, 1987.

Getting Well Program, 933 Bradshaw Terrace, Orlando, FL 32806, (407) 426-8662.

Levenstein, Mary Kerney. *Everyday Cancer Risks and How to Avoid Them*. Garden City, NY: Avery, 1992.

Moss, Ralph W., Ph.D. *Cancer Therapy: The Independent Consumer's Guide to Nontoxic Treatment and Prevention*. New York: Equinox Press/Moveable Type, 1992.

Quillin, Patrick, Ph.D., R.D., with Noreen Quillin. *Beating Cancer with Nutrition*. Tulsa, OK: Nutrition Times Press, 1994.

Rogers, Sherry A., M.D. *The Cure Is in the Kitchen: A Guide to Healthy Eating*. Syracuse, NY: Prestige Publishing, 1991.

———. *Wellness Against All Odds*. Syracuse, NY: Prestige Publishing, 1994.

Schardt, David. "Phytochemicals: Plants against Cancer." *Nutrition Action Health Letter* (Center for Science in the Public Interest): 21 (April 1994): 1, 9–11. April, 1994.

Siegel, Bernie, M.D. *Love, Medicine, and Miracles*. New York: Harper & Row, 1986.

Wainwright House, 260 Stuvyesant Ave., Rye, New York 10580, (914) 967-6080.

Walters, Richard. *Options: The Alternative Cancer Therapy Book*. Garden City, NY: Avery, 1993.

CERVICAL DYSPLASIA OR ABNORMAL PAP SMEAR

Butterworth, C. E., Jr., et al. "Improvement in Cervical Dysplasia Associated with Folic Acid Therapy in Users of Oral Contraceptives." *American Journal of Clinical Nutrition* (January 1982): 73–82.

Northrup, Christiane, M.D. *Women's Bodies, Women's Wisdom: Creating Physical and Emotional Health and Healing*. New York: Bantam, 1994.

Romney, Seymour L., et al. "Retinoids and the Prevention of Cervical Dysplasia." *American Journal of Obstetrics and Gynecology* (December 15, 1981): 890–894.

Wassertheil-Smoller, Sylvia, et al. "Dietary Vitamin C and Uterine/Cervical Dysplasia." *American Journal of Epidemiology* (November 1981): 714–724.

Whitehead, Nancy, et al. "Megaloblastic Changes in the Cervical Epithelium: Associated with Oral Contraceptive Therapy and Reversal with Folic Acid." *Journal of the American Medical Association* (December 17, 1973): 1421–1424.

CHRONIC FATIGUE SYNDROME (CHRONIC FATIGUE AND IMMUNE DYSFUNCTION SYNDROME)

The CFIDS Chronicle, CFIDS Association of America, P.O. Box 220398, Charlotte, NC 28222, (800) 442-3437.

CFIDS Treatment News, Chronic Fatigue Immune Dysfunction Syndrome Foundation, 965 Mission St., Suite 425, San Francisco, CA 94103, (415) 882-9986.

Journal of the Chronic Fatigue Syndrome. Haworth Press, 10 Alice Street, Binghamton, NY 13904-1580.

Bell, David S., M.D. *Curing Fatigue: A Step-by-Step Plan to Uncover and Eliminate the Causes of Chronic Fatigue*. Emmaus, PA: Rodale, 1993.

Berne, Katerina, Ph.D. *Running on Empty: Chronic Fatigue Immune Dysfunction Syndrome*. Alameda, CA: Hunter House, 1992.

Collinge, William, Ph.D., M.P.H. *Recovering from Chronic Fatigue Syndrome: A Guide to Self-Empowerment*. New York: Putnam, 1993. Also see the companion cassette tape series, "Recovering from Chronic Fatigue Syndrome: the Home Self-Empowerment Program," (707) 829-6813 or (800) 745-1837.

Cox, I. M. "Red Blood Cell Magnesium and Chronic Fatigue Syndrome." *Lancet* 337 (1991): 757–60.

Crook, William G., M.D. *Chronic Fatigue Syndrome and the Yeast Connection*. Jackson, TN: Professional Books, 1992.

Duff, Kate. *The Alchemy of Illness*. New York: BellTower/Harmony, 1993.

Durlach, J. "Chronic Fatigue Syndrome and Chronic Magnesium Deficiency" (CFS and CPMD). *Magnesium Research* 5 (1992): 68.

Hoffman, Ronald. *Tired All the Time*. New York: Poseidon Press, 1993.

Holvschlag, Molly E. "Q-10, Malic Acid and Magnesium May Improve CFIDS-FM Symptoms." *CFIDS Chronicle* (Chronic Fatigue Immune Dysfunction Syndrome Association of America) (Summer 1993): pp. 98–99.

Stoff, Jesse, M.D., and Pellegrino, Charles, Ph.D. *Chronic Fatigue Syndrome: The Hidden Epidemic*. New York: Random House, 1988.

CFIDS Buyer's Club (for nutritional supplements, products for the environmentally sensitive, and books about CFIDS), 1187 Coast Village Rd., #1-280, Santa Barbara, CA 93108-2794, (800) 366-6056.

Retreats and seminars: William Collinge, Ph.D., M.P.H., (707) 829-6813 or (800) 745-1837.

COLDS, FLU, SORE THROATS, and COUGHS

Rauch, Erich, M.D. *Naturopathic Treatment of Colds and Infectious Diseases*. Portland, OR: Medicina Biologica/Haug, 1993.

COLITIS

Ber, Abram, M.D., and Rothchild, Jonathan, M.A. "The Use of Sialic Acid Compounds in the Treatment of Inflammatory Bowel Disease." *Townsend Letter for Doctors* (August/September 1989): 433–439.

Gottschall, Elaine, B.A., M.Sc., *Food and the Gut Reaction: Intestinal Health Through Diet*. Kirkton, Ontario: Kirkton Press, 1987.

DEPRESSION

For an extensive list of books, articles, tapes, and seminars on nutritional/environmental/alternative approaches to the understanding and treatment of depression and other forms of mental illness, as well as in-patient treatment centers, contact:

- Carl Pfeiffer Treatment Center, 1804 Centre Point Dr., Naperville, IL 60563, (708) 505-0300.
- Princeton Bio-Center, 862 Rte. 518, Skillman, NJ 08558, (609) 924-8607.
- Schizophrenia Foundation—Canada, 16 Florence Ave., North York, Ontario, Canada M2N1E9, (416) 733-2117.
- The Well Mind Association, 4649 Sunnyside Ave. N., Seattle, WA 98103, (206) 547-6167.
- Well Mind Association of Greater Washington (D.C.), 11141 Georgia Ave., Suite 326, Wheaton, MD 20902, (301) 949-8282.

Pfeiffer, Carl C., M.D., Ph.D. *Nutrition and Mental Illness: An Orthomolecular Approach to Balancing Body Chemistry.* Rochester, VT: Healing Arts Press, 1987.

———. *Mental and Elemental Nutrients.* New Canaan, CT: Keats, 1975.

Philpott, William H., M.D., and Kalita, Dwight K., Ph.D. *Brain Allergies: The Psychonutrient Connection.* New Canaan, CT: Keats, 1987.

Sleigel, Patricia. *The Way Up from Down.* New York: Random House, 1987.

Werbach, Melvyn R., M.D. *Nutritional Influences on Mental Illness: A Sourcebook of Clinical Research.* Tarzana, CA: Third Line Press, 1991.

DIABETES MELLITUS

Anderson, James W., M.D. *Diabetes.* New York: Warner Books, 1987.

Barnes, Broda, M.D., Ph.D., and Galton, Lawrence. *Hypothyroidism: The Unsuspected Illness.* New York: Crowell, 1976.

Bernstein, Richard K., M.D. *Diabetes: The Glucograf Method for Normalizing Blood Sugar.* New York: Crown, 1981.

———. *Diabetes Type Two: Living a Long, Healthy Life Through Blood Sugar Normalization.* Englewood Cliffs, NJ: Prentice Hall, 1990.

Karjalainen, J. "A Bovine Albumin Peptide as a Possible Trigger of Insulin-Dependent Diabetes Mellitus," *New England Journal of Medicine,* July 30, 1992; 327(5): 302-307.

Koutsikos, D., et al. "Biotin for Diabetic Peripheral Neuropathy." *Biomedicine and Pharmacotherapy,* 1990 (44): 511–514.

Philpott, William, M.D. and Kalita, Dwight, Ph.D. *Victory Over Diabetes.* New Canaan, CT: Keats, 1983.

Pizzorno, Joseph, N.D., and Murray, Michael T., N.D. "Diabetes Mellitus." In *The Textbook of Natural Medicine,* Section VI, pp. 1–17. Seattle, WA: John Bastyr College Publications, 1985.

Suzuki, Y. J., et al. "Lipoate Prevents Glucose-Induced Protein Modifications." *Free Radical Research Communications* 17 (1992): 211–217.

Zahnd and Bever. "Plants with Oral Hypoglycemic Action." *Quarterly Journal of Crude Drug Research* 17 (1979): 139–196.

ENDOMETRIOSIS

Balweg, Mary Lou, and the Endometriosis Association. *Overcoming Endometriosis: New Help from the Endometriosis Association.* New York/Chicago: Congdon and Weed, 1987.

Northrup, Christiane, M.D. *Women's Bodies, Women's Wisdom: Creating Physical and Emotional Health and Healing.* New York: Bantam, 1994.

Also contact HERS (Hysterectomy Educational Resources and Services) for self-help information and newsletter, 422 Bryn Mawr Ave., Bala Cynwyd, PA 19004, (215) 667-7757.

FIBROCYSTIC BREAST DISEASE

Northrup, Christiane, M.D. *Women's Bodies, Women's Wisdom: Creating Physical and Emotional Health and Healing.* New York: Bantam, 1994.

Wright, Jonathan V., M.D. *Dr. Wright's Guide to Healing with Nutrition.* Emmaus, PA: Rodale Press, 1984.

FIBROIDS

Hufnagel, Vicki, M.D., with Susan Golant. *No More Hysterectomies.* New York: New American Library, 1988.

Northrup, Christiane, M.D. *Women's Bodies, Women's Wisdom: Creating Physical and Emotional Health and Healing.* New York: Bantam, 1994.

Also contact HERS (Hysterectomy Educational Resources and Services), 422 Bryn Mawr Avenue, Bala Cynwyd, PA 19004, (215) 667-7757.

FIBROMYALGIA

Backstrom, Gayle, with Bernard R. Rubin, M.D. *When Muscle Pain Won't Go Away.* Dallas: Taylor Publishing, 1992.

Davidson, Paul, M.D. *Chronic Muscle Pain Syndrome: How to Recognize and Treat It and Feel Better All Over.* New York: Berkley Books, 1989.

Holvschlag, Molly E. "Q-10, Malic Acid, and Magnesium May Improve CFIDS-FM Symptoms." *CFIDS Chronicle* (Chronic Fatigue Immune Dysfunction Syndrome Association of America) (Summer 1993): 98–99.

For more information, see:

Fibromyalgia Network. Newsletter for Fibromyalgia, Fibrocistis, Chronic Fatigue Immune Dysfunction Support Groups, 7001 School House Lane, Bakersfield, CA 93309.

HEART ATTACK and HEART FAILURE (CONGESTIVE HEART FAILURE)

Rath, Matthias, M.D. *Eradicating Heart Disease.* San Francisco, CA: Health Now, 1993.

See also ARTERIOSCLEROSIS.

HYPOTHYROIDISM

Barnes, Broda, M.D., Ph.D., with Lawrence Galton. *Hypothyroidism: The Unsuspected Illness.* New York: Crowell, 1976.

Langer, Stephen, M.D., with James F. Scheer. *Solved, the Riddle of Illness.* New Canaan, CT: Keats, 1984.

Wilson, E. Denis. *Wilson's Syndrome: The Miracle of Feeling Well.* Orlando, FL: Cornerstone, 1991.

For more information, contact the Broda O. Barnes, M.D., Research Foundation, Inc., P.O. Box 98, Trumbull, CT 06611, (203) 261-2101.

INFERTILITY

Schacter, A., et al. "Treatment of Oligospermia with the Amino Acid Arginine." *Journal of Urology* (September 1973): 311–313.

Wright, J. V. *Dr. Wright's Guide to Healing with Nutrition.* Emmaus, PA: Rodale Press, 1984: 413–416.

"Daily Vitamin C Protects Sperm from Genetic Damage." *Medical Tribune* (January 12, 1992): 23.

MEMORY IMPAIRMENT

Hoffer, Abram, M.D., Ph.D., and Walker, Morton, D.P. M. *Smart Nutrients.* Garden City, NY: Avery, 1994.

Ward, Dean, M.D., and Morganthaler, John. *Smart Drugs and Nutrients: How to Improve Your Memory and Increase Your Intelligence Using the Latest Discoveries in Neuroscience.* Santa Cruz, CA: B & J Publishing, 1990.

Ward, Dean, M.D., Morganthaler, John, and Fowles, Steven Wm. *Smart Drugs II The Next Generation: New Drugs and Nutrients to Improve Your Memory and Increase Your Intelligence.* Menlo Park, CA: Health Freedom Publications, 1993.

MENOPAUSE

Greenwood, Sadja. *Menopause, Naturally: Preparing for the Second Half of Life.* San Francisco: Volcano Press, 1989.

Kamen, Betty, Ph.D. *Hormone Replacement Therapy: Yes or No?* Novato, CA: Nutrition Encounter, 1993.

Lark, Susan, M.D. *Menopause Self-Help Book.* Berkeley, CA: Celestial Arts, 1990.

Lee, John R., M.D. *Natural Progesterone: The Multiple Roles of a Remarkable Hormone.* Sebastopol, CA: BLL Publishing, 1993.

Northrup, Christiane, M.D. *Women's Bodies, Women's Wisdom: Creating Physical and Emotional Health and Healing.* New York: Bantam, 1994.

Sheehy, Gail. *The Silent Passage.* New York: Pocket Books, 1992.

Van Eyck, Marian. *Transformation through Menopause.* Westport, CT: Bergin and Garvey/Greenwood, 1991.

Weed, Susan. *Wise Woman Ways for the Menopausal Years.* Hinesburg, VT: Upper Access Books, 1992.

MULTIPLE SCLEROSIS

Soll, Robert W., M.D., Ph.D. *MS: Something Can Be Done and You Can Do It.* Chicago, IL: Contemporary Books, 1984.

Swank, Roy, M.D. *The Multiple Sclerosis Diet Book.* New York: Doubleday, 1977.

OSTEOPOROSIS

Gaby, Alan, M.D. *Preventing and Reversing Osteoporosis: Every Woman's Essential Guide.* Rockland, CA: Prima Publishing, 1994.

Griffiths, J. "New Osteoporosis Treatment." *Medical Tribune* (November 29, 1990): 1.

Kamen, Betty, Ph.D. *Hormone Replacement Therapy: Yes or No?* Novato, CA: Nutrition Encounter, 1993.

Lee, John R., M.D. *Natural Progesterone: The Multiple*

Roles of a Remarkable Hormone. Sebastopol, CA: BLL Publishing, 1993.

OVERWEIGHT

Abravanel, Elliot, M.D. *Anti-Craving Weight-Loss Diet*. New York: Bantam, 1990.

Abravanel, Elliott, M.D., and King, Elizabeth A. *Dr. Abravanel's Body Type Program for Health and Fitness*. New York: Bantam, 1985.

Bates, Charles E., Ph.D. *Beyond Dieting: Relief from Persistent Hunger*. Olympia, WA/Courtenay, B.C., Canada: Tsolum River Press, 1994.

Ezrin, Calvin, and Kowalski, Robert. *The Endocrine Control Diet*. New York: Harper & Row, 1990.

Huebner, Hans F., M.D. *Endorphins, Eating Disorders and Other Addictive Behaviors*. New York: Norton, 1993.

Lad, Vasant. *Ayurveda: The Science of Self-Healing: A Practical Guide*. Wilmot, WI: Lotus, 1984.

Marsden, Kathryn. *The Food Combining Diet: Lose Weight the Hay Way*. San Francisco: Thorsons, 1993.

Ornish, Dean, M.D. *Eat More, Weigh Less*. New York: HarperCollins, 1993.

Powter, Susan. *Stop the Insanity*. New York: Simon and Schuster, 1993.

PREMENSTRUAL SYNDROME

Mabray, E. T., et al. "Treatment of Common Gynecologic/ Endocrinologic Symptoms by Allergy Management Procedures." *Obstetrics and Gynecology* 5 (May 1982): 560–64.

Northrup, Christiane, M.D. *Women's Bodies, Women's Wisdom: Creating Physical and Emotional Health and Healing*. New York: Bantam, 1994.

PROSTATE HYPERTROPHY

Champault, G., et al. "A Double-Blind Trial of an Ex- tract of the Plant Serenoa Repens in Benign Prostatic Hyperplasia." *British Journal of Clinical Pharmacology* 18 (1984): 461–462.

SEASONAL AFFECTIVE DISORDER (SAD)

Avery, D. "Bright-Light Therapy for Winter Depression." *Clinical Advances in the Treatment of Psychiatric Disorders* 2 (November–December 1988): 8–9.

Hyman, Jane Wegscheider. *The Light Book: How Natural and Artificial Light Affect Our Health, Mood, and Behavior*. Los Angeles: J. P. Tarcher, 1990.

Lewy, A. J. "Treating Chronobiologic Sleep and Mood Disorders with Bright Light." *Psychiatric Annals* 1987; *17*(10): 664–669.

Rosenthal, N. E. *Seasons of the Mind: Why You Get Winter Blues and What You Can Do About It*. New York: Bantam, 1989.

————. *Winter Blues: Seasonal Affective Disorder: What It Is and How to Overcome It*. New York: Guilford, 1993.

Rosenthal, N. E., and Wehr, T. A. "Seasonal Affective Disorders." *Psychiatric Annals* 17(10): 670–674.

SEIZURES

Higgins, Kathleen, M.S.W., A.C.S.W. *Living Well With Epilepsy: A Manual for Self Care*. Epilepsy Wellness, 6 Lake Bellevue Drive, Suite 209, Bellevue, WA 98005.

————. "Unlocking the Gifts Within," a guided relaxation tape (music by Marion Gerard). Epilepsy Wellness, 6 Lake Bellevue, Suite 209, Bellevue, WA 98005.

SURGERY, PREPARATION FOR

Moss, Richard, M.D. *How Shall I Live: Where Spiritual Healing and Conventional Medicine Meet*. Berkeley, CA: Celestial Arts, 1985.

PART FIVE

NEW AGE AND AGE-OLD APPROACHES

CHAPTER 18

FASTING, CLEANSING, REJUVENATION

For centuries health professionals oriented toward natural approaches have emphasized the importance of fasting in order to rest the gastrointestinal system and cleanse the body. They suggest that fasting enhances digestion and absorption and strengthens the body's detoxifying and eliminative capacities. They believe that during a fast the body burns up accumulated wastes—self-cleans, so to speak. This inner cleansing process facilitates cellular repair and building and general metabolic functioning. With improved nutrient absorption, toxin elimination, and cellular metabolism, our whole organism experiences a surge in health and well-being. We enjoy increased vitality, increased resistance to infections, less incidence of chronic degenerative disease, a slowing of the aging process, and a longer, healthier life.

FASTING, EVERY NIGHT

At first glance, you might consider these claims to be exaggerated, faddish, or extreme. In taking a closer look, however, we see that fasting is not a radical, outlandish practice. In fact, in its most conservative and common-sense form, fasting is what occurs every night when we're asleep. It's not without meaning that your morning meal is called "break-fast."

When the food supply to the body is temporarily curtailed, the entire digestive machinery takes a rest. There is a slowdown in hydrochloric acid and pepsin secretion from the stomach; protein-, carbohydrate-, and fat-digesting enzyme secretions from the pancreas; bile secretion from the liver and gallbladder; complex metabolic rearrangements of proteins, fats, and carbohydrates in the liver; and intestinal peristalsis. Thanks to

the reduction in these metabolic processes, we're able to build an energy reserve, some of which is used for the inner cleansing process.

ORIGINS OF TOXICITY

This vital self-cleaning activity can't really take hold when we eat three meals a day, seven days a week, especially when we commonly overeat and frequently snack between meals and late at night. How can an oven's self-cleaning mechanism get to work when the oven is continually cooking? Proteins and fats require three to five hours simply to work their way out of the stomach. When you go to bed an hour or two after dinner or a hearty bedtime snack, do you think that you'll actually be resting and rejuvenating in your sleep?

According to "nature cure" concepts, in an overburdened digestive and eliminative system, incompletely processed food is retained and stored as cell wastes. These accumulations impair normal metabolic processes, clog eliminative routes, and result in toxicity. This is how excesses do their damage and why so many of the common diseases in America today are the result of excess.

AUTOCLEANSING

Any machine will function more efficiently and last longer if it is turned off and cleaned periodically. In many ways, the body is a machine with delicately interrelated parts that need to cool down, rest, and be given a chance to recharge. According to such naturopathic writers as Paavo Airola, when you stop eating for a while, the body begins to digest and feed off its wastes.[1] In this way, the system cleanses itself and thereby continues to function efficiently.

Autocleansing, or self-cleansing, is a regularly self-maintained homeostatic function in organisms that eat sensibly. Consider the results of an experiment involving two identical groups of laboratory rodents, one fed several times a day and the other fed every other day. Both were fed identical types of food, but the group that was fed every other day had significantly fewer infections and tumors and a much longer life span. The researchers were so impressed by the results of this study that at least one has actually adopted the practice of fasting on fluids one or two days a week.[2]

Heed Nature's Warning

Given the documented association of several human cancers with high-caloric diets, it makes sense to think twice about all those huge sandwiches, full dinner plates, and frequent second helpings. Many of us plainly eat more than we need and in a style that does not allow an effective nightly fast.

Nevertheless, nature will attempt to enforce its laws when they are violated, ensuring that we cleanse and eliminate accumulated wastes by triggering an acute illness. We will lose our appetites, for example, and develop various kinds of body discharges—sinus and bronchial mucus, vomit, diarrhea, skin eruptions like boils, a coated tongue, dark, foul stools, dark urine, foul breath. Thus nature reacts to accumulated wastes by making use of all the eliminative routes: bowel, kidney, skin, and lungs.

When the toxin accumulation has exceeded the capacity of our eliminative routes, other symptoms emerge, such as nausea, fatigue, irritability, headache, and muscle and joint aches (see "Bowel Toxicity," pages 157–160). Most conventionally trained doctors lack an understanding of this concept and will rarely be alerted by the symptoms of toxicity to guide you to a cleansing regimen. More likely, they will prescribe a medication that suppresses your headache, joint ache, or nausea. In the short run, this will help you feel more comfortable, but over time, if done as a regular practice, it will continually diminish toxin elimination and it may contribute to a process of chronic illness.

CLEANSING WITHOUT FASTING?

The physiologic functions on which health depends, including the self-cleansing mechanisms, can be maintained by establishing a sensible way of eating. Having an early supper, avoiding regular between-meal snacks, and trying not to overeat will enable your self-cleansing mechanisms—and thus your digestive, eliminative, and metabolic systems—to operate at peak efficiency. Each night will indeed become a minifast, an opportunity for your body to avoid accumulating wastes. In this way, breakfast (if eaten twelve to thirteen hours after the previous night's dinner) will truly be "breaking a fast." Such a pattern minimizes an individual's need to adopt any special cleansing diets or lengthy fasts to maintain optimal health.

UNDOING THE DAMAGE THROUGH CLEANSING DIETS AND FASTING

Those of us who are unable to eat in an ideal way may benefit from a periodic cleansing diet or fast. Below are suggestions for a few of the options that can help you eliminate the digestive fatigue and accumulations to which our eating styles predispose us.

Cleansing or Purifying Diet

Periodically eat cleansing foods only—vegetables and/or fruits—for all the meals of a day. When heavy starches, proteins, and fats are eliminated, the digestive system is given a break and the self-cleaning mechanism has a chance to kick in.

One such regimen (discussed on pages 180–181) is the Liver Flush and Purifying Diet. Many individuals testify to a sense of lightness and increased energy and well-being after a few days' purification. Once they have experienced this, they turn to this diet whenever they feel an impending imbalance from dietary excesses. Cleansing diets can be undertaken safely for a day or two up to one week periodically. Of course, anyone with diabetes or some other significant metabolic ailment requiring medication or medical management should consult a physician first.

One-Day Fluid Fast

Fast for twenty-four to thirty-six hours on fluids once a week. Again, consuming only water, herb tea, vegetable broth, and vegetable and fruit juices for this period of time is quite safe for nearly everyone. However, unless your diet has been excessively contracting, building, and acidifying (see Chapter Four), relying primarily on fruit juice for a fast is inadvisable. Alternate the different choices of fluids. If you tend to be hypoglycemic, try using a hypoallergenic protein or meal replacement powder such as Ultra Clear Sustain or Ultra Balance (by Health Comm of Tacoma, Washington) several times throughout the day in addition to your fasting fluids. (See also Chapter Ten for the recognition and treatment of hypoglycemia.)

A one-day fast is relatively easy; give it a try. Your mind may not welcome it, but your body most likely will. If you are underweight or cannot afford to lose any weight, you could still manage a one-day fast, especially if you use a nutrient powder (as mentioned above) throughout the day. If you are unsure or if you have diabetes or other metabolic problems, get advice from a health professional first.

Three- to Seven-Day Fluid Fast

Consider a three-day fast every month or two, or a seven- to ten-day fast once or twice a year. The latter is most beneficial to individuals who have been chronically abusing their bodies and for those who have developed chronic health problems.

WORSE BEFORE BETTER: COMMON CLEANSING REACTIONS

It's important to realize that a fast of any length, or even a cleansing diet, may temporarily trigger a number of uncomfortable symptoms:

Sinus and bronchial mucus discharge
Coughing
Diarrhea
Dark, foul stools
Dark urine
Skin eruptions—rashes, boils, acne
Coated tongue
Foul breath and bad taste in mouth
Fatigue
Irritability
Anxiety
Poor concentration
Confusion
Headaches
Joint or muscle pains

These are often simple cleansing reactions, as excessive toxin accumulations seek a way to exit. Consider gradually reducing your toxin load prior to a fast to lessen the severity of such reactions. Again, if you have any chronic disorder requiring medical management, consult a health professional before attempting a fast of any length.

Many natural health practitioners speak of a "healing crisis," which is essentially the same as a cleansing reaction (although it can also refer to a more exaggerated response). According to "Herring's Law of Natural Cure" (named for Constantine Herring, 1800–1880), as your body heals itself, it may effect a temporary and usually minor recurrence of a previous illness. Anne-

marie Colbin offers a summary of Herring's law in her book *Food and Healing*:[3]

Herring's Law of Natural Cure

1. Symptoms move from the inside to the outside of the body (mucus in the lungs is coughed up; toxic matter from deep within the system comes out as boils or rashes).

2. Symptoms move from the upper part to the lower part of the body (medication that affects the kidneys, such as steroids, can be discharged by a rash on the legs).

3. Symptoms relating to chronic conditions disappear in the reverse order of their appearance. The ones that emerged last leave first. Then the other ones re-emerge and leave last.

This means that long after we set out on a healing path, we might relive symptoms of very old problems if these were suppressed or incorrectly treated. Their reemergence—sometimes known as retracing—if treated naturally and allowed to follow its course, would only mean that the body is healing itself. For example, if you used to cough a lot as a child and took medicine and then developed asthma, when you go into a healing mode, you may have a brief flare-up of the asthma and later—even several years later—have a coughing episode that is in fact a "retracing" of your childhood condition.

To these, Colbin adds:

4. A feeling of well-being precedes a healing crisis.

5. There is also a feeling of well-being at the core during the crisis; that is, deep down inside it feels OK.

Some of the symptoms in the list above may also reflect a withdrawal state. Many allergic foods are also addictive. When you eliminate them from your diet during a cleansing regimen, this may trigger a feeling of discomfort (see Chapter Thirteen). Buffered vitamin C and/or Alka-Seltzer Gold tablets can help minimize these symptoms (see page 247).

Another process that occurs during a cleansing regimen is the mobilization of stored drugs and chemicals in the body's fatty tissues. These often toxic substances, which have been either ingested, respired, or absorbed through the skin, may be released into the bloodstream during a fast or cleansing diet and trigger uncomfortable symptoms. The body's cleansing process will make every attempt to eliminate them one way or another. Enhancing elimination through the skin can be accomplished through skin brushing and saunas (see page 440).

There is one other reason for feeling worse during a fast: As chemicals are detoxified in the liver, the free radicals normally generated by this process in phase one reactions (see Chapter Nine) can make you feel ill, especially if your antioxidant nutrient stores are deficient.

Using vitamin C during the fast and a broad spectrum of antioxidants (see Chapter Three) in the weeks before fasting may help alleviate free radical stress and make your fast more comfortable.

FASTING—HOW OFTEN?

It's important to note that some individuals become extremists about cleansing and fasting. They fast too long and too frequently, until it becomes a regular way of life and they do damage to themselves. Health does not come primarily from any radical cleansing or fasting technique, but rather from our day-to-day practices that enhance living and eating in balance. Granted, cleansing techniques may be of extraordinary benefit, but carried too far they will become imbalancing and weakening.

Anyone who follows a sensible eating plan, gives the digestive system a rest, and allows the self-cleansing mechanism to operate nightly will have little need for extended fasting. Moreover, the enhanced feeling of well-being works in your favor: The better you feel from these practices, the easier it becomes to resist old cravings and harmful eating patterns.

In addition, while those who fast seven to ten days once or twice a year tend to be highly motivated to eat appropriately in the few weeks following the fast, they may slip back into their old habits as time goes on. Yes, extended fasts can accomplish great things—I have done them and have recommended them to others. Nevertheless, I believe that shorter and more frequent fasts tend to keep you more attuned to healthful eating.

THE PSYCHOLOGICAL BENEFITS OF FASTING

We create a wonderful opportunity to examine our relationship to food when we decide not to eat for one or several days. We learn how often we eat for reasons that have little to do with hunger or with sustaining the body through nutrition. We discover how frequently we eat out of boredom, loneliness, frustration, anxiety, depression, nervousness, guilt, anger, lack of love, or lack of joy. We may learn that we eat certain foods because we're addicted to them and would suffer from withdrawal symptoms if we stopped.

Eating can be an easy way to feel better emotionally. Depression, anxiety, and loneliness create a hunger. We often eat to suppress our feelings and slow the mind, make it less conscious—which may be useful at times. However, we don't resolve anything or allow ourselves to grow and change when eating is our way of dealing with stress. In fact, we can do damage to ourselves in this way, sometimes deadly damage. During a fast, we must confront our longings and repressed emotions in other ways. Through fasting we can learn to respect food and respect our bodies in new, healthier ways. We also learn more about self-control, about discipline.

When we fast, we realize how much time we devote to thinking about, preparing, eating, and digesting food. When this isn't a major focus of our day, we discover how much time we have for other pursuits and activities and how much more energy we have to do the things we've been putting off for so long. The process of digestion, particularly for overeaters and snackers, consumes extraordinary amounts of energy and can leave a person chronically fatigued. During a fast, some people experience a surge of energy and vitality they haven't felt in years. Fasting can also be a time of spiritual renewal. When we take time out from our involvement with food, it becomes much easier for our minds and hearts to open up in new ways. Fasting can help you raise your consciousness.

PREPARING FOR A THREE- TO TEN-DAY FAST

If you've been on a standard American diet and want to fast for three days or more, it would be wise to make some preparatory changes. Give yourself at least a week or two to make the transition:

1. Begin to minimize the health hazards in your diet: sugar, refined flour, caffeine, fried foods, and processed and packaged food that contains chemical additives. Include more whole grains, legumes, fresh vegetables and fruits, and eat somewhat smaller amounts of meat and dairy foods. If your diet is already relatively free of hazards, proceed to the next item.

2. Stabilize any hypoglycemic tendencies you may have (see Chapter Ten).

3. Improve the function of the bowel and detoxify your system of elimination through an intestinal cleansing program (pages 166–169).

4. Improve the function of the liver and detoxify it by using the Liver Flush and Purifying Diet (pages 180–181).

By following this approach, you will begin reducing the level of toxins in your body gradually and gently. Then the detoxification and eliminative systems will be primed to take on the more intense work of fasting. Such cleansing reactions as nausea, headache, joint pains, fatigue, and skin eruptions can be minimized in this way, and fasting can be made not only physically comfortable, but also a spiritually renewing experience. Even the preparations for a fast are significant moves toward better health, whether or not you decide to go ahead with the fast.

WHEN TO FAST

Extended fluid fasts are best done during the warmer months. If you choose to fast for seven days during the winter, you may have to take excessive measures to keep warm, and your body may have less energy available for cleansing. A brown rice fast (see below) may be more suitable for the colder season. Climate is less of an issue for short fluid fasts.

CHOOSING A FAST

In choosing a fast that is most appropriate for you, the principles outlined in Chapter Four for selecting the most appropriate diet may be helpful. How you see yourself within the traditional polar opposites—acid/alkaline, contractive/expanding, building/cleansing—may help determine what kind of fast and which kinds of fluids would be best for you.

Remember that one purpose of your fast is to counteract the excesses of your previous diet. Of the five fasts described later in this chapter, the first two—the Airola fast and the master cleanser lemonade fast—would be most useful for counterbalancing a standard American diet that has been excessive in the contractive, building, cooked, and acidic categories (too much meat, salt, grains, and legumes).

The next two—the bancha (kukicha or twig) tea fast and the brown rice fast—are more appropriate for those whose diets have been expansive, cleansing, raw, and alkaline (high in vegetables, fruits, sugar, and dairy). The tea and brown rice fasts are sometimes good choices for those who have excess fluid retention in their bodies or are often cold.

Of course, the foods I have listed here do not strictly fit all the corresponding polar categories, but they correspond well enough to the recommended fasts. Try some prudent experimentation; it sometimes proves more helpful than theory. You may find one type of fast more suitable for your body than another, regardless of your previous diet.

The last fast I'd like to suggest, the "Ultra Clear" program, is actually a metabolic clearing/detoxification program that nearly anyone could try. It involves a fortified rice-based powder beverage for three days, and then a gradual reintroduction of specific foods.

IMMEDIATELY PRECEDING THE FAST

Begin to reduce your caloric intake for half the number of days you intend to fast. For example, if you plan to fast for seven days, begin cutting down on your intake of food at least four days before the fast. Gradually reduce the heavier foods first—the animal proteins and fats. It's best to begin these reductions at your evening meals. As you approach your first fast day, you will drop your evening meal altogether and drink fluids instead.

At this point, your diet will be primarily vegetarian. Gradually reducing the amount of food you eat is actually more important than whether you eat vegetable or animal protein. In this way, your body will not be traumatized by the fast itself. In fact, you'll probably be surprised to find that after two to three days your hunger will subside. This period just before the actual fast should be considered part of the entire program. For a one-day fast, I do not feel it necessary to make any significant adjustments the day before.

DURING THE FAST

Following are some useful guidelines about fluids in general, as well as important information about enhancing your routes of elimination. These recommendations can heighten your fasting experience and create an optimal outcome.

Fluids

Water Use distilled, artesian, spring, or adequately filtered tap water. You can fast safely on pure water alone, although water fasts for more than a few days should be supervised professionally.

Vegetable and Fruit Juices Store-bought juices will suffice, but nothing can compare with the juice of fresh vegetables or fruits, made on the spot with your own juicer (see Chapter Four). The vitamins, minerals, and enzymes present in freshly made juices enhance the detoxification and cleansing processes. If possible, find organic produce for your juices and broths.

Vegetable Broths This warming, nutrient-rich drink is especially high in potassium (see recipe in Chapter Five).

Herbal Teas Health food stores, food co-ops, some supermarkets, and some public markets carry peppermint, spearmint, chamomile, rose hips, hibiscus, licorice root, red clover, and other varieties of herbal teas. Use herbs considered to be blood purifiers—red clover, echinacea root, sarsaparilla, and burdock root.

The Body's Eliminative Routes

Bowel Before your fast, do a bowel-cleansing program (as described in Chapter Eight) to minimize bowel toxicity. During a fast, peristalsis is extremely diminished, so bowel toxins can be absorbed into the circulation more easily. Therefore, if you are planning to fast for three or more days, a daily enema would be beneficial (see instructions on page 442). A saltwater purge (see pages 442–443) can also help clear the intestinal tract. The contractive fasts (bancha tea and rice) usually do not call for bowel cleansing.

Skin   Your skin absorbs and excretes in ways similar to the kidneys and bowel. Dry brushing helps you cleanse and stimulate your skin, increase its capacity to eliminate toxins, and relieve your kidneys and bowel of some of their burden. You will also be improving the tone, color, and texture of your skin.

Using a natural or vegetable bristle skin brush, vigorously brush your entire body—while your skin is dry—with all strokes going in the direction of your heart. Take five minutes each morning and, if possible, at night as well. Begin at your feet and come up both legs; then do hands and arms, and finally, the torso, back and front, using a reasonable amount of pressure. Avoid brushing irritated, damaged, infected, or particularly sensitive areas of your body, and avoid using stiffer brushes until your skin is less sensitive. Use a softer bristle brush made especially for the face. Your skin will positively glow and tingle. If you wish, you can continue dry brushing your skin even after the fast. Be sure to wash the brush every few weeks. I like to skin brush before showering.

Saunas or steam baths can also assist in eliminating toxins through the skin. Be particularly careful to do these in moderation; too many, especially during a fast, can leave you weakened.

Another method of stimulating the skin is to take hot and cold alternating showers. Stay under the hot water for several minutes, until you are warm. Then stand under water as cold as you can take for thirty to sixty seconds—don't allow yourself to get chilled. If you have a history of heart disease, consult your doctor before attempting this. Do a cycle of three hot/cold showers, always ending with cold, then towel dry vigorously. (See pages 466–469 for a more thorough explanation of the healthful effects of this hydrotherapy procedure.)

Lungs   Deep-breathing exercises center you and increase your vitality even as they encourage elimination through the lungs. A few exercises are offered on page 304. If possible, spend some time during your fast outside an urban environment, where the air is fresh.

Kidneys   The fluid you will be consuming in place of food will give your kidneys a good flushing. Cleansing the blood by enhancing the eliminative function of the liver, colon, and skin reduces the work the kidneys have to perform and helps preserve their optimum function.

Take any other measures you can to preserve these crucial filters, such as avoiding toxic chemicals and unnecessary drugs, as well as avoiding excess dietary protein. Naturopathic physicians often recommend the herbs uva ursi and nettles (*Uritoca dioca*), either in capsule or tincture form, to encourage elimination through the kidneys. Watermelon seed tea and watermelons are traditional kidney cleansers. Try a watermelon fast for one to two days. (You can juice watermelon, even the rind and skin—organic preferred.)

And be sure to use the most basic kidney cleanser—pure water—six to eight eight-ounce glasses daily.

Massage Therapy

Swedish massage, zone therapy, reflexology, acupressure, shiatsu, and various forms of energy massage are various types of bodywork that increase circulation and aid in the cleansing and elimination process. Massage is also worthwhile for the deep level of relaxation it brings. Your core vitality is thus strengthened, and more energy is made available for the cleansing process.

Exercise

Walking, yoga, stretching, swimming—any form of mild exercise—is beneficial during a fast, but don't overexert yourself. Vigorous exercise can burn muscle tissue, particularly if you're fasting for more than a few days.

Rest

Try to find the time to rest or nap at midday. During an extended fast of seven days or longer, it is best not to be engaged in any activity that is mentally strenuous or overly stressful. Try to insulate yourself from such demands during an extended fast, since your mental and physical energy and your ability to cope with stress may not be optimal—especially if you're new at fasting. On the other hand, some people experience a surge of mental and physical energy during a fast and feel able to carry out normal activities.

Sunbathing

Many authorities recommend brief sunbathing during a fast. The sun is the source of life on Earth. Unfortunately, the hazards of sunlight have been publicized far more than the benefits. However, an appropriate amount of sunlight has many documented healthful effects (see "Sunlight," pages 317–318).

Avoid Exposure to Negative Influences

You may become more open and vulnerable emotionally during a fast, so try to avoid difficult people and stressful situations.

Treat Yourself to Beauty

Spend some time in places of aesthetic beauty. Your appreciation of such things is often heightened during a fast, and, as you well know, an inspiring moment or experience will strengthen you on many levels.

BREAKING YOUR FAST

This aspect is as important as beginning a fast. Take at least half as many days as you fasted to return to a normal diet. Begin with one meal on the first day—breakfast—and take very small portions of food at first. Be sure to chew thoroughly, and by thoroughly I mean keep chewing until the food is nearly liquefied in your mouth. Some authors suggest chewing each mouthful over thirty times. If you consider your body sacred—and you likely will by the time your fast is over—you should be able to break your fast thoughtfully and respectfully.

Start with light, simple foods such as the fruits or vegetables you know you tolerate well. Then, gradually, over several days, add other foods you tolerate well: whole grains, well-cooked legumes, perhaps a few seeds and nuts, oils. Finally, if you are not vegetarian, add back animal protein last. If you suspect that you have food allergies, you may want to take advantage of this opportunity to test yourself (see Chapter Thirteen. You do not necessarily have to fast on water to test yourself for food allergies).

Breaking a Seven- to Ten-Day Fast

Note: You may need to substitute certain items listed below, depending on your own sensitivities and preferences. Although your food choices after a fast are important, portion sizes are even more crucial. Take very small amounts and chew thoroughly.

Day 1

BREAKFAST: 1 orange or 1 peeled apple or steamed grated carrots or rice cream without salt (see recipes in Chapter Five). Continue your fasting fluids the rest of the day.

Day 2

BREAKFAST: See day 1, or substitute soaked figs.
LUNCH: Vegetable salad (no oil) or vegetable soup or rice cream (no salt).

Day 3

BREAKFAST: See day 2. If you desire, add a small cup of yogurt.
LUNCH: See day 2. A little unrefined salt is okay at this point.
DINNER: Vegetable soup. Again, a little unrefined salt is okay.

Day 4

See day 3. Increase portion sizes a bit, and add a few raw nuts or seeds if you can tolerate them—best presoaked (see Chapter Two, "Peanuts and Nuts"). You can add a boiled or baked potato or yam, more whole grains, and a fruit snack.

Day 5

Begin to add back some protein foods and oil.

Day 6

Back to normal.

Once you break the fast, it may take a few days before your bowels begin to work normally. If enemas or saltwater purges have been part of your fast, continue them as necessary for two to four days after the end of the fast. Taking 1 to 2 teaspoons of flaxseed powder in a large glass of water, juice, or broth, and/or eating 3 to 5 soaked figs each day may also help get your bowels going again on their own.

SUGGESTED FASTS

The Airola Fast (up to ten days)[4]

(Reprinted from *How to Keep Slim, Healthy & Young with Juice Fasting*, by Paavo Airola, 1971, Health Plus Publishers, P.O. Box 1027, Sherwood, OR 97140.)

Upon arising	Enema
After enema	Dry brush massage, followed by hot and cold shower.
9:00 A.M.	Cup of herb tea—lukewarm, not hot. Health food stores carry a large assortment of herb teas. I recommend peppermint, chamomile, or rose hips. See the instructions on the package for preparing the teas.
11:00 A.M.	A glass of freshly pressed fruit juice, diluted fifty-fifty with water.

11:00 A.M. to   Walk or mild exercise, or sunbath-
1:00 P.M.   ing, if the weather permits.

1:00 P.M.   A glass of freshly made vegetable
juice or a cup of vegetable broth.*

1:30 to   Rest in bed
4:00 P.M.

4:00 P.M.   Cup of herb tea

4:15 to   Walk, therapeutic baths, exercises or
7:00 P.M.   other treatments.

7:00 P.M.   Glass of diluted vegetable or fruit
juice, or cup of vegetable broth.

Drink plain lukewarm water, or mineral water, when thirsty. The total juice and broth volume during the day should be between 1½ pints and 1½ quarts. Never dilute fresh juices with vegetable broth, only with pure water. The total liquid intake should be approximately 6 to 8 glasses—but don't hesitate to drink more, if thirsty.

Again, I suggest that, if possible, you have your fasting supervised by someone who is well initiated in it. Under expert supervision such a fast could be undertaken at home for up to 30 days if necessary. If you are ill, you should consult your doctor on advisability of fasting in your case. Show this chapter and the instructions to your own doctor and ask him to supervise your fasting and examine your condition as the fast progresses. Without expert supervision I would not advise fasting longer than one week to 10 days at a time. After a few weeks on a health-building diet (see Chapter 3), your fasting program may be repeated.

How to Take an Enema[5]

(Reprinted from *How to Keep Slim, Healthy & Young with Juice Fasting*, by Paavo Airola, 1971, Health Plus Publishers, P.O. Box 1027, Sherwood, OR 97140.)

To take an enema, you must have an enema can or bag with a rubber hose and a nozzle; it can be obtained at any drugstore.

Fill the enema bag with lukewarm water, about 99°F. Add a few drops of fresh lemon juice, or a cup of chamomile tea (can be bought at health food stores); however, the enema can be taken with plain water. For a do-it-yourself enema, 1 pint to 1 quart of water is sufficient.

The best position for taking an enema is on your knees, head down to the floor, with enema bag hanging

2½ to 3 feet above the anus, to get sufficient pressure in the flow of water. The flow can be regulated by squeezing the tube with the fingers; some enema bags have a special clamp to regulate the flow. Before inserting the nozzle into the anus make sure there is no air left in the tube; let water run out for a moment. Use some Vaseline, oil, or other lubricator on the nozzle to make insertion easier. If you feel discomfort or pain when water is running in, stop the flow for a while and take deep breaths, then continue again until the bag is empty.

If you can retain the water for a while and do not feel forced to empty the bowels at once, you may lie on a bed or soft rug for a few minutes, and let the water do its dissolving and washing work before letting it out. First lie on the back for a minute, then on the right side, then on the stomach and then on the left side. While you are doing this, gently massage your stomach with your hands. Then go to the toilet and let the water run out. Stay long enough to make sure that the bowels are empty.

The enema should be taken at least once each fasting day. The best time is the first thing in the morning. After the fast is broken, enemas should be continued until the bowels begin to move naturally without the help of the enemas. This usually takes two or three days. As soon as normal peristalsis is established, enemas should be discontinued.

Here are some additional points to watch:

- Make sure the enema water is not too cold or too hot. It should be of body temperature, or slightly above.
- Keep the equipment clean; wash it with soap and water. If several people use the equipment, also disinfect the nozzle with rubbing alcohol, then rinse with water.
- And finally, watch for copious amounts of debris and ill-smelling wastes coming out with the enema water, even after 5 weeks of fasting!

Note: The enemas are given in all European biological clinics that I am familiar with, and I am familiar with most of them.

But the number of enemas varies with various practitioners. At Buchinger Sanatorium, enemas are given once every morning or every second morning. At Sweden's Björkagarden Institute, as well as at Dr. Lars-Erik Essén's Vita Nova (both presented in detail in my book *THERE IS A CURE FOR ARTHRITIS*), enemas are administered 2 or 3 times a day—morning, noon and evening. Some clinics give enemas twice a day. My own recommendation is at least once a day, taken each morning.

Master Cleanser Lemonade Fast (up to ten days)

(Adapted from *Healing for the Age of Enlightenment* by Stanley Burroughs.)[6]

---

*Note: See Chapter 5 for a vegetable broth recipe.

1. Prepare for a fast.

2. Every night before retiring, take two to three herbal laxative tablets with warm water.

3. Every morning upon arising, drink one quart of warm water (preferably spring, distilled, or filtered tap) with one teaspoon of sea salt dissolved in it. This will stimulate a bowel purging in approximately thirty minutes and serve as a daily colon cleansing.

4. Do a dry skin brush.

5. To make lemonade: Per ½ gallon of filtered spring or distilled water, add 12 tablespoons of freshly squeezed lemon or lime juice and 12 tablespoons (less if you prefer, but this amount helps keep up your energy) of pure maple syrup. (Grade C maple syrup is best, as it is the least sweet and most mineral rich. Grade B is next best. Both are usually sold in bulk in health food stores and co-ops. Grade A will also do.) This fast seems to work for most people without the effect of sugar highs or lows. It's also recommended to add ½ teaspoon of cayenne pepper to the mix.

6. Drink ½ to 1 gallon of lemonade each day of your fast. You may also have pure water and peppermint tea. Be sure to rinse mouth out well with water and brush your teeth after each glass of lemonade—especially with baking soda—as the acidity of lemon juice is harmful to tooth enamel. Drinking through a straw helps to minimize some of the juice's contact with your teeth.

7. Break the fast.

Bancha or Kukicha (Twig) Tea Fast (up to seven days)

(Adapted from the teachings of Yasua Mori, shiatsu practitioner and instructor in Seattle, Washington.)

During the third day before the fast, have three meals a day of brown rice and vegetable-miso soup with about a teaspoon of light miso, like mugi (barley) miso, added to your bowl (not cooked)—(see page 108). Eat as much as you need. The following day, have only two meals (breakfast and lunch) of rice cream (see recipe, page 108) and vegetable soup with no miso or salt. Have moderate portions.

The day before the fast, eat as on the previous day, but only one meal—breakfast. Try to chew each mouthful of food at least fifty times before swallowing. Drink three to four cups of bancha or twig tea during the days preceding the fast. These teas are commonly available in health food or Japanese grocery stores. Simmer the twigs ten to fifteen minutes. Steep the bancha leaves ten to fifteen minutes.

The actual fast can last from four to seven days and consists of three to four cups of bancha or twig tea spaced throughout the day, and nothing else—not even water. I do not recommend more than four days for be-

ginners, as this fast is quite extreme. It is also not recommended during very hot or humid weather, due to the risk of dehydration from excessive sweating and insufficient fluid intake. For anyone on this fast who experiences profound fatigue lasting more than two days, I recommend drinking a little more fluid than usual and taking an enema or two. If the fatigue persists, break the fast. Traditionally, no enemas or other intestinal-cleansing measures are recommended for this fast, but an occasional enema may be done if you feel the need.

Break the fast with one small bowl of rice cream for breakfast, taking care to chew thoroughly. The following day, have breakfast and lunch (rice cream and vegetable soup), and on the third day, have three meals (the same fare). On the fourth day, add miso or salt. Continue drinking three to four cups of bancha or twig tea on these postfast days. On the fifth day, return to your regular diet. Since you may encounter profound fatigue on this fast, I advise you not to schedule any regular activities during this program. Take plenty of time to rest. However, it's also common to experience profound vitality in the few weeks following the fast.

Brown Rice Fast (up to four days)

(Adapted from *The Way of Herbs* by Michael Tierra. Copyright © 1980, 1983, 1990 by Michael Tierra. Reprinted by permission of Pocket Books, a division of Simon & Schuster, Inc.)[7]

Eat a small bowl of brown rice three times a day with no additional liquids. For a more effective fast, eat only one bowl of rice a day, taking a tablespoon of rice whenever you experience strong hunger. Chew very thoroughly, liquefying the rice in your mouth before swallowing. Do not take any other foods or drink any liquid during the three or four days of the fast. If constipation becomes a problem, however, eat a small bowl of stewed prunes once a day. Tierra advises taking an enema at the beginning of each day.

To break the fast, have only lightly cooked fruits and vegetables and soupy grains. Resume a normal diet in one or two days.

"Ultra Clear" Metabolic Detoxification

This program is described in Chapter Nine, page 180.

A SPRING CLEANING FOR BODY AND SPIRIT

The natural cleansing and detoxification systems of the human body are powerful and effective tools for maintaining our health. However, primarily through abusive eating patterns, the gastrointestinal system may become overburdened. Toxicity results, and because of this, multiple manifestations of ill health begin to develop. Periodic cleansing diets and fasts, lasting one to ten days, can mobilize the body's self-cleaning mechanisms, reverse toxicity, and give us back our natural sense of well-being.

SUGGESTED READING

Airola, Paavo. N.D. *Are You Confused?* Sherwood, OR: Health Plus, 1990, 104–147.

———. *How to Get Well.* Sherwood, OR: Health Plus, 1974: 214–243.

Burroughs, Stanley. *Healing for the Age of Enlightenment*, 3rd ed. Self-published—available from 5185 Meadowview Lane, Auburn, CA 95603, 1976, 1–34.

Kloss, Jethro. *Back to Eden.* Revised and updated—available from Back to Eden Books Publishing Co., P.O. Box 1439, Loma Linda, CA 92354.

O'Connor, T. P. "Dietary Fat, Calories, and Cancer," in *Contemporary Nutrition* 10:7, 1985: 1.

Poesnecker, G. E. *It's Only Nature.* Quakertown, PA: G. E. Poesnecker, Clymer Clinic, 1981: 228–238.

Shelton, H. *The Science and Fine Art of Fasting.* Tampa, FL: Natural Hygiene Press, 1978.

Tierra, Michael. *The Way of Herbs.* New York: Pocket Books, 1980: 63–64.

Walker, N. W. *Become Younger.* Prescott, AZ: Norwalk Press, 1949: 180–183.

Wolford, R. "Eating Longer Lengthens Life," in *Health and Longevity Report* 1:5, Baltimore, MD: Agora Publishing, 7.

HERBS AND THEIR
MEDICINAL USES

In this chapter we will briefly review the properties and medicinal uses of many common herbs. You may already be familiar with some of them—cayenne, chamomile, cinnamon, garlic, gingerroot, peppermint—that are used frequently in beverages and food. With such common ingredients, you can learn to relieve many ailments and even help prevent some major diseases. Other herbs that are not as common—those used primarily to treat illness by enhancing your body's natural healing capabilities—will also be discussed. Many are now more widely available, and safe guidelines for their use will be presented.

After an introductory discussion, we will offer an alphabetical listing of herbal agents. Over the centuries, herbal practitioners have found that some herbs enhance one another's properties. These are often combined for treating specific ailments. At the end of this chapter, you will find a list of common conditions, along with popular herbal combinations and the companies that produce them.

By giving herbs the opportunity to assist in your healing, you will reawaken your sense of wonder in and appreciation for nature's gifts and power.

HERBS AS BEVERAGES

Individual herbs or select combinations can be purchased in convenient, ready-to-use tea bags. Some commercially available blends are labeled for specific needs: sleep, stress reduction, improved digestion, and so on. If you want to create your own blends, you can purchase individual herbs in bulk in many health food stores and co-ops and from herb stores and distributors. Some herbs, such as the mints, lemon balm, and a few varie-

ties of sage, lend themselves to home growing. Others, such as chickweed, horsetail, rose hips, mullein, and chamomile, grow wild. All may be harvested fresh for use in teas. In Chapter Five, you will find two unusual recipes for herbal beverages.

HERBS AS MEDICINE

Taking herbs to overcome an ailment generally requires a more intense application than the occasional brewed tea. In fact, the various other forms in which herbs can be found—capsules, tablets, tinctures, fluid extracts, solid extracts, and syrups—are often more convenient and generally as effective, when the herb must be ingested several times a day for a week or more. In addition to oral use, herbs can be taken in the form of douches, suppositories, and enemas, and used externally as compresses, poultices, salves, liniments, and oils.

There are numerous excellent books detailing recipes and methods of application (see Suggested Reading list). The following suggestions are from Michael Tierra's *The Way of Herbs*.

(Adapted from *The Way of Herbs* by Michael Tierra. Copyright © 1980, 1983, 1990 by Michael Tierra. Reprinted by permission of Pocket Books, a division of Simon & Schuster, Inc.)

1. The more easily accepted medicinal teas are usually the ones brewed from mild-flavored herbs. However, if taste is not an issue, the stronger and more bitter-flavored herbs can also be taken in this form. The amount of herb for beverage use is ½ ounce, or approximately 1 to 2 teaspoons (the contents of a standard tea bag of dried herb) per 2 cups of water. The recom-

mended proportion for medicinal use is up to 1 ounce (7 teaspoons) per 2 cups of water. The dose for the latter is generally ½ to 1 cup three or more times a day.

INFUSION METHOD: After the water has boiled, add the herbs—or pour water over the herbs in a pot you have first rinsed with boiling water—and let steep ten to twenty minutes. It is best to use enamel, glass, or earthenware (nonmetallic pots), although stainless steel is an acceptable alternative.

If the herbs you use are freshly picked, use twice the amount in comparison to dried herbs. Immediately before using, rub the dried or fresh herbs between your hands for a moment to break up the tissue structure and to allow the release of active ingredients—an excellent tip for cooking with herbs as well. If you are using delicate plant parts, such as flowers (e.g., red clover blossoms, chamomile) or soft leaves, or you want to retain the volatile oils (such as in peppermint), cover the pot tightly while steeping. Leaves and flowers are generally prepared by steeping, not boiling.

DECOCTION METHOD: For stems and roots, bring the water to a boil, then simmer thirty minutes to one hour in an open pot; some volume loss should occur through evaporation. If volatile oils need to be preserved, such as in burdock root or cinnamon stick, gently simmer in a covered pot.

2. Encapsulated or tableted herbs are also available. Try to find out how fresh they are—over time, they lose potency. Some herbal companies use herbs that have been standardized for the potency of the active constituents (when known). This practice is quite common in Europe, where herbal medicines have for years been widely accepted. Without standardization you may not be getting the stated potency, which could account for the failure of an herbal treatment. Look for "standardized" on the label to ensure the potency of the active ingredient. If potency cannot be guaranteed, consider using freeze-dried tablets or capsules, which are usually reliable.

3. Tinctures and extracts (both fluid and solid) are not as subject to loss of strength as conventionally air-dried herbs. Tincture doses are generally 1 to 2 teaspoons three to four times a day diluted in fluid or taken straight, if tolerated. Those sensitive or intolerant to alcohol should avoid tinctures, as some have up to 80 percent grain alcohol content. Fluid extracts (sometimes alcohol-free) are more concentrated and potent and doses are generally lower: six to eight drops three times a day. Solid extracts are also very potent and doses are commonly ¼ to ½ teaspoon three times a day.

ADVANTAGES OF BOTANICAL MEDICINES

In general, herbs are whole-plant medicines and are less toxic and have fewer side effects than pharmaceutical medicines. Whole-plant medicines use primarily purified active ingredients. For example, the foxglove plant is far less toxic than its purified pharmaceutical component, digitalis.

Before the technology was available to isolate and standardize the primary constituent in a whole-plant extract, dispensing for an illness was pretty much a guessing game. This, of course, was what led eventually to the isolation, purification, and extract prescription of the active ingredients. Although there are many distinct advantages to such distillations, whole-plant medicines, now standardized for potency, present fewer hazards—and since the elements occurring in the whole plant often work synergistically with the active ingredients, the results are often superior.

THE GREATER SCHEME OF BALANCE

As you learn more about the general functions and specific properties of herbs, you enter a fascinating world of both art and science, one that reflects the greater scheme of balance that rules all life processes. Herbs have much to teach us about the balance of opposites: there are some that sedate and others that stimulate; some that are eliminative and cleansing and others that are building and toning; some that are cooling and others that are warming; some that are bitter and others that are sweet. Unfortunately, we can touch only briefly on this essence of traditional herbology, but several publications in the Suggested Reading list at the end of this chapter should be helpful.

THE MEDICINAL PROPERTIES OF SELECTED HERBS*

Aloe vera[1]

Reduces edema and promotes epithelial growth, differentiation, and revascularization, making it a great healer of the skin and mucous membranes. Available as juice or gel, aloe vera:

---

* I wish to acknowledge Joseph E. Pizzorno, N.D., and Michael T. Murray, N.D., authors and editors of "Pharmacology of Natural Medicines" in *A Textbook of Natural Medicine* (John Bastyr College Publications, 1985). Chapter Five of their book is the primary reference used for the preparation of this section of the chapter.

Note: Should any ailment persist or worsen, or if it is severe, be sure to seek professional help. Doses given throughout the following listing are primarily for adults. Children's doses need to be scaled down according to weight. Other than herbs specifically mentioned for children, none should be given internally to those younger than five years of age unless under the supervision of a health professional. During pregnancy, no herbal products should be used unless prescribed by an appropriate health professional.

1. Has bacteriostatic action and suppresses prostaglandin-induced inflammation.

2. Enhances protein digestion and assimilation and decreases bowel transit time.

3. Increases intestinal pH (an alkalinizer) and reduces Candida growth and bacterial overgrowth.

4. Has a tonic effect on the bowel, without being a laxative.

5. Can be used topically for burns and abrasions, and internally for indigestion, heartburn, ulcers, irritable bowel, colitis, constipation, bowel toxicity, and allergies.

Take 2 ounces of juice or 1 or 2 tablespoons of gel orally two or three times a day. The gel can be liberally applied topically several times daily. Simply squeeze the gel directly from a stalk of the plant.

Uses

TOPICAL: Burns, sunburn, abrasions

ORAL: Indigestion, heartburn, ulcers, irritable bowel, colitis, constipation, bowel toxicity, liver toxicity, allergies

Barberry

See GOLDENSEAL.

Bilberry (Vaccinium myrtillus)

Because of its flavonoid components (specifically anthocyanosides), this herb has several well-documented pharmacologic actions. Those most studied relate to collagen, the structural protein that gives strength and stability to the walls of veins, arteries (especially capillaries), intercellular matrices, cartilage, tendons, and ligaments. Bilberry:

1. Stabilizes collagen by enhancing and reinforcing the cross-linking of collagen fibers and promoting the biosynthesis of collagen and mucopolysaccharides.

2. Prevents destruction of collagen, which usually results from free radical damage or the release of destructive components of inflammation (enzymes, unfavorable prostaglandins, leukotrienes, histamines, etc.). The most common aging-related ailments in Western society occur in large part because of these pathophysiologic processes, so it is no surprise that bilberry has a wide clinical application.

3. Is commonly indicated for eye conditions. It has a particular affinity for the pigmented epithelium of the retina and is thus favored in the treatment of major ophthalmologic diseases—macular degeneration, glaucoma, cataract, and diabetic retinopathy—as well as for poor night vision and poor day vision.

4. Is often used in the treatment for the prevention of atherosclerosis, as well as rheumatoid and osteoarthritis, gout, periodontal disease, varicose veins, venous insufficiency, and microscopic hematuria caused by capillary fragility in the kidneys.

The usual dose is a 25 percent extract, 80 to 160 milligrams three times a day; or anthocyanosides (calculated as anthocyanidin), 20 to 40 milligrams three times a day; or fresh berries, 2 to 4 ounces three times a day. Bilberry and GINKGO have similar and synergistic actions and can be found formulated together.

Uses

Macular degeneration
Glaucoma
Cataract
Diabetic retinopathy
Poor night vision
Rheumatoid arthritis
Osteoarthritis
Gout
Periodontal disease
Varicose veins
Venous insufficiency
Microscopic hematuria
Atherosclerosis

Bromelain

This enzyme is extracted from pineapple. It:

1. Has numerous beneficial effects with minimal toxicity.

2. Can be used with meals as a digestive supplement, as it is primarily a protease (protein-digesting) enzyme.

3. It is a well-known anti-inflammatory, used for pain and swelling from trauma (including sports injuries, surgery, infections, and thrombophlebitis).

4. Quickens healing time and resolves bruises by preventing the accumulation of fibrin and inhibiting potent inflammatory substances, such as leukotrienes, neutrophilic lysosomal enzymes, and kinins.

5. Inhibits the aggregation (clumping) of platelets, thus preventing atherogenesis (plaque formation) and thrombosis (heart attacks, thrombophlebitis).

6. Is effective in the treatment of angina.

7. Is a smooth muscle relaxer, blocking unfavorable prostaglandin hormones (PGE-2) and helping to form more beneficial prostaglandins (PGE-1); used to treat menstrual cramps and similar disorders.

8. Improves the absorption of antibiotics and has its own antibiotic properties; effective in pneumonia, abscess, bronchitis, cutaneous staph, and kidney infections.

9. Helps thin mucus and has been helpful in cases of acute and chronic bronchitis and sinusitis; used for burn debridement.

10. If used synergistically with quercetin, the combi-

nation may help block a food allergy reaction if taken a half hour before eating.

Bromelain (250 milligrams) should be taken between meals, with the typical dosage one to two capsules three times a day. If used as a digestive aid, take with meals.

Uses
Digestive aid
Antibiotic
Anti-inflammatory (injuries, surgery, allergies, infections, phlebitis, thrombophlebitis)
Quickened healing time (wounds, injuries, bruises)
Inhibits platelet aggregation (prevention of arteriosclerosis, thrombosis, heart attack, angina)
Smooth muscle relaxer (menstrual cramps)
Thins mucus (respiratory infections)
Burn debridement

Buchu

A diuretic; very good for fluid retention and tissue bloating. Also excellent as an adjunct for bladder infections with UVA URSI, in equal parts.

Burdock root

A blood cleanser (used with ECHINACEA); good for skin eruptions due to impure blood. Use orally or topically.

Calendula

Excellent used topically for burns and skin infections, gum inflammation, infection, and sore throats. Available in salves, lotions, and liquid form. You can also make a tea from the flower petals, which can be used for swishing in mouth or gargling.

Cascara sagrada

A colon cleanser and laxative; can be used alone or in combination blends. *Warning: Like any laxative, cascara has abuse potential.*

Catnip

A mild sedative; useful for treating nervousness and restlessness. Excellent for children, especially mixed with chamomile, spearmint, and lemon balm teas.

Cayenne

Acts as a general tonifier and promotes circulation. Its traditional uses are broad: high blood pressure, gastrointestinal ulcers, constipation, poor circulation, cold extremities, feeble pulse. John Christopher, N.D., one of the fathers of herbal medicine in the United States, was an ardent promoter of this herb. Cayenne is useful in treating infections, particularly respiratory and sinus (in combination with other anti-infection agents: ECHINACEA, GARLIC, GOLDENSEAL, etc.). (See "Anti-infection," page 459.) One to two capsules of cayenne taken every few hours at the first sign of symptoms may forestall a cold. Cayenne is believed to help stop internal bleeding when taken orally, or when applied topically to cuts. Of course, direct pressure is indicated first for bleeding. Interestingly, cayenne can also dissolve unwanted clots.

Cayenne can also be taken mixed in food—but remember that it is very spicy hot. You can mix the powder in water—up to ½ to 1 teaspoon—depending on need and on one's tolerance. Such doses are best prescribed and supervised by an experienced herbalist. On an empty stomach, like any hot spice, it may cause a burning sensation; and it may also cause a temporary burning sensation when you pass a stool.

Chamomile

A mild sedative used for treating nervousness, restlessness, and insomnia. Very safe for children. Also used to treat colic (with CATNIP). Higher doses in the extract form may be helpful for spastic colon problems of adults. Use with YARROW to break a fever.

Chickweed

Used alone or in combination cough formulas with COMFREY (see warnings), (see LOBELIA, MARSHMALLOW ROOT, and MULLEIN). Available in combination capsules and tinctures (see COUGHS, page 460) as well as salves for skin irritations or rashes. Can be used internally or externally (crushed fresh sprigs make an excellent poultice, or use a chickweed-tea-soaked cloth). Can promote weight loss. Excellent eaten fresh in salads and as a substitute for any greens.

Chlorophyll

Available in liquid and capsule form; also as the fresh juice of greens. Chlorophyll:

1. Is an effective blood builder in treating anemia.
2. Has an antibiotic effect and can heal irritations and infections on the skin and in the mouth, throat, stomach, and intestines.
3. Can be used as an eyewash for conjunctivitis or eardrops for ear infections (if you are sure the eardrum

has not burst), or directly in wounds; can also be used as a vaginal douche.

4. Can be used as a rectal implant (retained enema) to build blood and cleanse the liver.

The enzymes from the fresh juice are most healing. Use any edible greens and preferably juice them or macerate in a blender with a small amount of water, and strain. Can be combined with COMFREY (for external use), also wheat grass and barley grass (for internal or external use). The green juice can be mixed with the pulp of the greens for a poultice (wheat grass is especially good) for external application for any skin irritation or infection, including mastitis. Use orally as a bowel and liver cleanser. In the fat-soluble form, chlorophyll is a good source of vitamin K to slow functional bleeding disorders such as heavy menstrual flow. Chlorophyll has also been used to chelate heavy metals from the body. The fresh juice is an effective source of folic acid. Chlorophyll is the main constituent of spirulina, chlorella, and blue-green algae. When fresh, bottled, or powdered, chlorophyll is a rich source of beta-carotene and other vitamins and minerals. Experiment to find the most palatable green drink.

Uses

TOPICAL: Cuts, sores, boils, abrasions, burns, mastitis, raw skin, conjunctivitis (pinkeye), ear infection, vaginitis, vulvitis

ORAL: Anemia, sore throats, respiratory infections, esophagitis, gastritis, ulcers, colitis, bowel and liver detoxification, heavy metal chelation

Cinnamon

For diarrhea, steep a teaspoon of powder in 1 or 2 cups of water with a touch of CAYENNE; or use a teaspoon in any fluid or in food three times a day.

Clove

The oil is used to treat toothaches. Apply to tooth and gum line.

Coltsfoot

Use to treat coughs and chest colds, generally as part of a formula with other lung herbs (see COUGHS, page 460).

Comfrey

Very high in allantoin, comfrey root:

1. Is an excellent healer for any mucous membranes, whether gastrointestinal, bronchial, or genitourinary.

Thanks to its high mucilage content, it has been used for esophagitis, gastritis, ulcers, colitis, any cough or bronchial infections, and genitourinary irritations, even in the healing phase of pelvic inflammatory disease. It can also help arrest internal bleeding from any of these systems.

2. Helps promote the secretion of pepsin in the stomach and aids digestion.

3. Has been frequently prescribed (sometimes with HORSETAIL, OATSTRAW, and IRISH MOSS) to help the healing of fractures.

4. Is useful as a poultice; a crushed fresh leaf can be applied to bruises, cuts, scrapes, and over the sites of closed cartilage and ligament injuries and closed fractures.

5. Is effective as a fomentation (a tea-soaked cloth for topical application).

Comfrey is very easy to grow, but watch out: It spreads.

Comfrey root is more potent than the leaf.

Warning: Because of its pyrolizidine alkaloid content, comfrey root has been banned for oral use in Canada, restricted in Germany and Australia, and the FDA has declared that the root cannot be sold for internal use.[2] Several cases of liver toxicity have been related to the use of comfrey, one involving a newborn whose mother ingested comfrey throughout the pregnancy. However, because hepatotoxicity is so rare, and successful results so common, some physicians continue to prescribe comfrey for oral use (not during pregnancy or infancy, however), but only for short periods of time. Other practitioners (myself included) are more conservative. We avoid the oral use of comfrey altogether and substitute other allantoin- and mucilage-containing herbs (ALOE VERA, MARSHMALLOW ROOT, PLANTAIN, SLIPPERY ELM).

Uses

TOPICAL:
Bruises
Abrasions, skin ulcers
Strains, sprains
Ligament and cartilage injuries (closed)
Fractures (closed)
ORAL: No longer recommended

Curcumin

See TURMERIC.

Dandelion root

As a stimulant for the flow of bile from the gallbladder, dandelion:

1. Is known as a liver cleanser and blood purifier.

2. Has been used in cases of hepatitis.

3. Is believed to stabilize both hypoglycemia and diabetes.

4. Is a diuretic, and is thus cleansing and clearing to the kidneys and bladder; because of its diuretic action, it can help in cases of high blood pressure.

Both the leaves (eaten young or used in tea) and the root are good sources of nutrients.

Uses

Liver cleanser
Blood purifier
Diuretic (leaf, especially)
Hypoglycemia
Hepatitis
Diabetes
High blood pressure

Dong Quai (or Tang-Kuei) (*Angelica sinensis* [Chinese] and *Acutilova* [Japanese])

Used traditionally in Asia to treat menstrual cramps, lack of menstrual periods, heavy menses, and menopausal symptoms. Used also for abdominal pain, headaches, and other symptoms. Many of dong quai's effects are attributed to its high coumarin content.

Containing highly active phytoestrogens (400 times less active in estrogen activity than animal estrogens), dong quai can be useful in both high- and low-estrogen conditions. If estrogen levels are low, it will exert a mild but needed estrogen-like effect—useful, therefore, in conditions such as amenorrhea (premature cessation of periods) and menopause. If estrogen levels are too high, it will fill up some of the estrogen sites, thereby exerting a decreased estrogen effect in the system. Such mechanisms may explain its usefulness in menstrual cramps and in some cases of premenstrual syndrome.

Dong quai has a potent calcium channel-blocking effect and acts to relax the smooth muscles of visceral organs, such as the intestines and the uterus. It can have the same effect on arteries, which lowers blood pressure. Dong quai has mild analgesic and tranquilizing effects, anti-allergy properties, and a stimulatory effect on the immune system, notably macrophage phagocytosis and interferon production and complement activation.

The European angelica herbs (*A. atropurpurea* and *A. archangelica*) are more useful for respiratory ailments, gas, and abdominal spasms. The more common Japanese and Chinese varieties are useful for disorders of menstruation, menopause (especially hot flashes), allergic conditions, and smooth muscle spasms (uterine cramps, migraines, intestinal spasms). Dong quai has also been used as an immunostimulant adjunct in can-

cer therapy (see MENOPAUSE, page 390, and MENSTRUAL CRAMPS, page 393).

Uses

Disorders of menstruation (menopause, menstrual cramps, amenorrhea, heavy menses, and premenstrual syndrome)
Muscle spasms (intestinal and uterine)
Allergies
High blood pressure
Immunostimulation
Sedative and tranquilizer
EUROPEAN SPECIES (ANGELICAS):
Respiratory ailments
Gas
Intestinal spasms

Echinacea root (purpurea, pallida, angustifolia, coneflower)

Used traditionally as a snakebite remedy, analgesic, antiseptic, and blood purifier, echinacea has been studied extensively and has been found to have immunostimulation, antiviral, wound-healing, and anti-inflammatory properties.

1. Due to its inulin component, which increases a serum globulin called properidin, echinacea mobilizes neutrophils, monocytes, and eosinophils, and promotes the neutralization of immune complexes, viruses, and bacteria.

2. Echinacea causes T-cell activation: transformation, induction of interferon, and secretion of lymphokines. It switches on the whole arm of cell-mediated immunity: increased macrophage phagocytosis (engulfing of foreign invaders), antibody binding, natural killer cell activity, and increased neutrophil counts.

3. Echinacea stimulates helper T cells. These in turn produce the interferon that causes the production of an intracellular protein that inhibits viral RNA transcription.

4. Echinacea is effective against influenza, herpes, and other viruses.

5. Echinacea has some antibacterial properties, but not as much in comparison with other herbs such as goldenseal.

6. Echinacea has some antitumor activity thanks to its content of (Z)-1-8-pentadecadiene.

7. The herb has also wound-healing and anti-inflammatory properties.

8. Echinacea has also been found to stimulate the adrenal-pituitary axis and is therefore useful for the stress response; however, supplemental vitamin C must be administered with it.

9. Echinacea root has some direct interferon-like activity.

Echinacea can be used alone or in combination formulas (see ANTI-INFECTION, ANTIVIRAL (ACUTE), and CANDIDA, page 471, and IMMUNE DEFICIENCY and IMMUNE ENHANCING, page 472).

Some herbalists suggest finding an echinacea product that contains all the species listed in the category head, preferably in a 300- to 500-milligram dose capsule to be taken three to five times a day (in tincture form, 1 to 2 teaspoons, three to five times a day). Large and frequent doses are necessary for clinical results. No toxicity is known over long-term use (more than three to four months consecutively). Echinacea is not in the same medicinal category as GINSENG (where long-term use is traditionally advised). Some herbalists suggest periodic discontinuance of echinacea for one to three months.

Uses
Immunostimulation
Antiviral
Antibacterial
Antiallergy
Antitumor
Anti-inflammatory
Enhanced stress response
Enhanced wound healing

Elder flowers

Taken with peppermint, good for treating onset of colds and fevers. Drink several cups, take a warm bath, go to bed immediately, and sweat. Do not allow yourself to become chilled.

Eyebright

Taken orally, helpful for eye conditions and irritations, as well as hay fever symptoms. Tea can be used as an eyewash or poultice with or without other herbs frequently formulated with it.

Fennel seed

Good for gas. Used to prevent gripping or cramping that laxative herbs may cause. Taken as a tea.

Flaxseed

Acts as a bowel lubricant when taken as tea. Seeds can also be used as a source of fiber. Soak 1 tablespoon overnight in water and either mix and drink or blend with the soaking water (not advised if you have diverticulosis). Flaxseed oil is one of the best sources of alpha linolenic acid, an essential fatty acid and crucial precursor to the beneficial prostaglandin hormone PGE-3 (see Chapter Three).

Garlic *(Allium sativum)*

Garlic is rich in a sulfur-containing compound called allicin, to which many of its benefits are linked. It also contains abundant selenium and germanium.

1. Garlic is most noted for its antimicrobial and cardiovascular effects. It possesses broad-spectrum antimicrobial properties effective against bacteria (staph, strep, bacillus, brucella, vibrio, *E. coli*, proteus, salmonella, klebsiella, mycobacterium), fungi (including *Candida albicans*, epidermophyton, and trichophyton), parasites, roundworms, and hookworms, and viruses (influenza). Garlic is very useful in cases where an organism has become resistant to conventional antibiotic therapy.

2. Garlic has many beneficial cardiovascular effects. It decreases levels of triglycerides and cholesterol (total and LDL), and raises HDL cholesterol. It lowers blood pressure, prevents excessive platelet aggregation (clumping), and minimizes the risk of thrombus formation (blood clots). Raw and cooked forms seem to work equally well in this capacity.

3. Because garlic increases available insulin by lessening insulin breakdown, it is used in the treatment of diabetes.

4. Garlic has impressive immunostimulatory and antitumor effects. Its ability to increase natural killer cell activity may be due in part to an antioxidant effect, which may be related to the herb's germanium, selenium, and glutathione content. Many of the studies showing the benefits of garlic indicate a dose in the range of three to eight fresh garlic cloves a day for a 125-pound person. Some nutritionists suggest taking 0.7 grams of raw garlic per kilogram of body weight daily, which is quite substantial.

Cooking or heating garlic will inactivate the antimicrobial effects, so use either raw cloves or cryogenically frozen, vacuum-dried, or cold-aged garlic capsules or tablets or vacuum distillation–derived garlic oil products.

Besides being used orally, garlic preparations can be used topically for skin infections, and the oil of garlic, commonly combined with olive oil, can be used for ear infections (provided the eardrum is intact).

Warning: Garlic toxicity is fairly rare. However, some reports suggest that excessive doses can trigger red blood cell destruction (hemolysis) and anemia (though I have never witnessed this). If you take more than three or four large cloves or more than nine capsules daily for more than a few months consecutively, have your doctor periodically check your blood.

To avoid gastrointestinal upset, take garlic with meals. Skin irritations may result from local applica-

tions, so garlic (fresh) is contraindicated for skin conditions such as acne, rosacea, and eczema when taken internally.

Uses
Antibacterial
Antiviral
Antifungal
Antiparasitic
Antitumor
Antioxidant
Ear infections
Decreased total and LDL cholesterol levels
Decreased triglyceride levels
Increased HDL cholesterol level
Decreased blood pressure
Decreased platelet aggregation (clumping)
Prevention of thrombosis
Increased insulin availability for diabetics
Immunostimulation

Ginkgo (*Ginkgo biloba*)

1. The ginkgo heterocide, terpene flavonoids, and other active constituents of ginkgo have been shown to be effective in treating diminished blood flow to the brain caused by arteriosclerosis, which is common in older individuals. It has also been useful in reducing such symptoms as vertigo, headache, tinnitus, short-term memory loss, depression, and senility. It has some applications in Alzheimer's disease.

2. Ginkgo relaxes smooth muscle in arteries (counters arterial spasm) and provides arterial tone where there is vasomotor paralysis. Because it inhibits platelet aggregation by preventing platelets from being excessively sticky, ginkgo diminishes the chance of transient ischemic attacks, stroke, angina, and heart attack.

3. It is used to treat muscle cramps due to poor blood supply in individuals with peripheral vascular insufficiency.

4. It is used to help halt the progression of macular degeneration and diabetic retinopathy.

5. It has also been used in cases of impotence (erectile dysfunction) due to impaired arterial flow.

6. Many of ginkgo's functions are mediated by its membrane-stabilizing, antioxidant, and free radical–quenching effects.

7. Ginkgo activates cellular membrane pumps that regulate exchange of fluid and electrolytes.

8. It also enhances oxygen utilization and glucose uptake, and increases tolerance (particularly for brain cells) to diminished supply of oxygen. It is likely for this reason that ginkgo is used in the treatment of head injuries.

Recommended dose is 40 milligrams three times a day of concentrated extract (20 to 24 percent ginkgo heterocide content). It may take up to twelve weeks before a response is observed.

Uses
Vertigo
Headache
Tinnitus
Cochlear deafness
Short-term memory loss
Senility
Depression
Alzheimer's disease
Macular degeneration
Diabetic retinopathy
Impotence
Brain injury
Prevention of excessive platelet aggregation
Prevention of transient ischemic attacks and strokes
Prevention of peripheral vascular insufficiency

Ginseng (*Panax schinseng*)

Known for centuries as a revitalizing agent, ginseng has come to be known as an effective adaptogenic agent. This term is applied to any innocuous substance that exhibits an ability to increase resistance to a wide range of adverse influences (physical, chemical, biochemical) and to normalize a wide range of pathologic states. Ginseng has many known properties:

1. It increases mental and physical capacity for work, can increase strength and speed, improves endocrine functioning, delays the alarm phase reaction to stress, stimulates the central nervous system with respect to hypothalamic and pituitary function, and enhances adrenal function. It also lowers cholesterol and protects the liver from toxins. Part of its benefits seem to derive from its ability to preserve glycogen utilization by enhancing fatty acid oxidation.

2. It enhances functions that are directly influenced by estrogen and other steroid hormones, such as fertility, libido, muscle strength, etc.

3. Alone or combined with other adrenal-enhancing agents, such as bupleurum, curcumin (see TURMERIC), LICORICE ROOT, and SIBERIAN GINSENG, panax ginseng may prove effective in restoring or preserving normal adrenal function or in blocking adrenal atrophy from the chronic use of prednisone and other cortisone-type medication.

4. Ginseng can provide some degree of protection against harmful radiation and hasten recovery from radiation sickness.

5. Ginseng exerts a positive effect on the immune

system; it increases cell-mediated immunity, natural killer cell activity, production of interferon, and reticuloendothelial system proliferative and phagocytic functions.

6. In the liver, ginseng increases the growth of Kuppfer cells and the folliculi in the spleen and lymph nodes, thereby increasing the body's ability to defend itself against many external assaults.

Most of the ginseng sold in the United States comes from the lowest-grade root and is diluted with excipients and adulterants. Thus, it may be totally devoid of its active components, such as the ginsenosides, which are 13-triterpenoid saponins. Look for ginsengs that are standardized at 5 percent. A high-quality ginseng root powder dose would be 500 milligrams taken one to three times a day for general tonic effects. For a standardized panax ginseng extract containing 14 percent saponin content, take 200 milligrams one to three times a day.

Warning: Ginseng toxicity is possible, with such symptoms as high blood pressure, nervousness, insomnia, skin eruptions, diarrhea, inappropriate euphoria, and inappropriate estrogen-like effects. Panax use should be under the supervision of a health professional.

Uses

Increased mental and physical capacity
Increased strength and speed
Improved endocrine function
Enhanced stress tolerance
Enhanced adrenal function
Protection of adrenals during steroid use
Protection against liver toxins
Protection from radiation
Improved recovery from radiation illness
Decreased blood cholesterol level
Immunostimulation
Greater resistance to infection and to carcinogens
Exerts estrogen-like effect useful for postmenopausal symptoms

Siberian Ginseng (*Eleutherococcus senticosus*)

Eleuthero has been used traditionally by the Chinese to increase longevity, improve general health and appetite, and to restore memory. It is an adaptogen like panax ginseng, but it has distinct and different active constituents and is felt to be not quite as strong as panax. Eleuthero:

1. Can increase general body resistance to stress, fatigue, and disease.

2. Can prevent adrenal atrophy and hyperplasia.

Like panax, it protects the adrenals by inhibiting the alarm phase of stress reactions.

3. Increases one's tolerance to the daily workload, noise, heat, and exercise. It can also increase mental alertness.

4. Prevents cortisone-induced shrinking of the thymus and lymphatics and subsequent immunosuppression caused by chronic stress or cortisone-type medications.

5. Prevents both thyroid atrophy and hyperplasia.

6. Normalizes both high and low blood sugar levels, high and low white blood cell and red blood cell counts.

7. Lowers serum cholesterol and has a favorable influence on blood pressure (both high and low), angina, kidney infections, craniocerebral trauma, and neuroses.

8. Increases resistance to infection, has anticarcinogenic properties, protects against radiation sickness and exposure, and stimulates the synthesis of DNA and cellular repair enzymes.

9. May increase reproductive capacity.

10. Functions as an antioxidant.

The recommended dose for fluid extract (1:1) is 2 to 4 milliliters one to three times a day for up to sixty days; dried root, 2 to 4 grams one to three times a day; tincture (1:5), 10 to 20 milliliters one to three times a day; solid (dry powder) extract (20:1), 100 to 200 milligrams one to three times a day.

Uses

See also uses for GINSENG
Stabilized blood sugar
Stabilized white blood cell count (low and high)
Stabilized red blood cell count (low and high)
Normalized blood pressure (low and high)
Increased fertility
Stimulation of DNA synthesis and cell repair enzymes
Antioxidant
Maintains immune function when one is under chronic stress or when on cortisone-type medications

Goldenseal (*Hydrastis canadensis*)

Because of its isoquinolone alkaloids, of which berberine is best known (also the active ingredient in BARBERRY and OREGON GRAPE ROOT), goldenseal:

1. Soothes and promotes healing of the mucous membranes of the respiratory, gastrointestinal, and genitourinary tracts for inflammatory conditions caused by both allergy and infections.

2. Is known to have potent broad-spectrum antibiotic activity and to be effective against staph, strep, chlamydia, *E. coli*, salmonella, shigella, *Vibrio*

cholerae, pseudomonas, diplococcus pneumonia, trichomonas, gonorrhea, syphilis, *Leishmania donovani, Giardia,* amoeba, and *Candida albicans.*

3. Is useful for respiratory infections, infectious diarrhea, and bladder infections.

4. Can be used as a prophylactic for travelers going to areas of questionable water quality.

5. Unlike conventional antibiotics, goldenseal kills bacteria without stimulating the growth of yeast. It inhibits bacterial and yeast decarboxylase enzymes involved in the toxic amine production associated with intestinal toxicity—"leaky gut" syndrome—and cirrhosis.

6. Is used for treating gastric and duodenal ulcers when combined with SLIPPERY ELM (two parts slippery elm to one part goldenseal).

7. Increases the blood supply to the spleen and activates macrophages.

8. Increases digestive secretions: hydrochloric acid, pancreatic enzymes, and bile.

9. Enhances the liver's Kuppfer cells' ability to trap bowel toxins.

10. Is a therapeutic agent in gallbladder disease.

11. Is sometimes useful as a throat gargle for persistent infectious sore throats.

12. Is used nasally for the treatment of sinusitis.

Because goldenseal is very bitter, it is often used in capsule form, although the liquid extract and tincture forms are also available. Use standardized 8 percent alkaloid content, with a dose of 400 to 1,000 milligrams three times a day for acute problems, 200 to 400 milligrams three times a day for chronic administration.

Warning: Goldenseal should not be used during pregnancy or for prolonged, continuous treatment, as it can deplete certain nutrients from the body and weaken the functions of the stomach and intestines.

Uses

Antibacterial, infections: respiratory, pelvic, skin, urinary tract, traveler's aid
Antiparasitic
Antifungal
Immunostimulation
Mucous membrane healer: peptic ulcers, gastritis, colitis, cystitis
Increased digestive secretions
Bowel detoxifier
Liver cleanser

Gotu kola (*Centella asiatica*)

Gotu kola is known for its longevity factor and is used as a nerve tonic and brain food. Because it enhances connective tissue integrity, it can be used in treating disorders related to weakened or defective connective tissue structures, such as varicose veins. Gotu kola has been shown to be effective for treating venous insufficiency, particularly when combined with *Aesculus hippocastanum* (horse chestnut), which has a toning effect on veins and decreases edema and inflammation, and *Ruscus aculeatus* (butcher's broom), which is antiinflammatory and vasoconstricting. It is also helpful in the treatment of cellulite and can stimulate cortisol production from the adrenal glands. Use the extract standardized for 70 percent triterpenic acids.

Uses

Longevity factor
Brain food
Nerve tonic
Strengthened connective tissues
Varicose veins
Venous insufficiency
Adrenal stimulator

Hawthorn berry (*Crataegus oxyacantha*)

Crataegus has very potent collagen-stabilizing properties, whether in the walls of arteries and veins or in cartilages, tendons, and ligaments:

1. It diminishes collagen destruction from any inflammatory process, including arthritis, periodontal disease, and arteriosclerosis.

2. Because it decreases the chance of cholesterol deposition by preventing injury or loss of integrity of the arterial wall, it thus indirectly prevents angina, heart rhythm disturbances, heart failure, and heart attacks.

3. It has pronounced direct effects on the myocardium (heart muscle), notably the strengthening of heart contraction and stabilizing of heart rhythm.

4. It inhibits angiotensin-converting enzyme and therefore helps prevent high blood pressure.

Hawthorn berry is a wonderful cardiovascular food that will help prevent and treat all these conditions. Use an extract standardized to contain 1.8 percent vitexin-4-rhamnoside, 250 milligrams one to three times a day.

Warning: Do not use hawthorn berry with beta blocker type medications, as it may antagonize them.

Uses

Heart rhythm disturbances
Angina
High blood pressure
Arteriosclerosis (especially coronary artery disease)
Arthritis
Periodontitis
Cartilage deterioration and ligament instability

Horsetail (shavegrass)

High in silicon and therefore used to improve bone strength and prevent cardiovascular disease. Useful for healing of skin and for hastening the suppurative (pus-forming) process during an infection. Also a mild diuretic. Available as tea, capsules, and cell salt.

Uses
Fractures
Osteoporosis
Cardiovascular disease
Skin wounds
Infections
Water retention

Licorice root (*Glycyrrhiza glabra*)

Used traditionally as a demulcent (soother), expectorant, and mild laxative; also for ulcers, asthma, pharyngitis, malaria, abdominal pain, insomnia, and infections. Major active components are glycyrrhizin and isoflavonoids.

1. Because licorice root enhances the mucosal lining of the digestive tract, the deglycyrrhizinated form is especially useful in the treatment of peptic ulcer disease, gastric and duodenal ulcers, gastritis and gastrointestinal inflammations or ulcerations, and colitis. It increases the amount and quantity of mucus, increases the life span of the surface epithelial cells, and enhances circulation to the mucosal lining. It also increases the number of mucus-secreting goblet cells.

2. It can be used prophylactically to prevent gastrointestinal inflammations and ulcers common with the long-term administration of steroids and nonsteroidal anti-inflammatory agents.

3. Due to its glycyrrhizin content, licorice root has a potent anti-inflammatory and anti-allergic effect, suppressing the enzyme 5-beta reductase and therefore delaying the normal degradation of the body's cortisone; useful in low cortisol states, and may possibly lessen the dose needed in corticosteroid therapy.

4. Licorice root can help normalize low blood pressure, particularly when due to depleted adrenal glands and low cortisol levels.

5. Like ginseng, it prevents cortisone-induced shrinking of the thymus and subsequent immunosuppression caused by chronic stress or cortisone-type medications.

6. It stimulates the production of interferon, which leads to significant antiviral activity, and produces activation of macrophages and enhanced natural killer cell activity.

7. It inhibits RNA and DNA viruses, including herpes simplex, Epstein-Barr virus, and hepatitis B virus. It can be used topically on oral and genital herpes lesions to decrease pain and speed healing.

8. Licorice root has some antimicrobial activity against staph, strep, and candida.

9. Licorice root can inhibit damage to the liver from chemical agents such as carbon tetrachloride.

10. It contains phytoestrogens that can help in both low estrogen states like menopause and high estrogen states like premenstrual syndrome.

11. Because it is much sweeter than sugar, it can mask the bitter flavor of medicinal herbs taken in tea form.

Recommended dose for oral use: powdered root, 1 to 4 grams a day; fluid extract, 1 teaspoon before meals three times a day; solid extract, ¼ teaspoon before meals; deglycyrrhizinated licorice powder or tablets, 250 milligrams three times a day.

Warning: Due to its cortisol-like effects, excessive doses of licorice can cause hypokalemia (low potassium levels), fluid retention, and high blood pressure (these side effects do not apply to the deglycyrrhizinated form).

Also, consult a qualified health professional if you have a condition for which estrogen is contraindicated.

Uses
DEGLYCYRRHIZINATED FORM
Ulcers
Gastritis
Colitis
Prevents ulcers when used prophylactically with ulcer-causing medicines (aspirin, prednisone, nonsteroidal anti-inflammatories)

WHOLE LICORICE
Increases tolerance to stress
Low blood pressure
Premenstrual symptoms
Menopause
Inflammation
Allergy
Antioxidant
Low immune states
Viral infections; herpes
Bacterial infections
Fungal infections
Low cortisol states (adrenal exhaustion)
Liver imbalances
Protects immune system during cortisone therapy
May reduce needed dose of cortisone

Lomatium

One of the more effective antiviral botanicals, used successfully for the common cold and influenza as well as for chronic viral states such as cytomegalovirus, Epstein-Barr virus, and other chronic viral states associated with chronic fatigue, malaise, and debility. Previously, the more commonly available freeze-dried form in capsules was associated with significant incidence of serious skin eruptions. However, the alcohol extract isolate form (from Eclectic Institute of Sandy, Oregon) has overcome this troublesome side effect. Use up to 5 to 10 drops twice a day.

Marshmallow root

A membrane soother. Use to relieve burning sensations associated with bladder infections, bronchitis, ulcers, gastritis, and other mucous membrane inflammations. It is commonly included in or taken with anti-infection, cough, bladder, gastrointestinal, and other formulas.

Milk thistle (*Silybum marianum*)

Contains silymarin, one of the most effective liver-protecting substances known. Milk thistle prevents free radical damage by acting as an antioxidant, stimulates the production of new liver cells, and combats the formation of damaging leukotrienes. This makes it useful for treating all liver disorders, such as chemically induced liver damage, viral hepatitis (acute and chronic), alcohol-induced liver disease (cirrhosis), cholangitis, and pericholangitis. Milk thistle has also been used in the treatment of psoriasis. (See Chapter Nine, page 179 for more discussion.)

Uses

Antioxidant
Enhances liver detoxification systems
Chemically induced liver damage
Viral hepatitis
Alcoholic hepatitis and cirrhosis
Pericholangitis
Liver cell regenerator
Psoriasis
Bowel toxemia

Mullein

Available in tea, tincture, and capsule form, mullein is good for treating coughs, upper respiratory problems, and glandular swelling. Often used in combination with lung and anti-infection herbs. Mullein oil can be used to treat earache, provided the eardrum is intact (see page 460).

Myrrh tea

Excellent for pyorrhea (infected gums) with or without pus. Use with a little GOLDENSEAL and a touch of CAYENNE as a mouthwash or gargle, or apply to skin infections. Extremely bitter.

Oatstraw

Extremely high in silicon, therefore used like horsetail (see HORSETAIL). Oatstraw tea or capsules can also help calm the nervous system.

Onion (*Allium cepa*)

Like GARLIC, onion has a number of sulfur-containing compounds that have multiple benefits:
1. Onion has an antibacterial and antimicrobial effect when consumed raw or as freeze-dried juice.
2. Onion is superior to garlic in inhibiting platelet aggregation.
3. It lowers blood sugar levels and can be used in the treatment of diabetes.
4. Onion has an effective antiasthmatic agent, and can inhibit the production of inflammatory prostaglandin hormones and leukotrienes. Because of this, onion also has uses in other inflammatory-related conditions, such as psoriasis and eczema, which again respond better to onion than to garlic.
5. It appears to be toxic to tumor cells.

Recommended dose of freeze-dried onion juice (Eclectic Institute of Sandy, Oregon) is up to 1 capsule (250 milligrams) every two to four hours for acute needs, and 1 to 2 capsules three times daily otherwise.

Regular inclusion of onions in salads and cooked dishes is recommended for preventive purposes.

Warning: Like garlic, onion is not recommended for those who have skin conditions such as acne, rosacea, and eczema.

Uses

Antibacterial
Antimicrobial
Anti-inflammatory
Antiasthmatic
Antitumor
Lowers blood sugar in diabetics
Psoriasis and eczema

Oregon grape root

See GOLDENSEAL.

Osha

See page 459, ANTI-INFECTION.

Parsley

The tea, made of fresh sprigs, acts as a diuretic. Can also be used topically in a compress to treat dry, irritated eyes and poison ivy. Eat whole or blend with celery leaves and pineapple juice for a nutritious drink.

Warning: When taken over a prolonged period, high doses of parsley can induce hepatitis-like syndrome, with elevated liver enzymes.

Passion flower (*Passiflora*)

Used as a sedative, alone or in combination (see page 461, SEDATIVE).

Pau d'arco (*also called la Pachol, Ipe Roxo, and taheebo*)

This herb has been used widely in South America to treat assorted ailments and diseases:

1. Pau d'arco has been studied extensively for its broad-spectrum antimicrobial activity against bacteria (including brucella, anthrax, dysentery, tuberculosis, and staph), viruses (including herpes types I and II, influenza, and polio), parasites (including malaria, schistosomiasis, and trypanosomiasis), and fungi (including candida and trichophyton).

2. It has also been studied for its anti-inflammatory properties.

Use bark that has been standardized at 2 to 4 percent la Pachol content if at all possible to be sure you are getting the real thing. Recommended dose: 1 teaspoon to 1 tablespoon of the bark per cup of water, boiled fifteen to twenty minutes, up to eight cups a day. Total daily ingestion should be 1½ to 2 grams. Douches or tampons soaked in the tea can be used to treat vaginitis and cervicitis. I prescribe this herb for intestinal and vaginal candidiasis. A 1:4 concentrated fluid tincture is commonly available, though it is considered mild. Use up to 2 dropperfuls up to four or five times daily.

Uses
Antibacterial
Antiviral
Antifungal
Antiparasitic
Anti-inflammatory

Pennyroyal oil

Used on clothing, in sheets, and perhaps a dab on skin to avert fleas. *Warning: Do not use during pregnancy. May cause liver/kidney damage if used in excess.*

Plantain

Used topically for burns, other skin irritations, and mastitis. Used orally in combination with MARSHMALLOW ROOT for ulcers and other gastrointestinal irritations. (G.I. Encap by Thorne Research of Sandpoint, Idaho.)

Quercetin

A pigmented flavonoid occurring in various fruits, vegetables, nuts, seeds, leaves, flowers, and barks. An average diet provides approximately 50 milligrams a day of this most valued plant constituent. Quercetin is best known as an anti-inflammatory/antiallergy agent:

1. Because it stabilizes mast cell membranes and prevents the release of histamine and other inflammatory agents, it is often prescribed for food and inhalant allergies, asthma, eczema, psoriasis, gout, and ulcerative colitis.

2. Due to its antioxidant effect, quercetin can inhibit inflammatory processes mediated by leukotrienes (inflammatory agents a thousand times more powerful than histamines), hyaluronidase (collagen-destroying enzymes), and lysosomal enzymes (other promoters of localized inflammation).

3. Quercetin is antiviral (including herpes type I, influenza, and polio).

4. It helps prevent diabetic cataracts, retinopathy, and neuropathy by inhibiting the enzyme aldose reductase and preventing the formation of polyols.

5. It protects the insulin-producing beta cells of the pancreas from free radical damage and enhances insulin secretion.

6. It functions like other bioflavonoids in enhancing the collagen network (structural integrity) of blood vessels.

7. Contrary to reports of its mutagenicity, quercetin is actually an antitumor agent.

Recommended dose for most conditions is 400 milligrams twenty minutes before meals, three times a day. As quercetin is not well absorbed—perhaps more than 50 percent is excreted in the stool—taking it along with BROMELAIN may greatly enhance its absorption.

Uses
Anti-inflammatory (asthma, eczema, colitis, psoriasis, gout)
Antiallergic
Antiviral
Antioxidant

Preserves pancreatic insulin producing beta cells
Antitumor
Collagen enhancing
Diabetic cataracts
Retinopathy
Neuropathy

Sarsaparilla

Known primarily as a blood purifier and tonic. Because of its saponin content (sarsaponin), which binds bowel endotoxins and prevents their escape to the liver and general circulation, this herb aids in the treatment of various inflammatory diseases triggered by bowel toxicity: psoriasis, arthritis, gout, fevers. In decreasing the escape of toxins to the liver, sarsaparilla also aids liver function.

Uses
Psoriasis
Arthritis
Gout
Fevers
General liver function

Saw palmetto (*Serenoa repens*)

Traditionally used by Native Americans to treat genitourinary disturbances. Pharmacologically it is known to have antiandrogen, immune-stimulating, and antiedema effects. The prime therapeutic application is benign prostate hypertrophy, a condition that develops when too much testosterone is converted to dihydrotestosterone (DHT). This compound causes cells in the prostate to multiply excessively and eventually causes the gland to enlarge. Saw palmetto blocks this conversion as well as the attachment of DHT to prostate cells, and facilitates DHT excretion. It has also been used to treat hirsutism and virilism in women.

The extract should be standardized to 85 to 95 percent fatty acids and sterols. Recommended dose: 80 to 160 milligrams in capsule form twice daily.

Uses
Benign prostate hypertrophy
Hirsutism and virilism in women

Slippery elm

For inflamed mucous membranes such as sore throats, colitis, ulcers, gastritis, and other digestive disturbances. Can be combined with GOLDENSEAL for an effective ulcer medication. Its effects are conveyed by direct contact with mucous membranes. Powder can be mixed in fluid and taken orally for use as an intestinal lubricant and stool softener. Comes in lozenge form for sore throats or the tea can be gargled. In conditions of severe nausea and vomiting (stomach flu, morning sickness), slippery elm tea can often be tolerated and therefore helps prevent dehydration.

Uses
Ulcers
Gastritis
Colitis
Sore throat
Stool softener/intestinal lubricant
Nausea

Stone root (*Collinsonia*)

Useful for hemorrhoids.

Taheebo

See PAU D'ARCO.

Tang-Kuei

See DONG QUAI.

Turmeric (curcumin)

A potent anti-inflammatory, its effect in acute inflammations may be comparable to that of pharmaceutical medications such as hydrocortisone and phenylbutazone, without any of the side effects of the latter. For chronic inflammatory conditions, it is about half as effective as these drugs. Combined with BROMELAIN, it is used to treat sprains, strains, muscular exertion, and tissue trauma (see TRAUMA).

Like LICORICE ROOT, because curcumin has both antibacterial and antifungal activity and liver-protecting effects, it has been used to treat jaundice, hepatitis, and other liver ailments. It is virtually nontoxic. Recommended dose is 300 milligrams three times a day.

Uses
Anti-inflammatory
Antibacterial
Antifungal
General liver function

Uva ursi

Best known for its urinary tract antiseptic and diuretic qualities, it can be extremely effective for treating urinary tract infections. Take one to two capsules standardized for arbutin, 10 percent, every few hours when acute, reduce dose gradually to three to four times a day for up to one week.

Warning: Do not acidify urine by drinking cranberry juice when using uva ursi. If back pain, fever, and malaise are present with bladder infection symptoms, antibiotics and professional care are indicated.

Valerian

Used most commonly as a sedative, alone or in combination (see page 461, SEDATIVE).

HERBAL COMBINATIONS FOR SPECIFIC APPLICATIONS AND AILMENTS

Ingredients are given in parentheses. Doses given apply only to adults. For company information, see Resources list at end of chapter.

Allergies (Inhalant)

Allerplex 1 (celandine, dandelion root, fenugreek seed, capsicum, thyme leaf, violet leaf): one to three capsules three to four times a day (Herb Technology/Khalsa Health Center).

Adrenal Strengthening and Conserving

Adren-Plus or Adren-Comp (bupleurum, panax ginseng, Siberian ginseng, Mexican yam, licorice root, turmeric): one to two capsules two times a day (Phyto-Pharmica/Enzymatic Therapy) or Ginkgo-Centella Compound (ginkgo, gotu kola, avena sativa, and Siberian ginseng): fifteen to thirty drops two or three times daily (Eclectic Institute).

Antibacterial

Bactoplex 1 (capsicum, echinacea root, black pepper, goldenseal root): two to four capsules four times a day (Herb Technology/Khalsa Health Center). Isatis Gold (see ANTIVIRAL). Opti Biotic (echinacea, myrrh, garlic, ginger, cayenne with vitamins A, C, and B-6, zinc, magnesium, and bioflavonoids): 1-2 tablets three times a day (Eclectic Institute). Berberine Complex or Phyto-Biotic (Oregon grape root, barberry, goldenseal): one to four capsules three times a day (Phyto-Pharmica/Enzymatic Therapy). Goldenseal Propolis Cream (propolis, goldenseal, myrrh, calendula): apply topically as needed (Eclectic Institute).

Anti-infection (colds, flu, sinus problems, chest colds, earache, sore throat, fever, malaise)

I mix a combination tincture consisting of echinacea (3 parts), osha (2 parts), goldenseal (1 or 2 parts), garlic (1 or 2 parts), mullein (1 part), white pine (optional, 1 part), cayenne (⅛ part), clove (¼ part), and lobelia (optional, ⅛ part): add horseradish (1 part) for sinus trouble; add marshmallow root for any burning sensations (1 part). Good-quality tinctures are available from Eclectic Institute and Herb-Pharm. Many health food and herb stores sell premixed anti-infection tinctures with a similar formula.

Antiviral (acute)

Isatis Gold (echinacea, platycodon, goldenseal, ligusticum): three tablets every two hours as tolerated (Health Concerns). Super Immuno-Tone or Super Immuno-Comp (echinacea, goldenseal, astragalus, licorice root, shiitake with beta-carotene, vitamins C and B-6, and zinc): one to four capsules four times a day (Phyto-Pharmica/Enzymatic Therapy). Immunoplex 3 (boldo leaf, jalapeño pepper, capsicum, onion bulb, rose hip, gingerroot, cubeb berry, garlic bulb): up to five per meal or one or two per hour as tolerated. Mixture is spicy, so take with food or a lot of water to avoid gastric irritation (Herb Technology/Khalsa Health Center).

Antiviral (chronic)

See CHRONIC FATIGUE SYNDROME and IMMUNE DEFICIENCY.

Arthritis (noninfectious)

Herbal Bromelain (devil's claw, black cohosh, bromelain/pineapple, ginger, turmeric, celery, quercetin/yellow onion, feverfew): two to four capsules three to four times a day (Eclectic Institute). Rheumatoplex (Chinese nardostachytis, myrrh gum, Chinese mastix, Chinese notopterygii root, Chinese achranthis root, Chinese poria): one to five capsules three times a day (Herb Technology/Khalsa Health Center). Bromelain and Curcumin (bromelain, turmeric): one to two capsules three or four times a day, twenty minutes or more before meals and at bedtime (Scientific Botanicals).

Candida

See "Herbal Antifungal Agents" (page 228) or try Candiplex (celandine, amur corktree bark, white oak bark, gum benzoin, myrrh, eleuthero root) and Mycoplex (celandine, echinacea, eleuthero root, white oak bark, cayenne): one to two capsules three to four times daily of either formula (Herb Technology/Khalsa Health Center).

Chronic fatigue syndrome

Astra Isatis (when chronic virus is suspected, see "Immune deficiency," next column). Immunoplex 4 (acumina, black walnut hull, gum benzoin, celandine): acute phase, work up to five capsules four times a day or as tolerated; long-term, four per day (Herb Technology/Khalsa Health Center).

Coughs

A mixture of mullein, chickweed, coltsfoot, horehound, marshmallow root, and licorice is one formula; or wild cherry, slippery elm, coltsfoot, marshmallow, licorice, cinnamon, yarrow, and ginger is another (The Herbalist, Seattle, Washington). Check your health food and herb stores. Formulas may vary. If a tea blend, steep 2 to 3 teaspoons per cup (or stronger) and drink four to eight cups a day. In tincture form, 1 to 3 dropperfuls four or five times a day.

Digestion

See "Herbal Digestive Remedies" (page 152).

Ear infection

Mullein Flower Compound (St. John's wort, mullein, calendula, garlic in olive oil): several drops in affected ear two to three times a day, provided ear drum is intact; warm up oil mildly before application (Herb–Pharm). Ear Drops (mullein in glycerin, Saint-John's-wort oil, garlic oil): instructions same as for Mullein Flower Compound (Eclectic Institute).

Fertility (for women)

Fertile Garden (loranthus, liqustrum, glehnia, cuscuto, pseudostellaria, shatavari, dong quai, white peony, lycium fruit, poria ashwagandha, melia, baked licorice, placenta): three tablets two to three times daily but not during a menstrual period (Health Concerns).

Fever

Elder flowers and peppermint in equal parts or chamomile and yarrow in equal parts, as tea.

Hemorrhoids

A rectal suppository made from asculus, hammameleis, and collinsonia (Earth's Harvest, Boerick and Tafel).

Immune deficiency (chronic viral states)

Astra Isatis (isatis extract, astragalus, bupleurum, laminaria, codonopsis, epimedium, lycium fruit, dioscorea, broussonetia, atractylodes, licorice root): three tablets three times a day (Health Concerns). D-Plex (echinacea, astragalus, dandelion root, gum benzoin, red raspberry leaf, garlic bulb, jalapeño pepper): work up to eight per meal or more as tolerated and as needed until results are seen; then two to five capsules per day long-term (Herb Technology/Khalsa Health Center). HIV Plex (Chinese astragalus root, licorice root, Chinese self-heal, Chinese violet leaf): use ten to twenty capsules daily (Herb Technology/Khalsa Health Center). Immunoplex 7 (jalapeño, capsicum, Saint-John's-wort): maximum dose, determined by digestive tolerance (Herb Technology/Khalsa Health Center). Enhance (ganoderma, isatis extract, and twenty-eight other Chinese herbs) along with Clear Heat (isatis extract and eight other Chinese herbs): protocol available to your health practitioner from Health Concerns.

Immune Enhancing

Astra 8 (astragalus, codonopis, ligustrum, licorice, ganoderma, atractylodes, eleuthero ginseng, schizandra): two to three capsules twice a day between meals (Health Concerns). Power mushrooms (ganoderma, shiitake, tremella or silver tree mushroom, poria, polyporus): three tablets once or twice a day between meals (Health Concerns); can use with Astra 8. Echimune (echinacea, astragalus, ligustrum, lentinus edodes, licorice): one to three capsules three to four times a day (NF Formulas). Mycelin 3 (reishi, shiitake, cordyceps): one or two capsules three to four times a day (Allergy Research/Nutricology).

Menopause

Fem-Tone or Femtrol (dong quai, licorice root, true unicorn root, black cohosh, fennel, false unicorn root, hesperidin [bioflavonoids], and vitamin C): one to three capsules three to four times a day as needed (Phyto-Pharmica/Enzymatic Therapy). Two Immortals (shizandra, oyster shell, epimedium, morinda, tang-kuei, ligustrum, eclipta, damania, gotu kola, pseudotellaria, red dates, anemarrhena, phellodendron, baked licorice, scrophularia, eight moon fruit): two or three tablets twice a day (Health Concerns).

Menstrual cramps

Utero-Tone or Fem-Care (dong quai, peony, black haw, blue cohosh, true unicorn root, black cohosh): one to four capsules three to four times a day as needed (Phyto-Pharmica/Enzymatic Therapy). Women's Balance (bupleurum, dong quai, peony, dan shen or salvia, poria, atractylodes, cyperus, citrus, moutan, gardenia, ginger, licorice root): three tablets two or three times a day between meals (Health Concerns). Heavenly Water (gotu kola, chaste tree berries, passionflower, pseudostellaria, scute, pinellia, poria, peony, tang keui, cypres, trichosanthes, red date, baked licorice, citrus, blue citrus): three tablets twice a day (Health Concerns).

Premenstrual syndrome (PMS)

Women's Balance (see MENSTRUAL CRAMPS). PMS Plex (Chinese polygonum multiflorum root, lady slipper root, blue cohosh): four to ten per day (Herb Technology/Khalsa Health Center). Women's Balance (bupleurum, dong quai, peony, dan shen or salvia, poria, atractylodes, cyperus, citrus, moutan, gardenia, ginger, licorice root): three tablets two or three times a day between meals (Health Concerns).

Sedative

Mix equal amounts of skullcap, hops, and passionflower (with or without valerian); for children, try a combination of pleasantly sweet-tasting chamomile, catnip, lemon balm, and licorice root. Try Sedaplex (valerian root, passionflower, hops, skullcap, wild lettuce with calcium, magnesium, vitamin B-6, and niacinamide): 2 to 4 capsules at bedtime (Tyler Encapsulations).

Stomachache (from overeating)

Equal parts slippery elm, cinnamon, ginger, cayenne, and goldenseal.

Trauma (sprains, strains, fractures, dislocations, bruises, hematomas, postsurgery)

Use Bromelain and Curcumin (bromelain and turmeric): one to three capsules three to four times a day between meals and at bedtime (Scientific Botanicals).

Urinary tract and bladder infections

Arbu-Tone (uva ursi, lespedeza, boldo, goldenrod, vitamin B-6, magnesium, and potassium): one to three capsules every two hours while acute, then three to four times a day (Phyto-Pharmical Enzymatic Therapy). Or try a tea, capsules, or tincture of uva ursi, buchu, juni-

per berries, parsley, marshmallow root, lobelia, ginger, and goldenseal: up to 8 cups a day of the tea, capsule doses as per Arbu-Tone above, or 25 to 30 drops of the tincture every two to three hours while acute. See also antibiotic formulas above, which may be necessary along with these kidney/bladder formulas. If any back pain or fever is present, pharmaceutical antibiotics and professional care are indicated.

RESOURCES

Allergy Research/Nutricology, 400 Preda Street, San Leandro, CA 94577-0489, (800) 782-4274.

Boerick and Tafel, 2381 Circadian Way, Santa Rosa, CA 95407, (800) 876-9505 or (707) 571-8202.

Earth's Harvest, 2557 N.W. Division, Gresham, OR 97030, (800) 428-3308 or (503) 666-7744.

Eclectic Institute, 14385 S.E. Lusted Road, Sandy, OR 97055, (800) 332-4372 or (503) 668-4120.

Health Concerns, 8001 Capwell Drive, Oakland, CA 94621, (800) 233-9355 or (510) 521-7401.

Herb-Pharm, 20260 Williams Highway, Williams, OR 97544, (800) 348-4372 or (503) 846-7178.

Herb Technology/Khalsa Health Center, 1305 N.E. 45th Street, Ste. 205, Seattle, WA 98109, (800) 659-2077 or (206) 547-2007.

NF Formulas, Inc. 9775 S.W. Commerce Circle, Suite C-5, Wilsonville, OR 97070, (800) 325-9326 (in Oregon); (800) 547-4891 (outside Oregon).

Phyto-Pharmica/Enzymatic Therapy, 825 Challenger Drive, Greenbay, WI 54311, (800) 553-2370 or (414) 469-1313.

Scientific Botanicals, Inc., P.O. Box 31131, Seattle, WA 98103, (206) 527-5521.

Thorne Research, Inc., 901 Triangle Drive, Sandpoint, ID 83864, (800) 228-1966 or (208) 263-1337.

Tyler Encapsulations, 2204-8 N.W. Birdsdale, Gresham, OR 97030, (800) 634-1051 (in Oregon); or (800) 869-9705 (outside Oregon).

SUGGESTED READING

Alstat, E. *Eclectic Dispensatory of Botanical Therapeutics.* Sandy, OR: Eclectic Medical Publications, 1989.

Badgely, Lawrence, M.D. *Healing AIDS Naturally.* San Bruno, CA: Human Energy Press, 1987.

Beinfield, Harriet, and Korngold, Efrem. *Between Heaven and Earth: A Guide to Chinese Medicine.* New York: Ballantine, 1991.

Christopher, J. *School of Natural Healing.* Provo, Utah: BiWorld Publishers, 1978.

Gaeddert, Andrew. *Chinese Herbs in the Western Clinic.* Dublin, CA: Get Well Foundation, 1994.

Hoffman, D. *The Herb User's Guide: The Basic Skills of Medical Herbalism*. Rochester, VT: Thorson's, 1987.

Kloss, J. *Back to Eden*. Revised and updated. Available from Back to Eden Press, P.O. Box 1439, Loma Linda, CA 92354.

Mindell, E. *Earl Mindell's Herb Bible*. New York: Simon & Schuster/Fireside, 1992.

Murray, M. T. *The Healing Power of Herbs: The Enlightened Person's Guide to the Wonders of Medicinal Plants*. Rockland, CA: Prima Publishing, 1991.

Pizzorno, J. E., and Murray, M. T. "Pharmacology of Natural Medicines." In *A Textbook of Natural Medicine*. Seattle, WA: John Bastyr College Publications, 1985.

Tierra, M. *The Way of Herbs*. New York: Pocket Books, 1980.

———. *Planetary Herbology*. Santa Fe, New Mexico: Lotus Press, 1988.

Weiss, R. F. *Herbal Medicine*. Beaconsfield, England: Beaconsfield, Ltd., 1988.

MORE NATURAL THERAPEUTICS

BEE VENOM THERAPY*

Used for centuries, bee venom has proven to be an effective and safe treatment for numerous common ailments. Extensive research and clinical work at university centers in Russia, Austria, Germany, France, England, Switzerland, and Czechoslovakia suggests that this simple therapy may be a treatment of choice for the following conditions:

Acute and chronic rheumatoid arthritis
Acute and chronic osteoarthritis
Gout
Tendonitis
Bursitis
Neuritis
Neuralgia
Fibrositis
Fibromyalgia
Myalgia and myositis (muscle soreness and inflammation)

Bee venom has also been used to treat acute rheumatic fever and endocarditis, multiple sclerosis, spondylitis, hypertension, migraines, and seizure disorders.

A natural product of the honeybee, bee venom contains several biologically active components, one of which is melittin, a peptide (protein) compound that stimulates the pituitary-adrenal axis to release both adrenaline and cortisol. Cortisol, as you know, is one of the body's most potent anti-inflammatory substances. Stimulating an appropriate physiologic anti-inflammatory response is always preferable to taking anti-inflammatory medications, as the former has virtually no adverse effects. In addition, melittin also stimulates the smooth muscle in the heart to contract; and it dilates peripheral capillary vessels, which lowers blood pressure.

Melittin is also gangliolytic—having the remarkable property of blocking transmission of nerve impulses from one cell to another in nerve ganglions—interrupting pain cycles and other central and autonomic nervous system transmissions.

Bee venom also contains phospholipase A, apamin, hyaluronidase, cardiopep, and other substances. Generally speaking, bee venom can be categorized as an immunologic agent that enhances the body's own protective mechanisms: it is anti-inflammatory, antipain, antihypertensive, antiarrhythmic, anticoagulating, myocardial enhancing, and immune enhancing.

Most health practitioners utilizing bee venom therapy give their patients injections from multiple-dose vials. The venom is scraped from the diaphragm of honeybees, processed, sterilized, and bottled for use. The traditional folk medicine approach used by beekeepers and by some health professionals today is to apply a honeybee (held in tweezers) to a specific area of the body, where the bee will sting and inject its venom. After the individual has been tested for bee venom allergy, a gradually increasing number of stings or injections are given on a regular schedule, usually two or three times a week for twelve to sixteen visits. In general, less severe conditions will begin to respond favorably before the fifth treatment. More difficult cases take longer. A follow-up series of treatments may be required. I have yet to have a patient with chronic tendonitis not re-

---

*My acknowledgment and thanks to Christopher M. Kim, M.D., and to Bradford S. Weeks, M.D., for their teaching and reference materials.

spond dramatically to this treatment. My personal experience with arthritis patients is limited, but results seem promising. Workshops and general information for the public and health professionals are available through the American Apitherapy Society, P.O. Box 124, Woodsville, NH 03785 (603) 747-2507. Ask for their "Questions and Answers" handout.

BUTYRIC ACID

Butyric acid, used as a primary fuel by the mucosal cells of the large intestine, is a short-chain fatty acid normally produced in the large intestine by friendly bacteria. It is no coincidence that butyric acid is present in mother's milk, as it is crucial in the initial maturation of the infant's intestinal cells. Intestinal cells are extremely fast-growing—they slough off regularly and need to be replaced often—and therefore have high energy demands that butyric acid helps fulfill. Butyric acid also promotes cellular differentiation (healthy cells the body needs) and inhibits abnormal undifferentiated cells (cancer cells, which of course the body does not need). For this reason, butyric acid falls into the class of agents called biologic response modifiers.

Butyric acid has a particularly beneficial effect on inflamed or compromised intestinal epithelial cells and is used often to treat cases of colitis. Although taking capsules of butyric acid orally would eventually deliver some of this agent to the colon, this route is not considered optimal. The most effective method is through a retention enema. Stir the contents of four to six capsules into four ounces of warm water and instill through a standard enema, retaining it as long as possible.

Patients with food allergies and intestinal yeast and parasite infections have also benefitted from using butyric acid.

Because low stool butyrate levels have recently been used as one predictive test for colon cancer, butyrate supplementation has been used to help prevent colon cancer. High-dose supplementation has also been used to treat some cancers, including childhood leukemias. Butyric acid is available in capsules as calcium/magnesium butyrate (Butyrex from T. E. Neesby, Fresno, California). It is also available in an enema kit (ButyCol from Tyler Encapsulations, Gresham, Oregon).

CASTOR OIL PACKS

Castor oil packs, made popular by Edgar Cayce and the Association for Research and Enlightenment (ARE)[1], involve the topical application of castor oil to treat a variety of symptoms and conditions: constipation, intestinal toxicity, intestinal and abdominal cramping,

liver congestion/sluggishness, ovarian cysts, menstrual cramps, fibroids and other female problems, hepatitis, tendonitis, bursitis and various joint pains, musculoskeletal injuries, bruises, plantar warts, varicose veins, phlebitis, bronchitis, pneumonia, and more. There is much anecdotal evidence on the effectiveness of a castor oil pack. Just how and why it works is uncertain, although a certain amount of lymphatic flow and perhaps T-cell stimulation has been suggested, in addition to generally enhanced circulation to the areas treated.

Take a soft cloth (flannel is preferred) and be sure it is large enough to cover the area intended for treatment. A 7-by-8-inch cloth is usually large enough for an abdominal pack. Obtain a piece of plastic (produce or garbage bag variety) slightly larger than the cloth, a heating pad or hot water bottle, a towel or other appropriate wrap, and tape or safety pins. Saturate the cloth with castor oil and apply the cloth to the area needing treatment. Cover the cloth with plastic to protect your towel, clothing, or heating pad, then place the hot water bottle or heating pad on top of the plastic for fifty to sixty minutes. If you want to sleep with the pack in place (on your abdomen, for example) and get additional effects from the oil, wrap a towel completely around your midsection to keep the pack in place and secure with tape or safety pins—depending on the body part being wrapped. This step can be taken before you apply the heat; just be sure to remove the heat after the hour is up.

Castor oil packs are usually administered daily for two to three weeks at a time. When you remove the pack, fold the cloth in the plastic, and it will be ready for reuse. You may not need to add more oil each time you apply the pack, but do so every several days. If you cannot find a cold- or expeller-pressed castor oil at a health or massage supply store, use any pharmacy brand.

CRANIAL ELECTROTHERAPY STIMULATION (CES)

Cranial electrotherapy stimulation (CES) uses mild electronic stimulation of the brain in the treatment of such conditions as depression, anxiety, substance abuse withdrawal syndrome, and insomnia. CES should NOT be confused with electroconvulsive shock therapy (ECT) or aversion therapy. In CES therapy, battery-powered electrodes are placed just behind the ears, and a charge is administered. This induces a pleasant and comforting experience. Individuals can use the unit at home or at work without interrupting their normal activity. CES therapy has no known negative side effects and can be effectively used therapeutically without drugs.

It is hypothesized that CES acts by direct stimulation of the brain in the hypothalamic area with specific electronic frequencies. Such stimulation causes the brain to manufacture its own neurochemicals, such as endorphins, norepinephrine, dopamine, serotonin, and acetylcholine, up to levels of pre-stress homeostasis.

Research findings compiled from several human subject studies support the hypothesis that a mild effect is produced in the hypothalamic area of the brain. CES-stimulated endorphins inhibit the increased levels of norepinephrine from unduly stimulating neuroreceptors on the locus ceruleus (the brain's endorphin-producing site). This effectively blocks anxiety and associated panic states. Recent findings also indicate that CES-stimulated acetylcholine improves cognitive functioning, increasing both short-term memory and the ability to retain new information over time.

Variations of CES therapy have been in use in Europe for almost thirty years under such labels as electrosleep, neuroelectric therapy, transcranial electrotherapy, and transcranial electrostimulation. Serious research with CES was initiated in the United States in the mid-1960s. One of the first in-depth studies of the technique was conducted at the Medical College of Wisconsin at Milwaukee. The focus of this study was to determine if quantifiable physiological changes take place when electrical stimulation is applied during periods of high stress or anxiety.

Initial testing was done on monkeys by measuring levels of gastric acidity during periods of high stress and again following application of CES. Results of repeated testing showed a significant decline in the amount of gastric acidity following the CES treatment. Carefully controlled tests and studies with human volunteers yielded the same results. It was the conclusion of the research committee involved with the project that, based on the findings, CES had definite therapeutic value as a nondrug/noninvasive treatment for stress- and anxiety-related illness problems.

The most dramatic evidence of the benefits of CES therapy entails use of computerized EEGs, or topographical brainmapping, which validates that CES alters the abnormal electrophysiology associated with drug/alcohol abuse and other organic brain diseases, as well as normalizing other dysfunctional brainwave patterns. This has major implications in the treatment of chronic fatigue and immune deficiency syndrome.

Studies show CES to be a highly effective adjunct to methadone withdrawal in heroin addictions and in the control of rebound stress reactions associated with other chemical substances. It helps the brain bring its own neurochemistry back to pre-trauma levels of homeostasis, allowing cognitive functioning to return to normal patterns within weeks instead of the usual months—or in some cases, years—which is often the case with substance abusers.

Because of the fundamental bias in American medicine on behalf of pharmaceuticals, CES and electromedicine as a whole have been slow to gain acceptance in this country. Recently, however, there has been a resurgence of interest in this field. There are now more than 25,000 units in use in the United States. The therapy is currently employed at a number of psychiatric facilities and in several major hospital chains treating alcohol and substance abuse. CES is fast becoming a treatment of choice for those physicians and mental health professionals wanting a nonpharmacological alternative for the treatment of stress-related disorders.

The most extensive work presently being done on CES is at CES Labs in Redmond, Washington. In addition to their current 100-Hz unit (the configuration upon which most of the research is based), they are developing a new prototype in conjunction with the Pavlov Institute of St. Petersburg, Russia, whose unit has shown dramatic results in clinical studies involving more than 10,000 patients. Promising areas of application include the treatment of myocardial infarction (heart attack), duodenal and gastric ulcers, pain, headache, and alcohol withdrawal syndrome. They have also employed a variation of the modality as electroanesthesia, employed not only during the operation but also during the pre- and postoperative stages.

CES has major implications in a number of areas. In the war on drugs, it is a formidable new weapon in the treatment of the symptoms accompanying and retarding withdrawal. For those suffering from depression and anxiety, it means relief with none of the unpleasant side effects or addiction potential of prescription drugs. For those seeking relief from insomnia, it's an alternative to habit-forming sedatives. For an American public paying increasing attention to the effects of stress on physical health and emotional well-being, it is a way of addressing that stress in a safe and effective manner.[2]

GINGER COMPRESS

A ginger compress, used in Japanese traditional healing, can be useful for conditions requiring heat and improved circulation, such as sinus inflammation, bronchial and other lung infections, sore throat, and stomach flu, to name a few.[3]

To make a ginger compress, wrap fresh-grated gingerroot in a cheesecloth and place in water in a moderately large saucepan. Heat the water just short of boiling. Squeeze the contents of the cheesecloth, then immerse a soft cloth into the ginger water and apply cloth to the area being treated. Have a second cloth in the ginger water to use as soon as your first cloth loses warmth. Alternate these two cloths. Do not get it in your eyes. Keep the pack on for up to ten minutes until the skin turns noticeably red. Repeat several times a day.

The ginger water can be refrigerated and reused for several days by reheating, but do not boil.

HYDROTHERAPY*

References to the use of water in the treatment or prevention of illness date back as early as 1500 B.C. More recently, the science of hydrotherapy has been furthered and popularized by Father Sebastian Kneipp and the health spas of nineteenth-century Germany and central Europe, and in the early 1990s in the United States by J. H. Kellogg, M.D., and O. G. Caroll, M.D. Bernard Jenson, N.D., has written much about water therapy in his books, and most recently André Saine, N.D., has helped revive its use in the naturopathic profession.

Everyone has at some time or other experienced the soothing and relaxing qualities of a hot bath, as well as the invigorating and stimulating effects of a cold dip or cold shower. Less well known, however, are the more technical benefits these water applications offer: An increase in localized white blood cell counts and corresponding increases in IgM antibodies, alpha-2 macroglobulin, and C-3 complement.

With such enhanced immune system factors, hydrotherapy can be beneficial in the treatment of sore throats, colds, bronchitis, pneumonia, abscesses, pelvic inflammatory disease, bladder infections, flu, and chronic fatigue syndrome.

Because of its salubrious effects on circulation and other physiologic parameters, hydrotherapy is also helpful for nervous conditions, insomnia, anxiety, prostate, uterine, and other organ and glandular congestions, traumatic edema, acute and chronic pain, poor circulation, headaches, muscle spasms, fever, arthritis, fatigue, and detoxification programs.[4]

The thermal (heating and cooling) effects of water are responsible for its therapeutic benefits. A hot compress (a cloth immersed in hot water, wrung out to the desired amount of moisture, and placed on the body) can open blood vessels and attract more blood to the area—useful for abscesses or other skin infections. Enhancing the circulation also improves organ function. For example, an abdominal compress can stimulate the liver and spleen. Moist heat also relaxes tense muscles or spasms (on the abdomen for intestinal cramps, for example). Adding Epsom salts, specific herbs, or other ingredients to the water can enhance its effects.

A compress using very cold water will constrict blood vessels and decrease circulation—useful in treating sprains and contusions. Cold also works to diminish pain caused by a congestive condition, like a vascular headache. In this instance, try using a cold compress on the forehead while soaking your feet in hot water, to draw circulation out of the upper body and to the feet.

It is quite common to alternate hot and cold compresses, starting with the hot phase for five to ten minutes, then the cold for a minute or two. A consecutive series of three hot and cold applications is recommended.

Treatment using a cold double compress covered by several layers of dry wool or flannel has the same vasoconstricting effect as a normal cold compress, but when allowed to remain in place until warmed by the body it brings about a paradoxical increase in circulation to the treated area. Of course, increased circulation means the mobilization of white cells and the enhanced removal of metabolic wastes. The cold double compress is thought to be even more effective as a healing therapy than a hot compress because in fighting the cold, the body's immune system is more actively engaged. Such an application can be very effective for sore throats, bronchitis, pneumonia, and swollen lymph glands.

A large double compress placed on the trunk from the collarbone to the groin and then on the entire back is a primary aspect of constitutional hydrotherapy, effecting improvements in digestive, eliminative, and immune functioning. Constitutional hydrotherapy can be beneficial for those acutely ill, weakened, or convalescing. It is also used to enhance the cleansing process during a fast or detoxification program.

Not everyone has access to a naturopathic physician offering a specialized course of constitutional hydrotherapy. Fortunately, the basic process is easy to replicate at home, using the wet sheet pack or saunas, showers, and baths. (See "Fashioning Your Own Constitutional Hydrotherapy," page 467.)

Another form of localized water application is the sitz bath. This involves sitting in a deep basin or tub so that the buttocks and pelvis are immersed. Hot sitz baths (105° to 115° F) are prescribed generally for pain in the uterus, ureter, or testes; hemorrhoids; urinary retention problems; and after cystoscopy and hemorrhoidectomy. The hot sitz baths are NOT indicated during the menstrual period. Chronic pelvic inflammatory disease may also respond favorably. Taking a sitz bath for three to ten minutes several times a day is recommended for PID, often accompanied by a hot foot bath. The foot bath is NOT advised for diabetics.

Neutral temperature (92° to 95° F) sitz baths tend to have a sedative, calming effect and are used for insomnia, anxiety, nervous irritability, exhaustion, and chronic pain. They also relieve acute inflammatory conditions, such as pelvic inflammatory disease, bladder in-

*Acknowledgments to Robert Barry, M.D., for his personal assistance and his article on hydrotherapy in the *Textbook of Natural Medicine*, ed. Pizzorno, J. and M. T. Murray. Seattle: John Bastyr College Publications, 1985, Section III, pp. 1–12.

FASHIONING YOUR OWN CONSTITUTIONAL HYDROTHERAPY*

WET SHEET PACK:

The wet sheet pack is one of the most useful of all hydrotherapy procedures. It may be done either in the office or as a home treatment, if adequate direction is provided. It requires from one to three hours, depending on the condition of the patient. The technique is common to most schools of hydrotherapy. It is important to understand the process completely before using this treatment.

1. Using either a bed or treatment table, place two wool blankets lengthwise on the table with a small pillow at the head. The blankets must be large enough to cover the person being treated. If wool is not available, acrylic is the next best choice.

2. The patient must be warm before the pack is applied. If not, they may be warmed by a hot bath or shower, dry blanket pack, diathermy of the back, or any other appropriate technique.

3. Once the patient is ready, a clean white cotton sheet (equal in length to the height of the patient) is wrung as dry as possible, after being soaked in cold water. It is much easier if two people are available to wring out the sheet. The sheet is opened and placed lengthwise along the table with equal amounts draped over each side of the table. The sheet should be one to two inches below the height of the blankets.

4. The patient now removes all clothing and lies on the wet sheet with shoulders four inches below the top of the sheet. Both arms are raised while the attendants quickly wrap one side of the sheet around the body, tucking it in on the opposite side, and carefully molding it to the body. Below the hips, the sheet is wrapped around the leg on the same side.

5. The arms are now lowered and the opposite side of the sheet is drawn over the body covering both arms. It is also wrapped around the opposite leg. The wet sheet is quickly smoothed over the body to ensure complete contact and is tucked in around the feet. As this is a shocking experience, it should be performed quickly and efficiently.

6. At this point, the blankets are quickly pulled over the body and tucked in firmly, ensuring no drafts around the neck or the feet. Additional blanket(s) may be laid over the patient and tucked in as appropriate. A stocking cap may be pulled over the head to increase the heating effect.

While the patient is in the pack, it is necessary to have someone nearby at all times. Sudden attacks of claustrophobia in some individuals can cause extreme anxiety. Should this occur, first remove the sheet from the feet, as this may allow enough movement to allay the attack. If this is unsuccessful, it may be necessary to stop the treatment.

Providing hot teas is very helpful throughout the treatment. If the patient complains of chilliness, add blankets, place a hot water bottle to the feet, or provide warm drinks.

The wet sheet pack proceeds through four stages: tonic or cooling, neutral, heating, and eliminative. Depending on the desired effect, the therapist may wish to prolong any one specific stage.

1. **Tonic stage:** This stage may last from two to fifteen minutes and is finished when the patient no longer perceives the sheet as being cold. This phase is intensely alterative to the body, due to the intense thermic reaction induced.

   The length of this stage is directly dependent on the amount of water left in the sheet. For weak or exhausted patients, the sheet should be wrung out as completely as possible. For young, strong individuals for whom a more tonifying treatment is desired, more water may be left in the sheet.

2. **Neutral stage:** Once the sheet reaches body temperature, the person no longer feels cold. At this time the neutral phase begins. It may last from fifteen minutes to an hour or longer, depending on the vitality of the patient. During this phase there is a sense of calm similar to that experienced during a neutral bath. Very often the patient will fall asleep during this phase. This stage is indicated in cases of insomnia, anxiety, and delirium. In order to prolong the neutral phase, provide only adequate covering to prevent the patient from feeling cool. Greater amounts of blankets will trap more heat and the neutral phase will finish sooner.

3. **Heating stage:** As heat accumulates beneath the blankets, the patient will gradually sense the warming, and eventually begin to show light perspiration on the forehead. Between the time the patient feels warm to the beginning of perspiration is the heating phase. This may last from fifteen minutes to an hour.

4. **Elimination stage:** The final stage begins when the body begins to perspire. In a febrile patient this stage will be reached sooner. This stage is especially beneficial for those patients in a detoxification process such as withdrawal from alcohol, tobacco, coffee, or other toxins. It may also be used with acute infections, such as colds, flu, or bronchitis. Certain skin conditions, such as jaundice, may also be benefited, as well as acute inflammatory conditions, such as arthritis.

During the elimination stage, it's important to provide adequate fluid to the patient. Herb teas, used either for their diaphoretic or therapeutic effects, are most appropriate.

This phase may last up to an hour. The treatment should be ended quickly if the patient begins to feel chilled or becomes uncomfortable.

The treatment ends by quickly removing the patient from the pack, frictioning the skin briskly with a dry towel, and having the patient dress. As this is often an intensive treatment, it should be followed with rest or appropriate activity. Lying down and resting in a warm room for an hour is an ideal follow-up to this treatment. If done at home, it is best done in the evening just before bedtime.

From "Hydrotherapy" by R. Barry, N.D., from Textbook of Natural Medicine, edited by J. Pizzorno and M. Murray, Bastyr College Publications, 1993, pp. III: Hydro-9, 10. Reprinted by permission of Bastyr College Publications, 144 N.E. 54th Street, Seattle, WA 98105.

fections, epididymitis, prostatitis, and itching of the anus or vulva.

A cold sitz bath (55° to 75° F) is given right after a short hot sitz bath and lasts from thirty seconds to eight minutes (the level of the cold water should be not quite as high as that used in a hot sitz bath). It is usually administered for its tonifying effect on prostatic congestion, weak bladder, metrorrhagia, and other conditions. As with alternating hot/cold compresses, the hot/cold sitz bath should be taken in a series of three, cold always following hot.

Neutral temperature baths can last for fifteen minutes to four hours. For the longer baths, hot water may need to be added periodically to keep the temperature stable. Because it's very important not to become chilled, you should take this bath immediately before bedtime.

Saunas, Showers, and Baths

Another way to fashion your own constitutional treatment is to alternate between a sauna and a cool shower, between a warm bath and a cool shower (if the shower stall is separate from the bath), between a warm bath and a cool bath (if you have access to two tubs), or between a hot shower and a cool shower.

Generally, three cycles are completed back to back, with cold always following hot. The hot phase should get you warm, even sweating if you're using a sauna, but nowhere near deliriously hot. And don't overdo. Although it is far more appealing and comfortable to take a hot bath than a cold shower or dip, prolonging the heat phase can actually weaken you. The cold phase, on the other hand, engages the healing response, but take care not to become chilled: the cold phase should simply cool you off.

The stronger and healthier you are, the more resistant you are and the colder and longer the cold phase can safely be. However, if you are weak or acutely ill, the temperature should not be as cold and the duration should be short. The therapy here needs to be gentle. So experiment, and gauge the time and temperature of each phase according to your needs. (If you have heart disease or high blood pressure, check with your doctor first before trying saunas or hot/cold therapy.)

MASSAGE AND BODYWORK

It was not in medical school that I first formally learned about bodywork and therapeutic touch and massage. It wasn't until the first year of my current practice, in Seattle in 1979. I was living and working out of my home, without a secretary or a receptionist, using a phone machine, doing the insurance and billing myself, making house calls, attending to patients in the hospital, and being on call twenty-four hours a day, seven days a week.

My neck soon began to feel tight. But with so many demands to meet, I ignored the tension until the pain became the most pressing issue in my life. Out of desperation for relief and at the prompting of friends, I began to see a massage therapist on a weekly basis. She used Swedish, acupressure, and muscle-releasing techniques that relaxed my muscles, restored circulation, and eased my pain.

The generalized tension and anxiety I'd been feeling for months began to lessen, and as a result I felt better able to cope with stress. In the process, I gained a new awareness of my body and a true sense of relaxation. In fact, I was soon feeling so good that I was stimulated to make some necessary and major changes in my life.

The massage treatments helped me see clearly that I'd simply been performing beyond my limits, trying to be everything to everybody. In so doing, I was sacrificing my main interests and talents. Over the course of several months, I began to practice yoga and take other self-care measures that minimized my need to see a massage therapist regularly and helped me to function at my best.

From the simple goal of reducing my neck pain, I grew to realize the depth of healing and self-knowledge inherent in bodywork.

The choices for bodywork are numerous. Swedish massage is a relatively gentle technique that, among other things, can increase circulation of blood and lymph and bring relaxation to tense muscles and nerves. Rolfing, on the other hand, is the deep and sometimes painful probing of underlying connective tissue and muscle sheaths to realign posture along true planes of movement, assist the body in finding its center line of gravity, increase efficiency of movement, and relieve many chronic or recurring musculoskeletal conditions.

Bodywork can also be employed to unlock "body armoring" and trigger the release of emotional blocks—an extremely effective psychotherapeutic tool that can give birth to personal and spiritual growth. Bioenergetics, Reichian therapy, and rebirthing incorporate specific breathing techniques to assist in this unlocking. SHEN (specific human energy nexus), Reiki, and therapeutic touch are primarily tactile-sensitive systems (although in some cases the practitioner's hands rest just above the skin without actually making contact). These modalities can also work psychotherapeutically and are known to decrease physical pain, fever, and anxiety, and speed physical healing.

For nearly a century now, chiropractic technique and osteopathy have both put forward the idea that structure regulates function. By means of manipulating the joints, especially on the spinal vertebrae, these techniques—sometimes forceful, sometimes gentle, depending on the practitioner's particular style—are said to restore and maintain nerve and circulatory function, ease pain, and help the body heal musculoskeletal conditions and such ailments as ulcers, infections, deafness, fatigue, nervousness, bowel problems, dizziness, and menstrual cramps.

Chiropractors, depending on the state in which they practice, may be licensed to practice nutrition, minor surgery, even primary health care, in addition to manipulation. Osteopaths today are licensed to practice as conventional medical doctors, but a growing number still make structural manipulation a primary part of their practice.

Craniosacral techniques employed by some chiropractors and osteopaths (and by other health professionals) involve the very gentle and subtle manipulation of the cranial bones and the sacrum. The cranial bones of the skull are movable joints that can be misaligned by trauma from birth, head injury, dental stress, and other factors. Impinging on the brain and the flow of cerebrospinal fluid, such misalignments can cause or contribute to headaches, temporomandibular joint (TMJ) dysfunction, spinal and other musculoskeletal pain, behavioral and learning problems, seizures, visual and hearing problems, vertigo, and a vast array of other conditions. Impingements of cranial bones on eustacian tubes and sinus passageways can trigger recurrent ear and sinus infections. Craniosacral technique is considered one of the more refined and specialized of the manipulation therapies.

I have directly experienced, either as a patient or as a practitioner, many bodywork therapies: acupressure, shiatsu, reflexology/zone therapy, polarity therapy, ginsin-do, Trager, Hellerwork, orthobionomy, strain/counterstrain, Feldenkrais, Alexander, touch for health/applied kinesiology, and naprapathy. Other techniques include Aston patterning, Lomi school, Rosenwork, Hakomi, postural integration, toning, and harmonics. (See William Leigh's *Bodytherapy: From Rolf to Feldenkrais to Tanouye Roshi*. Water Margin Press, 1989. See resources list following and Suggested Reading for further information.)

"Physical therapy," a form of bodywork long considered an extension of conventional medicine, is often effective for a variety of musculoskeletal conditions. I know several physical therapists who have gone beyond their formal training to study other forms of bodywork and then incorporate them into their practice. In so doing, they have greatly enhanced what standard physical therapy alone can achieve.

Human beings respond to touch, sometimes quite dramatically. Even without any of the special bodywork training or massage therapy techniques you have read or know about, there is much each of us can do to help others. Simply holding someone's hand can bring a feeling of security or trigger needed emotional release. Rubbing someone's back or neck can ease tight, tense muscles. Cradling someone's head can relieve a headache. Laying your hands gently on someone's stomach can reduce pain and anxiety. You may already be aware that your hands have the ability to bring great comfort. Technique and training are invaluable, certainly, but the untrained quality of loving touch can bring dramatic responses.

If bodywork is a new and appealing concept to you, you might try a session with a licensed massage therapist. In nearly all states that allow massage therapy, basic licensing requirements include a thorough knowledge of anatomy and physiology and Swedish massage techniques. Many therapists practice a combination of Swedish, shiatsu, deep tissue massage, Tragering, and other techniques that require advanced training. From such an experience with a massage therapist, you may get to know your body and mind in new ways and be drawn further into the field of bodywork.

Resources for Massage and Bodywork

Alexander Technique, The North American Society of Teachers of the Alexander Technique, P.O. Box 517, Urbana, IL 61801, (217) 367-6956. Alexander Technique International, 9605 Carriage Rd., Kensington, MD 20895, (202) 362-1649.

American Massage Therapy Association, 820 Davis St., Evanston, IL 60201, (312) 761-AMTA.

Cranial Academy, 3500 DePaul Blvd. Suite 1080, Indianapolis, IN 46268, (317) 879-0713.

Feldenkrais Guild, 706 SW Ellsworth St., P.O. Box 489 Albany, OR 97321-0143, (503) 926-0981.

Hakomi Institute, 1800 30th St., Suite 201, Boulder, CO 80301, (303) 443-6209.

Heller Work Inc., 406 Berry St., Mount Shasta, CA 96067, (916) 926-2500.

Rolf Institute, P.O. Box 1868, Boulder, CO 80306, (303) 449-5903.

Sutherland Institute, 4116 Hartwood Dr., Fort Worth, TX 76109, (817) 735-2498.

Trager Institute, 33 Millwood, Mill Valley, CA 94941, (415) 388-2688.

Upledger Institute, 1211 Prosperity Farms Rd., Palm Beach Gardens, FL 33410, (800) 233-5880.

STAPHAGE LYSATE VACCINE

The rationale behind vaccinations is as follows: if a weakened form of a bacteria is introduced into the body, the immune system will be stimulated to produce antibodies specific to fighting that bacteria. Should an individual then be exposed to the disease, the immune system will be primed to prevent it.

Staphage lysate (SPL), a lesser-known bacterial vaccine, is an immunizing agent that can augment the body's defense against *Staphylococcus aureus*. The serum is prepared from colonies of staph that are lysed (killed and fragmented) by bacteriophage viruses and finally sterilized by ultrafiltration. When standard antibiotic therapy, incision, drainage, and other medical-surgical approaches have been deemed ineffective, SPL can often be used effectively.

Given by injection or other routes, depending on the location of the infection, SPL engages the immune system through antibody production and macrophage stimulation and mobilization to specifically attack and protect the body from staph. It has been used to treat recurrent or chronic sinusitis, abscesses, bronchitis, pneumonia, ear infections, conjunctivitis, furunculosis, folliculitis, enterocolitis, osteomyelitis, and septicemia.

Because it can stimulate and mobilize other immune mechanisms, including nonspecific macrophages and bacterial/viral antibodies, recurrent or resistant infections from organisms other than staph may respond to SPL (nonspecific immune cells and antibodies will attack anything foreign). Thanks to other SPL-mediated changes in immune function, this agent has become known as a biological response modifier. Additional properties include stimulation of lymphoproliferation, lymphotoxin and interferon induction, the elicitation of other lymphokinins, increased production of circulating monocytes, increased production of prostacyclin (a favorable prostaglandin hormone), increased production of endorphins, decreased pain, increased appetite, weight gain, and wound healing.

SPL has also been used to treat bacterial infections, viral infections (flu, respiratory, and gastrointestinal viruses, chronic fatigue syndrome, Epstein-Barr virus, cytomegalovirus, AIDS), Candida overgrowth, hypersensitivity and allergic states, and asthma. It has also been used as a complementary therapy in cancer patients or others who can benefit from immune stimulation. As an approved pharmaceutical treatment for staph, it is available to practicing physicians. SPL is an attractive option for some individuals in need of immune support.[5] It is available from Delmont Laboratory in Swarthmore, Pennsylvania.

SUGGESTED READING

Bee Venom

Benjamin, B. E. "Bee Venom Therapy." *Massage Therapy Journal*, Summer (1990): 16–17.

Billigham, M. "An Anti-Inflammatory Peptide from Bee Venom." *Nature*, Volume 245, September 21 (1973).

Kim, C. M. "Bee Venom Therapy for Arthritis." *Rheumatologie* 41(3): 67–72 (1989).

———. "Bee Venom Therapy—Apitherapy." In *Managing Pain and Stress*. Available from Pain Institute, Union Square, Suite 9-C, 500 Hwy. 35, Red Bank, NJ 07701.

Kinghardt, D. "Bee Venom Therapy for Chronic Pain." *Journal of Neurological and Orthopedic Medicine and Surgery*, Volume 11, Issue 3, October (1990).

Weeks, B. "The Medicinal Uses of Honeybee Products." Apitherapy Workshop, Seattle, Feb. 22, 1992. Available from Bradford S. Weeks, M.D., American Apitherapy Society, P.O. Box 124, Woodsville, NH 03785, (603) 747-2507.

Weissman, G. "Effects of Bee Venom on Experimental Arthritis." *Annals of Rheumatologic Disease* 32, (1973): 466.

Butyric Acid

Cummings, J. H. "Short-Chain Fatty Acids in the Human Colon." *Gut* 22 (1981): 763–779.

Jass, J. R. "Diet, Butyric Acid, and Differentiation of Gastrointestinal Tract Tumors." *Medhypoth* 18 (1985): 113–118.

Watson, J. "Butyric Acid in the Treatment of Cancer." *Lancet* (April 8, 1933): 746–748.

Wright, J. V. "Butyrate Determination and Colon Cancer." *International Clinical Nutrition Review* 9(2): 1989.

Massage and Bodywork

Barlow, Wilfred. *The Alexander Technique: How to Use Your Body Without Stress*. Rochester, VT: Healing Arts Press, 1990.

Brennan, Barbara. *Hands of Light: A Guide to Healing Through the Human Energy Field*. New York: Bantam, 1987, 1988.

Feldenkrais, Moshe. *Awareness Through Movement: Easy-to-do Exercises to Improve Your Posture, Vision, Imagination, and Personal Awareness*. San Francisco: HarperCollins, 1991.

Feiss, George. *Mind Therapies, Body Therapies: A Consumer's Guide*. Millbrae, CA: Celestial Arts, 1975.

Hanna, Thomas. *Somatics: Reawakening the Mind's Control of Movement, Flexibility and Health*. Reading, MA: Addison-Wesley, 1988.

Heller, Joseph and Henkin, William. *Bodywise: Regaining Your Natural Flexibility and Vitality for Maximum Well-Being*. Los Angeles: J.P. Tarcher, 1986.

Kreiger, Dolores, R.N. Ph.D. *The Therapeutic Touch: How to Use Your Hands to Help or Heal*. Englewood Cliffs, NJ: Prentice Hall, 1979.

Leigh, William. *Bodytherapy: From Rolf to Feldenkrais to Tanouye Roshi*, 2nd ed. Vancouver, B.C.: Water Margin Press, 1989.

Lowe, Carl and Nechas, James W. *Whole Body Healing*. Emmaus, PA: Rodale Press.

Macrae, Janet. *Therapeutic Touch: A Practical Guide*. New York: Knopf, 1988.

Ohashi, Wataru. *Do It Yourself Shiatsu*. New York: NAL, 1976.

Pavek, Richard. *The Handbook of SHEN (Specific Human Energy Nexus)*. Sausalito, CA: SHEN Therapy Institute, 1987.

Stone, Randolph, M.D. *Polarity Therapy: The Complete Collected Works*. Reno, NV: CRCS Publications, 1986.

ENERGY MEDICINE: ACUPUNCTURE AND HOMEOPATHY

The term "energy medicine" is used to define a unique domain of healing practice that includes acupuncture and homeopathy. Unlike the nutritional, botanical, and physical modalities with which you are familiar, acupuncture and homeopathy cannot easily be explained in conventional physiologic terms.

The ancient Chinese practice of acupuncture, for example, is based on the philosophy that a cycle of energy flowing through the body controls health and that pain and disease develop when there is a disturbance in that flow. By inserting needles at specific points in the body, an acupuncturist can remedy that imbalance and effect a therapeutic response elsewhere in the body.

Homeopathy is based on the idea that an illness should be treated, not with drugs designed to suppress symptoms, but with an agent that in a healthy person would produce symptoms similar to the illness. Administering a minute (homeopathic) dose of the agent, however, will engage a response in the body to reverse the symptoms and cure the illness.

Because acupuncture and homeopathy work through subtle bioelectric mechanisms induced by "vibrational" and "energetic" influences, both of these techniques have had a difficult time gaining support from the scientific and medical communities. Yet both have proven effective and have gained many adherents in the East and in the West. They are time-tested practices that are worthy of consideration as tools which can support optimal wellness.

ACUPUNCTURE*

Acupuncture, as part of the oldest complete medical system, has probably been used to treat more people than any other method in the history of the world. Stone and iron needles have been found in South America and Egypt, as well as in China, suggesting the use of acupuncture in ancient civilizations. Yet acupuncture is but one of the modalities in a medical system that also features herbal and nutritional therapy, manipulation, massage, therapeutic, internal, and psychological exercises.

Acupuncture occupies a unique position in world medicine as a technology for direct physical adjustment of the nervous system in specific ways. Known as Traditional Chinese Medicine (TCM), the theoretical model of acupuncture, initially transmitted from the texts and academies of China to the West, is actually only a minimal representation of the vast, rich storehouse of Oriental medicine tradition. This traditional knowledge survives in the form of thousands of individual master hierarchies throughout China, Japan, Korea and Vietnam, preserving through oral transmission special techniques and systems of great practical benefit. American and European practitioners, unfettered by traditional loyalties to a particular master tradition, can now select from this multiplicity of styles to develop original syntheses, the East-West medical approaches that promise to propel acupuncture medicine into a new era.

Oriental medicine has traditionally been used for much more than simple pain, which is its common association in the West. Many specialized branches exist, including pediatrics, obstetrics and gynecology, and

*This section was written by Dr. Richard Kitaeff, Naturopathic Physician and Acupuncturist, Director of New Health Medical Center, Seattle, WA.

internal medicine. Today China's official policy is "letting the past serve the present," and encourages the integration of traditional Chinese and modern Western medicine in the training of medical personnel as well as in hospital practice.

How Acupuncture Works

Traditionally, the primary application of acupuncture and its associated therapies has been preventive rather than curative. In fact, the doctor who had to resort to curative procedures was considered inferior to the physician who succeeded in keeping a patient well. In the hierarchy of traditional Chinese medical practitioners, the most highly regarded and honored doctor was the one who counseled patients on their lifestyle. Next in rank was the practitioner who used physical interventions and medications. And least regarded was the purveyor of surgery, who was considered to be violating sacred human flesh. Furthermore, the physician was paid only so long as the patient remained well. One could well speculate on the implications of such a model for the way Western medicine is practiced.

The Scientific Mechanism Theory of Acupuncture Effects
Patients who have experienced this treatment describe it as both energizing and deeply relaxing, because it essentially balances and tonifies the nervous system. According to thousands of research studies carried out in China and the West, acupuncture regulates the nervous system by increasing the number of blood cells and circulating immune agents and by releasing anti-inflammatory and pain-relieving chemicals produced by the body. According to the "gate control" theory by Melzak and Wall,[1] pain messages can be suppressed or "gated" by the stronger nervous system stimuli produced by acupuncture, as well as by acupressure and electroacupuncture.

Yin and Yang Theory
Traditionally, acupuncture is explained in terms of yin and yang, the dual, complementary energy flows in the universe. Yin is the contractive, passive, cold, dark, damp, tendency associated with the feminine principle in nature. Yang is the expansive, active, hot, bright, dry masculine tendency. The balanced expression of these principles in the mind and body reflects an ideal condition of harmony and balance in the universe.

Disease represents an imbalance of the yin and yang tendencies in the body. Acupuncture, Chinese herbs, and related therapies can be used to correct the imbalance through a selection of a specific polarity and dosage of treatment. For example, cauterization therapy—the application of a heated, dry herbal substance at or near acupuncture points—provides an active hot yang tendency suitable for treatment of yin conditions such as paralysis (see box).

Treats a Wide Range of Medical Conditions
The World Health Organization recommends the use of acupuncture for such conditions as arthritis, bursitis, tendonitis, neuritis and neuralgia, back pain, sciatica, neck and shoulder strain, and migraine and tension headaches.

It has also been remarkably successful in treating functional disorders, such as infertility, impotence, epilepsy, diabetic neuropathy and endocrine imbalances, chronic fatigue syndrome, allergies, digestive disorders, asthma and bronchitis, urinary incontinence, constipation, high blood pressure, insomnia, nervousness, and depression. Because of its deep stress-relieving and energizing effects, acupuncture is known to control smoking, weight, and drug addictions. In China, acupuncture is commonly used for analgesia or control of pain in surgery and dental work.

In traditional Chinese medicine, acupuncture is also used to treat medical emergencies such as high fever, cardiac arrhythmias, heart attacks, sudden respiratory failure, unconsciousness, hemorrhage, and seizures. However, where Western medical technology is available, it should be the first treatment choice for all emergencies.

ACUPUNCTURE POINTS AND MERIDIANS

The acupuncture points are relatively sensitive areas often found at anatomical conjunctions and easily detected by their reactivity to pressure or electronic skin resistance measurement. According to Chinese legend, the points were discovered accidentally by soldiers in battle, who found they could ease the pain of wounds by pricking themselves at the sensitive points.

Eventually, these points were found to be organized along meridians, or energy pathways that governed various physiological and psychological functions and anatomical structures. There are twelve main meridians corresponding to such organs as the lung, liver, and kidneys, as well as additional meridians that follow the midline of the trunk, front, back, and other areas of the body.

The meridian of the heart and circulation, for example, which relates also to mental or nervous system balance, runs from the side of the chest down the inside of the arm to the little finger (see Fig. 21–1). In Western medicine, this is the pathway frequently found to manifest during the pain of a heart attack.

Unfortunately, the existence of meridians is not

YIN AND YANG

The qualities of yin and yang are projected to all levels of the cosmos through a system of correspondences. Some of the more general correspondences are listed here:

YIN	YANG
Earth	Heaven
Female	Male
Night	Day
Moon	Sun
Low	High
Heaviness	Lightness
Falling tendency	Rising tendency
Movement inward	Movement outward
Relative stasis	Clear action

It must be remembered that yin and yang are complementary and not contradictory. Nor is one regarded as "good," and the other "bad." Rather, a harmony is sought between them and any imbalance avoided. Because the yin/yang concept is all-pervasive in Chinese thought, it was naturally adopted by the founders of Chinese medicine. Distinguishing between the yin and yang qualities of a person's constitution, or the character of one's illness, is an important step in the process of synthesis necessary to making a traditional diagnosis. Some general medical correspondences are:

YIN	YANG
Interior	Exterior
Front	Back
Lower section	Upper section
Bones	Skin
Inner organs	Outer organs
Blood	Chi (vital energy)
Inhibition	Stimulation
Deficiency	Excess

All of these applications of yin and yang are relative. What is yin in relation to one thing may be yang in relation to another. For example, the front of the body is yin compared to the back. Yet on the front of the body itself, the chest is yang in relation to the abdomen. In traditional physiology, pathology, diagnostics, and treatment, yin and yang provide the broad parameters within which all other observations and conceptualizations are gathered.

widely recognized in Western biomedicine, since they do not correspond to known nerve pathways. However, numerous experimental studies carried out primarily in China and Japan appear to demonstrate acupuncture or bioelectronic effects along traditional meridian lines.

One demonstration occurred in Japan with a patient who had been struck by lightning and whose skin had become hypersensitive. This man could feel an "echo," or current running over the surface of his body from a single acupuncture needle insertion. With his finger, he was able to trace the pathways of the energy as it moved at a speed much slower than that of nerve impulses.[2] It was found that the pathways he traced corresponded exactly to those of the traditional meridian network throughout the body.

Besides the meridian system, acupuncture medicine includes certain microsystems that act as holograms of the whole body; for example, in the ear (see Fig. 21–2) and on the hand and the scalp. These microsystems have been found to be extremely valuable for both diagnosis and treatment of pain and functional disorders. Stimulation of lines on the scalp, for example, is remarkably effective in reversing the motor dysfunctions brought about by a stroke.

Acupuncture Diagnostic Procedures

An important part of the overall evaluation is the acupuncturist's assessment of the relative yin or yang balance of the patient's energic tendency, or *chi* (often spelled *Qi*). In fact, several specific types of chi are cited in traditional Chinese medical texts corresponding to different organs, areas of the body, energy channels or meridians, and physiological processes like respiration, digestion, and elimination. The fundamental organ systems of the body are thought to function in phase or in correspondence not only with yin and yang, but also with the energies represented by the five elements: earth, metal, water, wood, and fire.

Relationships of mutual reinforcement and suppression among these organs underlie states of health and disease. The causes of disease may be internal—emotions like anger, which correlates with the liver; fear, which is related to kidney function; and grief, which is related to the lungs. Or it may have the characteristics of external forces like cold, heat, wind, and dampness. Thus a typical pattern of energy imbalance might be described as liver/heat or kidney/yin deficiency (see the following table).

To diagnose such patterns, the acupuncturist examines the patient's pulses, as well as tongue, face, and physical features, and palpates test points for tenderness. The pulse system in Chinese medicine is highly developed. There are six positions on each wrist, and numerous differences in pulsebeats that a trained practitioner uses to determine the frequency, intensity, and quality of the pulse and thus the energy condition of the corresponding internal organ systems.

In recent years an electronic device, the AMI, was developed in Japan to measure the electrical resistance and potential at the acupuncture meridian terminal points on the fingers and toes. The AMI has been used for preliminary diagnostic screening of government employees, since its measurements of internal organ function have been shown to predict serious pathology, later corroborated by conventional Western diagnostic testing.[3]

Treating Conditions Through Acupuncture

Based on the diagnosis of an energy imbalance, the acupuncturist selects points in the local area of the problem, at a distance along the related meridian line or at other theoretically relevant points. The therapeutic strategy may be to surround an area of pain or inflammation, or to draw the excess energy away along the meridian to a remote terminal.

In general, the basic treatment principles are to tonify or stimulate in a case of deficient energy, and to sedate or disperse when the energy pattern is one of excess. Very fine needles of different lengths may be used. The sensation they produce is usually a brief pinprick or dull ache followed very shortly by the feeling of warmth, energy, and deep relaxation. Besides needle stimulation of the points, the acupuncturist may use finger acupressure, and heat or moxybustion. A mild, low-frequency tingling electronic current may be passed through the needles particularly for relief of severe pain.

Laser stimulation of acupuncture points is becoming a popular alternative, especially for patients who don't like needles. Some consider this treatment comparable to acupuncture. Laser stimulation given for fifteen to thirty seconds could have effects similar to those of acupuncture needles left in place for thirty minutes.

Acupuncture in the Modern World

The future of acupuncture seems to lie in an expansion of traditional medical philosophical concepts into the technological approach of a new energy medicine. The AMI computerized electronic assessment of the meridian energetic condition reflects this trend, as do the technologies of laser, magnetic, electronic, and ultrasonic stimulation of the acupuncture points.

Dr. Hiroshi Motoyama of Japan, who developed the AMI device, has also pioneered an instrument that surveys the electromagnetic energy field emitted from the body in the area of different organ systems. He correlates this data with the results of meridian measurement.

Another Japanese researcher, Dr. Yoshio Manaka,

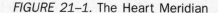

FIGURE 21–1. The Heart Meridian

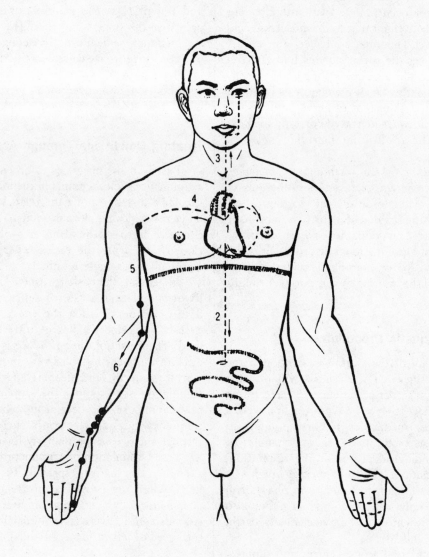

The heart meridian has three branches, each of which begins in the heart (1). One branch runs downward through the diaphragm (2) to connect to the small intestine. A second branch runs upward from the heart along the side of the throat (3) to meet the eye. The third branch runs across the chest from the heart to the lung (4), then descends and emerges in the underarm. It passes along the midline of the inside of the upper arm (5), runs downward across the inner elbow, along the midline of the inside of the forearm (6), crosses the wrist and palm (7), and terminates at the inside tip of the little finger, where it connects with the small intestine meridian.

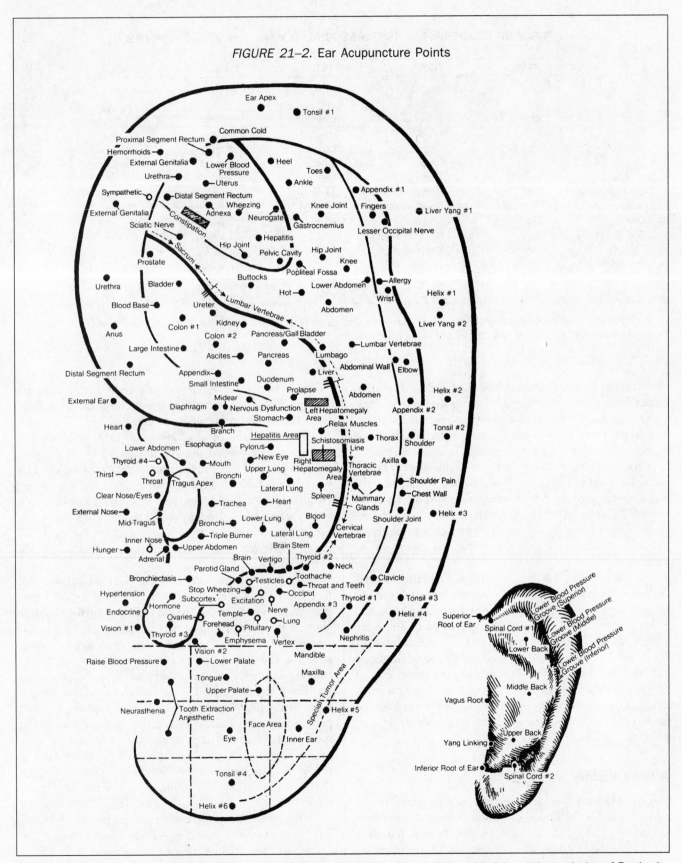

FIGURE 21–2. Ear Acupuncture Points

TABLE OF CORRESPONDENCES ASSOCIATED WITH THE FIVE ELEMENTS

	WOOD	FIRE	EARTH	METAL	WATER
Direction	East	South	Center	West	North
Season	Spring	Summer	Long summer	Autumn	Winter
Climatic condition	Wind	Summer heat	Dampness	Dryness	Cold
Process	Birth	Growth	Transformation	Harvest	Storage
Color	Green	Red	Yellow	White	Black
Taste	Sour	Bitter	Sweet	Pungent	Salty
Smell	Goatish	Burning	Fragrant	Rank	Rotten
Yin organ	Liver	Heart	Spleen	Lungs	Kidneys
Yang organ	Gallbladder	Small intestine	Stomach	Large intestine	Bladder
Opening	Eyes	Tongue	Mouth	Nose	Ears
Tissue	Sinews	Blood vessels	Flesh	Skin/Hair	Bones
Emotion	Anger	Happiness	Pensiveness	Sadness	Fear
Human sound	Shout	Laughter	Song	Weeping	Groan

Reprinted from Acupuncture: A Comprehensive Text, *Shanghai College of Traditional Chinese Medicine, with permission of Eastland Press, P.O. Box 99749, Seattle, WA 98199. All rights reserved.*

restores the balance between areas of excess and deficiency in the body by using a diode to direct bioelectric energy between acupuncture points connected by a simple cable. There is no input from an external electronic source—only the body's own energy is involved.[4]

Practitioners of the auricular medicine system developed by French physician Paul Nogier, M.D., use the pulse to measure the body's reaction to specific test substances "presented" through specialized filters to the reflex areas of the ear. The electromagnetic feedback provides practitioners with diagnostic and treatment information.

In Europe and America, electronic evaluation of meridians is becoming increasingly popular through the use of the Vega test, Dermatron, Computron, Interro, and Eclosian devices. These have the capacity to evaluate the effects on an individual of samples of medications, or food, or allergens placed in a circuit between the body and the test instrument.[5] This means that the effects of various foods, environmental toxins, microorganisms, drugs, vitamins, herbs, and homeopathic remedies can be assessed in relation to specific organ systems or acupuncture points in the body.

A Case History

Dr. Manaka has described the disease state as the product of an imbalance or subtle bias in the nervous system. It is this bias that can be detected by acupuncture methods of diagnosis. The stimulation of acupuncture points, by whatever means, then provides a counterbias that sets in motion the healing process.

When a person's lifestyle doesn't undo the rebalancing efforts, then homeostasis—the condition of physiological balance—is the ultimate result.

The methods of diagnosis and treatment used in acupuncture medicine may be illustrated by an example taken from a recent publication, *Acupuncture Case Histories from China.*[6] In a case of premenstrual pain in a twenty-two-year-old woman, cramps, beginning one week before the period, radiated to the lower back and upper abdominal regions. Chinese medical theory distinguishes between excess and deficiency types of painful menstruation.

In this case, the occurrence of pain several days before the onset of the period and the fitful nature of the pain were indications of the excess type. Further analysis showed that the condition was related to the liver organ system, which in traditional Chinese medicine is responsible for the storage of blood and has a regulating or calming influence on the emotions.

From the integrated mind-body perspective of Oriental medicine, low spirits in the patient, coupled with pain in the upper abdomen, clots in the dark-colored menstrual flow, the dark appearance and purple spots on the tongue, plus a "wiry" pulse could all be associated with "stagnant" energy in the liver. A connecting channel transmitted this influence to the uterus, causing pain.

Two of the acupuncture treatment points were chosen from the liver meridian—Liver-3 on the foot and Liver-14 in the area of the ribs overlying the liver. Stimulation of these points was intended to calm the liver and regulate the energy. The other points—CV-6 in the lower abdomen and SP-6 in the leg—were combined to regulate the flow of energy and blood to the area of the lower organs or "lower burner," of which the uterus is a part. The needling manipulation technique was one designed to sedate the excess liver energy.

Treatment was carried out daily, starting a week before the onset of the menstrual period and continuing until the end of the period. The needles were left in place for twenty minutes during each treatment session. After three treatments, the pain diminished and accompanying symptoms improved. When treatment was resumed a week before the next period, no pain was reported, except for slight discomfort in the lower abdomen, and menstrual flow was normal in color. A six-month follow-up indicated no relapse.

HOMEOPATHY

Like acupuncture, a state of homeostasis—physiologic balance—is a primary goal of homeopathy, a system of natural medicine developed in the late 1700s by the German physician Samuel Hahnemann. Hahnemann strove to develop remedies that were both safer and more effective than those employed by the medical profession in the late eighteenth century. In large part, he attained his goal. In fact, by the late 1800s, there were 110 homeopathic hospitals and 145 homeopathic dispensaries in the United States alone, successfully treating typhoid fever, yellow fever, cholera, and other diseases of the time that carried a significant mortality rate.

However, when modern medicine and the pharmaceutical industry emerged in the early 1900s, their politicking in this country all but destroyed homeopathic practice. Nevertheless, homeopathy's popularity abroad remained strong, and its growing reputation in England, where it has been incorporated into the British national health system, as well as in Europe, Greece, India, Mexico, and Argentina, has helped fuel its current renaissance in the United States.

How It Works

A homeopathic remedy for a symptom is a microdilution or microdose of the very same plant, mineral, or chemical substance that in its original concentration will bring on that illness. For instance, ipecac syrup induces nausea and vomiting, while homeopathic ipecac diminishes nausea and vomiting. Thus homeopathy embodies the principle of "like curing like."

Equally fascinating is the fact that the weaker the dilution, thus the smaller the microdose, the stronger and deeper-acting the remedy. In fact, the most dilute remedies have no detectable original active ingredient left. Their effect is created by the very "essence" or energy of the substance. Such concepts defy conventional medical precepts, which is why they engender much skepticism toward homeopathic practice.

Homeopathy has several distinct advantages over conventional drug therapy. Homeopathic remedies:

- Are nontoxic. They rarely cause any harm.
- Effect healing at levels deeper than the superficial suppression of symptoms common to conventional drug therapy, making them extremely useful in the treatment of chronic conditions.
- Are ideal for infants and children who cannot swallow pills, or who will balk at the taste of many medications or herbs. Youngsters seem to prefer the tiny, sweet-tasting homeopathic tablets, which dissolve easily in the mouth.
- Can be effective when other alternative approaches have failed, and for illnesses that are thought to be "untreatable."

A correctly prescribed homeopathic remedy will catalyze a defense response, stimulate heightened vitality, and bring an individual back to health. By restoring balance and strength at physical, mental, and emotional levels, homeopathy can effect true cures because the whole individual is being treated. A classical homeopath will take a very unusual medical history, scrutinizing all related symptoms while extracting the nature and characteristics of personality, emotions, and constitutional traits.

Common questions in a homeopathic case-taking may include:

- Are the symptoms worse or better in the night or day, from cold air or a warm room, from drinking hot or cold fluids, from movement or being still, from lying down or sitting up, from being touched or held or being left alone?
- Is there fear, irritability, whining, weeping, explosive anger, or apathy?
- Is there thirst, hunger, chills, sweats, a very red face, one cheek red and the other pale?
- Did symptoms come on suddenly or gradually?

Two individuals with the same diagnosis of bronchitis will have very different responses to the questions above (and the many other questions that are asked), and therefore would be prescribed different remedies. Thus, homeopathy differs from conventional medicine in that it treats the individual with the disease rather than the disease alone. Herein lies one of the reasons for homeopathy's success.

One of my patients was helped significantly with thyroid medication, supplemental hydrochloric acid, and the removal of wheat and several other allergy-causing foods from her diet. Soon many of her symptoms subsided, her energy and glow returned, and she was no longer susceptible to recurrent bronchitis. It was one of those patient-practitioner exchanges in which she was quite pleased and I was quite gratified.

Several months later, however, she returned and told me that she had felt somewhat burdened by the regimen. She had seen a homeopathic physician, and, under his treatment with remedies specific to her total person, she was able to discontinue both the hydrochloric acid and thyroid supplements and begin to eat what used to be allergy-causing foods. She retained her improved health. Although my approach had been successful, in comparison to the results with homeopathy it seemed only palliative.

Like any medical modality, homeopathy will appeal to some individuals and not to others. I have seen it work exceptionally well in some individuals, yet I have known others who found it ineffective. Human beings and their illnesses can be extraordinarily complicated, multilayered, and baffling. Selecting the right homeopathic remedy can be an enormous challenge. In some cases a treatment fails because of an incorrect remedy. In others, both the practitioner's and the patient's unwillingness to persevere may play a role. Constitutional homeopathic treatment can take many months, and some individuals find this approach difficult to deal with given their "magic bullet/quick cure" mentality.

Homeopathic Self-Care

Homeopathy lends itself extremely well to self-care, particularly in cases of common illnesses and injuries. Individuals can learn to treat minor problems before they require medical intervention. My wife has no medical background, yet through self-help homeopathy books and an astute sense of observation, she has successfully treated our children homeopathically for coughs, colds, sore throats, ear infections, headaches, fever, stomach flu, insect bites, bee stings, itching, sprains, contusions, injuries to fingers and toes, burns, cuts, head injuries, sleeplessness, irritability, teething, and colic.

After you become more knowledgeable about different remedies, your confidence will increase and the process becomes easier. Knowing the remedies is key. They have distinct characteristics, and the art is to observe the predominant features of the patient and of the illness and match them to a remedy. Sometimes the key indicator is a part of the person's mood, such as intense irritability (chamomile), or mild whining (pulsatilla). Sometimes the indicator is the color of the patient's face (bright red: belladonna) or the thick, sticky nature of the nasal discharge (kalibicrom). The next section lists a few common remedies to help get you started. For more in-

formation, consult the books in the Suggested Reading list at the end of this chapter.

Although individualizing a case and finding the single best remedy will bring the most gratifying results, such an endeavor requires time, patience, and learning. Prepared homeopathic combination formulas are easier to use and are often effective. Simply choose the formula that corresponds to your primary complaint, such as ear infection, sore throat, hay fever, sinus infection, anxiety, insomnia, etc. A combination is formulated to include several of the most common remedies indicated for the main complaint and associated symptoms, so there is a good chance that it will be effective even without individualization.

Homeopathic preparations for home use are usually low-potency and therefore useful for acute problems. Some are available through direct mail and health food stores; others are sold only to health professionals. The resources list on page 481 notes several companies that sell home remedy kits for personal use.

Homeopathic First Aid

Many homeopathic remedies can be used as first-aid measures. By knowing which remedies are specific to which ailments, appropriate first-aid treatment can be instituted. For 6x or 12x strength, take four tablets dissolved in the mouth every fifteen to sixty minutes as needed until symptoms improve, then reduce frequency of dose or discontinue the remedy when you note improvement. Take immediately or as soon as possible after symptoms appear. You can use stronger potencies and repeat doses less often. For persistent or serious symptoms, consult a physician.

Aconite napellus For sudden high fevers before fever breaks or any sudden and intense onset of chills, malaise, or other symptoms, especially when accompanied by fear, panic, anguish, or restlessness. Also good for croup.

Apis mellifica For bee sting or other insect sting or bite.

Arnica montana For any bruises, swellings, strains, sprains, concussion, pain from trauma. Arnica also comes in gel and ointment forms for topical applications.

Belladonna For fevers and infections when the person looks red-hot and burning, has a strawberry-looking tongue—red with stippled taste buds—is bothered by light, has dry, hot skin, but is not thirsty.

Cantharis For second-degree burns (those with blisters). Any burning symptoms from heel blisters, cystitis (bladder infections), insect bites, or stings.

Chamomile For cold, flu, earache, or other condition, when accompanied by irritability, unreasonableness, restlessness, irascibility, or general agitation that is difficult to comfort. This remedy is geared more toward calming the emotional and mental state accompanying many physical illnesses, and not so much toward the illness itself. Also good for insomnia, restlessness, and teething.

Hypericum perforatum For sharp neural pains (neuritis), especially in fingertips. Use if arnica does not work.

Ledum For any puncture-type injuries. Also useful for spider bites.

Rhus toxicodendron For poison oak or poison ivy.

Ruta graveolens For any joint injuries after one or two days of treatment with arnica.

Urtica urens For first-degree burn (sunburn); also, hives and any nonspecific itching.

RESOURCES

Acupuncture

For more information on acupuncture and for referrals, contact state acupuncture associations or the American Association of Acupuncture and Oriental Medicine, 433 Front Street, Catasauqua, PA 18032-2506, (610) 433-2448.

Institute for Advanced Training and Research in East-West Healing Arts, 23700 Edmonds Way, Edmonds, WA 98026, (206) 775-6001.
Medical Acupuncture for Physicians, UCLA Extension, 10995 LeConte Ave., Los Angeles, CA 90024-2883, (310) 794-7277.
Northwest Institute of Acupuncture and Oriental Medicine, 1307 N. 45th, Seattle, WA 98103, (206) 633-2419.

Homeopathy

Foundation for Homeopathic Education and Research, 2124 Kittredge St., Berkeley, CA 94704, (510) 649-8930.
Homeopathic Education Services, 2124 Kittredge St., Berkeley, CA 94704, (510) 649-0294.

International Foundation for Homeopathy, 2366 Eastlake Ave. E., #301, Seattle, WA 98012, (206) 324-8230.

Manufacturers of Homeopathic Remedies

Boericke and Tafel, 2381 Circadian Way, Santa Rosa, CA 95407, (707) 571-8202.
Biological Homeopathic Industries, Inc. P.O. Box 11280, Albuquerque, NM 87192, (505) 293-3843.
Boiron/Borneman, 1208 Amosland Road, Norwood, PA 19074, (215) 532-2035 or (800) 253-8823.
Dolisos, 3014 Rigel Ave., Las Vegas, NV 89102, (702) 871-7153.
Luyties Pharmacal Company Homeopathic Medicine, P.O. Box 8080 St. Louis, MO 63156, (314) 533-9600.
Standard Homeopathic Co. 210 W. 131st St., Box 61067, Los Angeles, CA 90061, (800) 624-9659 or (213) 321-4284.

SUGGESTED READING

Acupuncture

Beinfield, Harriet and Korngold, Efrem. *Between Heaven and Earth: A Guide to Chinese Medicine.* New York: Ballantine, 1991.
Bensky, Dan, and O'Connor, John, eds. *Acupuncture: A Comprehensive Text.* Chicago: Eastland, 1981.
Kaptchuk, Ted J. *The Web that Has No Weaver.* New York: Congdon & Weed, 1983.
Manaka, Yoshio, and Urquhart, Ian. *A Layman's Guide to Acupuncture.* New York: Weather Hill, 1972.

Homeopathy

Cummings, Stephen, and Ullman, Dana. *Everybody's Guide to Homeopathic Medicines: Taking Care of Yourself and Your Family with Safe and Effective Remedies.* Los Angeles: Tarcher/New York: St. Martin's Press, 1984.
Horvilleur, Alain, M.D. *The Family Guide to Homeopathy.* Arlington, VA: Health and Homeopathy Publishing, Inc., 1986.
Panos, Maesimund, and Heimlich, Jane. *Homeopathic Medicine at Home: Natural Remedies for Everyday Ailments and Minor Injuries.* Los Angeles: Tarcher/Boston: Houghton Mifflin, 1980.
Vithoulkas, George. *Homeopathy: Medicine of the New Man.* Englewood, NJ: Prentice-Hall, 1979.

PART SIX

YOU AND THE
MEDICAL PROFESSION

CHAPTER 22

CHOOSING AND RELATING TO YOUR DOCTOR

CHOOSING THE RIGHT HEALTH CARE PROVIDER

You may already be aware that the concept of self-care extends beyond what you can do for yourself directly. It also includes making appropriate choices and wise use of health care practitioners. As empowered as you might feel in learning and implementing self-care skills, it is also important to remember that others can be of great help and guidance to you, and that you may benefit from their knowledge, experience, and services. Therefore I would like to offer you some suggestions on the process, the pitfalls, and pointers of choosing and relating to a medical doctor, although much of this information will apply to other kinds of practitioners as well, whether they are chiropractic, osteopathic, naturopathic, or Ayurvedic physicians.

Even with the numerous options for alternative health care practitioners, and despite the known inadequacies of conventional medicine, a medical doctor is a vital member of your health care team. Although this professional may not be able to fill all your health needs, he or she may provide crisis care more effectively than anyone else for a serious illness or injury. Your doctor can establish a diagnosis for a chronic problem, perform screening tests for early detection of disease, and execute needed surgical or technological procedures. Furthermore, if your rapport and relationship with a physician is especially good, he or she may be willing, upon your request, to administer or supervise an alternative therapy. But without this strong relationship, a conventional medical doctor would probably not even consider such a deviation from standard care.

There are many excellent practicing physicians, and I advise you to find one and develop a close and contin-uing relationship with him or her. If you desire such a relationship and are interested in genuine healing and learning, you will need to learn several key pieces of information about the practitioner you have in mind.

- What are the specific skills and approaches offered: Is the physician and his or her associates skilled in the areas that are particularly related to your needs?
- Is the physician competent and effective? What is the degree of experience and success the physician and his or her associates have had with your problems and/or goals?
- How much time does the physician spend with each patient one-on-one initially and on subsequent visits? How many people does he or she see generally on any given day? Does the scheduling policy allow enough time for sufficient one-on-one consultation?
- What type of professional training does your physician have? What do you know about his standing in the profession?
- What types of services are offered? What services does the physician provide directly; which ones are provided by associates; and what is their level of expertise?
- What is the cost of the various services, including laboratory tests? Can he or she substitute recent test results you may have had done by other health care providers? What is the average cost of an initial visit and subsequent visits? Find out if your insurance plan is accepted and exactly what services are and are not covered by it.
- Assess the physician's inner qualities. Is he or she compassionate, genuine, and caring? Does he or she take the time to explain diagnoses and procedures to you,

and make certain you understand your options? What is the attitude of the entire office?

• Does the physician practice any complementary or alternative approaches or at least recognize their validity?

A good place to begin gathering this information is with a recommendation from a friend or health care professional who knows you well. However, you may need to resort to the Yellow Pages or a referral list from an organization or publication. Either way, you must find out for yourself if a physician is right for you.

You may be able to establish enough confidence in the "rightness" of a physician from a phone conversation with a staff member, either a receptionist or nurse, to schedule an initial visit. If not, ask to speak directly with the physician to get answers to any questions his or her staff cannot provide. If this isn't possible, you may need to talk with the physician in person before you can know if the chemistry between you is good. By scheduling a brief interview expressly to determine if you will be comfortable working with this doctor, you should be able to find out enough without accruing significant expense. If your experience is favorable, you can schedule an appointment.

In interviewing the physician, clearly state your goals and interests, how you want to be helped, and perhaps how you do not want to be helped. Ask if he or she can genuinely assist you in these ways. If the answer is yes, inquire a little further as to how. Assess the physician's reaction carefully. Would you want to be addressed in this way when asking about a part of your body, especially when you are ill or worried?

Keep the interview short. In five or ten minutes you should be able tell if you feel good or not working intimately with this person. Be honest and real. And be sure to ask if he or she would feel comfortable working with you. There are many physicians who, unfortunately, feel they should work with every well-meaning and good-paying person who seeks their services. Giving the physician the opportunity to be honest and real in this way—in essence, giving "permission" to refer you to a colleague if he or she feels uncomfortable working with you—may be a great gift to you both.

The whole process may have the additional effect on the physician of becoming more clear, more communicative, and accountable. And if you decide to go elsewhere because he/she does not genuinely offer a nutritional, preventive, or wellness focus (if that happens to be your interest), perhaps your request might stimulate the doctor to start educating him/herself in these areas.

Though not a surefire indicator, if your request for an interview is met with an unfavorable reaction, this may be a sign that this office does not value or recognize the interpersonal healing factors involved in the relationship between practitioners and their patients. It also may reflect an extremely busy and popular physician, but such a reaction is still noteworthy, for it may signal how you will be treated if you make any other "unusual" requests.

Keep in mind that some holistic and alternative physicians—just like some conventional physicians—are more interested in their techniques and tools than in the patients they treat. Sometimes, unfortunately, the physician in question is the only one in your area offering the techniques and competence you need, yet the chemistry between you is not the best. In such cases, you may still need to see this practitioner simply for the needed specialized treatment, but look elsewhere for a source of compassion.

When looking for the right helping professional, remember to be the same intelligent consumer you are when shopping for a car or a home. After all, your body not only gets you around, it's where you live.

HOLISTIC HEALTH CARE

"Holistic" is a much maligned and misunderstood term, partly because of its association with nonscientific practices and often nondegreed practitioners. It is derived from the Greek root *holos*, meaning "whole."

Holistic medicine is primarily concerned with the whole person, and encompasses both conventional care and complementary/alternative modalities. It focuses on treating illness and maintaining health on all levels—physical, mental, emotional, spiritual, and environmental.

Calling herbal or nutritional medicine holistic simply because it is "alternative" is as inaccurate as calling pharmaceutically based medicine not holistic simply because it is conventional. If either practice is applied without regard for all the levels on which an individual thrives, it cannot be considered holistic. Chemotherapy, for example, can be considered part of holistic care if a particular patient's fear, poor nutritional status, marital unhappiness, and need for an exercise program are recognized along with the cancer, and if measures are taken to meet these issues. A naturopathic colon- and liver-cleansing regimen can also be called holistic if that patient's lack of self-esteem and mismanaged stress are recognized along with the gastrointestinal toxicity. After all, the two former conditions fueled the patient's eating abuses, which in turn have most directly resulted in the physical illness.

Holistic, then, does not refer to any particular modality, but to the concept of considering the *whole* patient when analyzing an illness. A holistic practitioner certainly can't be expected to meet every need of a patient. But he or she can acknowledge that human beings

PRINCIPLES OF HOLISTIC MEDICAL PRACTICE*

1. Holistic physicians embrace a variety of safe, effective options in diagnosis and treatment, including:
     - education for lifestyle changes and self-care;
     - complementary approaches; and
     - conventional drugs and surgery.
2. Searching for the underlying causes of disease is preferable to treating symptoms alone.
3. Holistic physicians expend as much effort in establishing what kind of patient has a disease as they do in establishing what kind of disease a patient has.
4. It is preferable to diagnose and treat patients as unique individuals rather than as members of a disease category.
5. When possible, lifestyle modifications are preferable to drugs and surgery as initial therapeutic options.
6. Prevention is preferable to treatment and is usually *more* cost-effective. The *most* cost-effective approach evokes the patient's own innate healing capabilities.
7. Illness is viewed as a manifestation of a dysfunction of the whole person, not as an isolated event.
8. In most situations encouragement of patient autonomy is preferable to decisions imposed by physicians.
9. The ideal physician-patient relationship considers the needs, desires, awareness, and insight of the patient as well as those of the physician.
10. The quality of the relationship established between physician and patient is a major determinant of healing outcomes.
11. Physicians significantly influence patients by their example.
12. Illness, pain, and the dying process can be learning opportunities for patients and physicians.
13. Holistic physicians encourage patients to evoke the healing power of love, hope, humor, and enthusiasm and to release the toxic consequences of hostility, shame, greed, depression, and prolonged fear, anger, and grief.
14. Unconditional love is life's most powerful medicine. Physicians strive to adopt an attitude of unconditional love for patients, themselves, and other practitioners.
15. Optimal health is much more than the absence of sickness. It is the conscious pursuit of the highest qualities of the spiritual, mental, emotional, physical, environmental, and social aspects of the human experience.

*Reprinted by permission of the American Holistic Medical Association.

are complex and multilayered, and that a problem in one area can often cause an ailment in another. Treating only the ailment and not the underlying problem constitutes incomplete treatment. As a result, appropriate and timely referrals are very much a part of holistic total health care.

The American Holistic Medical Association, at 4101 Lake Boone Trail, Suite 201, Raleigh, NC 27607, (919) 787-5146, is the professional medical organization that has been my primary inspiration in moving toward the wholeness approach. The educational meetings of the AHMA have taught me to employ a broader and more complete perspective in the care I offer my patients. They have also taught me to apply this perspective to myself and my own personal health and happiness. Over the years, I've come to realize that the quality of care I provide for my patients depends on the quality of care I provide for myself. How can I examine a patient holistically, with insight and depth, if I'm not capable of ministering to myself this way?

The biblical proverb "Physician, heal thyself" remains the best advice for all helping professionals. No matter how many degrees acquired, diplomas mounted on the wall, or techniques mastered, only the individual who has embraced this self-healing philosophy can truly be considered a holistic practitioner. (For an excellent overview of holistic medicine, see *Holistic Medicine: A Meeting of East and West* by Henry Edward Altenberg, M.D.: Japan Publications, 1992).

RELATING TO YOUR DOCTOR

Once you have chosen or been assigned a doctor or other health care professional, or if you already have an established relationship with one, there is much you can do to enhance the outcome of your visits and the quality of your relationship. You may find the following suggestions helpful.

- Address your doctor by his or her first name, if you are comfortable with that, after asking if he or she is comfortable. This tends to remind the physician that he or she needs to be a genuine person, not just a genuine doctor. And if the doctor's delivery is stiff and couched in professional jargon, hearing his or her first name may soften that style.
- Toward the beginning of the visit, ask how the doctor is feeling, perhaps as part of your greeting. Show your concern. In this way you're acknowledging his or her humanness. The doctor may then treat you not just as another patient, but as more of an equal.
- Appearances can influence anyone, even your doctor, and can affect the quality of care you receive. If you consistently show up looking shabby, your doctor may relate the level of care you give to your own appearance to the level of expectation you have of the quality of your health care. I'm not suggesting that you dress up or wear clothes that are not you. If your illness or circumstances do not get in the way, simply be clean and reasonable in your appearance.
- Don't just call your doctor when you're sick. If you get better after treatment, let your doctor know by a note or through the receptionist that you're feeling better, and thank him or her. Most of the time doctors only hear from patients when something is wrong. It is a breath of fresh air to receive such a thank-you. When your doctor receives genuine appreciation from you, he or she may feel more motivated to go the extra mile for you in the future.
- Tell your doctor if his or her compassion, loving presence, or loving touch moved you or helped you in a special way. A doctor usually gets recognition for making the right diagnosis, prescribing an effective drug, or doing a successful procedure, and this only from colleagues. By acknowledging the quality of his or her presence, you may be reminding your doctor of the importance of that side of healing and giving him or her permission to nurture those qualities and show them more often.
- Let your doctor know that you do not expect complete expertise on every question or issue you raise, and that it comforts you to hear an honest "I don't know."
- Bring to your visit a list of concerns and questions so you can remember all your goals for the visit and get as much out of it as possible. Prioritize the list so you can cover the most important items. Don't save your main reason for coming until the last few minutes, or it won't get sufficient attention. On the other hand, if the issue is of a very sensitive nature, you may want to get to know the doctor better in order to determine whether or not you can trust him or her.
- Respect your doctor's time constraints, but respect even more your own need for his or her time and attention. Find the right balance. If you consistently feel shortchanged, bring this up in a responsible way. If you can't work things out to your satisfaction, or if you're made to feel that your concerns are excessive, perhaps you'd do better and be more comfortable with someone else.
- If you're feeling sick, weak, or not thinking clearly, bring along a close friend or family member as your advocate. Such a companion can also be useful if you tend not to ask for what you want, or find it hard to stick up for yourself, or are easily intimidated.
- Take careful note of any intimidation, arrogance, or condescension you feel from your doctor. These qualities often indicate a physician who needs supreme authority and a passive, obedient client and staff.
- If you don't understand a concept or a treatment recommendation, ask (or have your companion ask) to have it explained again. If there is resistance on your doctor's part, it may be because he or she is rushed. However, he or she may not realize that a thorough understanding of the treatment recommendations helps you maintain your role as an active participant in your own health care. Some doctors, in fact, don't want you to understand anything, or don't care whether you understand. They simply want you to comply with their recommendations.
- In making a decision about a treatment recommendation, always ask about the percentage of success for such a treatment, given someone in your particular state; any common side effects; and the likelihood of your experiencing them.
- If you do not like the implications of your doctor's recommendations, ask about other effective options. Do not be surprised if you're told that there are no other effective treatment options. You may need to see a different kind of health practitioner, one with a

different background and belief system, to find out about your range of options. Ask what the probable outcome would be if you followed no treatment at all. After all, some treatments may be worse than the ailment, and many ailments will subside on their own.

- If you're advised by your primary care doctor to see a specialist for a specific treatment or procedure that you don't quite feel comfortable with, try to engage his or her trust. Ask what he or she would do as a patient under the circumstances. Your doctor might be candid enough to tell you something off the record that's different from the original advice.

- If your doctor recommends a costly or controversial treatment or procedure and you don't feel quite comfortable about it, express your desire to seek a second opinion. If you encounter hostility or impatience, chances are a second opinion might reveal that you may not even require the treatment. In any case, the type of health insurance policy you have may require a second opinion, depending on the procedure in question.

- If you seek a second opinion, it's also important to consult someone who has no financial incentive bearing on the decision. Let that physician know that you will have the procedure done elsewhere if you decide to go ahead with it, that you are only asking for an opinion about whether or not the treatment is necessary. Select someone who is not a close colleague of your doctor.

- It may also prove worthwhile to consult a type of practitioner who offers alternative approaches. As an example, several women with Class II Pap smears (mildly abnormal cellular changes in the cervix) who consulted me had been advised by their gynecologists to undergo laser surgery "to prevent cervical cancer," or so they were told. I advised them to take folic acid, vitamin C, and vitamin A and to have a repeat Pap smear in three months before even considering surgery. All cases reverted to Class I (normal). I also advised them to be leery about physicians who seemed overenthusiastic about performing procedures.

- If you are diagnosed with cancer (or any other major illness) and are advised to undergo a specific treatment, ask your doctor how many patients with the same diagnosis at the same stage he or she has treated similarly. Ask about the doctor's percentage of success—in other words, how many of these patients were alive and well after five years, and after ten years, and with what side effects or complications.

You may feel more confident if, for example, you are told about four hundred other patients with a success rate between 80 and 90 percent, rather than twenty people, with a success rate of 50 percent. You must also weigh the side effects and complications of treatment along with the success rates as you make your decision.

- If you're dissatisfied with your doctor, write and tell him or her exactly why. Do it in a civil and responsible way that encourages a civil response. Often the problem involves a simple misunderstanding that honest communication will repair. You may be surprised to know how much your doctor honors you, and also how much you might be able to teach him or her.

I've written many thank-you letters in response to "hate mail"—letters from dissatisfied patients who cared enough and took the time to voice their complaints and point out my shortcomings. I've become a better doctor from such feedback, and I've also developed some deeply satisfying relationships as a result. If your letter is reasonable and you get back a defensive or condescending response—or no response at all—it may be that you would fare better with another physician.

- If your doctor has been unable to help you, and you find a cure or significant contributing factor to your well-being elsewhere, write your doctor and share your discoveries. While your doctor may not be open to learning something new, your letter may still encourage him or her to be more open in the future. Send photocopies of magazine or journal articles or a book chapter or whole books that you have found significant and would like to share.

Physicians cannot possibly keep current in more than a few areas. I have become aware of many new treatments and developments relevant to my practice through information sent by my patients. Take note if your doctor is above learning anything from you.

There is a transformative movement just now beginning to take root in U.S. medicine. Whereas traditionally, medical care dictated what was best for patients, now the tables are turning. Finally, there is a growing recognition that patients' experiences of their illnesses and care can influence and improve the standard of medical care. (See the article by Stanley Joel Reiser, M.D., "The Era of the Patient: Using the Experience of Illness in Shaping the Missions of Health Care," in the *Journal of the American Medical Association*, Volume 269, Number 8; pages 1012–1017, February 24, 1993.)

If you have a long-standing relationship with your doctor and have worked on some problems together that have not been adequately helped by recommended treatments, try telling your doctor the following:

"We both know you have helped me significantly, and I respect your medical judgment. But I still have a number of persistent symptoms that don't seem to be responding to the treatments we've tried. So I've done some research on my own since I know you don't have the time to look into all these things. Here's what I've come up with. [Explain what you've found and stress the safety or low toxicity of your choice, if that's the case.] I very much wish you'll consider giving me this test or this treatment."

Have some pertinent articles, photocopied chapters, or books with you. If your doctor isn't willing right then to help you in the way you've requested, but is willing to look at the literature, make it clear that you'd appreciate his or her professional review of these options. When you talk again, the fact that you've done your homework, coupled with your perseverance and goodwill—not to mention the persistence of your symptoms—may persuade your physician to try an alternative approach.

- Find an acceptable balance between knowing what to expect from your doctor (seeking the services and relationship he or she is capable of) and providing your input to make the relationship more to your liking.

MUTUAL RELATIONSHIP, MUTUAL RESPONSIBILITY

The patient–doctor relationship is like any relationship—it will have little chance of becoming mutually nourishing if only one party is held accountable for the content and quality of the association. Do not be afraid to fire your doctor if you must. If you have the courage and maturity to take at least equal responsibility in this relationship, you may find that your effect on your doctor is as powerful as, if not more so than, his or hers is on you. Even if you have a wonderful relationship with your doctor, always be aware of your doctor's particular expertise and build your expectations accordingly. No single practitioner can be expected to provide you with all the answers necessary to maintaining lifelong optimal wellness. It may be necessary for you to consult more than one health care practitioner in order to meet your personal health objectives.

THE WOES OF MANAGED HEALTH CARE

Physicians don't necessarily practice medicine solely on the basis of their particular views on health and disease. Economic and medicopolitical pressures often dictate a style of practice. In fact, the impact of such issues is so profound that your ability to find the kind of medical care you desire—even your medical freedom of choice—may be in jeopardy.

Take, for example, HMOs (health maintenance organizations) or "managed care" operations. Commonly, the organization pays a member physician working in such a context a certain set monthly fee to care for any one patient. This is known as "capitation." The patient or patient's employer, of course, pays the organization a certain premium for such care. The physician is entitled to his or her fee whether or not the patient requires any care—not a bad deal for the physician if the patient rarely comes in.

However, this easy money goes back to the organization if another patient requires excessive care and needs more visits or lab tests than a physician's set fee is meant to cover. The physician can end up working many extra hours without extra pay. If he or she orders what the organization considers to be too many tests and refers patients to too many specialists, such expenses are sometimes taken out of his or her year-end dividend. In some plans, doctors can even lose their jobs if they cost the organization too much money, even if these expenses result from necessary care. Thus, it's in the physician's best financial interest to minimize the number and length of patient visits, to order as few lab tests as possible, and to make minimal referrals to specialists.

It's often difficult in such plans for patients to make as many appointments as they feel necessary. Sometimes they must wait months to get an appointment and nearly have to strangle their primary care doctors to get a referral to a specialist.

The physicians also have to endure binding regulations by the system. For example, they may have to restrict routine patient visits to brief encounters even for complicated problems and even when they'd prefer to investigate with the patient underlying but time-consuming health issues. The inclusion of any alternative or complementary approaches is discouraged, if not outright forbidden, in many medical plans.

Such a system, considered by many to be "herd 'em in, herd 'em out" production-line medicine, is based first on cost-efficiency goals. From the standpoint of disease and symptom care, it's usually competent, but to patients—and to many physicians—it often feels substandard. Such bare bones medicine is likely to be the standard of care with ever-increasing government intervention.

From the point of view of true health care and preventive medicine, the HMO and many managed care systems are woefully inadequate. Doctors and patients alike who believe in a more comprehensive approach often cannot last long in such a system. Patients will promptly choose another health plan if they have a choice, or pay additional fees out of their own pockets for the care they prefer and need. Accordingly, disgruntled doctors may not renew their contracts or will find other places to work.

Private practice (fee for service) medicine can easily fall into the same "herd 'em in, herd 'em out" mentality. The more patients a physician sees in a day, the more money he or she will bring in. Only through increased volume and quicker patient visits can a physician realistically accept work through PPOs (preferred provider organizations) or other similar contracts that offer reduced compensation for services. "Preferred" doesn't imply any expertise or competence; it's simply a designation given to a doctor who has signed a contract that obligates him or her to accept less payment from the insurance company than a nonpreferred doctor would be paid for delivering the same service.

In addition, continually restrictive government lids on Medicare and Medicaid reimbursements to physicians have prompted many doctors to shorten patient visits even more and increase patient volume. Patient satisfaction aside, physicians are growing increasingly discontented with and resentful of such economic restraints.

LOST OPPORTUNITIES

Unfortunately, contemporary society has begun to sacrifice opportunities to be guided toward a deeper level of health by our doctors. The prevalent, corporate-style type of medicine practiced today and destined for tomorrow—symptomatic treatments/"this drug for that symptom"—can be dispensed competently in a single, lightning-fast visit. However, in such a context, medicine cannot foster the teaching and the thorough investigation of underlying issues that could be gleaned from spending more time with individual patients. Nor will it be able to help sustain the motivation or the commitment that people need in order to take deeper responsibility for their health. Ironically, this level of responsibility would in the end successfully reduce the nation's health care expenditures—the very goal of corporate-inspired medicine.

The policies of many health insurance companies reinforce such limitations. Insurance companies will nearly automatically pay out thousands of dollars for an approved surgical procedure, such as a coronary bypass operation, yet may refuse to pay for preventive-oriented laboratory tests, nutritional counseling, acupuncture, homeopathy, or orthomolecular treatment. Nor will they adequately reimburse physicians for time spent with patients on preventive approaches and health education—measures that can prevent the need for far more costly crisis intervention down the line. As much financial sense as it makes to cover such relatively inexpensive preventive measures, in general, insurers still choose to pay only for recognized and approved treatment of existing disease.

To make matters worse, there is talk of the development of a "great American medical cookbook," a list of practice guidelines that, in the interest of cost containment, will dictate to physicians what tests to order and what treatments to recommend. It is highly unlikely that such guidelines will urge physicians to focus on their roles as teachers of healthful practices so that they can influence their patients' lifestyle and self-care choices. Rather, such a manual will likely offer efficient rules on pathology management, detailing the most cost-efficient and approved protocols for early diagnosis, and symptom and disease care, while leaving no opportunity for innovation or implementation of new ideas.

ALTERNATIVE MEDICINE MAY BE ON THE ENDANGERED LIST

The politics of modern medicine will make it difficult for physicians to practice anything but mainstream disease and symptom care medicine. Several states have already taken disciplinary action (practice restrictions, license suspensions, license revocations, and jailings) against physicians simply for prescribing such "unapproved" remedies as vitamins, minerals, enzymes, herbs, and homeopathics, or for using standard medicines or techniques in innovative ways. Rarely have any patients complained to authorities, and fewer still have ever been harmed. In fact, in some cases where disciplinary action has been taken, the patients in question had refused conventional treatment and had actively chosen the alternative approaches that these physicians then administered.

Medical disciplinary boards are notorious for ignoring the worthiness of innovative approaches. They usually have little or no understanding of, nor direct experience with, the approaches they are judging. They commonly conduct their hearings like lynch mobs, violating physicians' constitutional rights, and even making up rules as they go along. Acting ostensibly to protect the public from worthless or dangerous "quacks," the boards often infuse their proceedings with prejudice, fear, retaliation, and territorialism. They have attempted to ruin the practices and lives of good men and women, and in many cases have succeeded. There has long been a history of such a mentality in the medical profession—condemning as quacks bold and pioneering individuals whose innovative practices often subsequently become part of mainstream medicine. *Medical Mavericks*, by Hugh Riordan, M.D. (Biocommunications Press, 1989), details some of these innovators.

In six states—Alaska, Arizona, New York, Nevada, North Carolina and Washington—physicians, together with a supportive public, have succeeded in enacting legislation that protects a physician's freedom to practice alternative medicine. In Arizona, for example, there is now a separate disciplinary board to hear complaints that have been made against practitioners using alternative approaches. In Alaska and Washington the law reads: "The board may not base a finding of professional incompetence solely on the [fact] that a licensee's practice is unconventional or experimental in the absence of demonstrable physical harm to the patient." Part of the Washington state law calls for a physician practicing alternative-holistic medicine to serve as a member of the medical disciplinary board.[1] In these states physicians can practice with less fear. As a result, patients there have a new medical freedom of choice, and can more easily seek alternative approaches.

To protect themselves legally, physicians often refuse to care for patients who refuse conventional care and request alternative approaches. Consequently, such patients often have to travel to other states or out of the country to find willing medical doctors. Many individuals are forced to seek alternative treatments from unlicensed practitioners who do not often have a medical background. Although licensing and disciplinary boards believe they are protecting the public with such limitations, in this instance they are actually endangering the public.

PRESERVING YOUR HEALTH CARE ALTERNATIVES

With such constraints imposed upon the medical profession, it's no wonder that a growing number of individuals are looking elsewhere for the health information and services they want and need. The virtual explosion of interest in alternative approaches and self-care has been created, in part, by what people have not been able to get from their doctors. The public's needs and interests are simply growing too fast for the consciousness of standard medicine.

It is your interest in alternative approaches, your demand for a greater level of health and well-being, that is making the alternative and self-care health movement so strong and successful. But do not be fooled into thinking that you will always be free to choose a particular treatment or therapy. Conventional medicine is perceiving a very real threat to its existence, and its opposition to this movement grows steadily. "Quack busting" is more popular—and less discriminating—than ever. Government-sponsored institutions also threaten our freedoms. In 1993/94, the FDA attempted to ban consumers' right to buy vitamins, minerals, and herbs without a prescription. It was due primarily to massive public outcry that Congress was influenced to halt such inappropriate use of FDA power.[2]

Under the new proposed governmental health care reform, it may be difficult for private practice doctors to stay in business. Doctors who use alternative approaches may be required to practice medicine that allows no deviation from conventional methods. Managed health care conglomerates and state or federal health plans might even separate you from your doctor. Such regulations eliminate basic freedoms for both doctors and patients alike.

To preserve medical freedom of choice, massive public support must be rallied. Such effort is continually needed to educate legislators and influence their votes. In fact, public support was influential in preserving our freedom to purchase nutritional supplements.[3] Alternative health care groups in six states have learned to make the political system work on their behalf, and it can be done elsewhere. In Washington state, the successful efforts to pass a law protecting physicians using alternative approaches were engineered on a shoestring budget without a paid lobbyist.[4]

Enough constituent pressure will change the mindset of almost any legislator. The political system in this country does respond to organized, united, collective efforts. Such action will contribute not only to your own personal medical freedom and health, but quite possibly to the unification and evolution of health care in this country.

SUGGESTED READING

Colfelt, Robert, M.D. *Together in the Dark: Mysteries of Healing.* Seattle, WA: Madrona Publishers, 1987.

Dan, Bruce, and Young, Roxanne, eds. *A Piece of My Mind: A Collection of Essays from the Journal of the American Medical Association.* New York: Ballantine, 1990.

Smith, Wesley J. *Getting the Best From Your Doctor: A Nuts and Bolts Guide to Consumer Health.* Washington, DC: Center for Study of Responsive Law, 1994.

Walker, Martin J. *Dirty Medicine: Science, Big Business, and the Assault on Natural Healthcare.* London, UK: Slingshot Publications, 1993.

NOTES

INTRODUCTION

1. J. C. Bailar and E. M. Smith, "Progress Against Cancer." *New England Journal of Medicine* 34(19) (May 8, 1986): 1226–1232.

2. H. M. Sharma, B. D. Triguna, and D. Chopra, "Maharishi Ayur-veda: Modern Insights into Ancient Medicine." *Journal of the American Medical Association* 265(20) (May 22, 29, 1991): 2633–2637.

3. The origin of *Optimal Wellness* was a self-published version entitled *Wholeperson Self-Health Care* (1982, 1983) and its expanded sequels, *Your Health Is in Your Hands: A Guidebook for Self-Health Care* (1984, 1985).

3: DIETARY HAZARDS AND EXCESSES

1. W. Price, *Nutrition and Physical Degeneration* (New Caanan, CT: Keats Publishing, 1989; originally published 1939).

2. F. M. Pottenger, *Pottenger's Cats*, ed. E. Pottenger and R. T. Pottenger. (Available through Price Pottenger Nutrition Foundation, 2667 Camino Del Rio South, Suite 109, San Diego, CA 92108-3767, 1983.)

3. D. P. Burkitt and H. C. Trowell, eds., *Refined Carbohydrate Foods and Disease: Some Implications of Dietary Fiber* (New York: Academic Press, 1975).

4. N. Pritikin with J. Leonard and J. L. Hofer, *Live Longer Now: The First 100 Years of Your Life* (New York: Grosset & Dunlap, 1974). See also N. Pritikin and P. M. McGrady, *The Pritikin Program for Diet and Exercise* (New York: Grosset & Dunlap, 1979).

5. S. B. Eaton, M. Shostak, and M. Konner, *The Paleolithic Prescription: A Program of Diet and Exercise and a Design for Living* (New York: Harper & Row, 1988).

6. C. E. Koop—U.S. Department of Health and Human Services, Public Health Service, *The Surgeon General's Report on Nutrition and Health*, DHHS pub. no. 88–50211 (Washington, D.C.: Government Printing Office, 1988).

7. C. Junshi, T. C. Campbell, L. Junyao, and R. Peto, *Diet, Lifestyle and Mortality in China: A Study of the Characteristics of 65 Chinese Counties* (Oxford University Press, Cornell University Press, People's Republic of China, People's Medical Pub. House, 1990).

8. U.S. Senate, Senate Select Committee on Nutrition and Human Needs, *Dietary Goals for the United States* (Washington, D.C.: Government Printing Office, 1977).

9. E. J. Kozora, *Nutritional Guidelines* (Raleigh, NC: American Holistic Medical Association, 1983; rev. 1987).

10. M. L. Pearce and S. Dayton, "Incidence of Cancer in Men on a Diet High in Polyunsaturated Fat," *Lancet* 1 (1971): 464–467. See also F. Ederer et al., "Cancer among Men on Cholesterol-Lowering Diets: Experience from Five Clinical Trials," *Lancet* 2 (1971): 203–206.

11. R. P. Mensink, and M. B. Katan, "Effect of Dietary Trans-Fatty Acids on High Density and Low Density Lipoprotein Cholesterol Levels in Healthy Subjects," *English Journal of Medicine* 323 (1990): 439–445; R. T. Holman et al., "Effects of Trans-Fatty Acid Isomers upon Essential Fatty Acid Deficiency in Rats," *Proceedings of the Society for Experimental Biology and Medicine* 93 (1956): 175; and R. H. Hall, *Food for Naught: The Decline in Nutrition* (New York: Harper & Row, 1974).

12. R. Finlayson, "Ischemic Heart Disease, Aerobic Aneurysms and Atherosclerosis in the City of London, 1858–1982," *Medical History Supplement* 5 (1985): 151–168. See also A. U. Mackinnon, "The Origin of the Modern Epidemic of Coronary Artery Disease in England," *Journal of the Royal College of Practitioners* (Apr. 1987): 174–176.

13. M. A. Antar et al., "Changes in Retail Market Food Supplies in the United States in the Last 70 Years in Relation to the Incidence of Coronary Heart Disease, with Special Reference to Dietary Carbohydrates and Essential Fatty Acids," *American Journal of Clinical Nutrition* 14 (1964): 169–179.

14. J. D. Hunter, "Diet, Bodybuild, Blood Pressure, and Serum Cholesterol Levels in Coconut-eating Polynesians," *Federal Proceedings*, Suppl. 11, 21 (1962): 36.

15. F. W. Lowenstein, "Epidemiological Investigations in Relation to Diet in Groups Who Show Little Atherosclerosis

and Are Almost Free of Coronary Heart Disease," *American Journal of Clinical Nutrition* 15 (1964): 175.

16. S. L. Malhotra, "Serum Lipids, Dietary Factors, and Ischemic Heart Disease," *American Journal of Clinical Nutrition* 20 (1967): 452–475.

17. M. Gsell and J. Mayer, "Low Blood Cholesterol Associated with High Calorie, High Saturated Fat Intakes in a Swiss Alpine Village Population," *American Journal of Clinical Nutrition* 10 (1962): 471.

18. H. O. Bang and J. Dyerberg, "Lipid Metabolism and Ischemic Heart Disease in Greenland Eskimos," *Advanced Nutrition Research*, vol. 3, ed. H. H. Draper (New York: Plenum Press, 1980).

19. L. Galland, "Fact Sheet on Dietary Fats and Disease," *Townsend Letter for Doctors* 75 (Oct. 1989): 518–519.

20. A. L. Gittleman, *Beyond Pritikin: A Total Nutrition Program That Goes Beyond the Pritikin Principles by Adding Essential Fats for Rapid Weight Loss, Longevity, and Good Health* (New York: Bantam, 1988).

21. U. Erasmus, *Fats and Oils: The Complete Guide to Fats and Oils in Health and Nutrition* (Burnaby/Vancouver: Alive Books, 1986).

22. D. F. Horrobin et al., "Effects of Essential Fatty Acids on Prostaglandin Biosynthesis," *Biochemistry Acta* 43 (1984): S114–S120.

23. S. Markus, *Clinicians Reference Manual* (1988) Meridian Valley Clinical Laboratory, Kent, WA: 9.

24. L. Galland, "Fact Sheet on Dietary Fats and Disease," *Townsend Letter for Doctors* 75 (Oct. 1989): 518–519.

25. For more information on free radicals, see S. A. Levine and P. M. Kidd, "Biochemical Pathologies Initiated by Free Radical Oxidant Compounds in the Etiology of Food Hypersensitivity Disease," *International Clinical Nutrition Review* 5 (Jan. 1985): 5–24; B. A. Freeman and J. D. Crappo, "Biology of Disease: Free Radicals and Tissue Injury," *Laboratory Investigations* 47 (1982): 412–426; A. Autor, ed., *Pathology of Oxygen* (New York: Academic Press, 1982); and T. M. Florence, "Cancer and Aging: The Free Radical Connection," *International Clinical Nutrition Review* 4 (1984): 6–19.

26. See, for example, E. Cranton and Frackelton, "Free Radical Pathology in Age-Associated Diseases: Treatment with EDTA Chelation, Nutrition, and Antioxidants," *Journal of Holistic Medicine* (Spring/Summer 1984); D. Harman, "Free Radical Theory of Aging: Nutritional Implications," *Age* 1 (1978): 143; and "Free Radical Theory of Aging: Consequences of Mitochondrial Aging," *Age* 6 (July/Sept. 1983): 86–94.

27. R. W. Hubbard et al., "Atherogenic Effect of Oxidized Products of Cholesterol," *Progress in Food and Nutrition Science* 13 (1989): 17–44.

28. D. A. Snowdon, Letter to the Editor, *Journal of the American Medical Association* 254(3): 356–357.

29. Committee on Diet, Nutrition, and Cancer, Assembly of Life Sciences, National Research Council, *Diet, Nutrition and Cancer* (Washington, DC: National Academy Press, 1982).

30. See, for example, B. K. Larsson et al., "Polycyclic Aromatic Hydrocarbons in Grilled Food," *Journal of Agricultural Food Chemistry* 31 (July/Aug. 1983): 867–873; and W. Davies and J. R. Wilmhurst, "Carcinogens Formed in the Heating of Foodstuffs: Formation of 3, 4-Benzopyrene from Starch at 370–390°C," *British Journal of Cancer* 14 (1960): 295. See also P. Rathy and N. Mondy, "The Potato Dilemma: To Bake or Fry?" *Science News* 4 (Feb. 1984): 72.

31. Andrew Weil, M.D., *Natural Health, Natural Medicine* (Boston: Houghton Mifflin, 1990), 21.

32. "Triglycerol Structure and the Atherogenicity of Peanut Oil," *Nutritional Review* 41 (10) (Oct. 1983): 322–323. See also D. Vesselinovitch et al., "Atherosclerosis in the Rhesus Monkey Fed Three Food Fats," *Atherosclerosis* 20 (2) (Sept.–Oct. 1974): 303–321.

33. D. Burkitt and H. C. Trowell, ed., *Refined Carbohydrate Foods and Disease: Some Implications of Dietary Fiber* (New York: Academic Press, 1975), 338–339.

34. B. Dismukes. Research Dept., Sugar Association, letter Aug. 29, 1985 (unpublished data based on Economic Research Service and USDA estimates).

35. For more information on the link between sugar and arteriosclerosis, see J. Yudkin, "Levels of Dietary Sucrose in Patients with Occlusive Atherosclerotic Disease," *Lancet* 2 (1964): 6, and "Dietary Factors in Arteriosclerosis: Sucrose," *Lipids* 13 (1978): 370; S. Szanto et al., "The Effect of Dietary Sucrose on Blood Lipids, Serum Insulin, Platelet Adhesiveness, and Body Weight in Human Volunteers," *Postgraduate Medical Journal* 45 (1969): 602; and J. Yudkin, S. S. Kang, and K. R. Bruckdorfer, "Effects of High Dietary Sugar," *British Medical Journal* 281 (1980): 1396.

36. A. Sanchez et al., "Role of Sugars in Human Neutrophilic Phagocytosis," *American Journal of Clinical Nutrition* 26 (1973): 180; and W. M. Risnsgsdorf, E. Cheraskin, and R. R. Ramsay, "Sucrose, Neutrophilic Phagocytosis and Resistance to Disease," *Dental Survey* 52(12): 46.

37. See S. Seely and D. F. Horrobin, "Diet and Breast Cancer: The Possible Connection with Sugar Consumption," *Medical Hypothesis* 11(3): 319–327; and K. K. Carroll, "Dietary Factors in Hormone-Dependent Cancers," *Current Concepts in Nutrition*, vol. 6, ed. M. Winick (New York: Wiley, 1977).

38. K. D. Israel et al., "Serum Uric Acid in Carbohydrate (Sucrose)-Sensitive Adults," *Annals of Nutrition and Metabolism* 32 (Nov. 1983): 1078–1081.

39. See, for example, H. M. Salzer, "Relative Hypoglycemia as a Cause of Neuropsychiatric Illness," *Journal of the National Medical Association* 58 (1966): 12; D. Anthony et al., "Personality Disorder and Reactive Hypoglycemia: A Quantitative Study," *Diabetes* 22 (1973): 664; L. Langseth and J. Dowd, "Glucose Tolerance and Hyperkinesis," *Federal Cosmetics Toxicology* 16 (1978): 129; A. Schauss and C. E. Simonsen, "A Critical Analysis of the Diets of Chronic Juvenile Offenders," *Journal of Orthomolecular Psychiatry* 8 (1979): 149; and S. Schoenthaler, "The Alabama Diet-Behavior Program: An Empirical Evaluation at the Coosa Valley Regional Detention Center," "The Los Angeles Probation Department Diet-Behavior Program: An Empirical Analysis of Six Institutional Settings," and "The Northern California Diet-Behavior Program: An Empirical Examination of 3,000 Incarcerated Juveniles," *International Journal of Biosocial Research* 5(2): 70–106.

40. S. S. Kang et al., "Renal Damage in Rats Caused by

Dietary Sucrose," *Biochemical Society Transactions* 5 (1977): 235.

41. J. Lemann et al., "Possible Role of Carbohydrate-Induced Calciuria in Calcium Oxalate Kidney-Stone Formation," *New England Journal of Medicine* 280 (1969): 232.

42. R. J. Wurtman, "Neurochemical Changes Following High-Dose Aspartame with Dietary Carbohydrates," *New England Journal of Medicine* (1983): 429–430. See also H. J. Roberts, "Neurologic, Psychiatric, and Behavioral Reactions to Aspartame in 505 Aspartame Reactors," in *Proceedings of the First International Congress on Dietary Phenylalanine and Brain Function*, ed. R. J. Wurtman and E. Ritter-Walker, May 8–10, 1987; and D. W. Remington and B. W. Higa, *The Bitter Truth about Artificial Sweeteners* (Provo, Utah: Vitality House International, 1987).

43. L. Goldfrank et al., "Caffeine," *Hospital Physician* 11(81): 41–59.

44. For more on caffeine and adverse conditions, see M. Binstock et al., "Coffee and Pancreatic Cancer: An Analysis of International Mortality Data," *American Journal of Epidemiology* 118 (Nov. 1983): 630–640; R. E. Christianson et al., "Caffeinated Beverages and Decreased Fertility," *Lancet* 1 (1989): 378; C. La Vecchia et al., "Coffee Consumption and Myocardial Infarction in Women," *American Journal of Epidemiology* 130 (1989): 481–485; and R. P. Heaney and R. R. Recker, "Effects of Nitrogen, Phosphorus, and Caffeine on Calcium Balance in Women," *Journal of Laboratory and Clinical Medicine* 99 (1982): 46–55.

45. See L. K. Massey and M. Strang, "Soft Drink Consumption, Phosphorus Intake, and Osteoporosis," *Journal of the American Dietetic Association* 80 (1982): 581; and H. H. Draper and C. A. Scythes, "Calcium, Phosphorus, and Osteoporosis," *Federal Procedures* 40(9): 2434–2438.

46. Adapted from J. S. Bland, *Selected Papers by Jeffrey Bland, Ph.D.* (Gig Harbor, WA: Healthcom, 1985–1986). The sections discussing the potential adverse health effects of chlorine and fluoride are not adapted from Dr. Bland.

47. J. M. Price, *Coronaries/Cholesterol/Chlorine* (Saginaw, MI: Alta Enterprises, 1969).

48. B. Hileman, "Fluoridation of Water," *Chemical and Engineering News* (Aug. 1, 1988): 26–42. See also "Fluoride Linked to Bone Cancer," *Medical Tribune*, 28, 1989; "New Rap Against Fluoride: P&G Study," *Medical Tribune*, 22, Feb. 1990: "NTP Technical Report on the Toxicology and Carcinogenesis Studies of Sodium Fluoride" (Research Triangle Park, NC: NTP Public Information Office, Dec. 1990); "Review of Fluoride Benefits and Risks: Report of the Ad Hoc Subcommittee on Fluoride of the Committee to Coordinate Environmental Health and Related Programs" (Washington, DC: Public Health Service, Dept. of Health and Human Services, Feb. 1991); and J. A. Yiamouyiannis, "National Institute of Dental Research Study Shows No Relationship Between Fluoridation and Tooth Decay Rate," *American Laboratory* (May 1989).

49. See, for example, M. Jacobsen, *The Complete Eater's Digest and Nutrition Scoreboard* (New York: Doubleday, 1986); and N. Freyberg and W. Gortner, *The Food Additives Book* (New York: Bantam, 1982).

50. J. S. Spika et al., "Chloramphenicol-resistant Salmonella Newport Traced through Hamburger to Dairy Farms," *New England Journal of Medicine* 316 (1987): 555–570; and S. B. Levy, "Playing Antibiotic Pool: Time to Tally the Score," *New England Journal of Medicine* 311 (1984): 663–664.

51. National Academy of Sciences, National Research Council, Food and Nutrition Board, *Recommended Dietary Allowances*, 9th ed. (Washington, DC: NAS, 1980), 178.

52. F. R. Shank et al., "FDA Perspective on Sodium," *Food Technology* 37 (1983): 73–79.

53. D. E. Grobbee and A. Hofman, "Does Sodium Restriction Lower the Blood Pressure?" *British Medical Journal* 293 (1986): 27–29. See also "Nonpharmacological Approaches to the Control of High Blood Pressure: Final Report of the Subcommittee on Nonpharmacological Therapy of the 1984 Joint National Committee on Detection, Evaluation, and Treatment of High Blood Pressure," *Hypertension* 8(5): 444–467.

54. O. Ophir et al., "Low Blood Pressure in Vegetarians: The Possible Role of Potassium," *American Journal of Clinical Nutrition* 37 (1983): 755–762; and K. T. Khaw and S. Thom, "Randomized Double-blind Cross-over Trial of Potassium on Blood Pressure in Normal Subjects," *Lancet* 2 (1982): 1127–1129.

55. L. M. Resnick et al., "Intracellular Free Magnesium in Erythrocytes of Essential Hypertension: Relationship to Blood Pressure and Serum Divalent Cations," *Proceedings of the National Academy of Sciences USA* 81(2): 6511–6515; T. Dyckner and O. Wester, "Effect of Magnesium on Blood Pressure," *British Medical Journal* 286 (1983): 1847–1849; and D. A. McCarron, "Is Calcium More Important than Sodium in the Pathogenesis of Essential Hypertension?" *Hypertension* 7(4): 607–627.

56. S. A. Whitescarver et al., "Salt-Sensitive Hypertension: Contribution of Chloride," *Science* 223 (1984): 1430; and T. W. Kurtz and R. C. Morris, Jr., "Dietary Chloride as a Determinant of 'Sodium-Dependent' Hypertension," *Science* 222 (1983): 1139.

57. J. de Langre, *Sea Salt's Hidden Powers: How to Tell Its Integrity and Use It Correctly* (Magalia, CA: Grain and Salt Society, 1985); and *Sea Salt: The Vital Spark of Life* (Magalia, CA: Happiness Press, 1991).

58. See, for example, V. M. Bowerman, "Milk and Thought Disorder," *Journal of Orthomolecular Psychiatry* 19(4): 263–267; D. J. Rapp, "Food Allergy Treatment for Hyperkinesis," *Journal of Learning Disabilities*, 12 (1979): 608; L. W. Mayron, "Allergy, Learning, and Behavior Problems," *Journal of Learning Disabilities* 12 (1979): 32; F. W. Scott, "Cow Milk and Insulin-Dependent Diabetes Mellitus: Is There a Relationship?" *American Journal of Clinical Nutrition* 51 (1990): 489–491; A. Kahn et al., "Insomnia and Cow's Milk Allergy in Infants," *Pediatrics* 76 (1985): 880; and J. Monro et al., "Food Allergy in Migraine," *Lancet* (July 1980): 1–4.

59. K. A. Oster, "Folic Acid and Xanthine Oxidase," *Annals of Internal Medicine* 86 (1977): 367.

60. A. J. Clifford et al., "Homogenized Bovine Milk Xanthine Oxidase: A Critique of the Hypothesis Relating to Plasmalogen Depletion and Cardiovascular Disease," *American Journal of Clinical Nutrition* 38 (Aug. 1983): 327–332.

61. F. A. Oski, *Don't Drink Your Milk* (Syracuse: Mollica Press, 1983), 59; and J. McDougall and M. McDougall, *The*

McDougall Plan (Piscataway, NJ: New Century Publishers, 1985): 68.

62. D. Broughton, "Pushing Synthetic Growth Hormone BST into the Dairies and into Our Milk," *PCC Sound Consumer* no. 219 (June 1991): 1–2, 11 (published by Puget Consumers' Co-op, 5828 Roosevelt Way N.E., Seattle, WA 98105).

63. "Triacylglycerol Structure and the Atherogenicity of Peanut Oil," *Nutritional Review* 41 (Oct. 1983): 322–323.

64. "The Nuttiest Peanut Butter," *Consumer Reports* 55 (9): 588–592.

65. A. Wigmore, *The Hippocrates Diet and Health Program* (Wayne, NJ: Avery, 1984); and *Recipes for Longer Life* (Wayne, NJ: Avery, 1978).

66. Hazel Richards–Griffen, *Ninety-two Years: Perfect Health in an Unpolluted Body.* (Available through Survival Ministries, 4415 Semoran Farms Rd., Kissimmee, FL 34744-9211).

67. B. Jensen, *Nature Has a Remedy* (Escondido, CA: Bernard Jensen International, 1978); and *My System* (Escondido, CA: Bernard Jensen International, 1980).

68. V. Kulvinskas, *Survival in the 21st Century— Planetary Healers Manual* (Wethersfield, CT: Omangod Press, 1975).

69. Based on Professor Louis C. Kervran's original unpublished paper of the same title and to be published by the Grain and Salt Society of Magalia, CA.

70. D. R. McLachlan et al., "Aluminum and Neurodegenerative Disease: Therapeutic Implications," *American Journal of Kidney Diseases* 6(5): 322–329; C. Moon et al., "Main and Interaction Effects of Metallic Pollutants on Cognitive Functioning," *Journal of Learning Disabilities* 18(4): 217–221; and H. Tomlinson, *Aluminum Utensils and Disease* (Essex, England: L. N. Fowler, Ltd., 1958, 1978).

71. R. Newsome et al., "Organically Grown Foods: A Scientific Status Summary by the Institute of Food Technologists' Expert Panel on Food Safety and Nutrition," *Food Technology* (Dec. 1990): 123–130.

72. R. Wolford, "Eating Lean Lengthens Life," *Health and Longevity Report* 1(5): 7, and A. Colbin, *Food and Healing: How What You Eat Determines Your Health, Your Well-Being, and the Quality of Your Life* (New York: Ballantine, 1986).

4: FINDING YOUR OPTIMAL DIET

1. P. D'Adamo, "The ABO Blood Groups and Other Polymorphic Systems," *Townsend Letter for Doctors* (Aug./Sept. 1990): 528–534.

2. D'Adamo Serotype Polymorphisms (DSP-1) available through Meridian Valley Clinical Laboratory, 24030 132nd Ave. S.E., Kent, WA 98042; (206) 631-8922 or (800) 234-6825.

3. For more information on seasonal implications on diet, see E. Haas, M.D., *Staying Healthy with the Seasons* (Berkeley, CA: Celestial Arts, 1981); and *Staying Healthy with Nutrition: The Complete Guide to Diet and Nutritional Medicine* (Berkeley, CA: Celestial Arts, 1990).

4. For more information on macrobiotics, see H. Aihara, *Basic Macrobiotics* (Tokyo: Japan Pub., 1988); M. Kushi, *The Book of Macrobiotics* (Elmsford, NY: Japan Pub., 1979);

S. Rogers, *The Cure Is in the Kitchen: A Guide to Healthy Eating* (Syracuse, NY: Prestige Publishing, 1991).

5. N. Pritikin with J. Leonard and J. L. Hofer, *Live Longer Now: The First 100 Years of Your Life* (New York: Grosset and Dunlap, 1974), and N. Pritikin with P. McGrady, *The Pritikin Program for Diet and Exercise* (New York: Grosset & Dunlap, 1979).

6. A. Wigmore, *The Hippocrates Diet and Health Program* (Wayne, NJ: Avery, 1984).

5: ALL-STAR FOODS

1. J. Budwig, *Flax Oil as a True Aid Against Arthritis, Heart Infarction, Cancer, and other Diseases* (Vancouver: Apple Publishing, 1992).

6: NUTRITIONAL DEFICIENCIES

1. USDA (United States Department of Agriculture): Continuing Survey of Food Intakes by Individuals (CSFII). Report #86–3. Hyattsville, MD, 1986. See also DHHS/USDA (Department of Health and Human Services/U.S. Dept. of Agriculture): Operational Plan for the National Nutrition Monitoring System: Report to Congress. Public Health Service. Bethesda, MD, 1987; Y. Touitou et al., "Prevalence of Magnesium and Potassium Deficiencies in the Elderly," *Clinical Chemistry* 33 (1987): 518; J. A. Driskell, A. J. Clark and S. W. Moak, "Longitudinal Assessment of Vitamin B-6 Status in Southern Adolescent Girls," *Journal of the American Dietetic Association* 87 (1987): 307–310; A. J. Clark, S. Mossholder and J. Spengler, "Folacin Status in Adolescent Females," *American Journal of Clinical Nutrition* 46 (1987): 302–306; C. W. Hutton and R. B. Hayes-Davis, "Assessment of the Zinc Nutritional Status of Selected Elderly Subjects," *Journal of the American Dietetic Association* 82 (1983): 148–153; P. L. Armstrong, "Iron Deficiency in Adolescents," *British Medical Journal* 298 (1989): 499; B. R. Bistrian et al., "Prevalence of Malnutrition in General Medical Patients," *Journal of the American Medical Association* 235 (1976): 1567; R. S. Gibson and C. A. Scythes, "Dietary Chromium, Selenium and Other Trace Element Intakes of a Sample of Canadian Menopausal Women," *Federal Proceedings* 42 (1983): 816; J. T. Kumpulainen et al., "Determination of Chromium in Selected United States Diets," *Journal of Agricultural and Food Chemistry* 27 (1979): 490; C. J. Lee, "Nutritional Status of Selected Teenagers in Kentucky," *American Journal of Clinical Nutrition* 31 (1978): 1453; K. J. Morgan et al., "Magnesium and Calcium Dietary Intakes of the U.S. Population," *Journal of the American College of Nutrition* 4 (1985): 195; J. M. Holden, W. R. Wolfe, and W. Mertz, "Zinc and Copper in Self-Selected Diets," *Journal of the American Dietetic Association* 75 (1979): 23; J. Azuma et al., "Apparent Deficiency of Vitamin B-6 in Typical Individuals Who Commonly Serve as Normal Controls," *Research Communication in Chemical Pathology Pharmacology* 14 (1976): 343; J. L. Gregor, "Prevalence and Significance of Zinc Deficiency in the Elderly," *Journal of the American Dietetic Association* 82 (1983): 148.

2. See, for example, B. Smith, "Organic Foods vs. Supermarket Foods: Element Levels," *Journal of Applied Nutrition* 45 (1993): 35–39.

3. H. A. Schroeder, "Losses of Vitamins and Trace Miner-

als Resulting from Processing and Preservation of Foods," *Journal of Clinical Nutrition* 24 (1971): 562.

4. For an overview, see P. Hausman and A. Dickinson. "Recipe for Risk: A Critique of the National Research Council's Diet and Health Report" (Washington, DC: Council for Responsible Nutrition, 1989).

5. See, for example, H. A. Rafsky and M. Weingorten, "A Study of the Gastric Secretory Response in the Aged," *Gastroenterology* (May, 1946): 348–352; and D. Davies and T. G. James. "An Investigation into the Gastric Secretion of a Hundred Normal Persons Over the Age of Sixty," *British Journal of Medicine* I (1939): 1–14.

6. D. J. Patterson et al., "Niacin Hepatitis," *Southern Medical Journal* 76 (1983): 234–241.

7. G. E. Mullin et al., "Fulminant Hepatic Failure after Injection of Sustained-Release Nicotinic Acid," *Annals of Internal Medicine* 111 (1989): 253–255; and Y. Henkin, "Rechallenge with Crystalline Niacin after Drug-Induced Hepatitis from Sustained-Release Niacin," *Journal of the American Medical Association* 264 (1990): 241–243.

8. G. J. Parry and D. E. Bredesen, "Sensory Neuropathy with Low-Dose Pyridoxine," *Neurology* 35 (1985): 1466–1468.

9. See, for example, B. Rimland, "The Use of Megavitamin B-6 and Magnesium in the Treatment of Autistic Children and Adults" (San Diego, CA: Autism Research Institute, 1987), and B. Rimland et al., "The Effect of High Doses of Vitamin B-6 on Autistic Children: A Double Blind Cross-over Study," *American Journal of Psychiatry* 135 (1978): 4–8.

10. M. Colgin, *Your Personal Vitamin Profile* (New York: Morrow, 1982): 139–140.

11. R. P. Henry et al., "Meal Effects on Calcium Absorption," *American Journal of Clinical Nutrition* 49 (1989): 372–376.

12. See, for example, M. E. Shils and V. R. Young, *Modern Nutrition in Health and Disease,* 7th ed. (Philadelphia: Lea & Febiger, 1988); F. Clark, "Drugs and Vitamin Deficiency," *Journal of Human Nutrition* 30 (1976): 333; and R. A. Buist, "Drug-Nutrient Interactions—An Overview," *International Clinical Nutrition Review* 4 (July 1984): 114–121.

13. For more information on vitamin C, see E. Cheraskin, W. M. Ringsdorf, and E. L. Sisely, *The Vitamin C Connection* (New York: Harper & Row, 1983); B. Leibovitz and B. Siegal, "Ascorbic Acid, Neutrophil Function, and the Immune Response," *International Journal of Vitamin Nutrition Research* 48 (1978): 159; B. Kennes et al., "Effect of Vitamin C Supplements on Cell-Mediated Immunity in Old People," *Gerontology* 29 (1983): 305; T. W. Anderson, D. Reid, and G. H. Beaton, "Vitamin C and the Common Cold: A Double-blind Trial," *Canadian Medical Association Journal* 107 (1972): 503–508; P. G. Shilotri and K. S. Bhat, "Effect of Megadoses of Vitamin C on Bacteriacidal Activity of Leukocytes," *American Journal of Clinical Nutrition* 30 (1977): 1077; M. Fox, "Protective Effects of Ascorbic Acid against Toxicity of Heavy Metals," *Annals of the New York Academy of Science* 258 (1975): 144; J. A. Scott and G. M. Kolodny, "Interaction of Ionizing Radiation and Ascorbic Acid on 3T3 Mouse Fibroblasts," *International Journal of Vitamin Nutrition Research* 51 (1981): 155–160; I. Jialal, G. L. Vega and S. M. Grundy, "Physiologic Levels of Ascorbate Inhibit the Oxidative Modification of Low-Density Lipoprotein," *Atherosclerosis* 82

(1990): 185–191; H. Sprince, C. Parker, and G. Smith, "Comparison of Protection by L-Ascorbic Acid, L-Cysteine, and Adrenergic-blocking Agents against Acetaldehyde, Acrolein, and Formaldehyde Toxicity: Implications in Smoking," *Agents Actions* 9 (1979): 407.

14. J. V. Wright, *Dr. Wright's Guide to Healing with Nutrition* (Emmaus, PA: Rodale, 1984), 74; and J. W. Piesse, "Nutritional Factors in Calcium Containing Kidney Stones with Particular Emphasis on Vitamin C," *International Clinical Nutrition Review* 5 (July 1985), 110–129.

15. For more information on vitamin E, see J. G. Bieri, L. Corash and V. S. Hubbard, "Medical Uses of Vitamin E," *New England Journal of Medicine* (1983): 1063–1071; S. Ayres and R. Mihan, "Vitamin E as a Useful Therapeutic Agent," *Journal of the American Academy of Dermatology* 7 (1982): 521–525; M. K. Horwitt, "Therapeutic Uses of Vitamin E in Medicine," *Nutrition Review* (1980): 105–113; N. C. Cavarocchi et al., "Superoxide Generation During Cardiopulmonary Bypass: Is There a Role for Vitamin E?" *Journal of Surgery Research* 40 (1986): 519; H. H. Klein et al., "Combined Treatment with Vitamins E and C in Experimental Myocardial Infarction in Pigs," *American Heart Journal* 118 (1989): 667; B. Hennig and G. A. Boissoneault, "The Roles of Vitamin E and Oxidized Lipids in Atherosclerosis," *International Clinical Nutrition Review* 8(1988): 134–139; K. Gey et al., "Inverse Correlation between Plasma Vitamin E and Mortality from Ischemic Heart Disease in Cross-Cultural Epidemiology," *American Journal of Clinical Nutrition* 53 (1991): 3245–3265; E. B. Rimm et al., "Vitamin E Consumption and the Risk of Coronary Heart Disease in Men," *New England Journal of Medicine* 328 (1993): 1450–1456; M. J. Stampfer et al., "Vitamin E Consumption and the Risk of Coronary Heart Disease in Women," *New England Journal of Medicine* 328 (1993): 1444–1449; S. Ayres and R. Mihan, "Is Vitamin E Involved in the Autoimmune Mechanism?" *Cutis* 21 (1978): 321–325; D. P. Muller, J. K. Lloyd, and O. H. Wolff, "Vitamin E and Neurological Function," *Lancet* 1 (1983): 225–228; M. Meydani, J. B. Macauley, and J. B. Blumberg, "Effect of Dietary Vitamin E and Selenium on Susceptibility of Brain Region to Lipid Peroxidation," *Lipids* 23 (1988): 405–409; M. Menkes et al., "Serum Beta-Carotene, Vitamin A and E, Selenium, and the Risk of Lung Cancer," *New England Journal of Medicine* 315 (1986): 1250; M. A. Brown, "Resistance of Human Erythrocytes Containing Elevated Levels of Vitamin E to Radiation-Induced Hemolysis," *Radiation Research* 95 (1983): 303–316; K. H. Calhoun et al., "Vitamins A and E Do Protect against Oral Carcinoma," *Archives of Otolaryngology Head Neck Surgery* 115 (1989): 115; C. Chow, "Dietary Vitamin E and Cellular Susceptibility to Cigarette Smoking," *Annals of the New York Academy of Science* 393 (1982); and L. Corwin and R. Gordon, "Vitamin E and Immune Regulation," *Annals of the New York Academy of Science* 393 (1982): 437–451.

16. For more information on vitamin A, see G. T. Keusch, "Vitamin A Supplements—Too Good Not to Be True," *New England Journal of Medicine* 323 (1990): 985–987; B. Cohen and R. Elin, "Vitamin A–Induced Nonspecific Resistance to Infection," *Journal of Infectious Diseases* 129 (1974): 597; W. Bollag, "Vitamin A and Retinoids: From Nutrition to Pharmacotherapy in Dermatology and Oncology," *Lancet* 1

(1983): 860–863; G. D. Hussey and M. Klein, "A Randomized Controlled Trial of Vitamin A in Children with Severe Measles," *New England Journal of Medicine* 323 (1990): 160; N. Nuwayri-Salti and T. Murad, "Immunologic and Anti-Immunosuppressive Effects of Vitamin A," *Pharmacology* 30 (1989): 255; and T. Byers et al., "Dietary Vitamin A and Lung Cancer Risk: An Analysis by Histologic Subtypes," *American Journal of Epidemiology* 120 (1984): 769–776.

17. For more information on beta-carotene, see E. R. Abril et al., "Beta-Carotene Stimulates Human Leukocytes to Secrete a Novel Cytokine," *Journal of Leukocyte Biology* 45 (1989): 255; M. Alexander, H. Newmark, and R. Miller, "Oral Beta-Carotene Can Increase the Number of OKT4+ Cells in Human Blood," *Immunology Letters* 9 (1985): 221; L. C. Higgins, "Beta-Carotene Protection Hinted," *Medical World News* (Aug. 28, 1989): 19; M. Mathews-Roth, "Antitumor Activity of B-Carotene, Canthaxanthin and Phytoene," *Oncology* 39 (1982): 33–37; G. Braubacher and H. Weiser, "The Vitamin A Activity of B-Carotene," *International Journal of Vitamin Nutrition Research* 55 (1985): 5; and G. Burton and K. Ingold, "B-Carotene: An Unusual Type of Lipid Antioxidant," *Science* 224 (1984): 569.

18. For more information on vitamin B-6, see D. B. Gridley et al., "In Vivo and in Vitro Stimulation of Cell-Mediated Immunity by Vitamin B6," *Nutrition Research* 8 (1988): 201–207; E. R. Yendt and M. Cohanim, "Response to a Physiologic Dose of Pyridoxine in Type 1 Primary Hyperoxaluria," *New England Journal of Medicine* 312 (1985): 953–957; W. J. Serfontein et al., "Vitamin B6 Revisited: Evidence of Subclinical Deficiencies in Various Segments of the Population and Possible Consequences Thereof," *South African Medical Journal* 66 (1984): 437–441; and K. Dalton and M. Dalton, "Characteristics of Pyridoxine Overdose Neuropathy Syndrome," *Acta Neurologica Scandinavica* 76 (1987): 8.

19. For more information on calcium, see B. Dawson-Hughes et al., "A Controlled Trial of the Effect of Calcium Supplementation on Bone Density in Postmenopausal Women," *New England Journal of Medicine* 323 (1990): 878–883; M. S. Sheikh and J. S. Fordtran, "Calcium Bioavailability from Two Calcium Carbonate Preparations," *New England Journal of Medicine* 323 (1990): 921; J. Miller et al., "Calcium Absorption from Calcium Carbonate and a New Form of Calcium (CCM) in Healthy Male and Female Adolescents," *American Journal of Clinical Nutrition* 48 (1988): 1291–1294; M. S. Sheikh et al., "Gastrointestinal Absorption of Calcium from Milk and Calcium Salts," *New England Journal of Medicine* 317 (1987): 532–536; G. W. Bo-Linn et al., "An Evaluation of the Importance of Gastric Acid Secretion in the Absorption of Dietary Calcium," *Journal of Clinical Investigation* 73 (1984): 640–647; and H. J. Roberts, "Potential Toxicity Due to Dolomite and Bonemeal," *Southern Medical Journal* 76 (1983): 556.

20. For more information on magnesium, see P. O. Wester, "Magnesium," *American Journal of Clinical Nutrition* 45 (1987): 1305; H. S. Rasmussen et al., "Intravenous Magnesium in Acute Myocardial Infarction," *Lancet* 1 (1986): 234–236; J. R. Dipalma, "Magnesium Replacement Therapy," *American Family Practice* 42 (1990): 173–176; N. Skobeloff et al., "Intravenous Magnesium Sulfate for the Treatment of Acute Asthma in the Emergency Department," *Journal of the*

American Medical Association 262 (1989): 1210; B. M. Altura and B. T. Altura, "Role of Magnesium in Hypertension, Atherosclerosis and Vascular Disease," *Journal of the American College of Nutrition* 8 (1989): 454; H. S. Friedman, "The Role of Magnesium in Congestive Heart Failure and Its Effects on the Cardiovascular System," *Journal of the American College of Nutrition* 8 (1989): 455; and G. Paolisso et al., "Magnesium and Glucose Homeostasis," *Diabetologia* 33 (1990): 511–514.

21. For more information on selenium, see S. A. Levine and J. Parker, "Selenium and Human Chemical Hypersensitivities: Preliminary Findings," *International Journal of Biosocial Research* 3 (1982): 44–47; G. Combs and L. Clark, "Can Dietary Selenium Modify Cancer Risk?" *Nutritional Review* 42 (1985): 325; G. Schrauzer et al., "Selenium in the Blood of Japanese and American Women with and without Breast Cancer and Fibrocystic Disease," *Japanese Journal of Cancer Research* 76 (1985): 374; B. Sheffy and R. Schultz, "Influence of Vitamin E and Selenium on Immune Response Mechanisms," *Federal Proceedings* 38 (1979): 2139; and S. Flora, S. Singh, and S. Tandon, "Role of Selenium in Protection against Lead Intoxication," *Acta Pharmacologica Toxicologica* 53 (1983): 28.

22. For more information on zinc, see A. S. Prasad, "Clinical, Biochemical and Nutritional Spectrum of Zinc Deficiency in Human Subjects: An Update," *Nutrition Review* 41 (1983): 197–208; J. D. Bogden et al., "Zinc and Immunocompetence in Elderly People: Effects of Zinc Supplementation for 3 Months," *American Journal of Clinical Nutrition* 48 (1988): 655; E. Grant et al., "Zinc Deficiency in Children with Dyslexia: Concentration of Zinc and Other Minerals in Sweat and Hair," *British Medical Journal* 296 (1988): 607–609; A. G. Schauss and D. Bryce-Smith, "Evidence of Zinc Deficiency in Anorexia Nervosa and Bulimia Nervosa," in *Nutrients and Brain Function*, ed. W. Essman (Farmington, CT: S. Karger, 1987); H. G. Petering, "Some Observations on the Interaction of Zinc, Copper, and Iron Metabolism in Lead and Cadmium Toxicity," *Environmental Health Perspectives* 25 (1978): 141; and S. Barrie et al., "Comparative Absorption of Zinc Picolinate, Zinc Citrate and Zinc Gluconate in Humans," *Agents Actions* 5/6 (1986): 1.

23. For more information on copper, see J. Bland, "Copper Salicylates and Complexes in Molecular Medicine," *International Clinical Nutrition Review* 4 (July 1984): 130–134; M. A. Johnson and S. E. Kays, "Copper: Its Role in Human Nutrition," *Nutrition Today* (Jan./Feb. 1990): 6–14; and J. Rothschild, "Therapeutic Uses of Copper Complexes," *Research Perspectives in Arthritis and Rheumatism* (Concord, CA: Cardiovascular Research/Ecological Formulas, 1989).

24. For more information on vitamin D, see Select Committee on GRAS Substances, *Evaluation of the Health Aspects of Vitamin D₂ and Vitamin D₃ as Food Ingredients* (Washington, DC: Food and Drug Administration, 1978); H. G. Ainsleigh, "Sunshine Prevents Cancer Deaths," *The Townsend Letter for Doctors* (June 1991): 441–442; R. C. Butler, P. A. Dieppe, and A. C. Keat, "Calcinosis of Joints and Periarticular Tissues Associated with Vitamin D Intoxication," *Annals of Rheumatic Diseases* 44 (July 1985): 494–498; L. M. Dalderup, "Ischaemic Heart Disease and Vitamin D," *Lancet* 14 (July 1973): 92; B. Dawson-Hughes et al., "Effect of Vitamin D Supplementation on Wintertime and Overall Bone Loss in

Healthy Postmenopausal Women," *Annals of Internal Medicine* 15 (Oct. 1, 1991): 505–512; C. Garland and F. Garland, "Do Sunlight and Vitamin D Reduce the Risk of Colon Cancer?" *International Journal of Epidemiology* 9 (1980): 227–231; C. Garland et al., "Geographic Variation in Breast Cancer Mortality in the United States: A Hypothesis Involving Solar Radiation." *Preventive Medicine* 19 (1990): 614–622; and P. Hausman, *The Right Dose: How to Take Vitamins and Minerals Safely* (Emmaus, PA: Rodale Press, 1987): 220–242.

25. A. R. Webb and M. F. Holick, "The Role of Sunlight in the Cutaneous Production of Vitamin D₃," *Annual Review of Nutrition* 8 (1988): 375–399.

26. For more information on chromium, see G. W. Evans and R. I. Press, "Cholesterol and Glucose Lowering Effect of Chromium Picolinate," *FASEB Journal*, Abstract 310 (1981); H. A. Schroeder et al., "Abnormal Trace Minerals in Man," *Journal of Chronic Diseases* 15 (1961): 941; R. Press et al., "The Effect of Chromium Picolinate on Serum Cholesterol and Apolipoprotein Fractions in Human Subjects," *Western Journal of Medicine* 152 (Jan. 1990): 41–45; R. A. Anderson et al., "Urinary Chromiun Excretion and Insulinogenic Properties of Carbohydrates," *American Journal of Clinical Nutrition* 51 (1990): 864–868; H. A. Schroeder, A. P. Nason, and I. H. Tipton, "Chromium Deficiency as a Factor in Atherosclerosis," *Journal of Chronic Diseases* 23 (1970): 123–142; J. F. Potter et al., "Glucose Metabolism in Glucose-Intolerant Older People during Chromium Supplementation," *Metabolism* 34 (1985): 199–204; and R. A. Anderson, "Chromium Supplementation of Human Subjects: Effects on Glucose, Insulin, and Lipid Variables," *Metabolism* 32 (1983): 894–899.

27. For more information on coenzyme Q-10, see K. Folkers and Y. Yamamura, eds., *Biomedical and Clinical Aspects of Coenzyme Q* (New York/Amsterdam: Elsevier, 1977–1986); and K. Folkers et al., "Biochemical Deficiencies of Coenzyme Q10 in HIV-Infection and Exploratory Treatment," *Biochemical Biophysical Research Communications* 153 (1988): 888–896.

28. Folkers et al., "Biochemical Deficiences."

29. For more information on iron, see C. J. Bates, H. J. Powers, and D. I. Thurnham, "Vitamins, Iron and Physical Work," *Lancet* 2 (1989): 313; "Iron Nutriture and Risk of Cancer," *Nutrition Review* 47 (1989): 176; J. A. Stockman, "Infections and Iron: Too Much of a Good Thing?" *American Journal of Diseases of Children* 135 (1981): 18–20; and P. Cutler, "Deferoxomine Therapy in High-Ferritin Diabetes," *Diabetes* 38 (1989): 1207–1210.

30. For more information on essential amino acids, see E. Braverman and C. Pfeiffer, *The Healing Nutrients Within: Facts, Findings and New Research on Amino Acids* (New Canaan, CT: Keats, 1987).

31. For more information on cysteine, see W. Banner et al., "Experimental Chelation Therapy in Chromium, Lead, and Boron Intoxication with N-Acetylcysteine and Other Compounds," *Toxicology Applied Pharmacology* 83 (1986): 142–147; O. I. Aruoma et al., "The Antioxidant Action of N-Acetylcysteine: Its Reaction with Hydrogen Peroxide, Hydroxyl Radical, Superoxide, and Hypochlorous Acid," *Free Radical Biologie Medicale* 6 (1989): 593–597; J. Wu, E. M. Levy and P. H. Black, "2-Mercaptoethanol and N-acetyl-cysteine Enhance T Cell Colony Formation in AIDS and

ARC," *Clinical Experimental Immunology* 77 (1989): 7–10; M. Roederer et al., "Cytokine-Stimulated Human Immunodeficiency Virus Replication Is Inhibited by N-Acetyl-L-Cysteine," *Proceedings of the National Academy of Science USA* 87 (1990): 4884–4888; and L. Borgstrom, B. Kagedal, and O. Paulsen, "Pharmacokinetics of N-Acetylcysteine in Man," *European Journal of Clinical Pharmacology* 31 (1986): 217–222.

32. D. Gavish and J. L. Breslow, "Lipoprotein(a) Reduction by N-Acetylcysteine," *Lancet* 337 (1991): 203–204.

7: POOR DIGESTION AND ASSIMILATION

1. J. H. Lenz et al., "Wine and Five Percent Alcohol are Potent Stimulants of Gastric Acid in Humans," *Gastroenterology* 85 (1983): 1082–1087; and M. V. Singer et al., "Beer and Wine but not Whiskey and Pure Ethanol Do Stimulate Release of Gastrin in Humans," *Digestion* 26 (1983): 73–79.

2. See, for example, H. Shelton, *Food Combining Made Easy* (San Antonio, TX: Dr. Shelton's Health School, 1951); V. Kulvinskas, *Survival into the 21st Century* (Wethersfield, CT: Omangod Press, 1975); A. Wigmore, *The Hippocrates Diet and Health Program* (Wayne, NJ: Avery, 1984); and H. Diamond and M. Diamond, *Fit for Life* (New York: Warner Books, 1985).

3. J. V. Wright, *Dr. Wright's Guide to Healing with Nutrition* (Emmaus, PA: Rodale Press, 1984): 31–41, 449–450; J. N. Hunt and C. Johnson, "Relationship between Gastric Secretion of Acid and Urinary Excretion of Calcium after Oral Supplements of Calcium," *Digestive Diseases and Science* 28 (1983): 417; and P. Ivanovich, H. Fellow, and C. Rich, "The Absorption of Calcium Carbonate," *Annals of Internal Medicine* (May 1967): 917–923.

4. D. T. Davies et al., "An Investigation into the Gastric Secretion of a Hundred Normal Persons Over the Age of Sixty," *Quarterly Journal of Medicine* 23 (Oct. 1930): 1–14.

5. G. W. Bray, "The Hypochlorhydria of Asthma in Childhood," *Quarterly Journal of Medicine* (Jan. 1931): 181–197.

6. L. E. Rosenthal and H. L. Mobley, "Campylobacter Pylori: An Infectious Cause of Peptic Ulcer Disease?" *Contemporary Gastroenterology* 2 (May 1988): 9–13.

7. See, for example, P. A. Gross et al., "Effect of Fat on Meal-Stimulated Duodenal Acid Load, Duodenal Pepsin Load, and Serum Gastrin in Duodenal Ulcer and Normal Patients," *Gastroenterology* 75 (1978): 357–362; C. T. Richardson et al., "Studies on the Mechanisms of Food-Stimulated Gastric Acid Secretion in Normal Human Subjects," *Journal of Clinical Investigation* 58 (1976): 623–631; and C. Owyang et al., "Nutrient and Bowel Segment Dependency of Human Intestinal Control of Gastric Secretion," *American Journal of Physiology* 243 (1982): G372–G376.

8. C. B. Beal and J. E. Brown, "A Simple Screening Test for Gastric Achlorhydria," *American Journal of Digestive Diseases* 13 (1968): 133.

9. W. T. Steinberg et al., "Heidelberg Capsule I: In Vitro Evaluation of a New Instrument for Measuring Intragastric pH," *Journal of Pharmaceutical Sciences* (May 1965): 772–776; and M. R. Andres, "Tubeless Gastric Analysis with a Radio-Telemetering Pill (Heidelberg Capsule)," *Canadian Medical Association Journal* (May 21, 1970): 1087–1089.

10. F. Lami et al., "A Single-Specimen Fecal Chymotryp-

sin Test in the Diagnosis of Pancreatic Insufficiency: Correlation with Secretin-Cholecytokinin and NBT-PABA Tests," *American Journal of Gastroenterology* 79 (1984): 697–700; and G. Cavallini et al., "The Fecal Chymotrypsin Photometric Assay in the Evaluation of Exocrine Pancreatic Capacity. Comparison with Other Direct and Indirect Pancreatic Function Tests," *Pancreas* 4 (1989): 300–304. For testing, have your doctor contact DiagnosTechs, Inc. P.O. Box 58948, Seattle, WA 98138-1948, (206) 251-0596.

11. C. Lang et al., "Assessment of Exocrine Pancreatic Function by Oral Administration of N-Benzoyl-L-Tyrosyl-P-Aminobenzoic Acid (Bentiromide): 5 Years of Clinical Experience," *English Journal of Surgery* 68 (1981): 771–775. For testing, have your doctor contact Meridian Valley Clinical Laboratory, 24030 132nd Ave. S.E., Kent, WA 98042, (800) 234-6825.

12. See, for example, E. Howell, *Enzyme Nutrition: The Food Enzyme Concept* (Wayne, NJ: Avery, 1985); A. Wigmore, *The Hippocrates Diet and Health Program* (Wayne, NJ: Avery, 1984); and H. Sommer and H. Casper, "Effective Long-Term Administration of Dietary Fiber on the Exocrine Pancreas in the Rat," *Hepato-Gastroenterology* 31 (1984): 176–179.

13. Examples are Polyzyme by Interplexus, Inc., Kent, WA 98032, (206) 251-0511; N-Zymes by National Enzyme Co., Forsyth, MO, (800) 825-8545; and Similase by Tyler Encapsulations, Gresham, OR, (800) 869-9705.

14. For laboratory testing, have your doctor contact DiagnosTechs, Inc., P.O. Box 58948, Seattle, WA 98138-1948, (206) 251-0596; or Great Smokies Diagnostic Laboratory, 18A Regent Park Blvd., Asheville, NC 28806, (704) 253-0621 or (800) 522-4762.

15. Ibid.

8: THE TOXIC BOWEL

1. For more information on lactobacilli, see A. G. Schauss, "Lactobacillus Acidophilus: Method of Action, Clinical Application, and Toxicity Data," *Journal of Advancement in Medicine* 3 (Fall, 1990): 163–178; A. G. Plaut, "Gut Bacterial Metabolism and Human Nutrition," in *The Role of the Gastrointestinal Tract in Nutrient Delivery*, ed. M. Green and H. L. Green (New York: Academic Press, 1984): 199–208; K. M. Shahani and B. A. Friend, "Nutritional and Therapeutic Aspects of Lactobacilli," *Journal of Applied Nutrition* 36 (1984): 125–152; K. M. Shahani, J. R. Vakil and A. Kilara, "Natural Antibiotic Activity of Lactobacillus Acidophilus and Bulgaricus," *Cultured Dairy Products Journal* 12 (1977): 8; and S. J. Bahatia et al., "Lactobacillus Acidophilus Inhibits Growth of Campylobacter Pylori in Vitro," *Journal of Clinical Microbiology* (Oct. 1989): 2328–2330.

2. R. Phillips and D. A. Snowdon, "Dietary Relationships with Fatal Colorectal Cancer among Seventh Day Adventists," *Journal of the National Cancer Institute* 74 (1985): 307.

3. D. Burkitt and H. Trowell, *Western Diseases: Their Emergence and Prevention* (Cambridge, MA: Harvard University Press, 1981); and *Refined Carbohydrates, Foods and Diseases* (New York: Academic Press, 1975).

4. J. O. Hunter, "Food Allergy—or Enterometabolic Disorder?" *Lancet* 338 (Aug. 24, 1991): 495–496.

5. E. Rauch, *Health Through Inner Body Cleansing: The Famous MAYR Intestinal Therapy from Europe* (Heidelberg, Germany: Carl F. Haug, 1988). U.S.A. distributor: Portland, OR: Medicina Biologica, 2937 N.E. Flanders St., Portland, OR 97232, (503) 287-6775.

6. B. Jensen and S. Bell, *Tissue Cleansing through Bowel Management: From the Simple to the Ultimate* (available from Bernard Jensen International, 24360 Old Wagon Rd., Escondido, CA 92027).

7. For information on iridology, see B. Jensen, *The Science and Practice of Iridology* and *Iridology: The Science and Practice in the Healing Art, Vol. II* (both are available from Bernard Jensen International, 24360 Old Wagon Rd., Escondido, CA 92027).

8. K. Stefansson et al., "Sharing of Antigenic Determinants between the Nicotinic Acetylcholine Receptor and Proteins in Escherichia Coli, Proteus Vulgaris, and Klebsiella Pneumoniae: Possible Role in the Pathogenesis of Myasthenia Gravis," *New England Journal of Medicine* 4: 221–225. See also A. Ebringer et al., "Klebsiella Antibodies in Alkylosing Spondylitis and Proteus Antibodies in Rheumatoid Arthritis," *British Journal of Rheumatology* 27 (suppl. 2): 72–85; and E. A. Deitch et al., "Bacterial Translocation from the Gut Impairs Systemic Immunity," *Surgery* 109 (3): 269–276.

9. Great Smokies Diagnostic Laboratory, 18A Regent Park Blvd., Asheville, NC 28806, (800) 522-4762. See also Meridian Valley Clinical Laboratory, 24030 132nd Ave. S.E., Kent, WA 98042, (800) 234-6825.

10. V. L. Hughes and S. Hiller, "Microbiologic Characteristics of Lactobacillus Products Used for Colonization of the Vagina," *Obstetrics and Gynecology* 75 (1990): 244.

11. For information on *Saccharomyces boulardii*, see C. M. Surawicz et al., "Treatment of Antibiotic-Associated Diarrhea by *Saccharomyces boulardii*: A Prospective Study," *Gastroenterology* 96 (1989): 981–988; Surawicz et al., "Treatment of Recurrent Clostridium Difficile Colitis with Vancomycin and *Saccharomyces boulardii*," *American Journal of Gastroenterology* 84 (1989): 1285–1287; and J. P. Buts et al., "Stimulation of Secretory IgA and Secretory Component of Immunoglobulins in Small Intestine of Rats Treated with *Saccharomyces boulardii*," *Digestive Diseases and Sciences* 35 (1990): 251–256.

12. For information on fructooligosaccharides, see R. C. McKellar and H. W. Modler, "Metabolism of Fructooligosaccharides by Bifidobacterium Species," *Applied Microbiology Biotechnology* 31 (1989): 537–541; H. Hidaku et al., "Effects of Fructooligosaccharides on Intestinal Flora and Health," *Bifidobacteria Microflora* 5 (1986): 37–50; and P. J. Perna, "Fructooligosaccharides, an All Natural Food which Promotes Bifidobacteria and Lactobacillus" (monograph from Center for Applied Nutrition, Zea Gen, Inc., 350 Interlocken Blvd., Broomfield, CO 80021, 1992).

13. See, for example, J. Bland, *Intestinal Toxicity and Inner Cleansing* (Connecticut: Keats Publishing, 1987); L. Berry, *Internal Cleansing: A Practical Guide to Colon Health* (available from Botanical Press, P.O. Box 742, Capitola, CA 95010); *Yerba Prima Internal Cleansing Program* (available from Yerba Prima Botanicals, P.O. Box 2569, Oakland, CA 94614); R. Gray, *The Colon Health Handbook: New Health through Colon Rejuvenation* (Oakland, CA: Rockridge Publishing,

1983); and *Sonne's or Veico Intestinal Cleansing Program* (available from Sonne's Organic Foods, Natick, MA 01760).

14. E. Rauch, *Health Through Inner Body Cleansing: The Famous MAYR Intestinal Therapy from Europe* (Heidelberg, Germany: Carl F. Haug, 1988). USA distributor: Portland, OR: Medicina Biologica.

15. B. Jensen and S. Bell, "Tissue Cleansing through Bowel Management: From the Simple to the Ultimate" (available from Bernard Jensen International, 24360 Old Wagon Rd., Escondido, CA 92027).

9: THE SLUGGISH LIVER

1. G. Jost et al., "Overnight Salivary Caffeine Clearance: A Liver Function Test Suitable for Routine Use," *Hepatology* 7(2): 338–344.

2. Contact DiagnosTechs, Inc., Clinical and Research Laboratory, P.O. Box 58948, Seattle, WA 98138-1948, (206) 251-0596, or National BioTech Laboratory, 3212 N.E. 125th Street, Seattle, WA 98125, (206) 363-6006.

3. Contact Meridian Valley Clinical Laboratory, 24030 132nd Ave. S.E., Kent, WA 98042, (206) 631-8922.

4. Eclectic Institute, 14385 S.E. Lusted Rd., Sandy, OR 97055, (503) 668-4120.

5. NF Formulas, 9775 S.W. Commerce Circle, Suite C-5, Wilsonville, OR 97070-9602, (503) 682-9755.

6. K. Nagai, "A Study of the Excretory Mechanisms of the Liver—Effect of Liver Hydrolysate on BSP Excretion," *Japanese Journal of Gastroenterology* 67 (1970): 633–638; S. Hirayama et al., "Therapeutic Effect of Liver Hydrolysate on Experimental Liver Cirrhosis," *Nisshin Igaku* 45 (1978): 528–533; and K. Fujisawa et al., "Therapeutic Effects of Liver Hydrolysate Preparation on Chronic Hapatitis—A Double-Blind, Controlled Study," *Asian Medical Journal* 26 (1984): 497–526.

7. D. S. Sachan, T. H. Rhew, and R. A. Ruark, "Ameliorating Effects of Carnitine and Its Precursors on Alcohol-Induced Fatty Liver," *American Journal of Clinical Nutrition* 39 (1984): 738–744.

8. M. T. Murray, *Phyto-Pharmica Review* 1 (fall 1987). Available from Phyto-Pharmica, P.O. Box 1348, Green Bay, WI 54305, (414) 435-4200.

9. Information on the benefits of lipoic acid is available from Cardiovascular Research, Ltd./Ecological Formulas, Product Information, 1061-B Shary Circle, Concord, CA 94518, (800) 888-2636.

10. V. V. Subbarao, "Effect of an Indigenous Drug Liv. 52 against Alcohol Induced Hepatic Damage: A Biochemical Study," *Proceedings of the 31st International Congress on Alcoholism and Drug Dependence*, Bangkok, Thailand, Feb. 23–27, 1975; and A. K. Kale et al., "Effect of Liv. 52 on Growth and Alcohol-Induced Hepatic Dysfunction in Rats," *Current Medical Practices* 10 (1966): 240.

10: HYPOGLYCEMIA

1. W. J. Hudspeth et al., "Neurobiology of the Hypoglycemia Syndrome," *Journal of Holistic Medicine* 3 (Spring/Summer 1981): 60–71; A. I. Arieff et al., "Mechanisms of Seizure and Coma in Hypoglycemia: Evidence for a Direct Effect of Insulin on Electrolyte Transport in the Brain," *Journal of Clinical Investigation* 54 (1974): 654–663; and D. D. John-

son et al., "Reactive Hypoglycemia," *Journal of the American Medical Association* 243 (1980): 1151–1155.

2. For more information on the role of the liver in hypoglycemia, see B. Barnes and C. W. Barnes, *Hope for Hypoglycemia: It's Not in Your Mind, It's Your Liver* (Ft. Collins, CO: Robinson Press, 1989).

3. R. J. Wurtman and J. J. Wurtman, "Caffeine: Metabolism and Biochemical Mechanisms of Action," in *Nutrition and the Brain*, vol. 6 (New York: Raven Press, Ltd., 1983); S. Bolton and G. Nall, "Caffeine, Psychological Effects, Use and Abuse," *Journal of Orthomolecular Psychiatry* 10 (3): 202–211; and J. D. Lane et al., "Caffeine Effects on Cardiovascular and Neuroendocrine Responses to Acute Psychosocial Stress and the Relationship to the Level of Habitual Caffeine Consumption," *Psychosomatic Medicine* 52 (1990): 320–336.

4. H. Selye, *Stress without Distress* (New York: Signet, 1975).

5. C. R. Scriver and L. E. Rosenberg, *Amino Acid Metabolism and Its Disorders* (Philadelphia: Saunders, 1973).

6. W. J. Hudspeth et al., "Neurobiology of the Hypoglycemia Syndrome," *Journal of Holistic Medicine* 3 (Spring/Summer 1981): 60–71; and D. D. Johnson, et al.; "Reactive Hypoglycemia," *Journal of the American Medical Association* 243 (1980): 1151–1155.

7. J. R. Kraft, "Detection of Diabetes Mellitus, In Situ (Occult Diabetes)," *Laboratory Medicine* 6 (2): 10–22. For interpretation and guidelines for the glucose-insulin tolerance test, contact Meridian Valley Clinical Laboratory, 24030 132nd Ave. S.E., Kent, WA 98042, (206) 631-8922.

8. For more information on treating hypoglycemia, see C. Fredericks and H. Goodman, *Low Blood Sugar and You* (New York: Constellation International, 1969); P. Airola, *Hypoglycemia: A Better Approach* (Phoenix: HealthPlus, 1977); E. Cheraskin and W. M. Ringsdorf with A. Brecher, *Psychodietetics: Food as the Key to Emotional Health* (New York: Stein & Day, 1974); and J. V. Wright, *Dr. Wright's Book of Nutritional Therapy* (Emmaus, PA: Rodale Press, 1979), 197–208.

9. F. Bornet et al., "Insulinemic and Glycemic Indexes of Six Starch-Rich Foods Taken Alone and in a Mixed Meal by Type II Diabetics," *American Journal of Clinical Nutrition* 45 (1987): 558–595; and S. W. Ross et al., "Glycemic Index of Processed Wheat Products," *American Journal of Clinical Nutrition* 46 (1987): 631–635.

11: ADRENAL EXHAUSTION

1. A. C. Guyton, "Adrenocortical Hormones," in *Textbook of Medical Physiology*, 4th ed. (Philadelphia: W.B. Saunders, 1971), Chap. 76, 890–895; and G. H. Williams, R. G. Dluhy, and G. W. Thorn, "Diseases of the Adrenal Cortex," T. R. Harrison, ed., in *Harrison's Principles of Internal Medicine*, 7th ed., M.M. Wintrobe et al., ed. (New York: McGraw-Hill, 1974), Chap. 86, 491–492, and W. M. Jeffries, "Cortisol and Immunity," *Medical Hypotheses* 34 (1991): 198–208.

2. J. P. Kahn et al., "Salivary Cortisol: A Practical Method for Evaluation of Adrenal Function," *Biological Psychiatry* 23 (1988): 335–349; M. H. Laudat et al., "Salivary Cortisol: A Practical Approach to Assess Pituitary-Adrenal Function," *Journal of Clinical Endocrinology and Metabolism* 66 (1988): 343–348; and Fahmy D. Riad et al., "Steroids in Saliva for As-

sessing Endocrine Function," *Endocrine Reviews* Fall 3(4): 367–395.

3. DiagnosTechs, Inc., Clinical and Research Laboratory, 6620 So. 192nd Pl., J-104, Kent, WA 98032-1948, (800) 878-3787 (outside of Washington); (206)521-0596 (in Washington).

4. E. Ilyia, "The New Definition of Stress Evaluation, Adrenal Stress Index" (Monograph). DiagnosTechs, Inc., Clinical and Research Laboratory, 6620 So. 192nd Place, J-104, Kent, WA 98032-1948, 1991, 7a-1 to 7d-5.

5. J. B. Jemmott, III et al., "Academic Stress, Power, Motivation and Decrease in Salivary IgA Secretion Rate," *The Lancet* (June 1983): 1400–1402; R. A. Daynes, D. J. Dudley, and B. A. Araneo, "Regulation of Murine Lymphokine Production in Vivo. II Dehydroepiandrosterene Is a Natural Enhancer of Interleukin 2 Synthesis by Helper T Cells," *European Journal of Immunology* 20(4) (April 1990): 793–802; and E. Ilyia, "The New Definition of Stress Evaluation, Adrenal Stress Index," (Monograph). DiagnosTechs, Inc., Clinical and Research Laboratory, 6620 So. 192nd Place, J-104, Kent, WA 98032-1948, 1991, 7a-1 to 7d-5.

6. J. Born et al., "Gluco- and Antimineralocorticoid Effects on Human Sleep: A Role of Central Corticosteroid Receptors," *American Journal of Physiology* 260 (1991): E183–E188; F. Horst, J. Born, "Evidence for the Entrainment of Nocturnal Cortisol Secretion and Sleep Process in Human Beings," *Neuroendocrinology* 53 (1991): 171–176; T. Kobayashi, Y. Tsuji, and S. Endo, "Sleep Cycles as a Basic Unit of Sleep," in *Ultradian Rhythms in Physiology and Behavior* (Experimental Brain Research Supplementum; 12), H. Schulz and P. Lavie, eds. (Berlin: Springer-Verlag, 1985) 260–269; and J. Born, W. Kern, K, Bieber, G. Fehm-Wolfsdorf, M. Schiebe, and H. L. Fehm, "Night-Time Plasma Cortisol Secretion Is Associated with Specific Sleep Stages," *Biological Psychiatry* 21(14) (Dec. 1986): 1415–1424.

7. E. Ilyia, "The New Definition of Stress Evaluation, Adrenal Stress Index" (Monograph), DiagnosTechs, Inc., Clinical and Research Laboratory, 6620 So. 192nd Pl., J-104, Kent, WA 98032-1948, 1991, 7a-1 to 7d-5; B. E. Nordin et al., "The Relation Between Calcium Absorption, Serum Dehydroepiandrosterone, and Vertebral Mineral Density in Postmenopausal Women," *Journal of Clinical Endocrinology and Metabolism* 60(4) (Apr. 1985): 651–657.

8. I. E. Nestler et al., "Dehydroepiandrosterone Reduces Serum Low Density Lipoprotein Levels and Body Fat But Does Not Alter Insulin Sensitivity in Normal Men," *Journal of Clinical Endocrinology and Metabolism* 66(1) (Jan. 1988): 57–61.

9. P. de Feo et al., "Contribution of Cortisol to Glucose Counter Regulation in Humans," *American Journal of Physiology* 257 (1989): E35–E42.

10. I. E. Nestler et al.

11. J. Guechot et al., "Simple Laboratory Test of Neuroendocrine Disturbance in Depression: 11 p.m. Salivary Cortisol," *Neuropsychobiology* 18 (1987): 1–4.

12. H. P. Schwarz, "Conversion of Dehydroepiandrosterone Sulfate (DHEA-S) to Estrogens and Testosterone in Young Non-Pregnant Women," *Hormone and Metabolic Research* 22(5) May, 1990: 309–310.

13. R. A. Daynes, D. J. Dudley, and B. A. Araneo, "Regulation of Murine Lymphokine Production in Vivo. II. Dehydroepiandrosterone Is a Natural Enhancer of Interleukin 2 Synthesis by Helper T Cells," *European Journal of Immunology* 20(4) (April, 1990): 793–802.

14. E. Ilyia, "The New Definition of Stress Evaluation, Adrenal Stress Index," monograph by DiagnosTechs, Inc., Clinical and Research Laboratory, 6620 South 192nd Pl., J-104, Kent, WA 98032-1948, 1991, 7a-1 to 7d-5.

15. V. Felt, and L. St'arka, "Metabolic Effects of Dehydroepiandrosterone and Atromid in Patients with Hyperlipemia," *Cor Et Vasa* (8)1 (1966): 40–48; and I. E. Nestler et al., "Dehydroepiandrosterone Reduces Serum Low Density Lipoprotein Levels and Body Fat but Does Not Alter Insulin Sensitivity in Normal Men," *Journal of Clinical Endocrinology and Metabolism* 66(1) (January 1988): 57–61.

16. B. Zumoff, "Abnormal hormone levels in men with coronary artery disease," *Arteriosclerosis* 2 (1982): 58. See also B. Zumoff et al., "Age Variation of the 24-Hour Mean Plasma Concentrations of Androgens, Estrogens, and Gonadotropins in Normal Adult Men," *Journal of Clinical Endocrinology and Metabolism,* 54(3) (Mar. 1982): 534–538; and Barrett et al., "A Prospective Study of Dehydroepiandrosterone Sulfate, Mortality, and Cardiovascular Disease," *New England Journal of Medicine* 315(24) (Dec. 11, 1986): 1519–1524.

17. I. E. Nestler et al., "Dehydroepiandrosterone Reduces Serum Low Density Lipoprotein Levels and Body Fat but Does Not Alter Insulin Sensitivity in Normal Men," *Journal of Clinical Endocrinology and Metabolism* 66(1) (January, 1988): 57–61.

18. D. Nerozzi et al., "Early Cortisol Escape Phenomenon Reversed by Phosphatidyl Serine in Elderly Normal Subjects," *Clinical Trials Journal* 26(1) (1989): 33–38.

19. R. H. Kimberlin, "An Overview of Bovine Spongiaform Encephalopathy," *Developmental Biology Standards—Scrapies and Related Diseases Advisory Service* 75 (1991): 75. See also M. H. Groschup, and E. Psaff, "Studies on a Species Specific Epitope in Murine, Ovine, and Bovine Prion Protein," *Journal of Virology* 74 (1993): 1451; and F. X. Meslin, "Surveillance and Control of Emerging Zoonoses," *World Health Statistics Quarterly* (Division of Communicable Diseases World Health Organization) 45 (1992): 200; M. H. Laudat et al., "Salivary Cortisol: A Practical Approach to Assess Pituitary-Adrenal Function," *Journal of Clinical Endocrinology and Metabolism* 66 (1988): 343–348.

20. W. M. Jeffries, *Safe Uses of Cortisone* (Springfield, IL: Charles C. Thomas, 1981).

12: YEAST OVERGROWTH

1. See M. S. Seelig, "Role of Antibiotic in the Pathogenesis of Candida Infections," *American Journal of Medicine* 40 (1966): 887–917; C. M. Allen et al., "Role of Tetracycline in Pathogenesis of Chronic Candidiasis of Rat Tongues," *Infection and Immunity* 47 (1985): 480–483.

2. A. Shanchez et al., "Role of Sugars in Human Neutrophilic Phagocytosis," *American Journal of Clinical Nutrition* 26 (1973): 180; and W. M. Ringsdorf, E. Cheraskin, and R. R. Ramsay, "Sucrose, Neutrophilic Phagocytosis, and Resistance to Disease," *Dental Survey* 52 (12):46.

3. L. Galland, "Nutrition and Candidiasis," *Journal of Orthomolecular Psychiatry* 15 (1985): 50–60; L. P. Samarana-

yake, "Nutritional Factors and Oral Candidosis," *Journal of Oral Pathology* 15 (1986): 61–65; J. Edman et al., "Zinc Status in Women with Recurrent Vulvovaginal Candidiasis," *American Journal of Obstetrics and Gynecology* 155 (1986): 1082–1085; and R. Boyne and J. R. Arthur, "The Response of Selenium-Deficient Mice to *Candida Albicans* Infection," *Journal of Nutrition* 116(5) (1986): 816–822.

4. J. P. Trowbridge and M. Walker, eds., *The Yeast Syndrome* (New York: Bantam, 1986), 60–62.

5. M. Boero et al., "Candida Overgrowth in Gastric Juice of Peptic Ulcer Subjects on Short- and Long-Term Treatment with H-2-receptor Antagonists," *Digestion* 28 (1983): 158–163. See also R. Kochhar et al., "Invasive Candidiasis Following Cimetidine Therapy," *American Journal of Gastroenterology* 83 (1988): 102–103.

6. C. O. Truss, "Tissue Injury by Candida Albicans: Mental and Neurological Manifestations," *Journal of Orthomolecular Psychiatry* 7 (1978): 17–37; and C. O. Truss, "The Role of Candida Albicans in Human Illness," *Journal of Orthomolecular Psychiatry* 10 (1981): 228–238.

7. Ibid.

8. C. O. Truss, M.D., *The Missing Diagnosis*, 2nd ed. (available from P.O. Box 26508, Birmingham, AL 35226).

9. E. Carlson, "Synergistic Effect of Candida Albicans and Staphylococcus Aureus on Mouse Mortality." Infection and Immunology 38 (1982): 921–924; E. Carlson, "Enhancement by *Candida Albicans* of *Staphylococcus Aureus, Serratia Marcescens, and Streptococcus Faecalis* in Establishment of Infection in Mice," *Infection and Immunology* 39 (1983): 193–197; and "Effect of Strain of Staphylococcus Aureus on Synergism with Candida Albicans Resulting in Mouse Mortality and Morbidity," *Infection and Immunology* 42 (1983): 285–292.

10. C. O. Truss, "Metabolic Abnormalities in Patients with Chronic Candidiasis—The Acetaldehyde Hypothesis," *Journal of Orthomolecular Medicine* 13 (1984): 63–93.

11. H. Kaj, Y. Asonuma, H. Saito et al. "The Autobrewery Syndrome—the Repeated Attacks of Alcoholic Intoxication Due to the Overgrowth of Candida (Albicans) in the Gastrointestinal Tract," Materia Medica Polona 8 (1976): 429–435; K. Iwata, "Review of the Literature on Drunken Symptoms Due to Yeasts in the Gastrointestinal Tract," in *Yeasts and Yeast-like Microorganisms in Medical Science* K. Iwata, ed. (Tokyo: University of Tokyo Press, 1976) 260–268; and A. Hunnisett, J. Howard, and S. Davies, "Gut Fermentation (or the 'Auto-brewery') Syndrome: A New Clinical Test with Initial Observations and Discussion of Clinical and Biochemical Implications," *Journal of Nutritional Medicine* 1 (1990): 33–38.

12. P. L. Saifer and N. Becker, "Allergy and Autoimmune Endocrinopathy: APICH Syndrome" in *Food Allergy and Intolerance*, J. Brostoff and S. J. Challacombe, eds. (Philadelphia: Balliere Tindall, 1987), 781–793.

13. C. O. Truss, *The Missing Diagnosis*, 2nd ed. (available from P.O. Box 26508, Birmingham, AL 35226).

14. Contact DiagnosTechs, Inc., P.O. Box 58948, Seattle, WA 98138-1948 (206) 251-0596; Great Smokies Diagnostic Laboratory, 18A Regent Park Blvd., Asheville, NC 28806 (800) 522-4762; Meridian Valley Clinical Laboratory, 24030-132nd Ave. S.E., Kent, WA 98042 (206) 631-8922,

(800) 234-6825.; and Physicians Clinical Laboratories, 15613 Bellevue-Redmond Rd., Bellevue, WA 98008 (206) 881-2446.

15. Contact DiagnosTechs, Inc., P.O. Box 58948, Seattle, WA 98138-1948 (206) 251-0596.

16. Ibid.

17. Contact Meridian Valley Clinical Laboratory, 24030-132nd Ave. S.E., Kent, WA 98042 (206) 631-8922 or (800) 234-6825; Physicians' Clinical Laboratories, 15613 Bellevue-Redmond Rd., Bellevue, WA 98008 (206) 881-2446; Antibody Assay Laboratories, 1715 E. Wilshire, #1715, Santa Ana, CA 92705 (714) 972-9979 or (800) 522-2611; and Immunodiagnostic Laboratories, 488 McCormick St., San Leandro, CA 94577 (800) 888-1113.

18. Dioxychlor is available from American Biologics of 1180 Walnut Ave., Chula Vista, CA 91911.

19. Echo (Box 126, Delano, MN 55328) promotes the use of food-grade hydrogen peroxide.

13: FOOD ALLERGIES

1. A. H. Rowe and A. Rowe, Jr., *Food Allergy: Its Manifestations and Control and the Elimination Diets, A Compendium* (Springfield, IL: Thomas, 1972).

2. T. G. Randolph and R. W. Moss, *An Alternative Approach to Allergies* (New York: Lippincott/Crowell, 1980).

3. Ibid.

4. Sources for food allergy intolerance: J. C. Breneman, *Basics of Food Allergy* (Springfield, IL: Thomas, 1978); Robert R. Buist, *Food Intolerance: What It Is and How to Cope with It* (Houston: Prism Press, 1986); S. Faelton, and the editors of *Prevention* magazine. *Allergy Self-Help Book* (Emmaus, PA: Rodale, 1983); M. Mandell, and L. W. Scanlon. *Dr. Mandell's 5-Day Allergy Relief System* (New York: Crowell, 1979); K. Mumby, *Allergies: What Everyone Should Know* (London: Unwin Paperbacks); T. G. Randolph, and R. W. Moss. *An Alternative Approach to Allergies* (New York: Lippincott/Crowell, 1988); D. J. Rapp, *Allergies and Your Family* (New York: Sterling, 1982); D. Sheinkin, M. Schacter, and R. Hutton. *Food, Mind and Mood* (New York: Warner Books, 1987; original title: *The Food Connection*).

5. J. Barret, *Textbook of Immunology* (St. Louis: Mosby, 1983); S. Barrie, "Food Allergy," in *A Textbook of Natural Medicine*, ed. J. E. Pizzorno and M. T. Murray. (Seattle: John Bastyr College Publications, 1985); P. M. Donovan, "The ELISA/ACT Test: Its Role in Identifying Time-Delayed Reactive Environmental Toxicants (Parts I and II)," *Townsend Letter for Doctors* 94 (May 1991): 326–328, and 95 (June 1991): 480–484; P. Gel, R. Coombs, and P. Lachman, eds. *Clinical Aspects of Immunology* (1975) (Oxford, UK: Blackwell Scientific Publications; Philadelphia: distributed by J. B. Lippincott); and I. Roit, J. Brostoff, and D. Male, *Immunology* (New York: Mosby, 1986).

6. W. T. K. Bryan and M. P. Gryan, "The Application of the In Vitro Cytotoxic Reactions to Clinical Diagnosis of Food Allergy," *Laryngoscope* 70 (1960): 810.

7. S. Barrie, "Food Allergy," in *A Textbook of Natural Medicine*, ed. J. E. Pizzorno and M. T. Murray (Seattle: John Bastyr College Publications, 1985); A. L. de Weck, *Pathophysiologic Mechanisms of Allergic and Pseudo-Allergic Reactions to Foods, Food Additives, and Drugs, Ann. All.* 53 (1984): 583–586; and P. M. Donovan, "The ELISA/ACT Test: Its Role

in Identifying Time-Delayed Reactive Environmental Toxicants (Parts I and II)," *Townsend Letter for Doctors* 94 (May 1991): 326–328, and 95 (June 1991): 480–484, L. Perelmutter, "Non-IgE Mediated Atopic Disease," *Annals of Allergy* 52 (1984): 640–68; and J. Egger et al., "Are Migraines Food Allergies?" *Lancet* ii (1983): 8355–63.

8. See notes 5 and de Weck from 7.

9. E. Benjamini, and S. Leskowiski, *Immunology: A Short Course* (New York: Alan Liss, 1988); E. Braunwald, K. Issel-bacher, R. Petersdorf, et al., eds., *Harrison's Principles of Internal Medicine*, 11th ed. (New York: McGraw-Hill, 1987), 354–364; P. M. Donovan, "The ELISA/ACT Test: Its Role in Identifying Time-Delayed Reactive Environmental Toxicants (Parts I and II), *Townsend Letter for Doctors* 94 (May 1991): 326–328, and 95 (June 1991): 480–484; R. Hall, T. Lawley, J. Heck, and S. Kats, "IgA-Containing Circulating Immune Complexes in Dermatitis Herpetiformis, Henoch-Schonlein Purpura, Systemic Lupus Erythematosis, and Other Diseases," *Clinical Experiments in Immunology* 40 1980: 431–437; R. Jaffe, "Immune Defense and Repair System: II. Clinical Expression of Impaired Immune Competence," in *Clinical Chemistry and Nutrition Guidebook* 1, ed. P. Yanick and R. Jaffe (Reston, VA: HSC Press, 1989); R. Levinsky, "The Role of Souble Immune Complexes in Disease," *Archives of Disease in Childhood* 53 (1978): 96–99; T. Soderstrom, G. Hansson, and G. Larson, "The Escherichia Coli K1 Capsule Shares Antigenic Determinants with the Human Gangliosides GM3 and GD3," *New England Journal of Medicine* 310 (1984): 726–727; and K. Stephansson, M. Dieperink, D. Richman et al., "Sharing of Antigenic Determinants between the Nicotinic Acetylcholine Receptor and Proteins in *Escherichia Coli, Proteus Vulgaris* and *Klebsiella Pneumoniae*," *New England Journal of Medicine* 312 (1985): 221–225.

10. J. Ely, "Allergic Dysautonomia: The Role of Dehydro-ascorbic Acid," unpublished paper. University of Washington Radiation Studies (FM 15), Seattle. See also J. W. Patterson, "Diabetogenic Effect of Dehydroascorbic and Hydroisoascorbic Acid," *Journal of Biological Chemistry* 183 (March 1950): 183–188.

11. Randolph and Moss, op. cit.

12. Ibid. See also R. J. Rinkel, "Food Allergy: IV. The Function and Clinical Application of the Rotary Diversified Diet," *Journal of Pediatrics* 32: 266; and S. Rockwell, *The Rotation Game* and *Sally Rockwell's Allergy Recipes*, 1991. Also "The Rotation Diet," and "Yes, There's Food Left to Eat," a sixty-minute videotape, and "Overcoming Allergies," an audiocassette tape. Available from Sally Rockwell's Diet Design, P.O. Box 31065, Seattle, WA 98103.

13. R. Buist, Ph.D. *Food Chemical Sensitivity* (Houston: Prism Press, 1987).

14. B. Feingold, *Why Your Child Is Hyperactive* (New York: Random House, 1975). See also B. Feingold with H. S. Feingold, *The Feingold Cookbook for Hyperactive Children and Others with Problems Associated with Food Additives and Salicylates* (New York: Random House, 1979).

15. Randolph and Moss, op. cit.

16. I. Bjarnason, A. Ward., and T. J. Peters, "The Leaky Gut of Alcoholism: Possible Root of Entry for Toxic Compounds," *The Lancet* (Jan. 28, 1984): 179; J. S. Sandhu, and D. R. Frazier, "Assessment of Intestinal Permeability in the Experimental Rat with Celibiotol and Mannitol," *Clinical Science* 63 (1982): 311–316; and F. A. Wilson and A. N. Hoyumpu, "Ethanol and Small Intestinal Transport," *Gastroenterology* 76 (1979): 388–403.

17. J. Miller, *Food Allergy, Provocative Testing and Injection Therapy* (Springfield, IL: Thomas, 1972).

18. W. A. Commings and E. W. Williams, "Transport of Large Breakdown Products of Dietary Protein through the Gut Wall," *Gut* 19 (1978): 715. See also W. Walker, "Transmucosal Passage of Antigens," in *Food Allergy*, ed E. Schmidt (New York: Vevey/Raven Press, 1988); L. Mayron, "Portals of Entry—A Review," *Annals of Allergy* 40 (1979): 399–405; M. C. Reinhardt, "Macromolecular Absorption of Food Antigens in Health and Disease," *Journal of Allergy* 53 (1984): 597.

19. C. Andre, F. Andre et al., "Measurement of Intestinal Permeability to Mannitol and Lactulose as a Means of Diagnosing Food Allergy and Evaluating Therapeutic Effectiveness of Disodium Chromoglycate," *Annals Allergy* 59(2): 127–130; C. Dupont et al., "Diagnosis of Food Allergy by Measurement of Intestinal Permeability in Children with Cows' Milk Sensitivity Enteropathy and Atopic Dermatitis," *Journal of Pediatric Gastroenterology and Nutrition* 8 (1989): 459; M. Elia, R. Behrens, C. Northrop et al., "Evaluation of Mannitol, Lactulose, and 51Cr-EDTA as Markers of Intestinal Permeability in Man," *Clinical Science* 73 (1987): 197–204; S. O. Ukabam et al., "Small Intestinal Permeability of Sugars in Patients with Atopic Eczema," *British Journal of Dermatology* 110 (1984): 649–652; P.G. Jackson et al., "Intestinal Permeability in Patients with Eczema and Food Allergy," *The Lancet* (June 13, 1981): 1285; S. Strobel et al., "Sugar Permeability Test Complements Biopsy Histopathology in Clinical Investigation of the Jejunum," *Gut* 25 (1984): 1241–1246. Intestinal permeability test is available from Diagnos-Techs, Inc., P.O. Box 58948, Seattle, WA 98138-1948 (206) 251-0596; and from Great Smokies Diagnostic Laboratory, 18A Regent Park Blvd., Asheville, NC 28806 (704) 253-0621 or (800) 522-4762.

20. S. O. Ukabam et al., "Abnormal Small Intestinal Permeability to Sugars in Patients with Crohn's Disease of the Terminal Ileum and Colon," *Digestion* 27 (1983): 70–74; I. R. Sanderson et al., "Improvement of Abnormal Lactulose-Rhamnose Permeability in Active Crohn's Disease of the Small Bowel by an Elemental Diet," *Gut* 128 (1987): 1073–1076; and S. Strobel et al., "Sugar Permeability Test Complements Biopsy Histopathology in Clinical Investigation of the Jejunum," *Gut* 25 (1984): 1241–1246.

21. P. G. Jackson et al., "Intestinal Permeability in Patients with Eczema and Food Allergy," *The Lancet*, (June 13, 1981): 1285; and L. D. Juby et al., "Lactulose-Mannitol Test: An Ideal Screen for Celiac Disease," *Gastroenterology* 96 (1989): 79–85.

22. Chris M. Reading, M.D., and Ross S. Meillon, *Your Family Tree* (New Canaan, CT; Keats, 1988).

23. C. Andre, F. Andre et al., "Measurement of Intestinal Permeability to Mannitol and Lactulose as a Means of Diagnosing Food Allergy and Evaluating Therapeutic Effectiveness of Disodium Chromoglycate," *Annals Allergy* 59(2): 127–130.

24. S. Rockwell, *Coping with Candida Cookbook*, rev. 1990. Available from Design, P.O. Box 31065, Seattle, WA 98103 (206) 547-1814.

25. Mandell and Scanlon, op. cit.

26. A. F. Coca, M.D., *The Pulse Test: The Secret of Building Your Basic Health* (New York: Lyle Stuart, 1956).

27. R. Jaffe, "Antigen Detection (ELISA/ACT) Immunology Procedure," in *Clinical Chemistry and Nutrition Guidebook*, vol. 1, ed. P. Yanick and R. Jaffe (Santa Barbara, CA: TMH Publishing, 1988); and R. Jaffe, *Health Studies Collegium Information Handbook*, 10th ed. (Reston, VA: Health Studies Collegium, 1989).

28. J. J. Tsuei, C. W. Lehman et al., "A Food Allergy Study Utilizing the EAV Acupuncture Technique," *American Journal of Acupuncture* 12 (1984): 105–116. See also Biosource Listen System, Biosource Inc., 1388 W. Center St., Orem, UT 84057 (801) 226-1117; Computron Health Enhancement Services, (305) 365-9000; Eclosian, Eclosian Corporation, 4970 Unit A, Monaco St., Commerce City, CO 80022; and Occidental Institute Research Foundation, P.O. Box 5507, Bellingham, WA 98227-5507 (604) 946-7211. Research, publications, and training for electronic screening devices.

29. A. Ber, "Neutralization of Phenolic (Aromatic) Food Compounds in a Holistic General Practice," *Journal of Orthomolecular Psychiatry* 12(4): 283–291.

30. J. Miller, *Food Allergy, Provocative Testing and Injection Therapy* (Springfield, IL: Thomas, 1972); and H. J. Rinkel, "The Diagnosis of Food Allergy," *Archives of Otolaryngology* 79 (1964): 71–79.

14: CHEMICAL HYPERSENSITIVITY AND ENVIRONMENTAL ILLNESS

1. D. E. Root, D. B. Catzin, and D. W. Schnare, "Diagnosis and Treatment of Patients Presenting Subclinical Signs and Symptoms of Exposure to Chemicals Which Bioaccumulate in Human Tissue," from the *Proceedings of the National Conference on Hazardous Wastes and Environmental Emergencies*, May 1985, Cincinnati, OH. Complete proceedings can be obtained from Hazardous Materials Control Research Institute, 9300 Columbia Boulevard, Silver Spring, MD 20910.

2. S. A. Rogers, *The EI Syndrome: An Rx for Environmental Illness* (Syracuse, NY: Prestige Publishing, 1988); and *Tired or Toxic?* (Syracuse, NY: Prestige Publishing, 1990).

3. B. Feingold, *Why Your Child Is Hyperactive* (New York: Random House, 1975).

4. S. A. Rogers, *The EI Syndrome: An Rx for Environmental Illness.* (Syracuse, NY: Prestige Publishing, 1988); and "Diagnosing the Tight Building Syndrome," *Environmental Health Perspectives* 76: (1987) 195–198.

5. Randolph, T. G., M.D., and R. W. Moss, Ph.D. *An Alternative Approach to Allergies.* (New York: Harper Collins, 1990).

6. Liver detoxification capacity test: DiagnosTechs, Inc. (caffeine clearance), Seattle, WA (206) 251-0596, 800-87 TESTS; MetaMetrix, Inc. (caffeine and hippurate clearance), Norcross, GA (800) 221-4640.

7. For the ELISA-ACT test, contact Serammune Physicians Lab, 1890 Preston White Dr., 2nd Floor, Reston, VA 22091 (800) 553-5472.

8. A. Broughton, J. D. Thrasher and Z. Gard, "Immunological Evaluation of Four Arc Welders Exposed to Fumes from Ignited Polyurethane (Isocyanate) Foam: Antibodies and Immune Profiles," *American Journal of Industrial Medicine* 13: (1988) 463–472; E. C. Ward, M. J. Murray, and J. H. Dean, "Immunotoxicity of Nonhalogenated Polycyclic Aromatic Hydrocarbons," in *Immunotoxicology and Immunopharmacology*, J. H. Dean et al., eds. (New York: Raven Press, 1985); *Low-Level Environmental Contamination and Immune Response*, Research Bulletin of the foundation for Advancements in Science and Education, Nov. 1986; A. Broughton, *Laboratory Diagnosis of the Environmentally Compromised Patient*. Santa Ana, CA: Antibody Assay Laboratories, 1715 E. Wilshire #715, (714) 972-9979, and J. Thrasher et al., "Evidence for Formaldehyde Antibodies and Altered Cellular Immunity in Subjects Exposed to Formaldehyde in Mobile Homes," *Archives of Environmental Health* 42 (Nov./Dec. 1987); and A. Broughton, J. D. Thrasher, and R. Madison, "Chronic Health Effects and Immunological Alterations Associated with Exposure to Pesticides," *Comments Toxicology* 4 (1990): 59–71.

9. Root et al., op cit.; Z. R. Gard, E. J. Brown, and G. DeSanti-Medina, "The Biotoxic Reduction Program: Eliminating Body Pollution," *The Townsend Letter for Doctors* 46, April 1987 (available from 911 Tyler St., Port Townsend, WA 98368); D. W. Schnare, M. Ben, and M. G. Shields, "Body Burden Reductions of PCBs, PBBs and Chlorinated Pesticides in Human Subjects," *Ambio* (A Journal of the Human Environment) 13 (1984); D. W. Schnare, and P. C. Robinson, *Reduction of Hexachlorobenzene and Polychlorinated Biphenyl Human Body Burdens*. From International Symposium on Hexachlorobenzene; IARC Scientific Publication Series, Vol. 77, Oxford University Press; and T. G. Randolph, and R. Wisner, "Detoxification: Personal Survival in a Chemical World" (available from Healthmed Detox, 5501 Fauer Inn Rd., Suite 140, Sacramento, CA 98520; (916) 387-8252).

10. A. Bocchetta, and G. U. Corsini, "Parkinsonism and Pesticides" (letter) *Lancet* (Nov. 1986): 1163. See also J. J. Chapman, and H. A. Peters, "Parkinsonism and Industrial Chemicals" (letter) *Lancet* (Feb. 1987): 332–333; and K. L. Davis, "Possible Organosophate-induced Parkinsonism," *Journal of Nervous and Mental Diseases* 166 (1978): 222–225.

11. Ward et al., op cit.; A. Broughton, *Laboratory Diagnosis of the Environmentally Compromised Patient*. Santa Ana, CA: Antibody Assay Laboratories, 1715 E. Wilshire, #715 92705 (714) 972-9979; J. Vos, "Dioxin-induced Thymic Atrophy and Suppression of Thymus-Dependent Immunity," *Branbury Report 18: Biological Mechanisms of Dioxin Action*. Author's address: Laboratory for Pathology, National Institute of Public Health and Environmental Hygiene, P.O. Box 3720 BA Bilthoven, The Netherlands; D. McConkey et al., "2,3,7,8-Tetracholorodibenzo-p-dioxin Kills Immature Thymocytes by CA^{2+}-mediated Endonuclease Activation," *Science* 242 (Oct. 1988): 256–259; P. A. Bertazzi et al., "Cancer Mortalities of Capacitor Manufacturing Workers," *American Journal of Industrial Medicine* 11 (1987): 165–176; M. Wasserman et al., "Organochlorine Compounds in Neoplastic and Adjacent Apparently Normal Gastric Mucosa," *Bulletin of Environmental Contaminants and Toxicology* 20 (1978): 544–553; J. D. Thrasher, A. Broughton, and R. Madison, "Immune Activation and Autoantibodies in Humans with Long-Term Inhalation Exposure to Formaldehyde," *Archives of Environmental Health* 45 (July-Aug. 1990): 217–223; and

A. Broughton, J. D. Thrasher, and R. Madison, "Chronic Health Effects and Immunological Alterations Associated with Exposure to Pesticides," *Comments Toxicology* 4 (1990): 59–71.

12. L. R. Hubbard, *Clear Body, Clear Mind: The Effective Purification Program* (Los Angeles: Bridge Publications, Inc., 1990).

13. D. W. Schnare, M. Ben, and M. G. Shields, "Body Burden Reductions of PCBs, PBBs and Chlorinated Pesticides in Human Subjects," *Ambio* (A Journal of the Human Environment) 13 (1984); See also Gard et al., op cit.; and D. E. Root and G. T. Lionelli, "Excretion of Lipophilic Toxicant through the Sebaceous Glands: A Case Report," *Journal of Toxicology—Cutaneus and Ocular Toxicology* 6 (1987): 13–17.

14. D. L. Dadd, *Nontoxic, Natural, and Earthwise: How to Protect Yourself and Your Family from Harmful Products and Live in Harmony with the Earth* (Los Angeles: J. T. Tarcher, 1990); and *The Nontoxic Home* (Los Angeles: J. T. Tarcher/St. Martin's Press, 1986).

15. R. M. Jaffe, *Toxic Minerals ELISA-ACT: Description of Items Tested* (Monograph) (Reston, VA: Serammune Physicians Lab, 1993).

16. C. W. Svare, "Dental Amalgam Related Mercury Vapor Exposure," *California Dental Association Journal* (Oct. 1984); 55–60; M. J. Vimy, and F. L. Lorscheider, "Intra-Oral Air Mercury Released from Dental Amalgam," *Journal of Dental Research* 64 (Aug. 1985): 1069–1071; M. J. Vimy, and F. L. Lorscheider, "Intra-Oral Air Mercury: Estimation of Daily Dose from Dental Amalgam," *Journal of Dental Research* 65 (Aug. 1985): 1072–1075; B. F. Emler, and M. Cardone, Sr., "An Assessment of Mercury in Mouth Air," *Journal of Dental Research* 64 (1985): 247, IADR Abstract no. 652; and J. E. Patterson, B. G. Weissberg, and P. J. Dennison, "Mercury in Human Breath from Dental Amalgams," *Bulletin of Environmental Contaminants and Toxicology* 34 (1985): 459–468.

17. R. Kupsinel, "Mercury Amalgam Toxicity: A Major Common Denominator of Degenerative Disease," *Journal of Orthomolecular Psychiatry* 13 (1984): 240–257; S. Ziff, and M. Ziff. *Infertility and Birth Defects: Is Mercury from Silver Dental Fillings a Hidden Cause?* Orlando, FLA: BioProbe 1990; W.F. Oettingen, *Poisoning: A Guide to Clinical Diagnosis and Treatment* (Philadelphia: Saunders, 1958); and *Environmental Health Criteria: Volume 1. Mercury* (Geneva: World Health Organization, 1976), pp. 1–131.

18. NIDR Workshop: "Biocompatibility of Metals in Dentistry," *Journal of the American Dental Association* 109 (1984): 469–471.

19. W. A. Banks and A. J. Kastin, "Aluminum Increases the Permeability of the Blood-Brain Barrier to Labled DSIP and Beta-Endorphin: Possible Implications for Senile and Dialysis Dementia," *Lancet* 2 (1983): 1227–1229.

20. Doctors' Data, Inc., P.O. Box 111, West Chicago, IL 60185, (800) 323-2784.

21. P. Donovan, and R. M. Jaffe, *Health Assurance: Your User Guide* (Reston, VA: HSC Press, 1995).

22. J. H. Graziano, "Role of 2,3-Dimercaptosuccinic Acid in the Treatment of Heavy Metal Poisoning," *Metal Toxicology* 1 (1986): 155–162.

15: PSYCHONEUROIMMUNOLOGY: THE BODY-MIND CONNECTION

1. M. Borysenko, "Area Review: Psychoneuroimmunology," *Annals of Behavioral Medicine* 9(2): 3–10; R. Ader and N. Cohen, "CNS-Immune System Interaction: Conditioning Phenomena," *Behavioral and Brain Sciences* 8 (1985): 379–394; Candace B. Pert, "The Wisdom of the Receptors: Neuropeptides, the Emotions and Bodymind," *Advances*, 3(3): 8–16; and J. Marx, "Anxiety Peptide Found in Brain," *Science* 227 (1985): 934; and Kenneth R. Pelletier and Denise L. Herzing, "Psychoneuroimmunology: Toward a Mindbody Model," *Advances*, Institute for the Advancement of Health, 5(1): 27–56.

2. Ibid.

3. R. W. Bartrop, E. Luckhurst, L. Lazarus, L. G. Kilch, and R. Penny, "Depressed Lymphocyte Function after Bereavement," *Lancet* 1 (1977): 834–836.

4. J. Kiecolt-Glaser, W. Garner, C. Speicher, G. Penn, J. Holiday, and R. Glaser, "Psychosocial Modifiers of Immunocompetence in Medical Students," *Psychosomatic Medicine* 46(1): 7–14.

5. K. Goodin et al. "Stress and Hopelessness in the Promotion of Cervical, Intraepithelial Neoplasia to Invasive Squamous Cell Carcinoma of the Cervix," *Journal of Psychosomatic Research* 30 (1986): 67–76; and Kranz et al., eds., *Handbook on Psychology and Health: Vol. 3 Cardiovascular Disorders and Behavior* (Hillside, NJ: Erlbaum, 1983).

6. T. H. Holmes and R. H. Rahe, "Booklet for Schedule of Recent Experience (SRE): Social Readjustment Rating Scale," *Journal of Psychosomatic Research* 11 (1967): 213–218.

7. F. Alexander, *Psychosomatic Medicine* (New York: Norton, 1950). See also H. S. Freidman and S. Booth-Kewley, "The Disease-Prone Personality," *American Psychologist* 42 (1987): 539–555.

8. W. F. Fry, "Benefits of Stress," *Healthline* 3(1): 6–8. Available from the Robert A. McNeil Foundation for Health Education, 2855 Campus Dr., San Mateo, CA 94403.

9. S. C. Kobasa, "The Hardy Personality: Toward a Social Psychology of Stress and Health," in *Social Psychology of Health and Illness*, ed. G. S. Sanders and J. Suls (Hillsdale, NJ: Erlbaum, 1982). See also S.C. Kobasa, "Stressful Life Events, Personality, and Health: An Inquiry into Hardiness," *Journal of Personality and Social Psychology* 37 (1979): 1–11.

10. F. Cohen and R. S. Lazarus, "Coping and Adaptation in Illness," in *Handbook of Health, Healthcare, and the Health Professions*, ed. D. Mechanic (New York: Free Press, 1983).

11. D.W. Orme-Johnson and J. T. Farrow, eds., *Scientific Research on the Transcendental Meditation Program*, vol. 1, Maharishi European Research University Press Publication no. G. 1181, Maharishi International University; A. Dalal and T. Barber, "Yoga, Yogic Feats, and Hypnosis in the Light of Empirical Research," *American Journal of Clinical Hypnosis* 11 (1969): 155–166; A. Elson et al., "Psychological Changes in Yoga Meditation," *Psychophysiology* 14 (1977): 52–57; "Mind over Matter in Tibet: Meditation Gives Monks Hot Feet," *Tarrytown Newsletter* Feb. 1983; R. Gundu et al., "Some Experiments on a Yogi in Controlled States," *Pratibha: Journal of the All India Institute for Mental Health* 1 (1958): 99–106; R. Wallace, "The Physiological Effects of

Transcendental Meditation," *Science* 167 (1970): 1751–1754; H. Benson and R. Wallace, "Decreased Blood Pressure in Hypertensive Subjects Who Practiced Meditation." *Circulation* Supp. 2 (1972), pp. II-130; H. Benson et. al., "Decreased Blood Pressure in Hypertensive Subjects Who Practiced Meditation," *Journal of Chronic Diseases* 27 (1974): 163–169; and Jeanne Achterberg, O. Carl Simonton, and Stephanie Mathews-Simonton, *Stress, Psychological Factors, and Cancer.* Available from Cancer Counseling and Research Center, 1300 Summit, Suite 710, Fort Worth, TX 76102.

12. Carl O. Simonton, and Stephanie S. Simonton, "Belief Systems and Management of the Emotional Aspects of Malignancy," *Journal of Transpersonal Psychology* (1974): 29–47. See also Jeanne Achterberg, O. Carl Simonton, and Stephanie Mathews-Simonton, *Stress, Psychological Factors, and Cancer.* Available from Cancer Counseling and Research Center, 1300 Summit, Suite 710, Fort Worth, TX 76102.

13. Hans Seyle, *Stress without Distress* (New York: NAL/Dutton, 1975).

14. E. Stauffer, *Unconditional Love and Forgiveness* (Burbank, CA: Triangle Publishers, 1987). Audiotapes are also available through Psychosynthesis International, Box 279, Ojai, CA 93024-0279 (805) 646-7041, and through Northwest Health Foundation, Edmonds, WA (206) 776-9355.

15. Feiss, *Mind Therapies, Body Therapies: A Consumer's Guide* (Berkeley, CA: Celestial Arts, 1979).

16. Gayle Delaney, *Breakthrough Dreaming: How to Tap the Power of Your 24-Hour Mind* (New York: Bantam Books, 1991). See also J. Taylor, *Dreamwork: Techniques for Discovering the Creative Power in Dreams* (Mahwah, NJ: Paulist Press, 1983).

17. W. Hart, *The Art of Living: Vipassana Meditation as Taught by S. N. Goenka* (New York: Harper & Row, 1987). See also *Vipassana Newsletter*, Vipassana Meditation Center, Box 24, Shelburne Falls, MA 01370 (413) 625-2160.

18. Kenneth R. Pelletier and Denise L. Herzing, "Psychoneuroimmunology: Toward a Mindbody Model," *Advances*, Institute for the Advancement of Health, 5(1): 27–56.

19. B. L. Spaulding, *Life and Teaching of the Masters of the Far East*, vol. 1 (Marina Del Ray, CA: DeVorss & Co., 1972).

20. E. E. Miller, Source: *Cassette Learning Systems, Inc.: Software for the Mind*, P.O. Box W, Stanford, CA: 94305 (415) 328-7171 or (800) 528-2737. A tape catalog for stress management, relaxation, guided imagery, affirmations, self-hypnosis, optimal performance, habit modifications and other subjects. See also Ragini Elizabeth Michaels, "Volume I: Answers Rest Within" and "Volume II: Awareness Arising" (cassette recordings). Facticity Trainings, Inc., P.O. Box 22814, Seattle, WA: 98122 (206) 462-4369; Louise Hay's tapes, Hay House, Inc., 501 Santa Monica Blvd., Santa Monica, CA 90401; (310) 394-7445 or (800) 888-6565; Shakti Gawain's tapes, P.O. Box 13257, Northgate Station, San Rafael, CA 94913. Bernie Siegel's *Prescription for Living* series, available through Hay House, Inc., 501 Santa Monica Blvd., Santa Monica, CA 90401, (310) 394-7445 or (800) 888-6565; Edith Stauffer's tapes, "Unconditional Love and Forgiveness," and others, Psychosynthesis International, Box 297, Ojai, CA 93024-0279 (805) 646-7041 or Northwest Health Foundation, Edmonds, WA (206) 776-9355.

21. J. Levey, *The Fine Arts of Relaxation, Concentration, and Meditation: Ancient Skills for Modern Living* (London: Wisdom Publications, 1987).

22. H. Benson, and M. Klipper, *The Relaxation Response* (New York: Avon, 1976).

23. Meditation adapted from A. Weil, *Natural Health, Natural Medicine* (Boston: Houghton Mifflin, 1990), 117.

16: THE TEN COMMON DENOMINATORS OF ILLNESS AND THE IMMUNE SYSTEM

1. J. David, "Organs and Cells of the Immune System"; C. Terhorst, and J. David, "Antigens, Antibodies, and T Cell Receptors"; J. David, "Immune Response Mechanisms"; D. Fearon and J. David, "The Complement System," Section 6, Immunology, in *Scientific American Medicine*, E. Rubenstein and D. D. Federman, eds., Scientific American, Inc., 1978 –1992; see also D. Fearon, and J. David, "The Complement System," ibid., and *Understanding the Immune System*, National Institute of Allergy and Infectious Diseases, National Institutes of Health Publication no. 85–529, reprinted July 1985.

2. Antibody Assay Laboratories, 1715 E. Wilshire # 715, Santa Ana, CA 92705 (800) 522-2611; Meridian Valley Clinical Laboratory, 24030 132nd Avenue S.E., Kent, WA 98042 (800) 234-6825 or (206) 631-8922; and Immunosciences Laboratory, 8730 Wilshire Blvd., Suite 305, Beverly Hills, CA 90211 (800) 950-4686.

3. W. R. Beisel, R. Edelman, K. Nauss, and R. M. Suskind, "Single-Nutrient Effects on Immunological Functions: Report of a Workshop Sponsored by the Department of Food and Nutrition and Its Nutrition Advisory Group of the American Medical Association," *Journal of The American Medical Association* 245 (Jan. 1981): 53–58; A. Bendich and R. K. Chandra, eds., *Micronutrients and Immune Function* vol. 587 (New York: New York Academy of Sciences, 1990); see also R. K. Chandra, ed., *Nutrition and Immunology* (New York: Allen Lis, 1988); "Can You Boost Your Immune System?" University of California, *Berkeley Wellness Letter* 5 (Dec. 1988); R. K. Chandra, "Nutrition: The Changing Scene. Nutrition, Immunity, and Infection: Present Knowledge and Future Directions," *Lancet* (March 1983): 688–691; "Nutrition and Immunity: Basic Considerations, Part I," *Contemporary Nutrition* 11 (1986), available from General Mills, Inc., P.O. Box 1172, Minneapolis, MN 55440; "Nutrition and Immunity: Practical Applications, Part II," *Contemporary Nutrition* 11 (1986); L. C. Corman, "Effects of Specific Nutrients on Immune Response: Selected Clinical Applications," *Medical Clinics of North America* 69 (July 1985): 759–791; "Does Diet Affect the Immune System?" *Bostonia in Depth*, (Jan. 1984): 51–53; S. Dreizen, "Nutrition and the Immune Response: A Review," *International Journal of Vitamin and Nutrition Research* 49 (1979); M. E. Gershwin, *Nutrition and Immunity* (Orlando, FL: Academic Press, 1985); S. J. Gregory, *A Holistic Protocol for the Immune System, HIV/ARC/AIDS, Candidates, Epstein/Barr, Herpes, and Other Opportunistic Infections* (Joshua Tree, CA: Tree of Life Publications, 1989); P. Gunby, "Closing in on the Nutrition-Immunity Link," *Journal of the American Medical Association, Medical News*, 244 (Dec. 1980): 2715; D. Kipp, "Stress and Nutrition," *Contemporary Nutrition*, 9 (July 1984); B. L. G. Morgan, "How

Does Stress Affect the Body's Nutritional Status?" *Nutrition and Health* 6 (1984) (Institute of Human Nutrition, Columbia University College of Physicians and Surgeons, Broadway and 116th Street, New York, NY). "How Nutrition Affects Your Resistance to Infection," *Nutrition and Health* 7 (1985); National Dairy Council, "Nutrition and the Immune Response," *Dairy Council Digest* 56 (Mar.–Apr. 1985), (NDC, 6300 N. River Rd., Rosemont, IL 60018-4233); "Nutritional Demands Imposed by Stress," *Dairy Council Digest* 51 (Nov.–Dec. 1980); Vitamin Nutrition Information Service, "Vitamin Nutrition and Stress," *Vitamin Issues* 3(3); and "Zinc and Immunocompetence," *Nutrition Reviews* 38 (Aug. 1980).

4. See, for example, B. Smith, "Organic Foods vs. Supermarket Foods: Element Levels," *Journal of Applied Nutrition* 45 (1993): 35–39; and R. H. Hall, *Food for Naught: The Decline in Nutrition* (New York: Harper & Row, 1974).

5. I. Bogdanov, *Observations of the Therapeutic Effect of the Anticancer Preparation from Lactobillus Bulgaricus LB-51: Test on 100 Oncologic Patients 1982.* Laboratory for the Research and Production of Biologically Active Substances, P.O. Box 272, Sofia, Bulgaria. (Available through ProBiologic, Bellevue, WA (206) 882-8218.)

6. "Beta Carotene Regresses Tumors in Animal Model," *Medical Area Focus: News from Harvard Medical, Dental, and Public Health Schools.* (June 1986): 1, 4–5; J.L. Schwartz and G. Shklar, "Regression of Experimental Oral Cancer by Beta Carotene and Algae Extract, *Journal of Oral and Maxillofacial Surgery* 45 (510).

7. Y. Jianzhe, *Icones of Medicinal Fungi from China* (Beijing: Science Press, 1987); N. Sugano et al., "Anticarcinogenic Actions of Water-soluble and Alcohol-insoluble Fractions from Culture Medium of Lentinus Edodes Mycelia," *Cancer Letters* 17 (1982); See also E. Alstat, *Eclectic Dispensatory of Botanical Therapeutics* (Sandy Oregon: Eclectic Medical Publications, 1989, Section 5, p. 23), "Lentinus Edodes." (Eclectic Institute, Sandy, OR)

8. G. Valensi, V. Barnaba, R. Benvenuto et al., "A CalfThymus Lysate Improves Clinical Symptoms and T-Cell Defects in the Early Stages of HIV Infection: Second Report." *European Journal of Cancer and Clinical Oncology* 23 (1987): 1915–1919; P. Berressem, "Application of Glycopeptide-Fractions in the Treatment of Tumor Patients Suffering from Immunodeficiency." Die Mediz Welt 40 (1989): 565–568; W. Kuhlmey, "Fifteen Years of Experimental and Clinical Experience with 'P'. In: *Cancer Research and Treatment* (Bock HE, ed). (Urban and Schwarzenber: Munich, Berlin, 1967); and H. Holzgartner: "The Application of 'P' in the Oncological Practice," *Der Bayerische Internist* 5: (1987): 57–59.

9. Echo, Box 126, Delano, MN 55328. (Send $3 for an information packet on the use of hydrogen peroxide including a sample newsletter and distributors); C. H. Farr, "Physiological and Biochemical Responses to Intravenous Hydrogen Peroxide in Man," *Journal of Advancement in Medicine* 1 (Summer 1988): 113–129. W. Forest, "Cancer, AIDS Cured by Hyperoxygenation?" Write Waves Forest, P.O. Box 768, Monterey, CA 93942; E. McCabe, *Oxygen Therapies: A New Way of Approaching Disease* (Morrisville, NY: Energy Publications, 1988); International Bio-Oxidative Medicine Foundation, P.O. Box 891954, Oklahoma City, OK 73189-1954 (405) 478-4266. (Offers a physician referral list to the public and ed-

ucational seminars for health professionals); *The Medical Complications of Ozone*, The International Ozone Association, 83 Oakwood Avenue, Norwalk, CT 06850 (203) 847-8169; S. Rilling, and R. Viebahn, *The Use of Ozone in Medicine*. (Heidelberg, West Germany: Karl F. Haug, Publishers, 1987), (U.S. Distributor: Medicina Biologica, Portland, OR 97211.)

10. R.O. Becker, *Cross Currents* (Los Angeles: J. P. Tarcher, 1990). Also see R. O. Becker and A. A. Marino, *Electromagnetism and Life*. (Albany, NY: University of New York Press, 1982), and R. O. Becker and G. Seldon, *The Body Electric: Electromagnetism and the Foundation of Life* (New York: William Morrow, 1986); A. R. Davis, and W. Rawls, *The Magnetic Effect*, and *Magnetism and Its Effect on the Living System* (Kansas City, MO: Acres USA, 1979, 1975, 1976); *The Journal of the Bio-Electric-Magnetics Institute*, Bio-Electric-Magnetics Institute, c/o John Zimmerman, 2490 West Moana Lane, Reno, NV 89509-3936 (702) 827-9099; W. H. Philpott and S. Taplin, *The Biomagnetic Handbook. A Guide to Medical Magnetics, The Energy Medicine of Tomorrow* (Choctaw, OK: Enviro-Tech, 1990). Magnetic products, books, and other information related to magnetic therapy are available through Enviro-Tech, 17171 S.E. 29th St., Choctaw, OK 73020 (405) 390-3499; Also see: W. H. Philpott, *Cancer, the Magnetic Oxygen Answer: The Magnetic Oxygen Answer for Infection, Inflammation and Toxicity* (Choctaw, OK: Philpott Medical Services, 1994). Available through Philpott Medical Services, 17171 S.E. 29th St., Choctaw, OK 73020 (405) 390-3009; and H. Hanneman, *Balancing Your Body's Energy Flow for Self-Healing* (New York: Sterling Publishing Co., 1990).

11. M. Friedman, "From Poland with Prana. Mietek Wirkus Brings Bioenergy Healing to America," *New Realities* (July/Aug. 1987): 11–15. Also contact the Wirkus Bioenergy Foundation, Margaret and Mietek Wirkus, 4803 St. Elmo Ave., Bethesda, MD (301) 652-3480.

12. P. Brodeur, *Currents of Death: Power Lines, Computer Terminals, and the Attempt to Cover Up Their Threat to Your Health* (New York: Simon and Schuster, 1989). Also see: C. Blackman, "Do Electromagnetic Fields Cause Health Problems?" *Frontier Perspectives* 2(2): 11–16 (The Center for Frontier Sciences of Temple University, Philadelphia, PA); Bethwatte et al., "Electromagnetic Fields and Cancer: An Ongoing Debate," *New Zealand Journal of Medicine* (June 1991): 225–226.

13. D.W. Black, "Laughter," *Journal of the American Medical Association* 252 (Dec. 1984): 2995–2998; K. M. Dillon, "Positive Emotional States and Enhancement of the Immune System," *International Journal of Psychiatry in Medicine* 15 (1985–1986): 13–17; B. Goldman, "How Humor Can Help Heal Patients," *Canadian Medical Association Journal* 131, (July 1984): 73–74.

14. T. Monte, "Healer John Diamond's Soul Music," *East West, The Journal of Natural Health and Healing* (July 1988): 38–45.

15. See also: Institute for Music, Health and Education, P.O. Box 1244, Boulder, CO 80306; American Association for Music Therapists, 66 Morris Ave., Springfield, NJ 07801; International Arts-Medicine Society, 1721 Pine St., Philadelphia, PA 19103; International Society for Music and Medicine, Sportkrankenhaus Hellersen, Paulmannshoher Strasse

17, 5880, Ludenscheidk, Germany; and National Music and Health Conferences, Department of Music, 101 Foster Building, Richmond, KY 40475.

16. H. G. Ainsleigh, "Sunshine Prevents Cancer Deaths," *The Townsend Letter for Doctors* (Port Townsend, WA, June 1991): 441–42.

17. C. Garland et al., "Geographic Variation in Breast Cancer Mortality in the United States: A Hypothesis Involving Solar Radiation," *Preventive Medicine* 19 (1990): 614–622.

18. C. Garland and F. Garland. "Do Sunlight and Vitamin D Reduce the Risk of Colon Cancer?" *International Journal of Epidemiology* 9 (1980): 227–231. See also C. Garland et al., "Vitamin D and Calcium and Risk of ColoRectal Cancer: A 19-Year Prospective Study in Men," *Lancet* 1 (1985): 307–309; C. Garland et al., "Serum 25-Hydroxy Vitamin D and Colon Cancer: 8-year Prospective Study," *Lancet* 2 (1989): 1176–1178.

19. F. L. Apperly, "The Relation of Solar Radiation to Cancer Mortality in North America," *Cancer Research* 1 (1941): 191.

20. H. K. Koh et al., "Sunlight and Cutaneous Malignant Melanoma: Evidence For and Against Causation," *Photochemical Photobiology* 51 (1990): 765–779.

21. I. K. Crombie, "Distribution of Malignant Melanomas on the Body Surface," *British Journal of Cancer* 43 (1981): 842–849; D. Vagero et al., "Melanoma and Other Tumors of the Skin Among Office and Other Indoor and Outdoor Workers in Sweden, 1961–1979," *British Journal of Cancer* 53 (1986): 507–512.

22. R. Jaffe et al., "Photobiology: Trigger of Brain Rhythms" in *Health Studies Collegium Information Handbook for Use with Your Immune Enhancement Program* 113th ed. (Reston, VA: Health Studies Collegium, 1987, 1993): 45.

23. K. Pelletier, *Longevity: Fulfilling Our Biological Potential* (New York: Dell, 1982).

24. R. Leichtman and C. Japikse, "The Way to Health," in *The Art of Living, Vol. 4* (Winchester, OH: Ariel Press).

18: FASTING, CLEANSING, REJUVENATION

1. P. Airola, *Are You Confused?* (Sherwood, OR: Health Plus, 1990), 104–147.

2. R. Wolford, "Eating Lean Lengthens Life," *Health and Longevity Report* 1 (5): 7 (Baltimore, MD: Agora Publishing).

3. A. Colbin, "Herring's Law of Natural Cure," in *Food and Healing* (New York: Ballantine Books, 1986), 218.

4. P. Airola, *Are You Confused?* (Sherwood, OR: Health Plus, 1990), 104–147.

5. Ibid: 128–129.

6. S. Burroughs, *Healing for the Age of Enlightenment*, 3rd ed. 1976, 1–34. (Self-published—available at 5185 Meadowview Lane, Auburn, CA 95603.)

7. M. Tierra, *The Way of Herbs* (New York: Pocket Books, 1980), 63–64.

19: HERBS AND THEIR MEDICINAL USES

1. J. Bland, "Aloe Vera," in *Selected Papers by Jeffrey Bland, Ph.D., 1985–1986*, Stewart Seminar Series (available from Health Comm, 3215-56th St. N.W., Gig Harbor, WA 98335).

2. P. M. Ridker and W. V. McDermott, "Comfrey Herb Tea and Hepatic Veno-Occlusive Disease," *Lancet* (March 25, 1989): 657–658; and D. J. Brown "Phytotherapy Review and Commentary," *Townsend Review for Doctors* 88 (November 1990): 736.

20: MORE NATURAL THERAPEUTICS

1. Association of Research and Enlightenment (ARE), P.O. Box 595, Virginia Beach, VA 23451 (804) 428-3588. See also H. Reilly and R. H. Brod, *The Edgar Cayce Handbook for Health through Drugless Therapy* (New York: Jove/Harcourt Brace Jovanovich, 1978), 338–346.

2. J. P. Feighner, S. L. Brown, and J. E. Olivier, "Electrosleep Therapy: A Controlled Double Blind Study," *Journal of Nervous and Mental Disease* 157 (1973): 121–128; E. Gomez and A. Mikhail, "Treatment of Methadone Withdrawal with Cerebral Electrotherapy (Electrosleep)," *British Journal of Psychiatry* 134: 111–113; J. Ryan, and G. Souheaver, "Effects of Transcerebral Electrotherapy (Electrosleep) on State Anxiety According to Suggestibility Levels." *Biological Psychiatry* 11(2): 233–237; R. Schmitt, T. Capo, and E. Boyd, "Cranial Electrotherapy Stimulation as a Treatment for Anxiety in Chemically Dependent Persons," *Alcoholism: Clinical and Experimental Research* 10(2): 158–160; R. Smith, and L. O'Neill, "Electrosleep in the Management of Alcoholism," *Biological Psychiatry* 10(6): 675–680; G. S. Wharton, C. E. McCoy, and J. Cofer, "The Use of Cranial Electrotherapy Stimulation in Spinal Cord Injury Patients," paper presented at the meeting of the American Spinal Injury Association, New York, 1982.

3. N. Muramoto. *Healing Ourselves* (New York: Avon/Swan, 1973), 110–111.

4. W. Boyle, and A. Saine, *Lectures in Naturopathic Hydrotherapy* (East Palestine, OH: Buckeye Naturopathic Press, 1988). D. Buchman, *The Complete Book of Hydrotherapy* (New York: Dutton, 1979). B. Jensen, *Nature Has a Remedy* (available from Bernard Jensen International, 24360 Old Wagon Rd., Escondido, CA 92027). F. B. Moor et al., *Manual of Hydrotherapy and Massage* (Mountain View, CA: Pacific Press, 1964).

5. J. S. DeCorsey, "Staphage Lysate (SPL)—A Safe Biological Response Modifier," (Swarthmore, PA: Delmont Laboratories, Inc., 1983). Also see D. J. Canfield, "Staphage Lysate (SPL)—A Safe Immune Response Potentiator," (Swarthmore, PA: Delmont Laboratories, Inc., 1984); T. Aoki et al., "Staphage Lysate and Lentinan as Immunomodulators and/or Immunopotentiators in Clinical and Experimental Systems," in *Augmenting Agents in Cancer Therapy*, ed. E. M. Hersh et al. (New York: Raven Press, 1981), 101–111; and C. E. Pitard, "Cancer Combination-Therapy Utilizing Licensed, Low Cost, Effective and Universally Available Members of That Class of Biologicals and Biological Response Modifiers Constituting the Fourth Conventional Modality of Cancer Treatment," self-published by Dr. Pitard, Clinical Associate Professor, Ear Nose and Throat, Head and Neck Surgery, Department of Surgery, University of Tennessee School of Medicine, Knoxville, TN 37920.

21: ENERGY MEDICINE: ACUPUNCTURE AND HOMEOPATHY

1. R. Melzack and P. D. Wall, "Pain Mechanisms: A New Theory," *Science* 150 (1965): 971–979.

2. H. Motoyama with R. Brown, *Science and the Evolution of Consciousness* (Boston: Autumn, 1978): 113–114.

3. Ibid: 117–119.

4. K. Matsumoto and S. Birch, *Hara Diagnosis: Reflections on the Sea* (Brookline: Paradigm, 1988): 354–361.

5. J. Kenyon, *Modern Technologies of Acupuncture* vols. I–III (Wellingborough: Thorsons, 1985).

6. J. Chen and N. Wang, eds., *Acupuncture Case Histories from China* (Seattle: Eastland, 1988) 270–271.

22: CHOOSING AND RELATING TO YOUR DOCTOR

1. For more information on the Washington State legislation, contact Citizens for Alternative Health Care, P.O. Box 8518, Kirkland, WA 98034.

2. For more information on protecting your health freedoms, contact Citizens for Health, P.O. Box 1195, Tacoma, WA 98401 (206) 922-2457 or (800) 357-2211 (there are over 165 local and regional chapters of this organization in forty-nine states). Also, contact Nutritional Health Alliance (800) 226-4642.

3. Ibid.

4. For more information on the Washington State legislation, contact Citizens for Alternative Health Care, P.O. Box 8518, Kirkland, WA 98034.

About the Author

RALPH GOLAN specializes in Preventative and Wellness medicine. Dedicated to self-care and to guiding his patients to a healthier way of living, Dr. Golan works with individuals as both a diagnostician and teacher to uncover underlying causes of recurring symptoms or chronic illness. Dr. Golan lives and works in Seattle, Washington.